Color Atlas and Text of

Clinical Medicine

Charles D. Forbes DSc, MD, FRCP, FRSE

Professor of Medicine,
Ninewells Hospital and Medical School,
Dundee,
Scotland, UK

William F. Jackson MA, MB, BChir, MRCP

Medical Writer and Television Producer;
Formerly Honorary Consultant,
Department of Medicine,
Guy's Hospital,
London,
England, UK

M Mosby-Wolfe

London Baltimore Bogotá Boston Buenos Aires Caracas Carlsbad, CA Chicago Madrid Mexico City Milan Naples, FL New York Philadelphia St. Louis Sydney Tokyo Toronto Wiesbaden

Mosby, Inc.
11830 Westline Drive
St. Louis, MO 63146

10   9   8   7   6   5   4

ISBN 0-8151-3271-9

English edition first published in 1993 by Mosby–Wolfe, an imprint of Times Mirror International Publishers Limited, Lynton House, 7–12 Tavistock Square, London WC1H 9LB, England.

Library of Congress Cataloging-in-Publication Data:
Forbes, C.D. (Charles Douglas). 1938–
      Color atlas of clinical medicine / Charles D Forbes, William F Jackson.
         p. cm.
    Includes Index.
    ISBN 0-8151-3271-9
      1. Symptomatology—Atlases. 2. Clinical Medicine—Atlases.
I. Jackson, William F. (William Francis) II. Title.
    [DNLM: 1. Clinical Medicine—atlases. WB 17 F692c]
RC69.F65 1992
616—dc20
DNLM/DLC
for Library of Congress   92-8667
                                          CIP

Contents

Preface

There are many textbooks of medicine, and many colour atlases concentrating on specific subjects, but as far as we know no-one has previously attempted to put together a colour atlas encompassing the whole of clinical medicine. Yet the need for such a book is clear. Clinical medicine has a strong visual content. From early student days onwards, doctors learn to interpret a vast range of visual appearances—on examination of patients and in assessing the results of a wide range of specific investigations. The importance of rapid visual identification or interpretation is recognised in the content of undergraduate and postgraduate examinations in medicine: long cases, short cases, and picture tests of various kinds all depend upon the interpretation of clinical appearances.

In most parts of the world, however, it is becoming increasingly difficult for the clinical or postgraduate student to experience at first hand the full spectrum of clinical abnormalities. Diseases are often detected and treated at an earlier stage than previously; treatment for many conditions is more effective than in the past; and far fewer patients with medical disorders are now admitted to hospital—the traditional main teaching ground for students. When patients are admitted to teaching hospitals, their admission is often brief. As a result, many students complete their training without seeing patients with many of the less common diseases 'in the flesh'.

In this book we try to combine the best features of the colour atlas and the medical textbook. We have gathered together a comprehensive range of pictures to illustrate the clinical signs of most major medical disorders, and we have supplemented these with high quality radiological, ultrasound, endoscopic and other images whenever this adds to the clinical value of the book. To keep the book to a manageable size we have not included illustrations of pathological specimens; and we have included histopathology or other microscopic appearances only where these are the key to classification and diagnosis—as, for example, in many renal and haematological disorders.

Each chapter has a similar structure: we start with an illustrated guide to symptoms, signs and investigations, and continue with a systematic coverage of common and rare disorders. Extensive cross-referencing should aid the effective use of the illustrations in the book.

Our aim in the text has been to match the depth of the shorter medical textbooks, so that this book can be used alone as an introduction to clinical medicine and for revision purposes. We also intend that it should be used as a companion to any of the major textbooks of medicine; in this setting it should provide both a useful visual review of most disorders and a concise summary of their key features.

Our intended readership includes clinical medical students worldwide, but we have pitched the book at a level which should also meet the needs of candidates for higher post-graduate examinations, such as those for the membership of the Royal Colleges of Physicians (MRCP) and the North American specialist boards, and equivalent examinations in the rest of the world. We hope that the book will also be of interest and use to a wide range of medical and paramedical staff in other clinical specialties.

We are grateful to the many colleagues who have contributed to this book. Much of the text was drafted by colleagues in Dundee and, while most of this has been substantially rewritten by us to ensure a common style and content, and to integrate text with pictures, we are very grateful for their help, without which our task might have proved just too daunting. Their contributions are acknowledged on p. 6.

Some of the illustrations in the book come from our personal collections, but no two individuals could hope to illustrate the broad range of clinical medicine from their own experience alone. We are indebted to many colleagues for the full range of pictures we have included. Our largest sources were the slide collections at Guy's Hospital, London and in Dundee, and we are grateful to The Dean, UMDS, Guy's Campus and to many colleagues in Dundee for granting permission for us to use these illustrations in the book, and to past and present physicians and medical photographers in these centres for their skilled observations and photography. Many other colleagues gave generous help in our search for illustrations, and Dr Jill Belch, Dr Leslie Jackson, Dr Mary Kerr, Dr Alex Paton and Dr John Winter were particularly far-reaching in their assistance. Further illustrations have been loaned to us by the authors of many established Wolfe atlases, and we are grateful to all these authors for their help and support, especially to Dr Malcolm Parsons for allowing us to use a number of his illustrations of neurological disorders. A full list of picture contributors appears on p. 7.

We carried out much of our collaborative editorial work within Mosby–Year Book Europe offices in London, and we were greatly encouraged by the constant help and support we received from the many staff there. Finally we must thank our families, who have cheerfully accepted our many absences from home in the interest of this book!

Charles Forbes
William Jackson

Text contributors

Jill J F Belch MD, FRCP (Edin, Glas),
Reader in Medicine,
University of Dundee,
Ninewells Hospital,
Dundee, UK

Allan B Bridges MB ChB, MRCP,
Research Fellow (Cardiology),
University of Dundee,
Ninewells Hospital,
Dundee, UK

Duncan L W Davidson BSc, MB ChB,
 FRCP (Edin),
Consultant Neurologist,
Dundee Royal Infirmary,
Dundee, UK

Charles D Forbes DSc, MD, FRCP
 (Glas, Edin, Lond), FRSE,
Professor of Medicine,
University of Dundee,
Ninewells Hospital,
Dundee, UK

Jennifer L Hanslip MB ChB, MRCP,
Lecturer in Ageing and Health,
University of Dundee,
Ninewells Hospital,
Dundee, UK

Iain S Henderson MB ChB, FRCP
 (Glas),
Consultant Nephrologist,
Ninewells Hospital,
Dundee, UK

William F Jackson MA, MB BChir,
 MRCP,
Medical Writer and Television Producer,
Harwell, Oxford, UK
(Formerly Honorary Consultant,
Department of Medicine,
Guy's Hospital,
London, UK)

Paul Jennings MD, MRCP,
Consultant Physician (Diabetes),
York District Hospital,
York, UK
(Formerly Lecturer in Medicine,
University of Dundee,
Ninewells Hospital,
Dundee, UK)

Mary R Kerr MB ChB, FRCP (Edin),
Consultant Physician in Infectious
 Diseases,
King's Cross Hospital,
Dundee, UK

Chak Lau MD, MRCP,
Lecturer in Medicine,
Queen Mary Hospital,
Hong Kong
(Formerly Research Fellow in
 Rheumatology,
Ninewells Hospital,
Dundee, UK)

Marion E T McMurdo MD, MRCP,
Senior Lecturer in Ageing and Health,
University of Dundee,
Ninewells Hospital,
Dundee, UK

Graeme P McNeill PhD, MB ChB,
 FRCP (Edin),
Consultant Cardiologist,
Ninewells Hospital,
Dundee, UK

Robert A MacTier MD, MRCP,
Consultant Nephrologist,
Glasgow Royal Infirmary,
Glasgow, UK
(Formerly Senior Registrar in
 Nephrology,
Ninewells Hospital,
Dundee, UK)

Susan M Morley MD, MRCP, FRACP,
Research Fellow in Dermatology,
University of Dundee,
Ninewells Hospital,
Dundee, UK

John Pears MB ChB, MRCP,
Research Fellow (Endocrinology and
 Diabetes),
University of Dundee,
Ninewells Hospital,
Dundee, UK

Christopher R Pennington BSc, MD,
 FRCP (Edin),
Consultant Physician and
 Gastroenterologist,
Ninewells Hospital,
Dundee, UK

Martin J Pippard BSc, MB ChB,
 MRCPath, FRCP (Lond),
Professor of Haematology,
University of Dundee,
Ninewells Hospital,
Dundee, UK

Richard C Roberts MA, DPhil, BM
 BCh, MRCP,
Senior Lecturer in Neurology,
University of Dundee,
Dundee Royal Infirmary,
Dundee, UK

William K Stewart PhD, MD, FRCP
 (Edin),
Formerly Reader in Medicine,
University of Dundee,
Ninewells Hospital,
Dundee, UK

John H Winter BSc, MD, MRCP,
Consultant Physician in Respiratory
 Medicine,
King's Cross Hospital,
Dundee, UK

Acknowledgements

We gratefully acknowledge the generosity of the many colleagues and institutions listed below, who lent us single, or in some cases, multiple pictures. In all cases, the final responsibility for picture selection, relevance and description rests with us. Also acknowledged in this list are a number of individuals who helped by reviewing sections of the book at draft stage.

CDF and WFJ

The estate of the late C W M Adams, London, UK
M C Allison, Glasgow, UK
J Anderson, Frostrup, Denmark
M A Ansary, Rochdale, UK
B M Ansell, Harrow, UK
E Asbrink, Stockholm, Sweden
J Baillie, Durham, NC, USA
Bailliere Tindall (7 tables modified from Kumar, PJ and Clark, ML (eds): *Clinical Medicine* 2nd edn, London, 1990)
M Baraitser, London, UK
G Barr, Safat, Kuwait
N R Barratt, Richmond, UK
A C Bayley, Lusaka, Zambia
D W Beaven, Christchurch, New Zealand
M A Bedford, London, UK
J S Beck, Dundee, UK
J F Belch, Dundee, UK
M Berger, Sydney, Australia
C M Black, London, UK
A Bloom, London, UK
S L Bloom, Oxford, UK
D Borislow, Durham, NC, USA
B J Boucher, London, UK
U Boundy, London, UK
A C Boyle, London, UK
A B Bridges, Dundee, UK
R L Broadhead, Liverpool, UK
J C Brocklehurst, Manchester, UK
S E Brooks, Christchurch, New Zealand
S E Brown, London, UK
A Bryceson, London, UK
T R Bull, London, UK
J F Calder, Glasgow, UK
Sir Roy Calne, Cambridge, UK
C Campbell, Dundee, UK
R Capildeo, Romford, UK
R Cerio, London, UK
Charing Cross and Westminster Medical School Department of Medical Illustration, London, UK
G S J Chessell, Aberdeen, UK
C Chintu, Lusaka, Zambia
R A Chole, Davis, California, USA

G M Cochrane, London, UK
W B Conolly, Sydney, Australia
N Conway, Southampton, UK
R A Cooke, Brisbane, Australia
P Cotton, Durham, NC, USA
A Cuschieri, Dundee, UK
D R Davies, London, UK
J Dequeker, Leuven, Belgium
V Dubowitz, London, UK
Dudley Road Hospital, Birmingham, UK
K Duguid, Aberdeen, UK
M Dynski-Klein, London, UK
D L Easty, Bristol, UK
P Ell, London, UK
A El-Rooby, Cairo, Egypt
C F Farthing, New York, USA
D C Ferlic, Denver, Colorado, USA
R J Flemans, Cambridge, UK
H Fuglsang, Copenhagen, Denmark
N J R George, Manchester, UK
H M Gilles, Liverpool, UK
J D Gillett, Bourne End, UK
J G Gow, Liverpool, UK
H W Gray, Glasgow, UK
B M Greenwood, Banjul, Gambia
W Guthrie, Dundee, UK
K H Harinasuta, Bangkok, Thailand
I A Harper, Perth, UK
C A Hart, Liverpool, UK
A R Harvey, Leeds, UK
F G J Hayhoe, Cambridge, UK
I S Henderson, Dundee, UK
R Hendrickse, Liverpool, UK
S M Herber, Sheffield, UK
S K Hira, Lusaka, Zambia
G J Hunter, London, UK
K A Hussein, Dundee, UK
M P Hutchinson, Carhampton, UK
The estate of the late J Ireland, Glasgow, UK
F L Jackson, Edmonton, Alberta, Canada
L K Jackson, Swindon, UK
M J Jamieson, Aberdeen, UK

1. Infections

Introduction

Infections are the most common cause of morbidity and mortality worldwide. The most common infections are the diarrhoeal diseases, respiratory infection, malaria, measles, hepatitis, schistosomiasis, whooping cough and neonatal tetanus. The course and severity of infection depends on a variety of factors, including the virulence of the strain of infecting organism, the resistance of the population or individual—which may be reduced by famine or intercurrent disease (**Table 1.1**)—social factors such as lack of sanitation, poor housing and a contaminated water supply, and the availability of medical facilities to provide vaccination or diagnosis and treatment.

In the past 30 years the availability and cheapness of air travel has allowed 'new' diseases to appear rapidly and unexpectedly in new places. The latest example of this 'jet age' transmission is HIV infection, which has rapidly crossed international boundaries, both by population movement (homosexual and heterosexual carriers) and also in blood products, notably factor VIII for haemophilia treatment.

Many (but not all) of the infections to be considered in this chapter present with fever, and the investigation of a patient with unexplained fever is a medical challenge that requires careful history taking, a meticulous examination and appropriate planned investigations.

To take an effective history it is important to understand reservoirs of infection and potential routes of transmission.

Reservoirs act as a source of infection within which the infective agent may often divide and multiply and from which it may be disseminated.

Animal reservoirs are particularly important, as it is often impossible to eliminate them; public health measures aim to stop spread into the human population. Examples of **animal reservoirs** include:

- **Viral:** rabies virus in infected domestic and wild animals.
- **Bacterial:** *Salmonella* species in contaminated eggs and poultry.
- **Fungal:** *Histoplasma capsulatum* in infected bird and bat droppings.
- **Protozoal:** *Leishmania* species in infected rodents
- **Helminthic:** toxocariasis in dogs and cats.

Human reservoirs are important, especially in virus infections. Examples include:

- **Viral:** upper respiratory tract virus infections (**1.1**) and HIV.
- **Bacterial:** acute streptococcal pharyngitis (**1.2**) and sexually transmitted diseases such as gonorrhoea and syphilis.
- **Fungal:** candidiasis and dermatophyte infections (**1.3**).
- **Protozoal:** *Trichomonas vaginalis* (transmitted sexually).
- **Helminthic:** *Enterobius vermicularis* (threadworms).

Table 1.1 Factors which may affect the course of infections.

Immune disturbances	Prosthetic devices and procedures
HIV infection	Indwelling urinary catheter
Intravenous drug abuse	Arterial and venous
Immunosuppression with	cannulae
steroids, cytotoxic drugs	Artificial valves
Immune deficiency –	Joint prostheses
hypogammaglobulinaemia	Vascular grafts
and neutropenia	Chronic ambulatory
Leukaemia and lymphoma	peritoneal dialysis
Various cancers	Intracranial shunts
Malnutrition	
Alcoholism and chronic liver	
disease	
Diabetes mellitus	
Post-splenectomy	

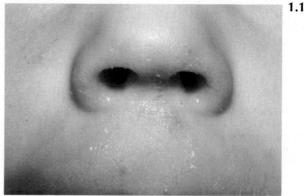

1.1

1.1 The nose is a reservoir of infection in the common cold. The mucoid nasal discharge contains viruses that may spread to others in droplets disseminated by sneezing or by direct contact.

Natural reservoirs include soil, water and vegetation. Many infecting organisms are found in nature, and some infect man via intermediate hosts.

- **Viral:** hepatitis A in faecally contaminated water (**1.4**).
- **Bacterial:** cholera in faecally contaminated water (**1.4**).
- **Fungal:** *Aspergillus* spores are ubiquitous in soil and vegetation, and are often released when old buildings are demolished.
- **Protozoal:** amoebae may live for weeks or months in the encysted form.
- **Helminthic:** schistosomes spend part of their life cycle in an intermediate host (water snail).

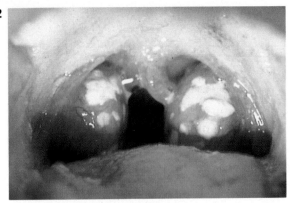

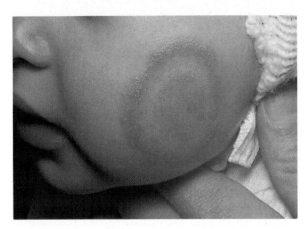

1.2 Acute streptococcal pharyngitis. There is pus in the tonsillar crypts, and some palatal petechiae are also seen. The patient acts as a reservoir of *Streptococcus pyogenes*: the organisms multiply in the pharynx and may be disseminated to others by coughing, sneezing or direct contact with oral secretions.

1.3 Tinea (ringworm). Patients with dermatophyte infections act as reservoirs of infection, and ringworm may also sometimes be 'caught' from contact with infected animals. This florid case results from infection with *M. canis.*

1.4

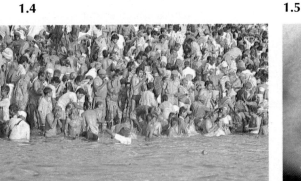

1.5

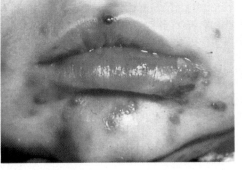

1.6

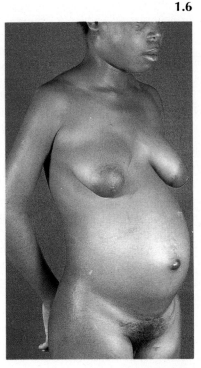

1.4 The river Ganges—an ancient epicentre of cholera. Mass bathing leads to a constant risk of faecal/oral transmission of hepatitis, cholera and other infections. Patients with mild and asymptomatic infections are very important in the epidemiology of cholera.

1.5 Primary herpes simplex in and around the mouth. The infection is usually acquired from siblings or parents, and is readily transmitted to other contacts. The infection commonly persists in a dormant phase, but the 'secondary' lesions that occur on reactivation (*see* p. 28) are also a common source of infection.

1.6 Mother-to-child transmission is important in a number of infections. This African patient had AIDS, with some Kaposi's sarcoma lesions on her face and generalised lymphadenopathy. If her child had lived, it would probably have had HIV infection; however, it died at birth and she died a few days later.

Transmission of infection can take many forms and understanding these is the key to public health measures to stop the spread of diseases. Routes of importance include:

- **Contact:** person-to-person as in sexually transmitted diseases, herpes simplex (**1.5**), chickenpox, impetigo, etc.;
  from animal reservoirs as in anthrax, orf, etc.;
  on fomites (books, crockery, towels, etc.), many bacteria, especially tuberculosis, yaws, etc.
- **Parent-to-child transmission:** rubella, syphilis, toxoplasmosis, hepatitis B, HIV infection (**1.6**), etc.
- **Aerosols:** from human reservoirs—common cold, influenza, streptococci and meningo-cocci, tubercle bacilli; from the environment—*Legionella, Aspergillus,* etc.; from animals or their excreta—histoplasmosis, psittacosis, etc.
- **Faecal/oral:** infective diarrhoeas, hepatitis A, typhoid, amoebiasis, giardiasis.
- **Via a vector:** malaria (**1.7**), leishmaniasis, plague, viral encephalitis, Lyme disease, trypanosomiasis, etc.
- **Direct entry:** through intact skin—leptospirosis, schistosomiasis;
  by bites—rabies;
  by transfusion—hepatitis B, cytomegalovirus, HIV, malaria, leishmaniasis, syphilis, etc. (**1.8**);
  by ingestion—*Salmonella, Listeria,* hydatid disease, tapeworms;
  traumatic and surgical infections.

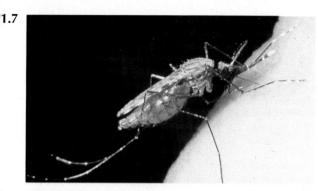

1.7 Malaria is transmitted by female *Anopheles* mosquitoes. Insect vectors are also important in a number of other infections.

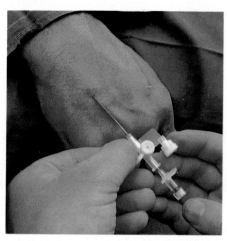

1.8 Intravenous infusion is an important route of direct entry infection, especially if blood or blood products are transfused. Blood-borne infections may be introduced in a medical setting or through illicit intravenous drug abuse. Local infection may also be introduced by any puncture of the skin, unless careful aseptic technique is used.

History

A careful history will often localise the site of a possible infection and may suggest its nature. Viral infections are the most common worldwide. They occur in epidemics, often initially in school age children, and are passed on to adults. Upper respiratory and diarrhoeal illnesses are most common. Points to be elicited in the history include:

- Recent contact with infected persons.
- Previous exposure to infections.
- Vaccination status. Occupation/social pursuits and hobbies.
- Contact with animals—wild or domestic.
- Recent foreign travel—types of endemic and epidemic diseases.

- Immigrants should be asked details of country and place of origin.
- Recent dietary history, especially type/source of food and water.
- Insect bites.
- Previous surgery/accidents/presence of prosthetic devices (**1.9**).
- History of intravenous drug abuse (**1.10**).
- Sexual activity and proclivity.
- Tattooing.
- Blood transfusion and injections.
- Recent drug history—especially documentation of native remedies and generic content of foreign or branded drugs.

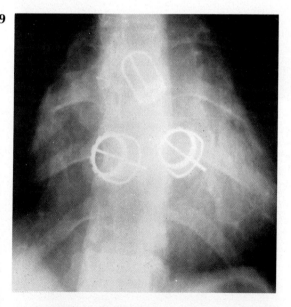

1.9 Prosthetic surgical devices are associated with an increased risk of systemic or local infection. This patient has had triple valve replacement with Starr–Edward's valves, and—like all those who have had heart valve surgery—is at increased risk of infective endocarditis. Similarly, patients with joint prostheses or other implants are at greater risk of systemic and local infection.

1.10 Intravenous drug abuse typically leads to this appearance, which results from repeated superficial thrombophlebitis of accessible veins in the arm or elsewhere in the body. The sharing and re-use of syringes and needles, together with the lack of aseptic technique, puts these patients at special risk of a wide range of infections, including bacterial septicaemia (sometimes with unusual organisms), hepatitis B and HIV infection.

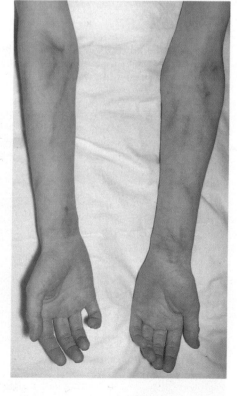

Clinical examination

Careful and complete clinical examination often provides clues to the nature and site of infection. Special attention should be paid to the skin (for nodules, rashes, bites), eyes, lymph nodes (enlargement of which may be local or generalised), and the liver and spleen. Especially in sexually transmitted disease, it is important to examine the genitalia, the perineum, the anus and the mouth. Thorough examination should include:

- Taking the temperature and plotting any fever (**1.11**).
- General examination for signs of jaundice, dehydration, weight loss, nutritional status, anaemia, oedema.
- Mouth, pharynx and throat for ulcers, membranes.
- Conjuntiva and retina for petechiae, inflammation and choroidal deposits (**1.12**).
- Tympanic membrane for otitis media (**1.13**).
- Skin for rashes, nodules, ulcers, scratching (**1.14**).
- Lymph nodes (**1.15**) and spleen (**1.16**) which may be tender to touch.
- Liver for tender and non-tender local swellings and generalised enlargement.
- Heart for evidence of endocarditis, failure.
- Genitalia for ulcers, discharge of pus.
- Lungs for production of sputum and consolidation or cavitation.
- Central nervous system for meningism, impairment of conscious level or focal neurological signs.
- Urine for evidence of infection or bleeding.

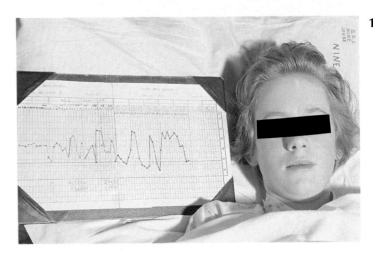

1.11 High swinging fever, plotted in a patient who presented with pyrexia of unknown origin (PUO). On blood culture she was found to have *Brucella abortus*. She had recently returned from a holiday in the Greek islands.

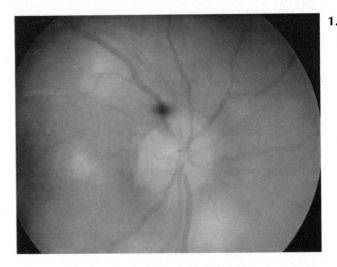

1.12 Choroidal tubercles in acute miliary tuberculosis. This appearance is virtually diagnostic so it is essential to examine the fundi of any patient in whom miliary tuberculosis is a possibility.

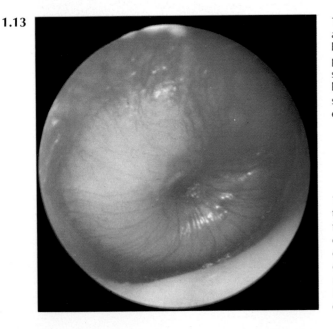

1.13 Acute otitis media, with bulging and hyperaemia of the tympanic membrane. The middle ear is filled with purulent fluid. Otitis media is usually symptomatic, but the young child may be unable to communicate his earache, so examination with the auriscope is essential.

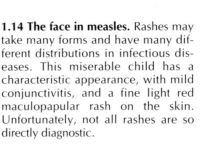

1.14 The face in measles. Rashes may take many forms and have many different distributions in infectious diseases. This miserable child has a characteristic appearance, with mild conjunctivitis, and a fine light red maculopapular rash on the skin. Unfortunately, not all rashes are so directly diagnostic.

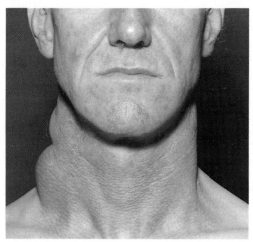

1.15 Enlarged lymph nodes in the posterior triangle on the neck. Lymphadenopathy is a feature of many infectious diseases, and aspirational biopsy of the enlarged nodes is sometimes helpful in diagnosis. This patient had no other clinical clues to the diagnosis, but histology demonstrated the typical caseating granulomas of tuberculosis (*see* p. 46).

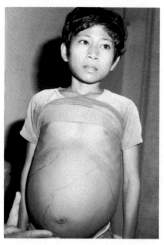

1.16 Gross splenomegaly has been marked on the abdomen of this Filipino boy who has schistosomiasis.

Investigations

A number of non-specific tests are often needed to give clues to the cause, site and extent of the disease. Many may also be of value in following its progress and the effects of therapy. Useful investigations include:

- Full blood count with a differential count. Eosinophilia is an important finding in parasitic infections (**1.17**). Lymphocytosis is usually found in viral infections.
- Erythrocyte sedimentation rate—a non-specific test which may be of value in monitoring the course of diseases.
- Examination of thick blood films for parasites, especially malaria (**1.187**), trypanosomiasis (**1.18**) and filariasis (**1.198**).
- Examination of smears with direct staining (**1.19**) or dark-field illumination or with fluorescent antibodies.
- Urinalysis for blood, bile, protein, pus cells and ova of schistosomiasis.
- Stool examination for amoebae, cysts (**1.20**), ova and parasites.

- Renal and liver function tests.
- Lumbar puncture for CSF examination in suspected meningitis (**1.21**).
- Cultures of blood, urine, stools, throat swab, CSF, pus, etc. for viruses, bacteria and fungi.
- Immunoglobulin levels.
- Serological tests for specific infections.
- Chest and abdominal X-ray.

Further specific investigations may be needed to localise the site of the infection, including tomography, ultrasound, isotope scanning with gallium, CT scanning (**1.22**) or MRI.

Biopsy may be required for a tissue diagnosis. Endoscopy is valuable in obtaining tissue from lung and alimentary tract, and laparoscopy allows direct inspection and biopsy of the abdominal contents.

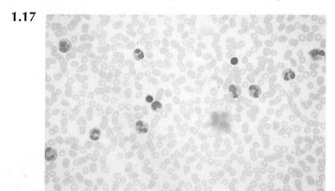

1.17 Eosinophilia is a common and important finding in parasitic worm infections. Allergies and drug reactions may also cause eosinophilia, but rarely to the same extreme degree as parasite infections, which should always be considered and often searched for when eosinophilia is found.

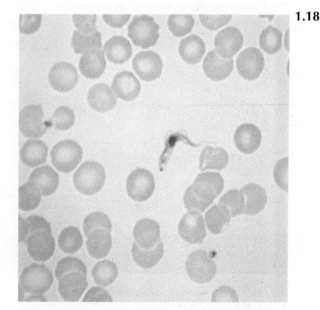

1.18 Blood smear showing *Trypanosoma brucei,* one of the causes of African trypanosomiasis. This finding is diagnostic.

Tissues which may provide a diagnosis include:
• Bone marrow—direct cytology and culture.
• Skin—fresh preparations and histology.
• Liver—histology and aspiration of abscess.
• Lung—transbronchial biopsy (**1.23**) or aspiration of bronchial washings.
• Lymph node or spleen.
• Colon and small intestine.

Failure to find the cause or type of infection is not uncommon, in which case a 'best guess' trial of appropriate chemotherapy is often used. Indeed in the very sick patient, treatment should be started immediately, with supportive measures and 'blind' drug therapy, which should be continued until the results of investigations dictate a change.

It is important to remember that multiple infections may occur in the same patient. It is common for secondary bacterial infections to occur in patients with primary viral infections, for example; and in patients with gross immunosuppression, such as those with AIDS, several infections may often co-exist.

The rest of this chapter is subdivided according to the nature of the infecting organisms. Because some infections are strongly organ-specific, they are covered in other chapters. The tables which appear at the start of each section of this chapter allow rapid reference to the correct page, while reminding the reader of the classification and inter-relationship of the causative organisms.

1.19

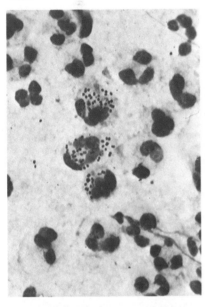

1.19 Intracellular gonococci in a smear of urethral discharge. This appearance is strongly suggestive of gonorrhoea, but definitive diagnosis depends on culture and identification of the organism.

1.20　　　　　　　　　　　　　**1.21**

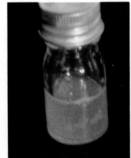　　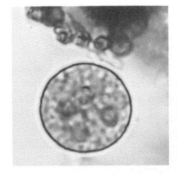

1.20 The mature cyst form of *Entamoeba histolytica*, on stool microscopy, showing the typical appearance with four nuclei. (*Iodine × 1800*)

1.21 Purulent cerebrospinal fluid, allowing a provisional diagnosis of pyogenic meningitis. Culture is required for confirmation, although the combination of this finding with the sudden onset of meningitis in a young person or with a rash is strongly suggestive of the diagnosis of bacterial meningitis, due to *N. meningitidis*, *H. influenzae* or *S. pneumoniae* (*see* p. 479, 492).

1.22

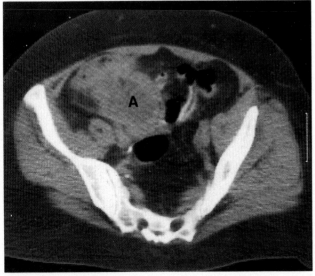

1.22 CT scan showing an appendix abscess (A) in a patient who had a pyrexia of unknown origin (PUO) following a rather vague episode of abdominal pain. Modern imaging techniques are very valuable in locating suspected abscesses and in many other ways in infectious conditions.

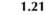

1.23 *Pneumocystis carinii*, dark stained by the Grocott method, in a transbronchial biopsy of the lung. Diagnosis of infections by tissue biopsy is necessary where the organisms are difficult or impossible to culture, as is the case with a number of the secondary infections which occur in AIDS, and with protozoal and helminthic infections.

Viral infections

Family	Important human viruses	Relevant human disease	Page reference
RNA viruses			
Retroviridae	Human immune deficiency virus (HIV 1 and 2)	Acquired immune deficiency syndrome (AIDS)	16
	Human T-cell leukaemia virus I and II (HTLV I and II)	Lymphoma/leukaemia	444, 451
Picornaviridae	Rhinovirus	Common cold	20
	Enterovirus		
	Poliovirus	Poliomyelitis	21
	ECHO viruses and coxsackieviruses	Herpangina, skin eruptions, pericarditis, hand–foot–mouth disease, myocarditis, pleurodynia, aseptic meningitis	21
	Hepatitis A	Hepatitis	398
Reoviridae	Orbivirus	Colorado tick fever, etc.	
	Rotavirus	Gastroenteritis	379
Togaviridae	Rubella virus	Rubella	22
	Encephalitis viruses	Encephalitis	23, 493
Flaviviridae	Yellow fever virus	Yellow fever	23
	Dengue	Dengue haemorrhagic fever	23
	Encephalitis viruses	Encephalitis	23, 493
Paramyxoviridae	Measles virus	Measles	24
	Mumps virus	Mumps	25
	Respiratory syncytial virus	Respiratory infections	174, 186
	Parainfluenza viruses	Respiratory infections	174, 186
Orthomyxoviridae	Influenza viruses A, B, C	Influenza	25
Rhabdoviridae	Rabies virus	Rabies	26
Arenaviridae	Lassa fever virus	Lassa fever	26
	Lymphocytic choriomeningitis virus	Meningitis	492
Filoviridae	Marburg virus	Haemorrhagic fever	27
Coronaviridae	Coronavirus	Respiratory infections	174
Bunyaviridae	Bunyavirus	Haemorrhagic fever	27
Caliciviridae	Norwalk agent	Gastroenteritis (winter vomiting)	379
DNA viruses			
Parvoviridae	Parvovirus (B19)	Erythema infectiosum	27
Papovaviridae	Papillomavirus	Warts	81, 98
Hepadnaviridae	Hepatitis B virus	Hepatitis	398
Adenoviridae	Adenovirus	Respiratory infections, diarrhoea	174, 379
Herpesviridae	Herpes simplex virus	Cold sore, genital infection	28, 493
	Varicella-zoster virus	Chickenpox, shingles	29, 30
	Cytomegalovirus	Generalised infection	31
	Epstein–Barr virus	Infectious mononucleosis	32
		Burkitt's lymphoma	33
		Nasopharyngeal carcinoma	
	Herpes 6 virus	Roseola infantum	33
Poxviridae	Smallpox virus	Smallpox (now eradicated)	
	Cowpox and orf viruses	Milker's nodules, orf	33
	Molluscum contagiosum virus	Skin papules	98

HIV Infection and AIDS

AIDS is the end result of infection with human immune deficiency virus (HIV). Transmission of the virus, human to human, is by sexual intercourse (homosexual or heterosexual), by inoculation of infected blood or blood products, by use of contaminated needles (drug abusers) and by vertical transmission from mother to infant (**1.6**). The virus infects and destroys CD4 lymphocytes (T-helper cells), causing impairment of the immune system which exposes infected people to a variety of ordinary and opportunistic infections and predisposes them to the development of certain tumours. Many millions of people worldwide are infected with HIV and the number of deaths from end-stage disease (AIDS) is increasing exponentially.

The usual inexorable progression of HIV infection is shown in **1.24**. The incubation period is usually between one and three months at the end of which seroconversion to the antibody positive state occurs. At the time of seroconversion the patient is often asymptomatic, but there may be a transient glandular fever-like illness with malaise, pyrexia, sore throat, rash (**1.25**), generalised adenitis and occasionally aseptic meningitis and encephalopathy.

Next is a latent period lasting for several years (on average about eight) during which the patient is asymptomatic but is infective and can transmit the virus.

Deterioration in health usually starts with **persistent generalised lymphadenopathy (PGL)**, which is characterised by painless lymphadenopathy (**1.26**), tonsillar enlargement (**1.27**), mild fever, sometimes general malaise, sweating and some weight loss.

1.24

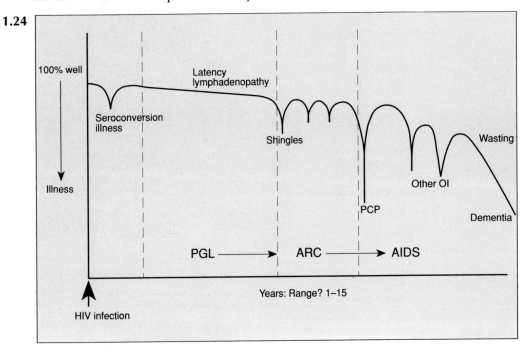

1.24 AIDS is a 'state of risk' rather than a single continuous illness. The patient suffers episodes of severe infection, being well for much of the intervening time. For the first few years, most patients with HIV infection remain well. After this latent period, they may enter the phase of persistent generalised lymphadenopathy (PGL) and subsequently AIDS-related complex (ARC), often heralded by the onset of shingles. This may be followed by several minor infections before the first presentation of AIDS, which is often with *Pneumocystis carinii* pneumonia (PCP). If the patient survives this infection, other opportunistic infections (OI) may follow, leading ultimately to death from a wasting syndrome or progressive HIV encephalopathy. The timescale for the full progression may range from 1 to 15 or more years.

1.25

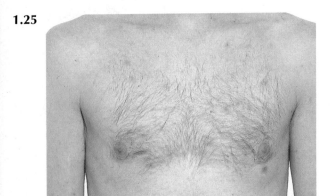

1.25 HIV-related rash in a 22-year-old man. In addition to this rash, he presented with fever, sore throat and headache. HIV serology was negative at this time, but seroconversion was noted 5 weeks later.

1.26

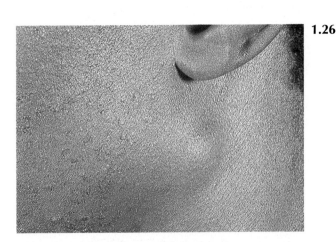

1.26 Painless lymph node enlargement at the PGL stage in a patient with HIV infection.

Table 1.2 Cutaneous manifestations which may be associated with HIV infection*

- Seborrhoeic dermatitis
- Folliculitis
- Acne vulgaris
- Xeroderma
- Fungal infections
- Herpes simplex
- Impetigo
- Drug eruptions
- Urticaria
- Vasculitis
- Alopecia
- Severe psoriasis
- Granuloma annulare
- Yellow nail syndrome

*Note that most of these conditions are common and benign in the absence of HIV infection.

The next stage is that of **AIDS-related complex (ARC)**, the features of which include marked malaise, fever, adenitis and significant weight loss. Skin lesions are common at this stage and may take many forms (**Table 1.2**). Seborrhoeic dermatitis is particularly common (**2.30, 2.31**). Patients may present with oral candidiasis (**1.28**), hairy leukoplakia (**1.29**), herpes simplex (**1.30**), herpes zoster (**1.31, 2.43**) or other secondary infections at this stage (**Table 1.3**). The number of CD4 cells in peripheral blood falls and the CD4:CD8 ratio usually falls below 1.0. There is also usually anaemia, thrombocytopenia, leucopenia and elevated serum globulins. Patients classified as ARC will almost invariably progress to AIDS.

1.27

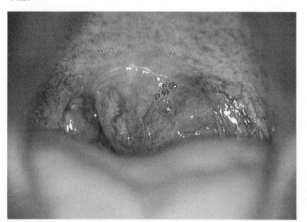

1.27 Gross tonsillar enlargement in an HIV-infected patient with PGL.

1.28

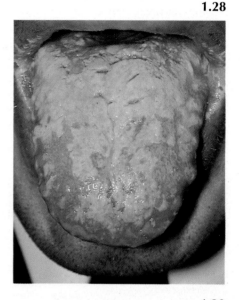

1.28 Extensive oral infection with *Candida albicans* in a patient at the ARC stage of HIV infection. Note the gross changes in the tongue and the angular chelitis.

1.30

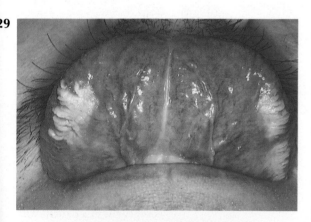

1.29 Hairy leukoplakia in a patient with ARC. Note the appearance of a ribbed whiteness along the sides of the tongue. The term 'hairy' refers to the histopathological appearance, and the cause appears to be a proliferation of Epstein–Barr virus in the superficial layers of the squamous epithelium of the tongue.

1.30 Severe perianal herpes simplex is a common problem in homosexual patients with ARC and AIDS. It may cause great discomfort, but often responds to oral acyclovir treatment.

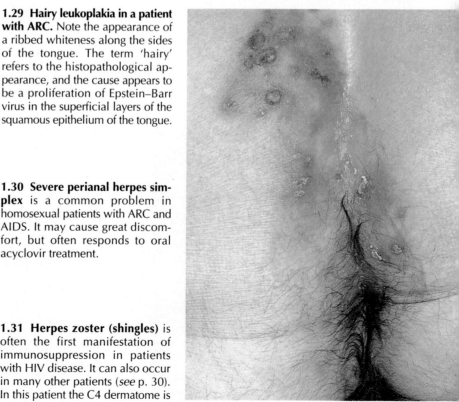

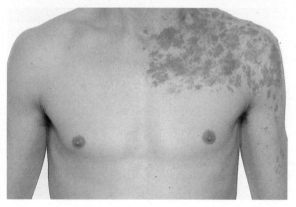

1.31 Herpes zoster (shingles) is often the first manifestation of immunosuppression in patients with HIV disease. It can also occur in many other patients (*see* p. 30). In this patient the C4 dermatome is affected.

For the diagnosis of AIDS the patient must have developed one or more major opportunistic infections or certain malignancies for which no other cause is identified. By this stage the immune system has been almost completely destroyed and

Table 1.3 Secondary infections associated with HIV infection at the ARC stage

- Oral candidiasis, especially in men
- 'Seborrhoeic dermatitis'
- Folliculitis and/or papular eczema
- Herpes zoster
- Herpes simplex, especially anal infection
- Molluscum contagiosum
- Impetigo contagiosa
- Cellulitis

opportunistic infection poses a major risk to life. Pneumocystis pneumonia (**1.32, 4.80**) is the most common opportunistic infection, but other organisms are also a threat. The target organs for major opportunistic infection depend on the organism involved. For example:

- Lungs—*Pneumocystis carinii*, Cytomegalovirus (CMV—**1.83**), atypical mycobacteria.
- CNS—*Cryptococcus neoformans* (**1.167**), *Toxoplasma gondii* (**1.33**), CMV.
- Gut—*Cryptosporidium*, *Isospora belli*, CMV and *Candida albicans* (**1.34**).
- Eyes—CMV (**1.35**) and *Toxoplasma gondii*.

Many opportunistic infections will respond to appropriate therapy, but life-long suppressive treatment will almost certainly be required to prevent relapse or recrudescence.

1.32

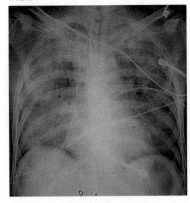

1.32 *Pneumocystis* pneumonia is the most common life-threatening opportunistic infection in patients with AIDS and in other immunocompromised patients. There is a significant mortality in AIDS patients in their first episode of *Pneumocystis* pneumonia, but the combination of intensive care and appropriate chemotherapy may achieve complete resolution of the infection. Prophylactic chemotherapy with co-trimoxazole or nebulised pentamidine reduces the risk of this complication.

1.33

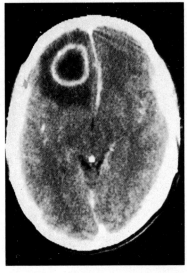

1.33 Cerebral abscess in the left frontal region on a CT scan. In patients with AIDS, the most common cause of cerebral abscess is *Toxoplasma gondii,* and the abscesses are often multiple.

1.34

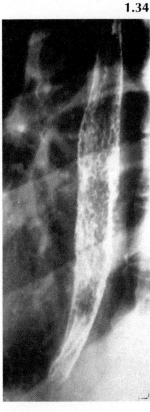

1.34 Candidiasis of the oesophagus in a patient with AIDS, demonstrated by barium swallow. Note the mottled appearance, which results from multiple plaques of candidiasis on the oesophageal mucosa.

1.35

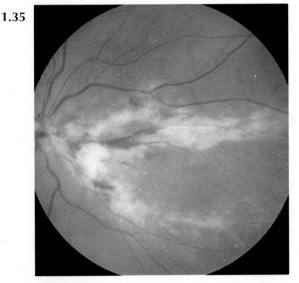

1.35 Cytomegalovirus (CMV) retinitis in a patient with AIDS. This serious opportunistic infection can rapidly progress to irreversible blindness. CMV causes a retinal vasculitis which leads to areas of infarction.

The common malignancies that develop in patients with AIDS include Kaposi's sarcoma (1.36–1.41) of skin, mucous membrane or internal organs and non-Hodgkin's lymphoma of lymph nodes (1.42), internal organs or brain. Direct involvement of the central nervous system in HIV infection causes dementia (1.43), encephalopathy and myelopathy.

A variant of AIDS has appeared in East and Central Africa, in which the dominant features are severe diarrhoea (not of bacterial origin, but often associated with protozoal infection), gross wasting (1.44) and often an itchy rash. This has been called **Slim disease**, and is rapidly fatal, even in the absence of the other complications of AIDS.

Diagnosis of HIV infection and AIDS depends on detection of antibody in serum or antigen in affected T-cells. Tests for HIV infection should not be carried out without prior counselling of the patient and provision of full support services for patients found to be infected. When opportunistic infection or malignancy is suspected, efforts must be made to establish the exact diagnosis.

Specific antiviral therapy may slow down disease progression, especially if given at a reasonably early stage of the illness; but current therapy is associated with a large number of side effects which include general malaise, gastrointestinal upset, rashes, anaemia, muscle weakness and occasionally seizures. Opportunistic infections require additional specific therapy. As with all serious illnesses, patients with AIDS require full medical, social and psychological support and support of the family and friends of patients is also important.

Prevention of the spread of HIV infection includes screening of blood donors, advice on safer sexual practices, measures to curtail intravenous drug abuse and the provision of syringe and needle exchange centres. It is hoped that eventually a safe and effective vaccine will become available for prevention of the disease.

1.36

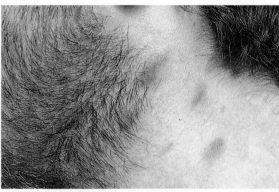

1.37

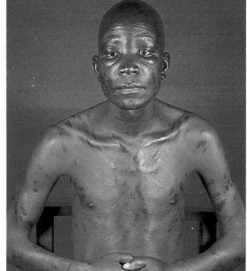

1.38

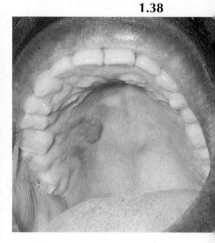

1.39

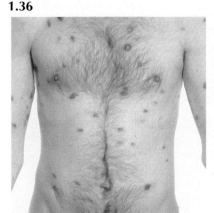

1.41

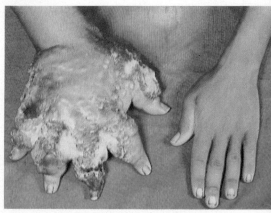

1.40

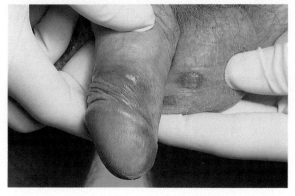

1.36–1.41 Kaposi's sarcoma is a common complication in AIDS patients, especially in those who contracted the disease by sexual transmission. In **1.36** note the generalised lesions, many of which show peripheral bruising. **1.37** shows the appearance of similar involvement in a black African patient. Kaposi's sarcoma may also affect mucous membranes, as seen in **1.38**, where there are two obvious plaques of Kaposi's sarcoma on the palate. The lesions are often aligned with skin creases, as shown on the neck of the patient in **1.39**. Kaposi's sarcoma lesions may occur anywhere on the surface of the body, including the penis and scrotum (**1.40**). In some cases the tumour may infiltrate extensively and rapidly, as seen in the hand of an African patient in **1.41**.

19

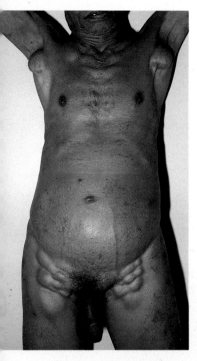

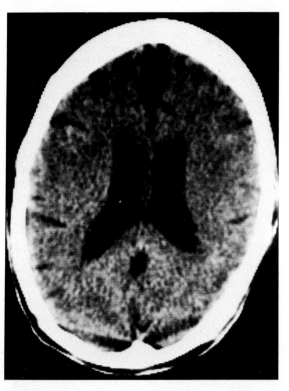

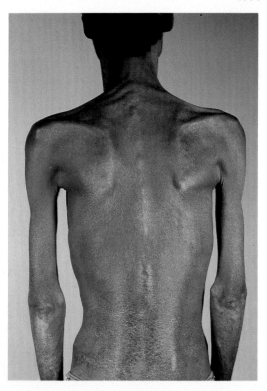

1.42 Non-Hodgkin's lymphoma in a patient with HIV infection. There is massive axillary and inguinal lymphadenopathy. He also had gross hepatosplenomegaly and ascites.

1.43 AIDS dementia. The CT scan shows cerebral atrophy with enlarged lateral ventricles.

1.44 Slim disease in which chronic diarrhoea is accompanied by gross weight loss and an itchy skin rash.

The common cold

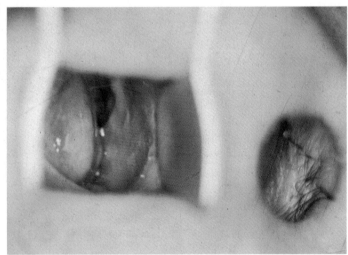

The common cold (acute coryza) is the most common disease caused by infection in the developed world, and the most frequent symptomatic manifestation of upper respiratory tract infection (URTI). URTIs may be caused by a range of viruses, including rhinoviruses, respiratory syncytial virus, parainfluenza viruses, coronaviruses and adenoviruses.

Uncomplicated acute coryza leads to nasal congestion (**1.45**), a watery nasal discharge (**1.1**), which may become purulent, and often a sore throat. Most cases resolve spontaneously, but the common cold may be complicated by secondary bacterial infection, leading to sinusitis, otitis media and infection of the lower respiratory tract.

1.45 Acute rhinitis in the common cold. The nasal mucous membrane is oedematous, so the inferior turbinate abuts against the septum causing obstruction, as seen here in a view through a nasal speculum.

Enterovirus infections

The enteroviruses can be subdivided into three main sub-groups—polioviruses, coxsackieviruses and ECHO viruses (hepatitis A, p. 398 is also caused by an enterovirus). All infect man by the faecal/oral route. Initial viral replication takes place in the gut mucosa, with subsequent shedding of virus in the stools. If host immunity is poor, virus enters the blood stream and may be disseminated to target organs such as the meninges, nervous tissue, heart and skin.

Poliomyelitis has an incubation period of up to 14 days and is characterised by an initial 'flu'-like illness followed, if host immunity is poor, by aseptic meningitis. Virus then enters nervous tissue, the main attack being on the anterior horn cells of the spinal cord, causing flaccid paralysis of limb muscles that tends to be asymmetrical and is usually permanent (**1.46, 1.47**). In severe cases, muscles of swallowing and respiration may be involved.

Management is symptomatic, but paralytic poliomyelitis requires skilled physiotherapy. Patients may also need long-term ventilation and, later, the provision of mechanical aids and/or corrective surgery.

An injectable killed virus vaccine (Salk vaccine) and a live attenuated oral vaccine (Sabin vaccine) are available for prevention of poliomyelitis. This disease is now very rare in the western world, but still occurs in developing countries where indigenous children and non-immunised expatriates of all ages are vulnerable.

Coxsackieviruses (Groups A&B) and ECHO viruses produce a wide variety of clinical syndromes, after a short but variable incubation period, including non-specific febrile illness, rashes (**1.48**), myocarditis, pericarditis, meningitis, meningo-encephalitis and, rarely, paralytic disease. **Herpangina** (ulcer-ative lesions on the palate and fauces) and hand–foot–mouth disease (**1.49, 1.50**) are caused by Group A coxsackieviruses.

Epidemic myalgia (Bornholm disease) is a common presentation of infection with Group B coxsackieviruses. Both ECHO viruses and coxsackieviruses can cause severe generalised infection in neonates. The post-viral fatigue syndrome may follow coxsackievirus infection.

Enteroviruses can be isolated from stool, pharyngeal secretions, CSF, pericardial fluid and, occasionally, from blood in severe neonatal infections. Rising antibody titres may be demon-strated to specific enteroviruses. Treatment of enterovirus in-fections is symptomatic.

1.46

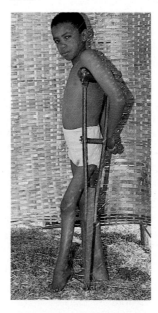

1.47

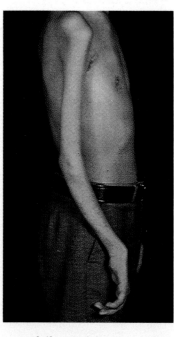

1.46 Paralysis of the left leg following poliomyelitis in an Ethiopian boy. The disease is still a major problem in developing countries.

1.47 Flail arm following polio-myelitis in infancy.

1.48

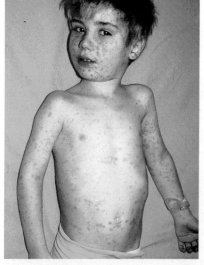

1.48 ECHO virus type 19 infection causing a maculopapular rash. Rashes of this kind may be very difficult to distinguish from rubella (*see* p. 22), and antibody studies may be required for a firm diagnosis.

1.49

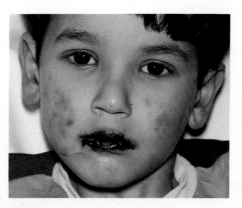

1.49 Hand–foot–mouth disease. This shows the typical rash of bright red macules, with small vesicles on an erythematous base on both cheeks and the lips. Similar lesions occur inside the mouth. This patient has been treated by the topical application of gentian violet.

1.50

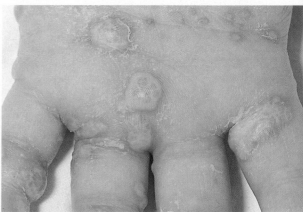

1.50 Hand–foot–mouth disease. Many of the lesions are distributed on the lateral aspects of the fingers, but in this young patient several lesions were also present on the palm.

Rubella

The causal agent is a togavirus, which causes a mild illness and is spread by droplets from the respiratory tract. The incubation period is 18–19 days. A pink maculopapular rash appears on the second day of illness (1.51, 1.52). On the trunk, the rash becomes confluent and may resemble the rash of scarlet fever. There is usually mild inflammation of the throat and palate, and the posterior cervical lymph nodes become enlarged and tender. The rash fades in about 48 hours and recovery, especially in children, is rapid. Complications include arthralgia (more common in adults), thrombocytopenia and very rarely encephalitis.

The diagnosis is confirmed by the detection of rising titre of IgM antibody in the serum. Treatment is not usually necessary but arthralgia requires relief of pain with analgesics.

Rubella in either childhood or adult life is usually a trivial, self-limiting illness, but the virus can cause serious damage to the developing fetus. Fetal infection can occur at any stage of pregnancy, but the damage tends to be most marked in the first trimester. The sequelae may include signs of infection at birth (1.53), microcephaly, deafness, blindness (1.54) and congenital cardiac malformations (*see* p. 234).

Suspected rubella in early pregnancy should be confirmed serologically; appropriate advice on risk to the fetus and availability of abortion should be given to the parents, if the disease is confirmed. If there is contact with rubella in early pregnancy, it is important to establish the diagnosis in the index case and to check the antibody status of the pregnant contact as soon as possible. A non-immune contact in early pregnancy should be given the option of abortion if rubella develops. If abortion is not performed, hyperimmune globulin can be given and is protective in about 40% of cases.

Prevention may be accomplished by live attenuated vaccine, used on its own or combined with measles and mumps vaccine (MMR). Rubella vaccine should not be given during pregnancy.

1.51

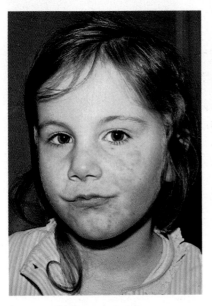

1.51 Rubella, showing the early stage of the rash on the face. Note that the patient shows no signs of catarrh or conjunctival discharge, in contrast to the typical patient with measles.

1.52 Rubella rash on the trunk. On the first day, the rash consists of discrete, delicate pink macules. These may coalesce on the second day, as here, but the severity of the rash varies considerably, and it may be missed altogether when the lesions are sparse.

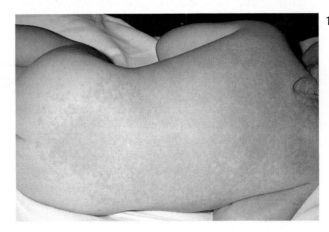

1.

1.53

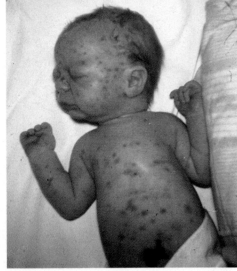

1.53 Congenital rubella presenting as a small-for-dates baby with a purpuric rash caused by thrombocytopenia. Children born with congenital rubella are a potential source of infection to others, and it is important that appropriate steps are taken to protect other patients and staff.

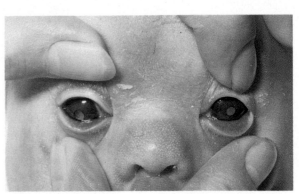

1.

1.54 Cataracts causing blindness in this newborn baby with congenital rubella.

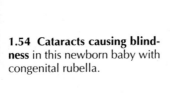

Yellow fever

This is an acute mosquito-borne infection caused by a flavivirus which results in a pyrexial illness, with liver and renal involvement and disseminated intravascular coagulation (DIC—*see* p. 463). It is found in both Africa and Central/Southern America in a narrow band about the Equator, but not in Asia. There are two important cycles of transmission: in the urban type the yellow fever virus is transmitted from an infected person to a non-immune recipient by mosquito (*Aedes* spp.); in the sylvan (or jungle) type there is a monkey reservoir and the vector is the *Aedes* spp. in Africa or *Haemagogus* spp. in America.

The spectrum of clinical illness varies from a very mild, transient, pyrexial illness to a rapid, progressively fatal form. The incubation period is short (4–6 days). The appearance of jaundice (not usually severe), proteinuria and haemorrhage give clues to the diagnosis. Haemorrhage is often apparent initially in the skin but haematemesis may occur and is a poor prognostic sign (**1.55**). In fulminant cases there is progression of liver and renal failure to coma and death. The mortality rate is about 40% in these severe cases.

There is no specific antiviral therapy, and general supportive measures are required for severely ill patients. Yellow fever vaccine gives protection for up to 10 years.

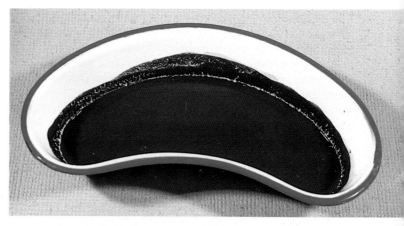

1.55 'Coffee ground' vomit in yellow fever has severe implications. As in other conditions, it is a sign of major upper gastrointestinal bleeding.

Dengue haemorrhagic fever

This is one of the haemorrhagic fevers found in Africa, South East Asia and India. It is transmitted by the mosquito *Aedes aegypti*, which is itself infected by the dengue virus (or one of six subtypes). The incubation is short (1–2 days), and the clinical presentation is abrupt with extreme nausea, vomiting and fever. Purpura appears on the second or third day and disseminated intravascular coagulation with bleeding from a variety of sites dominates the clinical picture (**1.56**, p. 463). Viraemia and blood loss produce a profound state of shock.

There is no specific treatment, but symptomatic treatment with oxygen and blood volume expanders is often essential. Despite this, there is a mortality rate of up to 50% in severe cases. Public health measures for mosquito control are important. The severe nature of this disease results from sequential infection with two subtypes of virus.

Classic dengue fever is not so severe in presentation and has a lower mortality.

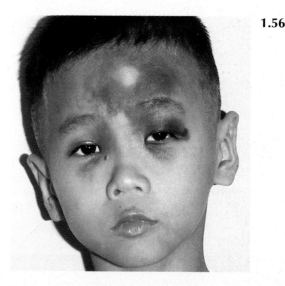

1.56 Dengue haemorrhagic fever causing marked ecchymoses associated with DIC in an infected 8-year-old boy in Vietnam.

Epidemic encephalitis

Several flaviviruses and togaviruses cause mosquito-transmitted encephalitis in various parts of the world. These include several forms of equine encephalitis in the American continent, Japanese encephalitis (**1.57**) and St Louis encephalitis. Russian spring-summer encephalitis and Powassan are similar diseases transmitted by ticks. Encephalitis results rapidly, and the patients present with fever and rigors. There is often rapid deterioration of mental status (*see* p. 493). Mortality is high (up to 40%) and there is a high morbidity in the survivors (up to 30%), with residual and neurological deficits. There is no specific treatment. Vaccination against Japanese B encephalitis is now available for those travelling to endemic areas.

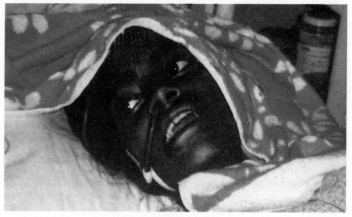

1.57 Encephalitis caused by Japanese B virus can be severe, resulting in serious sequelae such as mental retardation. Other encephalitis viruses may lead to similar consequences.

Measles

The causal agent is a paramyxovirus, and the disease is highly infectious. It is spread by droplets from the respiratory tract and preschool children are particularly at risk.

After an incubation of 10–11 days, the illness starts with fever and coryzal symptoms. Small white spots (Koplik's spots) appear on the buccal mucosa (**1.58**) on the second day. A red, blotchy, maculopapular rash starts on the neck, usually on the fourth day of illness. Thereafter, the rash spreads to the face (**1.14**), trunk and finally to the limbs (**1.59**). As the rash fades, there may be temporary purplish haemorrhagic staining of the skin.

Complications of measles include pneumonia, croup, otitis media, gastroenteritis and, rarely, encephalitis. In the third world, these complications lead to a high morbidity and mortality, especially in under-nourished children (**1.60**, **1.61**).

The diagnosis is usually made on clinical grounds, but if necessary can be confirmed by viral isolation or by serology. Treatment is symptomatic in uncomplicated cases. Appropriate antibiotic therapy is required for bacterial complications such as pneumonia and otitis media.

Active immunisation is available: combined with mumps and rubella vaccine (MMR), it should be offered to all children aged between 1 and 2 years. Passive immunisation with normal human immune globulin can prevent the disease if given early in the incubation period, but immunity is short-lasting.

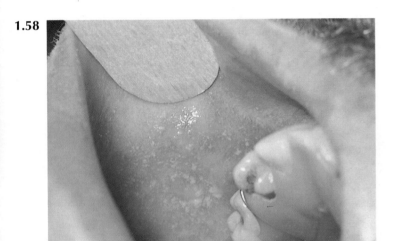

1.58 Koplik's spots in measles are most commonly seen opposite the molars or on the buccal surface of the lips and cheeks. They precede the main rash by several days.

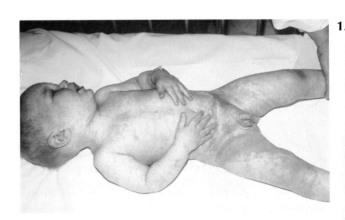

1.59 Measles. The typical maculopapular, morbilliform rash starts on the neck and face and spreads to involve the trunk and the limbs. This infant also had typical catarrh and conjunctivitis.

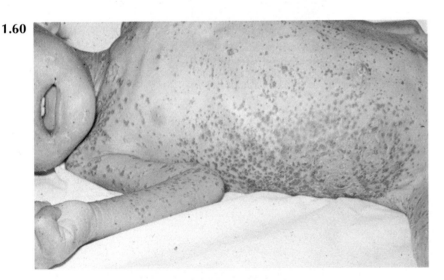

1.60 Measles in an under-nourished child in Guatemala. The rash is florid, and is likely to be associated with serious complications, including the development of overt kwashiorkor (*see* p. 343).

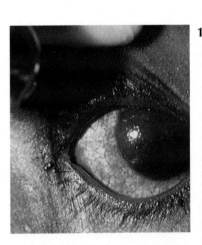

1.61 Measles keratoconjunctivitis and xerophthalmia are common complications of the infection in the malnourished child. The corneal light reflex is distorted, and the pre-ocular tear film is lacking.

Mumps

The causal organism is a paramyxovirus which spreads by droplets and saliva. The incubation period is 18–21 days. Most patients with mumps present with swelling of the salivary glands (**1.62**), but other glands may be involved, including the pancreas, the gonads (adults only) and the thyroid gland. The virus may also attack the meninges or the brain, causing aseptic meningitis or encephalitis. Transient deafness can occur during the course of mumps, but permanent nerve deafness is a rare complication.

Salivary gland swelling usually subsides within two weeks. About 10–15% of post-pubertal males will develop orchitis (**1.63**) which may be unilateral or bilateral. Breasts and ovaries are occasionally involved in females.

The diagnosis can be confirmed if necessary by viral isolation and by serology. This is important in patients who present without salivary gland involvement.

No specific therapy is available. If there is salivary gland involvement, attention must be paid to oral hygiene and fluid intake. Diet should be bland. The pain and swelling of orchitis usually responds to a short course of steroid therapy. Anti-emetics and intravenous fluids may be required for pancreatitis. Mumps meningitis is a benign illness and needs only bed rest and symptomatic treatment.

Active immunisation is available (alone or combined in MMR) and it should be offered to children and adults without a history of the disease.

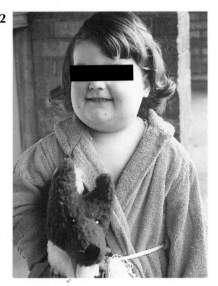

1.62 Mumps. There is marked bilateral enlargement of the parotid glands, which are usually tender, associated with generalised facial oedema. This girl was convalescent when photographed.

1.63 Mumps orchitis is the most serious complication of the disease in the adult, though it does not usually damage the pre-pubertal testis. It may be unilateral or bilateral and usually causes severe tenderness.

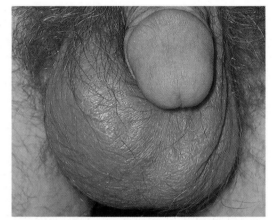

Influenza

This is an acute viral infection which is spread by droplets from person to person. It is caused by three groups of related myxo-viruses which produce fever, prostration, myalgia, headache and anorexia. The viruses undergo fequent antigenic changes, do not produce cross-immunity to each other and give rise to epidemics and pandemics. Five pandemics have occurred in the twentieth century with massive mortality. For example, up to 20 million people died in 1918, with millions more having continued morbidity from respiratory and neurological sequelae (postencephalitic parkinsonism, p. 502).

Acute infection may present with a spectrum of symptoms ranging from a very mild pyrexia which is rapidly self-limiting to an overwhelming infection with severe myalgia, headache, fever, sore throat, acute tracheitis and even pleurisy. In addition, encephalitis, myositis and myocarditis may supervene, especially in the elderly. Secondary bacterial infection, often with *Staphylococcus aureus, Haemophilus influenzae* and *Streptococcus pneumoniae,* is a common complication in the debilitated elderly patient (**1.64**, p. 186). Vaccination may give partial immunity, but only to the current antigenic type of virus. Treatment is usually symptomatic.

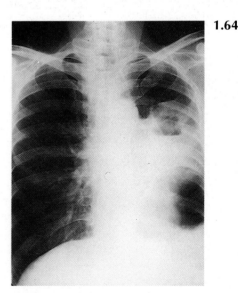

1.64 Secondary bacterial chest infection is the most frequent serious consequence of influenza. In this elderly patient, there is a left mid-zone cavitating pneumonia (note the fluid level in the cavity) and an accompany-ing left pleural effusion. The causative organism was *Staphylococcus aureus.*

Rabies

Rabies is caused by an RNA virus of the Rhabdoviridae family. Man is infected through bites from a rabid animal (1.65). The incubation period may be as short as two weeks, but in some cases may be as long as one year. The virus, once in the body, spreads via peripheral nerves to the central nervous system causing encephalomyelitis which is almost uniformly fatal.

Initial symptoms include pain and tingling at the inoculation site, extreme restlessness followed by severe spasms of the larynx and pharynx which are brought on by attempts to swallow, giving rise to the term hydrophobia (1.66). Eventually flaccid paralysis develops (1.67) and the patient lapses into coma. Some patients, especially those bitten by vampire bats, present initially with flaccid paralysis which often begins in the bitten limb, but which rapidly becomes generalised.

If possible, the diagnosis should be confirmed in the animal by histopathological examination of the brain. In humans the virus can be identified by immunofluorescence on skin or corneal impression smears or by brain biopsy. Serological tests may also be diagnostic, but may be difficult to interpret if post-exposure vaccination has been given.

Patients must be nursed in an intensive care unit. Heavy sedation and positive pressure ventilation are required. The disease is usually fatal but there have been several documented cases of recovery.

Prevention includes regular immunisation of domestic animals in endemic areas and pre-exposure immunisation of people at risk.

Post-exposure management of bitten people includes thorough cleaning of the bite, passive immunisation with human rabies immunoglobulin and an immediate course of human diploid cell rabies vaccine.

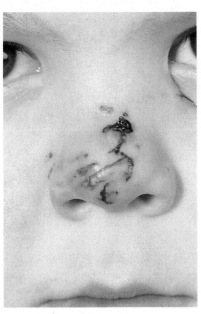

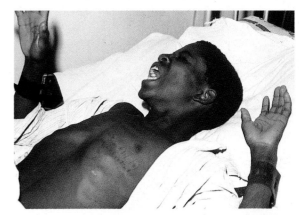

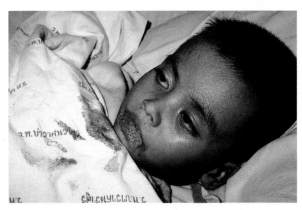

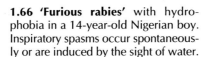
1.65 An infected dog bite is the usual route through which rabies virus gains access to the nervous system. Even in a rabies-free country such as the UK, the possibility of an illegally imported rabid animal should be considered.

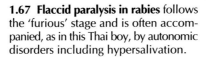
1.66 'Furious rabies' with hydrophobia in a 14-year-old Nigerian boy. Inspiratory spasms occur spontaneously or are induced by the sight of water.

1.67 Flaccid paralysis in rabies follows the 'furious' stage and is often accompanied, as in this Thai boy, by autonomic disorders including hypersalivation.

Lassa fever

This is caused by infection with an arenavirus (Lassa fever virus) and is found predominantly in West Africa. Infection with similar viruses causes Argentine and Bolivian haemorrhagic fevers in South America. The vector is the rodent, *Mastomys natalensis.*

Onset of the clinical disease is gradual, with fever, headache and myalgia, which particularly affects the legs. In addition there may be conjunctivitis, aphthous ulceration of the mouth, a fine generalised petechial rash and facial oedema (1.68). As the platelet count falls, haemorrhage may occur from a variety of sites. A combination of viraemia and haemorrhage produces shock and this may be associated with evidence of viral myocarditis. Encephalitis and permanent cranial nerve impairment may also occur. In severe cases a mortality of up to 20% has been found.

There is no specific treatment for the disease, but specific anti-viral agents (e.g. ribavirin) are promising. Symptomatic control of haemorrhage and shock are important. Prevention of spread of the disease depends on public health measures to control contact with rodents and with the virus-laden rodent excreta. Hospital outbreaks involve careful handling of all blood and excreta of patients.

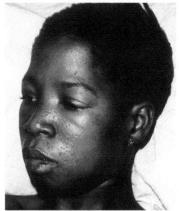

1.68 Facial oedema in Lassa fever is a common feature of severe cases and carries a poor prognosis.

African haemorrhagic fever

This is an acute onset fever, characterised by papular rash (**1.69**), proteinuria, pancreatitis, hepatitis and haemorrhage. It is caused by infection with either Marburg or Ebola viruses. Marburg disease was originally found in people in contact with green monkeys (*Cercopithecus aethiops*) which were obtained from Uganda. Subsequently there was evidence of transmission by needles and directly person-to-person. Both viruses cause acute disseminated intravascular coagulation (DIC, p. 463), and profound haemorrhage is the usual cause of death. There is no specific treatment, but the patients require intensive circulatory support and control of the DIC with heparin; and they may benefit from plasma containing virus-specific antibodies. Extensive precautions are needed to prevent spread of infection.

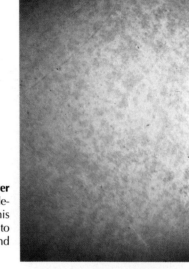

1.69 African haemorrhagic fever is often accompanied by a widespread papular rash, though this non-specific sign may progress to more serious petechiae and haemorrhage.

Erythema infectiosum

This acute self-limiting disease, also known as fifth disease or slapped cheek disease, is caused by human parvovirus B19. It occurs in outbreaks, most often in spring and summer. Any age may be affected but it is most common in children, in whom the usual presentation is a mild febrile illness followed by marked erythema of the cheeks and the appearance of a pink maculo-papular rash (**1.70**). The rash may become confluent and is most marked on the limbs; as it fades, it takes on a lace-like appearance. The rash may come and go over about 2–3 weeks. Adenopathy, arthralgia and arthritis are common especially in adults infected with the virus. Joints most involved are wrists and knees. The arthritis may, if prolonged, be mistaken for other forms of rheumatism. Transient marrow depression may occur during the course of the illness. In patients with congenital haemolytic anaemia, an aplastic crisis may be induced (*see* p. 433).

The diagnosis can be confirmed by finding a specific IgM antibody in the serum.

As the disease is self-limiting, children require no therapy. Analgesics and anti-inflammatory drugs may be needed for relief of joint pain in adults. If there is an aplastic crisis, blood transfusion is indicated. No vaccine is available for this disease.

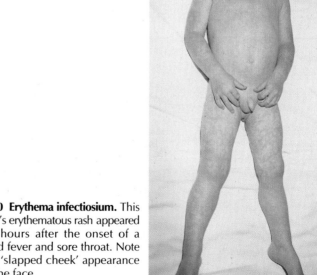

1.70 Erythema infectiosium. This boy's erythematous rash appeared 24 hours after the onset of a mild fever and sore throat. Note the 'slapped cheek' appearance of the face.

Herpes simplex

The causal agents are herpes simplex virus types I and II. Type II is associated with sexually transmitted genital infection, whereas most other infections are caused by type I. Following the primary infection, the virus remains latent in the tissues and may re-emerge at a later stage to produce local lesions.

Primary infection with type I virus usually occurs in childhood and takes the form of acute gingivostomatitis with multiple painful, shallow ulcers on the tongue, buccal mucosa and lips (1.5, 1.71). In genital herpes, ulcers are on the vulva, vagina, cervix or penis (1.72). In both instances, the primary lesions are self-limiting and clear in about 10 days. The local eruption may be accompanied by fever and malaise and, in the case of children, refusal to eat or drink. Other sites of primary infection are the fingers (herpetic whitlow) and the cornea (dendritic ulcer, 1.73). Herpes simplex encephalitis is a rare but very serious presentation. In the neonate, disseminated herpes simplex is a life-threatening illness. Patients with eczema may present with widespread lesions on the eczematous areas (eczema herpeticum, p. 93).

Reactivation of latent herpes simplex usually occurs in sites related to the primary infection (1.74). In the immuno-compromised patient, reactivation of virus may cause very severe local lesions (1.30), with generalised viraemia and encephalitis.

Virus can be cultured from vesical fluid or from swabs from genital or mouth ulcers. Viral particles can also be identified with the electron microscope. Rising antibody titres may be found in primary herpes simplex.

Most primary lesions are self-limiting and specific therapy is not usually required. If applied very early, idoxuridine paint or acyclovir cream may abort the development of 'cold sores'. Intravenous acyclovir should be used to treat herpes encephalitis and severe infections in the immunocompromised host and in the neonate. An ophthalmological opinion should be sought when there is involvement of the eye.

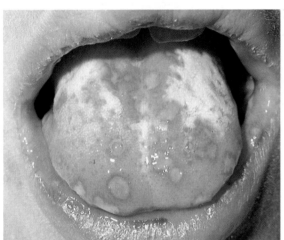

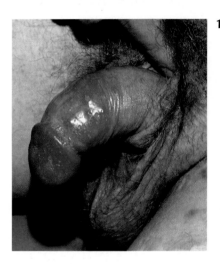

1.71 Severe herpetic gingivostomatitis. This young child was acutely ill with a high fever and had multiple vesicular lesions on the tongue, lips and buccal mucosa. In adult patients, a more common manifestation of herpetic stomatitis is the cold sore—usually a reactivation of latent infection.

1.72 Primary genital herpes. Note the numerous lesions on the penis and the associated tissue reaction.

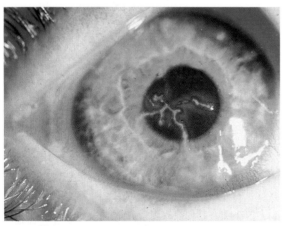

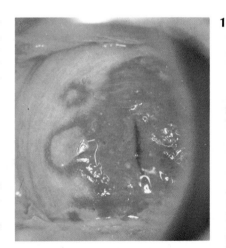

1.73 A primary herpetic dendritic ulcer, stained with fluorescein. Herpes simplex virus proliferates in the epithelial layer of the cornea. Urgent treatment with antiviral drops or ointment is indicated.

1.74 Recurrent herpes simplex on the cervix. The ulcers have recurred in a common primary site for genital infection. Other common sites include the external genitalia and the lips.

Herpes zoster

Varicella zoster causes two distinct diseases—chickenpox (varicella) and shingles (herpes zoster).

Chickenpox

This is a highly infectious disease caused by the *Varicella zoster* virus. It is usually mild in children but can be severe in adults and in immunocompromised patients. The incubation period is usually 14–15 days. In adults especially, there may be a short prodromal illness with fever, malaise, headache and occasionally a transient erythematous rash. The true rash is vesicular with a central distribution in the body (**1.75**). The spots are elliptical and come out in crops over a few days (**1.76**). Mucous membranes may also be affected (**1.77**). Scabs form rapidly and most have separated in 10–14 days. The commonest complication, especially in children, is skin sepsis, usually due to superinfection with *Staphylococcus aureus* or *Streptococcus pyogenes*. Varicella pneumonia, which can be life-threatening, occurs mainly in adults and in the immunocompromised (**1.78**,

10.63). Other rare complications include encephalitis and haemorrhagic chickenpox.

The diagnosis is usually made on clinical grounds but electron microscopy, viral culture and serology may be required in difficult cases.

No specific therapy is usually required. Children should be prevented, if possible, from scratching the spots. If the disease is severe, especially in the immunocompromised patient, the antiviral drug acyclovir may be used either parenterally or orally.

There is no active vaccine against *Varicella zoster*. Varicella zoster immune globulin may modify or prevent the disease if given within 48 hours of contact. Acyclovir may also be given prophylactically to immunocompromised patients who have been exposed to the disease.

1.75

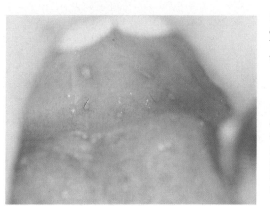

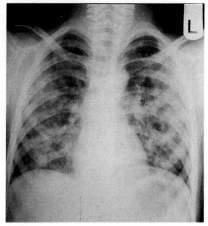
1.76

1.75 Chickenpox in a child, showing the predominantly central distribution of the rash (which used to be of great importance in differentiating chickenpox from the now-eradicated smallpox, where the rash is predominantly peripheral).

1.76 Chickenpox can be a severe disease, especially in adult patients. After several days, the rash is pleomorphic, as the lesions emerge in crops at irregular intervals. The rash in this patient shows vesicles at different stages of development.

1.78

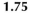
77

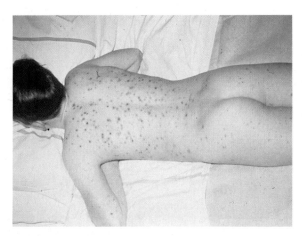

1.77 Vesicles on the palate in chickenpox often add to the discomfort of the disease. The vesicles rupture and ulcerate, but heal without scarring.

1.78 Chickenpox pneumonia affects mainly adults, and produces a severe illness with the characteristics of acute inflammatory pulmonary oedema. Chest X-ray shows widespread soft, nodular opacities throughout both lungs. The complication varies in severity from mild to life-threatening.

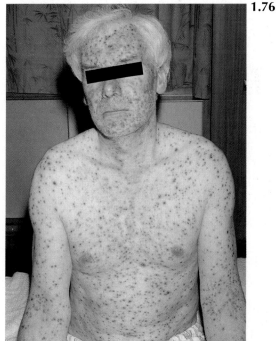

Shingles

This is caused by reactivation of latent varicella virus in sensory root ganglia in patients previously infected with chickenpox. Reactivation is common in the elderly and in immunocompromised patients (**1.31**). The skin eruption, which is always unilateral, appears along the line of one or two dermatomes (**1.79, 2.43**). The lesions are vesicular on an erythematous base. In ophthalmic herpes (**1.80**), especially if the nasociliary branch of the nerve is affected, there may be corneal ulceration (as in herpes simplex, **1.73**) and iridocyclitis. Ophthalmic herpes zoster is a medical emergency: corneal scarring (**1.81**) and other serious complications may occur. Dissemination of virus in the blood stream may result in the appearance of scattered chickenpox lesions elsewhere on the body. Viraemia may be overwhelming in immunocompromised patients. Pain may precede the skin rash, and post-herpetic neuralgia can be prolonged and severe especially in the elderly.

The most common complication is bacterial super-infection of the skin lesion. Occasionally there may be motor nerve involvement as in the Ramsay Hunt syndrome when seventh nerve paresis occurs (**1.82**). Meningo-encephalitis is a more serious but rarer complication.

Acyclovir given orally, or in severe cases intravenously, along with local applications of acyclovir skin cream may hasten healing and reduce viral shedding but there is little evidence that acyclovir prevents or reduces post-herpetic neuralgia. Analgesics are almost always required for pain control. If there is involvement of the eye, an ophthalmological opinion should be sought.

1.79

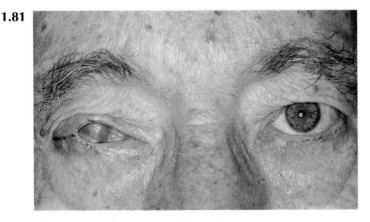

1.79 Herpes zoster affecting the L5 dermatome. The rash shows the characteristic 'band' distribution, starting from the midline, where some vesicles can be seen.

1.

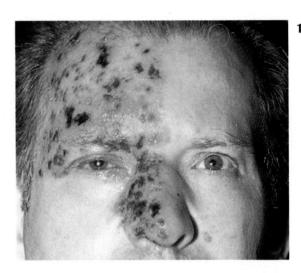

1.80 Ophthalmic herpes. The vesicular skin eruptions are in the distribution of the ophthalmic division of the fifth cranial nerve. Serious opthalmic complications are a real threat, especially when the tip of the nose is affected (this indicates involvement of the nasociliary nerve, which also supplies the cornea).

1.81

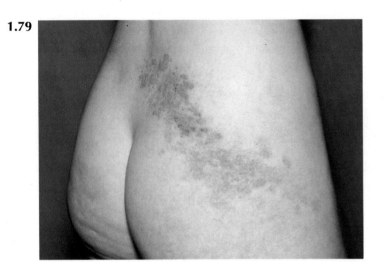

1.81 Corneal scarring is a late complication of ophthalmic herpes, resulting from corneal anaesthesia. In this patient a protective lateral tarsorrhaphy has been carried out.

1.

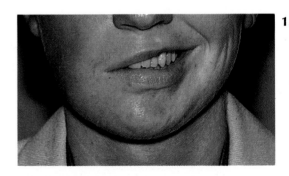

1.82 Ramsay Hunt syndrome (geniculate zoster). The patient has a right seventh nerve paresis. Full recovery occurs in about 50% of cases.

Cytomegalovirus

Like other herpes viruses, CMV remains latent in the body after primary infection and may only reactivate if the patient is stressed or becomes immunocompromised. The virus may be transmitted by respiratory secretions, sexually, by blood transfusion or by organ transplantation. Maternal infection spreads transplacentally or perinatally to the fetus.

Most CMV infections in the immunocompetent are subclinical, but there may be a glandular fever-like syndrome with fever, generalised lymphadenopathy, abnormal liver function tests and atypical mononuclear cells in the blood. Primary infection or reactivation of latent infection in the immunocompromised patient may cause serious illness with pneumonia (1.83), chorioretinitis (1.35), gastroenteritis, involvement of the central nervous system, haemolytic anaemia and thrombocytopenia. Intrauterine infection may cause fetal death. Severe neonatal CMV infection causes jaundice, hepatosplenomegaly (1.84), purpura, neurological damage and chorioretinitis. The infected infant may, however, appear normal at birth, and develop symptoms later.

The finding of specific IgM in serum is diagnostic of acute infection. Isolation of virus from urine or sputum may simply indicate prolonged excretion from past infection.

CMV inclusion bodies in biopsy specimens from the lung or gastrointestinal tract are diagnostic, so biopsy provides definitive diagnosis in the immunocompromised patient.

Most acquired infections are self-limiting but severe disease, especially in the immunocompromised, should be treated with intravenous ganciclovir or phosphonoformate. Treatment may have to be prolonged; relapses are common unless maintenance therapy is continued on a long-term basis.

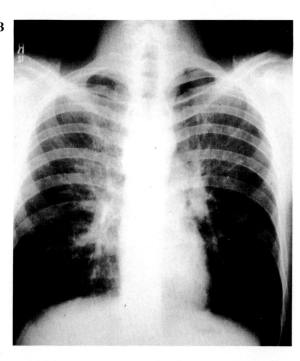

1.83 CMV pneumonia is often known as CMV pneumonitis, as the infection is generalised, and consolidation is not usually seen on X-ray. CMV is second only to *Pneumocystis* as a cause of pulmonary disease in patients with HIV infection, but CMV pneumonia cannot be diagnosed on clinical grounds or X-ray appearances alone.

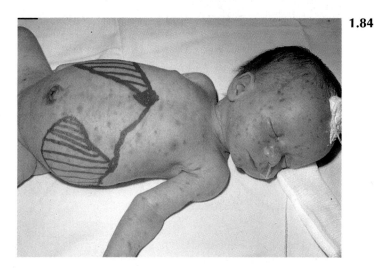

1.84 Congenital CMV infection. This infant has massive splenomegaly, hepatomegaly and a purpuric rash. A similar picture may be caused by a number of prenatal virus infections.

Epstein–Barr virus infections

Infectious mononucleosis

The Epstein–Barr virus (EBV) is the causal agent of infectious mononucleosis (IM). Primary infection with EBV is often sub-clinical, especially in young children. Older children and young adults usually present with symptoms of glandular fever.

In the most common form of the disease, there is enlargement of glands both in the anterior and posterior triangles of the neck, and usually in the axillae and groins. The fauces and palate become inflamed and oedematous. There may be palatal haemorrhages and a whitish or yellow pseudomembrane appears on the tonsils (**1.85**). There is usually marked nasopharyngitis and often puffiness of the face.

In the more generalised form of the disease, throat involvement is less marked. Presenting features are fever, generalised adenitis, splenomegaly and occasionally jaundice. There may also be a pink, maculopapular rash on the trunk and limbs (**1.86**). A rash is more often seen in patients who have been given ampicillin or related drugs (**1.87**).

Complications of IM include myocarditis, auto-immune haemolytic anaemia, thrombocytopenia and meningo-encephalitis. Splenic rupture is a rare complication which is usually associated with trauma. Post-viral fatigue syndrome may follow EBV infection.

The diagnosis is aided by the identification of atypical mononuclear cells in peripheral blood (**1.88**). The Paul–Bunnell test for heterophile antibodies usually becomes positive in the second or third week of the illness. In children under about 7 years, the Paul–Bunnell test is rarely positive, and diagnosis should be confirmed by EBV serology.

Treatment is symptomatic. Antibiotics are not indicated and ampicillin and related drugs should not be prescribed because of the high incidence of allergic reactions. Steroid therapy may be indicated if there is respiratory obstruction or auto-immune manifestations.

1.85

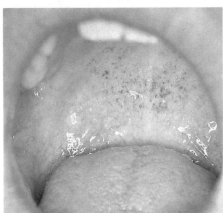

1.85 Infectious mononucleosis. Numerous petechial haemorrhages are seen in the hard palate. In many patients there is also a tonsillitis, indistinguishable from that seen in acute streptococcal pharyngitis (**1.2**).

1.86 Rash in infectious mononucleosis may be the result of the infection itself, as here. The maculopapular rash usually emerges during the second week of illness, and it is often indistinguishable from that of rubella (**1.52**).

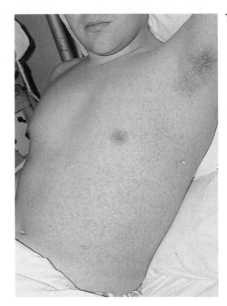

1.

1.87

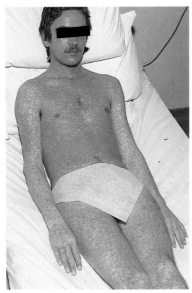

1.87 Rashes in infectious mononucleosis are most commonly caused by the administration of ampicillin or related penicillin compounds (these are often administered early in the disease on the presumption that the patient has bacterial pharyngitis). Ampicillin rashes occur more commonly in patients with infectious mononucleosis than in other patients, so the appearance of this kind of rash in a patient with typical symptoms points strongly to the diagnosis of infectious mononucleosis.

1.88 Blood film in infectious mononucleosis containing large numbers of atypical mononuclear cells. The cells vary greatly in size and shape and mitotic activity is greatly enhanced, but the cellular structure is not fundamentally deranged.

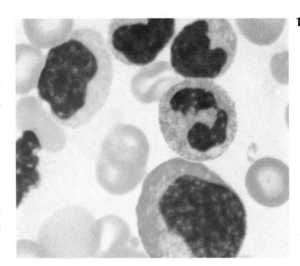

1.

Burkitt's lymphoma and nasopharyngeal carcinoma

EBV has been implicated in the aetiology of Burkitt's lymphoma, a transmissible neoplastic tumour particularly involving the head and neck (**1.89**), which is found in tropical Africa. The disease has a similar range of distribution to malaria, and it is thought that the virus may be transmitted via mosquitoes.

EBV has also been implicated in some nasopharyngeal carcinomas, and it may play a role in the genesis of hairy leukoplakia (**1.29**) and in other pre-malignant and malignant disease.

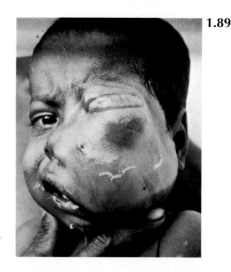

1.89 Burkitt's lymphoma, apparently originating in the maxilla and causing gross facial swelling in an African child.

Roseola

Roseola infantum is a common, benign exanthematous disease of young children. After a rapid-onset high fever, which lasts for a few days and then resolves, a generalised rubelliform rash appears (**1.90**). The rash fades after 24–48 hours, and the patient usually makes a complete and uncomplicated recovery.

The disease is now known to be caused by Herpes 6 virus (and the disease is also known as sixth disease).

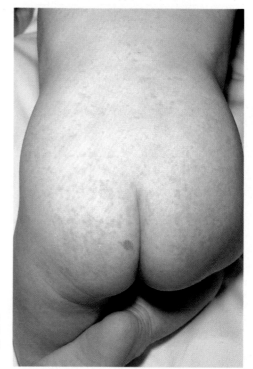

1.90 Roseola infantum. An erythematous macular or rubelliform rash appears. It is often particularly prominent on the buttocks and fades within 2 days. If the child has been treated with an antibiotic for the fever, the rash may be mistaken for drug sensitivity.

Orf

Orf (contagious pustular dermatitis) is a pox virus infection of sheep and goats, which causes an eruption on the animal's lips. It is sometimes contracted by those who work with these animals, and in man it usually causes a single papule on the skin of the hand, which develops from a flat vesicle to a haemorrhagic bulla (**1.91**). The lesions are usually self-limiting, but may act as a trigger for the onset of erythema multiforme. Milker's nodules are similar lesions, caused by cowpox virus and seen in farm workers dealing with cattle.

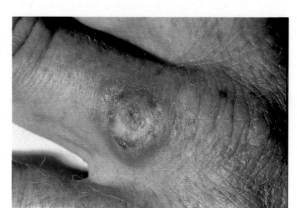

1.91 Orf. Three to seven days after inoculation from an infected sheep or goat, a firm, painless, dark papule may appear on the finger or hand. This develops into a pustule, but the condition is self-limiting, usually clearing within 4–8 weeks.

Bacterial infections

Family	Genus and species		Relevant human disease	Page reference
Cocci: Gram-positive				
Micrococcaceae	*Staphylococcus:*	*S. aureus* *S. epidermidis*	Skin infections, abscesses, toxic shock syndrome, food poisoning, toxic epidermal necrolysis, septicaemia, pneumonia, osteomyelitis and arthritis, meningitis, etc.	36, 97, 137, 158, 186, 242, 330, 379, 492
Streptococcaceae	*Streptococcus:*	*S. pyogenes* *S. pneumoniae* *S. viridans*	Skin infections, pharyngitis, pneumonia, otitis media, sinusitis, septicaemia, rheumatic fever,	38, 97, 186, 229, 242,
	Enterococcus:	*E. faecalis*	glomerulonephritis, meningitis, postpartum sepsis, urinary tract infection, dental caries, etc.	279, 297, 492
Cocci: Gram-negative				
Neisseriaceae	*Neisseria meningitidis*		Meningitis, pneumonia, septicaemia, arthritis	40, 137, 186, 463, 492
	N. gonorrhoeae		Urethritis, cervicitis, proctitis, urinary tract infection, septicaemia, arthritis, ophthalmitis, pelvic inflammatory disease	81, 137
	Branhamella catarrhalis		Respiratory infection, conjunctivitis, otitis media	186
Bacilli: Gram-positive				
Bacillaceae	*Bacillus:*	*B. anthracis* *B. cereus*	Anthrax Gastroenteritis, panophthalmitis	41 379
	Clostridium:	(*C. perfringens C. welchii*)	Bacteraemia, gas gangrene, food poisoning, necrotic enteritis	42
		C. tetani *C. botulinum* *C. difficile* *C. species*	Tetanus Botulism Pseudomembranous colitis Myonecrosis, soft-tissue infection	43 44 379 42
Corynebacteriaceae	*Corynebacterium diphtheriae*		Diptheria	44
Propionibacteriaceae	*Propionibacterium acnes*		Acne	105
Actinomycetaceae	*Actinomyces israelii*		Actinomycosis	45
Nocardiaceae	*Nocardia*		Nocardiasis, pneumonia	46, 186
Mycobacteriaceae	*Mycobacterium: M. tuberculosis*		Tuberculosis	46, 97, 137, 158, 188, 249, 298, 313, 379, 492
	Other mycobacteria		A range of infections in immuno-compromised patients	49
	M. leprae		Leprosy	49
Unclassified	*Listeria monocytogenes*		Neonatal disease, septic abortion, meningitis, septicaemia	51
	Erysipelothrix rhusiopathiae		Erysipeloid, septicaemia	39

Family	Genus and species		Relevant human disease	Page reference
Bacilli: Gram-negative				
Enterobacteriaceae	*Escherichia:*	*E. coli*	Multiple organ infections	180, 186, 297, 379
	Salmonella:	*S. typhi*	Typhoid	51
		S. paratyphi		
		S. enteritidis		379
	Shigella		Gastroenteritis/Bacillary dysentery	379
	Klebsiella		Pneumonia, urinary tract infection, septicaemia	186, 297
	Proteus		Urinary tract infection	297
	Yersinia:	*Y. pestis*	Plague	52
	Y. enterocolitica		Gastroenteritis, arthritis, septicaemia	137, 379
Vibrionaceae	*Vibrio:*	*V. cholerae*	Acute gastroenteritis	52
Spirillaceae	*Campylobacter*		Acute gastroenteritis	379
	Helicobacter pylori		Gastritis, ? peptic ulcer	362, 366
Pseudomonadaceae	*Pseudomonas*		Respiratory tract	186
			Urinary tract	297
Pasteurellaceae	*Haemophilus:*	*H. influenzae*	Respiratory tract infection	180, 186
		H. para-influenzae	Meningitis, urinary tract infection	297, 492
		H. ducreyi	Chancroid	82
Legionellaceae	*Legionella:*	*L. pneumophila*	Pontiac fever, Legionnaire's disease	53, 187
Bacteroidaceae	*Bacteroides*		Multiple organ infections	54
	Fusobacterium			
Miscellaneous	*Brucella:*	*B. abortus*	Septicaemia, arthritis, osteomyelitis, hepatitis	54
		B. mellitensis		
		B. suis		
	Bordetella:	*B. pertussis*	Whooping cough	55
	Francisella:	*F. tularensis*	Tularaemia	56
	Calymmatobacterium		Granuloma inguinale	83
Miscellaneous bacteria				
Spirochaetaceae	*Treponema:*	*T. pallidum*	Syphilis	83
		T. pertenue	Yaws	56
		T. carateum	Pinta	56
			Bejel	57
	Borrelia:	*B. vincentii*	Cancrum oris	57
		B. recurrentis	Louse-borne relapsing fever	
		B. burgdorferi	Lyme disease	58
	Leptospira:	*L. interrogans*		
	(i.e. *L. icterohaemorrhagiae*)		Leptospirosis	58
		L. canicola	Usually meningitis, renal and liver impairment	
		L. pomona		
Chlamydiaceae	*Chlamydia:*	*C. trachomatis*	Trachoma, conjunctivitis, blindness	59
			Non-specific urethritis (non-gonococcal)	86
			Reiter's syndrome	135
			Lymphogranuloma venereum	86
		C. psittaci	Psittacosis	60
Mycoplasmataceae	*Mycoplasma:*	*M. pneumoniae*	Pneumonia, pharyngitis	60, 187
		M. hominis	Urinary and genital tract infection	86
	Ureaplasma:	*urealyticum*	Non-specific urethritis	86
Rickettsiaceae	*Rickettsia*		Typhus	61
			Q fever	61
			Rocky Mountain spotted fever	61
			Rickettsialpox	61

Staphylococcal infections

Staphylococcus aureus, a Gram-positive coccus, causes a wide variety of community-acquired and nosocomial infections. The emergence of strains of the organism with multiple resistance to antibiotics is causing major problems of management and infection control. Certain areas of the body, especially the nasal mucosa and the skin of the axilla, groin and perineum, may become colonised by staphylococci and, given favourable circumstances, the organisms may invade the skin and subcutaneous tissue. Tissue breakdown and abscess formation are characteristic of staphylococcal lesions (1.92). Staphylococci may also enter the blood with subsequent involvement of other organs such as bone (p. 158), joints, lungs (1.64, 1.93, 4.31, 4.32), heart valves (p. 242), brain or meninges.

In addition to causing local sepsis, *Staphylococcus aureus* produces a number of toxins. Epidermolytic (exfoliative) toxin is responsible for the syndrome of **toxic epidermal necrolysis** (Lyell's disease, scalded skin syndrome). In this, there is sudden onset of fever and marked generalised erythema of the skin, followed by loss of large areas of the superficial layers of the epidermis, which produces an appearance resembling severe scalding. This condition occurs mainly in children (1.94). Ritter's disease is a neonatal form of the same condition.

Staphylococcal toxic shock syndrome, a rare, life-threatening illness, is seen mainly in young women who use tampons. The condition is caused by the production of an exotoxin by Staphylococcus aureus in the vagina. The patient presents with fever, hypotension, acute myalgia, profuse diarrhoea and usually a bright erythematous rash which resembles that of streptococcal scarlet fever (1.98). A similar illness may occur when erythrogenic toxin is released by staphylococci in other sites.

Most *Staphylococcus aureus* organisms are resistant to penicillin and ampicillin, so the drugs of choice for most infections are penicillinase-resistant antibiotics, such as cloxacillin and flucloxacillin. Flucloxacillin may be combined with fucidic acid to treat severe infections. In cases where there is allergy to the penicillins, and especially if the organisms have multiple resistance to antibiotics, choice of appropriate antibiotic therapy must depend on sensitivity testing; therefore, close co-operation with microbiologists is essential. Staphylococcal abscesses should be drained (1.95, 1.96), and full supportive measures are required for all serious infections including toxic epidermal necrolysis and toxic shock syndrome.

Staphylococcus epidermidis and related coagulase-negative staphylococci are important causes of infection in patients with prosthetic devices (especially heart valves (1.9), joints, shunts and vascular grafts) and in patients undergoing chronic peritoneal dialysis. Infection can also occur on heart valves which have been damaged as a result of acute rheumatism or are congenitally abnormal (p. 242).

1.92

1.92 A massive staphylococcal carbuncle, in which the infection has caused tissue breakdown and multiple inter-connected abscesses. Lesions of this kind are found most commonly in diabetic patients.

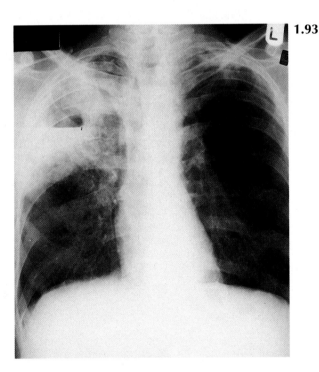

1.93

1.93 Staphylococcal pneumonia in a 20-year-old intravenous drug abuser. The organisms were introduced by a contaminated intravenous injection, but a similar picture may occur in debilitated or immunocompromised patients secondary to staphylococcal skin infection. Note the presence of a large cavity (septic infarct) in the right upper zone.

1.94 Toxic epidermal necrolysis (scalded skin syndrome), in which the skin is extremely painful, and large patches of necrotic epidermis slide off the underlying layers at the slightest pressure, leaving extensive raw areas. The condition occurs mainly in children, but a similar syndrome may occur at any age as a consequence of drug hypersensitivity (**2.126**).

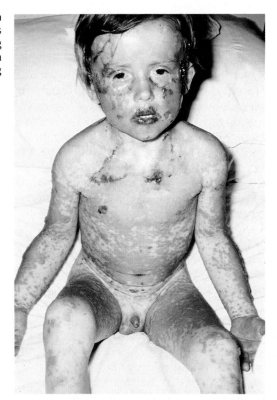

1.94

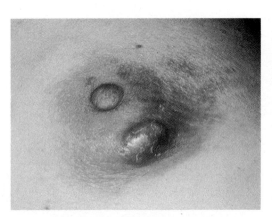

1.95

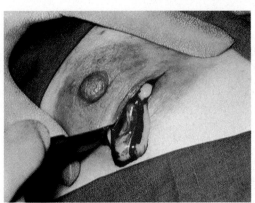

1.96

1.95, 1.96 Staphylococcal abscesses should be drained, as they are very unlikely to respond to antibiotic treatment alone. On the surface, this breast abscess did not appear large, but a large volume of pus was released when it was incised. After evacuation of the pus, the wound should be packed and left open.

Streptococcal infections

Streptococcus pyogenes causes a wide variety of infections in man, including tonsillitis, scarlet fever, skin lesions (impetigo, erysipelas and cellulitis), puerperal sepsis and septicaemia. The organisms are transmitted by direct contact, by droplets from the respiratory tract or indirectly through food, dust or fomites. Late complications of *Streptococcus pyogenes* infections include acute rheumatic fever, post-streptococcal glomerulonephritis, Henoch–Schönlein purpura and erythema nodosum.

Streptococcal tonsillitis is an acute illness with fever, marked general malaise and pain on swallowing. There is inflammation and oedema of the palate and fauces with spotty exudate on the tonsils (1.2, 1.97). The anterior cervical lymph nodes are enlarged and tender. Local complications include otitis media, streptococcal rhinitis, sinusitis and peritonsillar abscess (quinsy). As with all streptococcal infections, late complications may appear about 10 days after the onset of the illness, especially in patients not treated with antibiotics. The diagnosis of streptococcal tonsillitis can be confirmed by culture of throat swabs. There is usually a marked polymorph leucocytosis in peripheral blood. The diagnosis may be confirmed in retrospect, by the finding of a raised anti-streptolysin 0 titre (ASOT).

Scarlet fever is a streptococcal infection characterised by the appearance of an erythematous rash (1.98). The disease is seen mainly in children, who are susceptible to streptococcal erythrogenic toxin. Scarlet fever is usually associated with streptococcal tonsillitis but it may also follow infection of wounds or burns (surgical scarlet fever). The rash is a generalised punctate erythema which affects the trunk and limbs. As the rash fades, there may be desquamation of skin. Other characteristics of the disease are circumoral pallor (1.98) and white strawberry tongue (1.99). Complications of scarlet fever are similar to those of streptococcal tonsillitis.

1.97

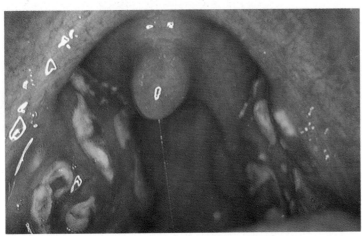

1.

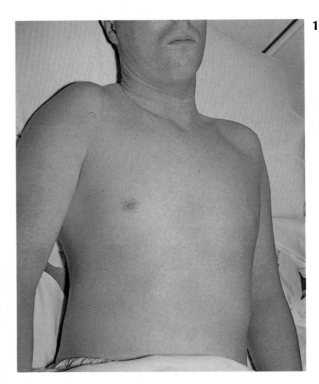

1.97 Acute tonsillitis. The appearance may vary from simple hyperaemia of the tonsils to a diffuse exudate resembling that found in infectious mononucleosis (**1.85**). The punctate appearance seen here is not uncommon in streptococcal tonsillitis. Penicillin is the treatment of choice, but ampicillin and related drugs may cause a drug rash if the true diagnosis is infectious mononucleosis rather than steptococcal sore throat (**1.87**).

1.98 Scarlet fever showing a typical erythematous rash on the trunk and a hint of the classical circum-oral pallor, with some oedema of the face.

1.99

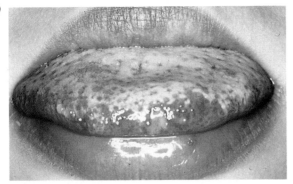

1.99 White strawberry tongue in scarlet fever. The oedematous red papillae protrude through a thick, white, furry membrane. This appearance is typical of the first two days, but later the white fur peels off, to leave a deep red strawberry tongue.

Streptococcal infections of skin and tissues

Erysipelas and **cellulitis** are skin and tissue infections with *Streptococcus pyogenes* which are usually found in patients in older age groups. Sites most often involved are the face (**1.100**) the legs, the hands and the arms (**1.101**). General symptoms include fever, malaise, rigors and sometimes delirium. The local lesion consists of an area of spreading erythema with a well-demarcated edge. Regional lymph nodes become tender and enlarged. There is a tendency for erysipelas to recur in a previously affected area.

A similar clinical picture, **erysipeloid**, may be produced by infection with *Erysipelothrix rhusiopathiae* (**1.102**), though systemic symptoms are rare. This is an occupationally-acquired infection in farmers, meat and fish processors and veterinary surgeons.

Impetigo is most commonly seen in children and is a superficial infection of skin, usually caused by either *Streptococcus pyogenes* or *Staphylococcus aureus*. It may occur de novo or as a secondary infection in areas of eczema or in pediculosis of the scalp. The lesions, which are often on the face, start as thin-walled vesicles that rupture, forming yellowish crusts (**1.103**). Infection is often spread by scratching.

Penicillin is the drug of choice for infections with *Streptococcus pyogenes*. Antibiotic therapy should be continued for 10 days in order to lessen the risk of rheumatic fever. In cases of allergy to penicillin, erythromycin is the second choice drug. Impetigo usually responds to topical antibiotic therapy.

1.100

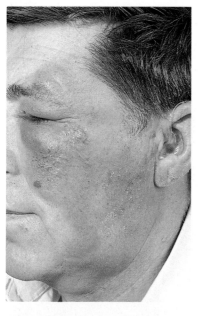

1.100 Erysipelas of the face. During the acute stage, the eyelids may become so swollen that they cannot be opened. The entire face may become erythematous, and this appearance is accompanied by an unpleasant sensation of tightness and burning.

1.101

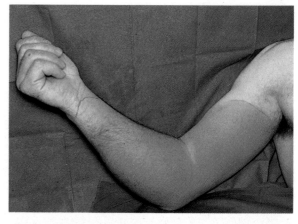

1.101 Cellulitis caused by streptococcal infection which entered through an apparently trivial knuckle injury. Other common sites of entry for the bacteria are areas of infected eczema and fungal infections of the toe-web with fissuring.

1.102

1.102 Erysipeloid (fish handler's disease) produces a similar clinical picture to erysipelas, although the systemic reaction is usually relatively slight.

1.103

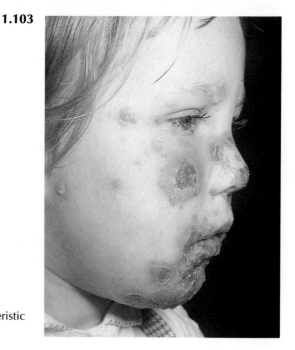

1.103 Impetigo of the face. The superficial nature of the infection and the characteristic honey-coloured serous crusting are typical.

Meningococcal infection

The causal agent is *Neisseria meningitidis,* a Gram-negative diplococcus with a number of serogroups. Infection results from inhalation of droplets. Meningococci colonise the pharynx, often giving rise to a carrier state; but they may spread from the pharynx to the blood and meninges. No age is exempt from meningococcal disease but young children and young adults are most at risk, especially those in a closed environment such as a school or camp.

The incubation period is usually less than one week. Infection produces a wide spectrum of illness from fulminating septicaemia, which can kill in a few hours, to a subacute illness with intermittent fever and a 'flea-bite' type rash. The most common presentation is **meningitis** (*see* p. 492) with or without septicaemia—the main features of which are high fever, severe headache, signs of acute meningeal irritation, often a purpuric rash and rapid deterioration of consciousness (**1.104**). **Fulminating septicaemia** (Waterhouse–Friderichsen syndrome) is a devastating illness with extensive skin haemorrhage (**1.105**,

1.106), disseminated intravascular coagulation (DIC—**10.103**, **10.106**) and circulatory failure due to adrenal haemorrhage. These patients usually do not live long enough to develop meningitis.

Meningococci can be cultured from blood, pharynx, skin lesions and CSF. If examined, the CSF is purulent (**1.21**) with a marked polymorph leucocytosis. Lumbar puncture may, however, be hazardous because 'coning' of the brain stem may occur with disastrous consequences. If the clinical diagnosis is not in doubt, therapy can be started without CSF examination.

Antibiotic treatment must be started promptly. Intravenous benzylpenicillin is still the drug of choice and should be given for 5–7 days. Intensive care nursing with full supportive therapy is required, especially for fulminating septicaemic cases.

Close contacts of the index case should receive prophylactic therapy—usually with rifampicin or ciprofloxacin. Vaccines against groups A and C meningococci are available, but as yet there is no vaccine for group B infection.

1.104

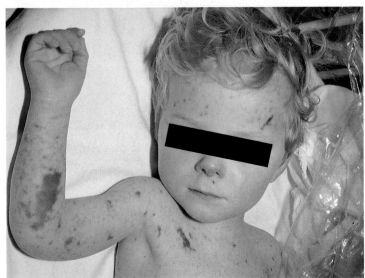

1.104 Meningococcal meningitis and septicaemia. This child is unconscious and has extensive petechiae and ecchymoses. Similar findings occur in meningitis from other causes.

1.105

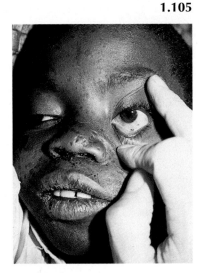

1.105 Meningococcal septicaemia in a Nigerian boy, with meningitis, repeated nose bleeds and petechial haemorrhages in the conjunctivae and skin.

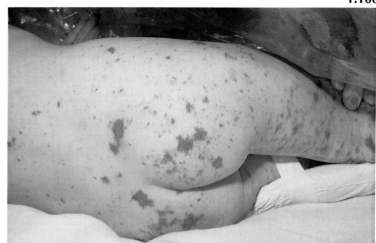

1.106 Fulminating meningococcal septicaemia is characterised by extensive purpuric lesions, a high fever, shock and evidence of disseminated intravascular coagulation (DIC—*see* p. 463).

Anthrax

The causal agent is *Bacillus anthracis,* a spore-bearing organism. Most human infections result from contact with animals or animal products, such as hides, wool or bones, and therefore most cases occur in farmers, vets and abattoir workers. Anthrax has an unfortunate potential for use in germ warfare, and anthrax spores may persist in an infected environment for many years.

Cutaneous lesions are usually single and are most common on exposed sites, especially hands, arms, head or neck. The classical anthrax lesion is the malignant pustule (**1.107**). This starts as a red papular lesion that vesiculates and becomes necrotic in the central area and finally dries up to form a thick, blackish scab which may take several weeks to separate. There is usually marked erythema and oedema of the surrounding tissues. Fever, headache and malaise accompany most lesions. Anthrax septicaemia is much less frequent in humans than in animals. Pulmonary anthrax (inhalation of spores) and gastrointestinal anthrax (ingestion of spores) are rare forms of the disease and carry a high mortality.

Anthrax bacilli can be identified in stained smears from the lesion. Confirmation is by culture or animal inoculation. Benzyl-penicillin is the treatment of choice. Erythromycin can be used if there is penicillin allergy. A killed vaccine is available for human use, but this is reserved for people in high-risk occupations. Other preventive measures include improvement of working practices, animal vaccination, proper disposal of animal carcases and sterilisation of animal products such as bone meal.

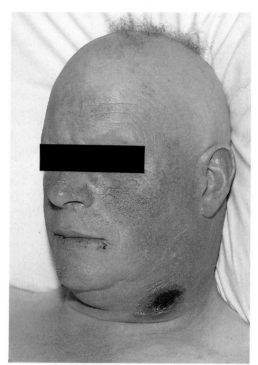

1.107

1.107 Anthrax. A single malignant pustule in a typical position on the neck. The patient was a porter who carried animal hides over his shoulders.

Clostridial tissue infections

Deep, penetrating wounds are often contaminated by a range of *Clostridium* spp. (including *C. tetani, perfringens, septicum* and *novyi*). These organisms may produce two main syndromes:

- Clostridial cellulitis
- Clostridial myonecrosis with the release of gas into the tissues ('gas gangrene').

Clostridial cellulitis may be superficial and of relatively minor consequence, but it may lead to rapidly progressive tissue destruction. In anaerobic conditions, associated with large amounts of devitalised tissue, clostridia may produce extensive myonecrosis and release gas, which tracks along the tissue planes. Gas gangrene has also been recorded at the site of intramuscular injections.

The clinical features of myonecrosis occur within a few days of injury especially in wounds with muscle damage, fractures, retained foreign bodies and impairment of the arterial supply. Patients present with severe pain in proximity of the wound, which rapidly becomes swollen with 'woody hard' oedema (**1.108**). A thin, watery, sweet-smelling discharge is often noted, and this becomes brown or frankly bloody later. Gas in the tissue planes may be apparent on X-ray before it can be felt (**1.109**). If a limb is involved, the part distal to the infection rapidly becomes cold, oedematous and pulseless before frank gangrene appears. The patient remains conscious during this time and has few other features, the clinical state being dominated by great pain at the site. There may be a slight fever. Progression of the condition leads to anorexia, profuse diarrhoea, circulatory collapse and renal and hepatic failure. There may be massive haemolysis.

Treatment consists of extensive early surgical debridement of the affected part under penicillin cover. The use of specific anti-toxins and hyperbaric oxygen is controversial. Circulatory support is necessary to prevent renal failure. Death is inevitable if treatment is not available, and often occurs suddenly and unexpectedly during surgery.

1.108

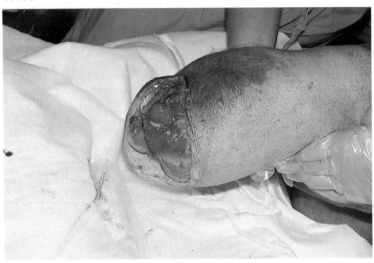

1.108 Clostridial cellulitis following amputation in a 45-year-old man who had been injured in a railway accident. The necrosis of skin and muscle is clearly seen.

1.109

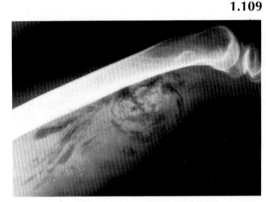

1.109 Gas gangrene in the soft tissues of the thigh following a penetrating injury. The combination of myonecrosis and gas results in swelling and impaired circulation distally.

Tetanus

Clostridium tetani is a spore-bearing organism which produces a powerful exotoxin which acts on the central nervous system, preventing feedback inhibition of neural discharges. Spores are present in the soil, and humans may be infected by inoculation of spores, usually into a deep wound, but sometimes even through minor breaks in the skin. Agricultural workers, athletes and road traffic accident casualties are particularly at risk. Neonates are also at risk (**1.110**), especially where the umbilicus is handled in an unclean manner (e.g. dung dressings which are used in parts of the developing world).

After an incubation period ranging from a few days to about three weeks, muscle rigidity develops. This is often first noted as jaw stiffness (trismus), but later becomes generalised, producing opisthotonos (**1.111**). Painful muscle spasms occur and these are often triggered by sensory stimuli such as loud noises (**1.112**). There may also be involvement of the autonomic nervous system. The severity of the disease is inversely proportional to the length of the incubation period.

The diagnosis is made on the history and clinical features of the disease. Patients with tetanus require intensive care nursing. Obvious wounds should be cleaned and debrided. Human tetanus immunoglobulin and penicillin should be administered as soon as possible. Moderate spasms can be controlled by diazepam, but severe tetanus may require full muscle relaxation and intermittent positive pressure ventilation.

Primary immunisation should be achieved in early childhood with three doses of diphtheria, pertussis and tetanus (DPT) vaccine. Booster doses of tetanus toxoid are required every 10 years to maintain immunity. After a penetrating injury an additional booster dose of toxoid should be given unless the previous booster dose was within five years. If the history of previous immunisation is uncertain and if wounds are heavily contaminated, anti-tetanus human immunoglobulin should be given and a course of tetanus toxoid started.

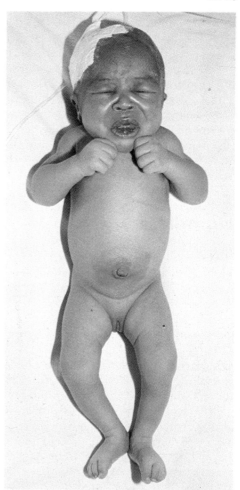

1.110 Neonatal tetanus. All the key diagnostic features are seen. Tetanus has resulted from unclean handling of the umbilical cord; note the inflammation around the umbilicus. The classical features of tetanus—trismus, risus sardonicus and muscle spasms of the arms and legs—are all present.

1.111

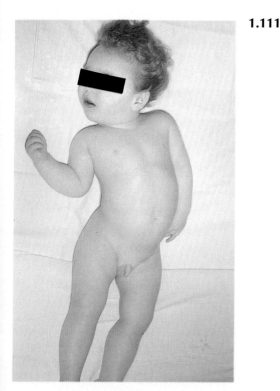

1.111 Tetanus causing opisthotonos in an infant. Contraction of all muscle groups leads to arching of the back and rigidity of the limbs. The attacks are frightening for the patient and those caring for him, and patients remain fully conscious throughout .

1.112

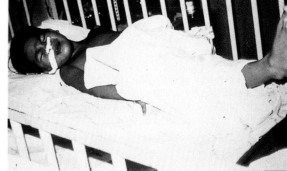

1.112 Tetanic spasms are painful, and the appearance of pain is accentuated by spasm of the facial muscles, giving a characteristic 'grin' (risus sardonicus).

Botulism

Botulism results from ingestion of the endotoxin of *Clostridium botulinum* or, in some cases, from the release of endotoxin by surviving ingested organisms in the gut. This is usually caused by bacterial or spore contamination of improperly canned or preserved meat and meat products, which allows growth of the organism and toxin production. Rarely, wounds may be infected with *C. botulinium*. The toxin interferes with the release of acetylcholine at the neuromuscular junction, and as a result progressive descending muscle paralysis dominates the clinical picture with diplopia, laryngeal and pharyngeal palsy and generalised symmetrical paralysis of muscles, especially those of the cranial and respiratory systems. Loss of the pupillary reflex is an early sign.

The diagnosis is confirmed by finding toxin in the food, gastric contents or faeces. Airway support with assisted ventilation is the keystone of treatment. Antitoxin is of value and antibiotics may have a role where organisms survive in the gut. Mortality is about 50%. Public health measures are aimed at prevention during food preparation for preservation, especially when this is done at home.

Diphtheria

Diphtheria is now rare in the developed world, as a result of effective immunisation campaigns. The causal agent is *Corynebacterium diphtheriae*. The most common type of diphtheria is faucial-pharyngeal in which the local lesion takes the form of a greyish white, translucent membrane, which may start on the tonsils (**1.113**), but which tends to spread to the palate, uvula and pharynx. Other sites of the local lesion include anterior nares, larynx and occasionally skin. The organisms multiplying in the local lesion produce a powerful exotoxin which especially affects the heart and the central nervous sytem.

Toxic complications include cardiogenic shock (**1.114**), cardiac arrhythmias and sudden cardiac arrest. Nervous sytem damage is due to demyelination of motor nerves. This may lead to paralysis of extraocular muscles, palate and pharynx and more rarely to paralysis of limbs and respiratory muscles (**1.115**). Obstruction of the airway by a membrane is a life-threatening complication of laryngeal diphtheria, in which exhaustion due to respiratory muscular effort is rapidly followed by death (**1.116**).

The diagnosis is confirmed by culture of the organism from the local lesion. Diphtheria antitoxin must be given with penicillin or erythromycin. Bed rest is important, especially in the presence of cardiac involvement. Laryngeal obstruction may require intubation or tracheotomy.

Infants should be immunised against the disease with combined diphtheria/pertussis/tetanus vaccine (DPT). The Schick test can be used to determine immune status.

1.113

1.114

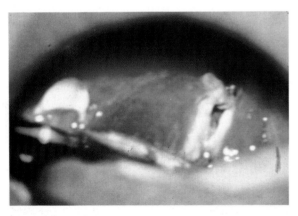

1.113 Diphtheria membrane in the pharynx. The membrane is usually white or greyish-yellow in colour, and the child may have relatively few symptoms at this stage.

1.114 Diphtheritic myocarditis led to cardiac failure and acute pulmonary oedema in this child (*see also* p. 244).

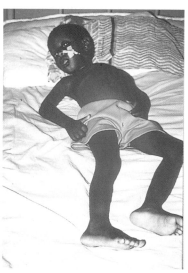

1.115 Polyneuritis is a relatively rare complication of diphtheria. In this Sudanese child, it has led to a generalised flaccid paralysis.

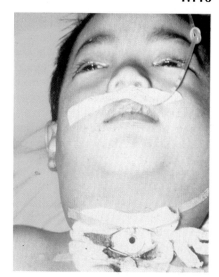

1.116 Respiratory obstruction was a life-threatening complication of diphtheria, and the need for urgent tracheostomy was the reason that most doctors carried a small penknife before the advent of effective immunisation. This child has a palatal palsy (hence the nasogastric tube), and a 'bull neck' (a characteristic appearance of cervical oedema).

Actinomycosis

Infection with *Actinomyces israelii*, an anaerobic filamentous bacterium, is uncommon in the West. The organism can be found as a commensal in the mouth and intestine, and it may invade any part of the body when immunity is suppressed. Three sites are commonly involved:

- **Cervicofacial actinomycosis**, in which the presentation is a reddish indurated subcutaneous mass in the anterior triangle of the neck or submandibular region. There may be slight tenderness with low-grade fever and general symptoms of malaise.
- **Pulmonary actinomycosis** usually involves previously damaged lungs, e.g. cavitation following pulmonary tuberculosis (*see* p. 188).
- **Abdominal actinomycosis** usually involves the appendix and caecum and presents with lower abdominal pain, low-grade fever and a slow-growing abdominal mass. It may occasionally be seen in association with an intrauterine device.

In all these sites, the infection may ultimately discharge through the skin, forming sinuses (**1.117**). Classically, these sinuses discharge typical sulphur granules (**1.118**).

A prolonged course of high-dose penicillin is the treatment of choice.

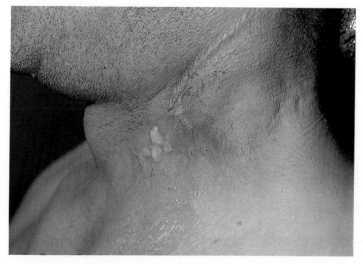

1.117 Cervical actinomycosis. The patient presented originally with an indurated subcutaneous mass in the anterior triangle of the neck. The chronic nature of the condition is demonstrated by the signs of a previous sinus higher up in the neck, which has healed, and an actively discharging sinus below it.

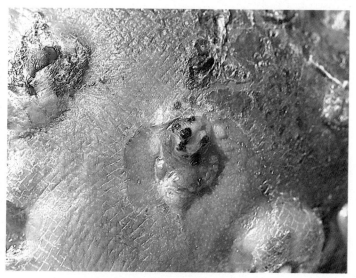

1.118 Sulphur granules discharging from multiple sinuses in the foot of a patient with actinomycosis.

Nocardiasis

This can be an acute, subacute or chronic infection by a family of Gram-positive filamentous 'higher' bacteria. These are usually inhaled, but occasionally may enter via penetrating wounds of the skin (usually the foot). The organisms have a worldwide distribution and are soil saprophytes. Most infections occur in people who have pre-existing immunosuppression resulting from cancer, cancer therapy, steroid therapy, alcoholism or HIV infection. Pulmonary nocardiasis presents like any other pneumonia, with fever, productive cough and progressive signs of lung consolidation. Despite antibiotics the disease progresses to cavitation, and there may be direct spread to the pleural cavity with empyema formation. Blood-borne spread to the brain and other organs occurs. Surgical drainage of the abscesses is required, along with prolonged therapy with a sulphonamide.

Tuberculosis

The incidence of tuberculosis (TB) has declined markedly in the developed world in recent years. Various factors have contributed to this, including improved social conditions, mass miniature radiography, good contact tracing, BCG vaccination of schoolchildren and the use of effective anti-tuberculous therapy. People now at special risk of developing tuberculosis include those in or from developing countries, the elderly, the debilitated, alcoholics, diabetics and immunocompromised patients. Tuberculosis may become more common again in the future, as it is a frequent (and treatable) complication of HIV infection.

Mycobacterium tuberculosis is spread mainly by droplets, and the organisms gain entry to the body by inhalation, ingestion or occasionally by inoculation through the skin. Primary infection usually involves the lungs (**1.119**, **1.120**), but parts of the gastrointestinal tract may also be affected, and there is usually also lymph node involvement. The organisms provoke granuloma formation, often with caseation and cavitation.

Occasionally, primary infection may lead directly to more widespread disease—usually by haematogenous spread, which may occur at any stage of the disease. More commonly, the primary focus of infection in the lung heals, but the healed

1.119

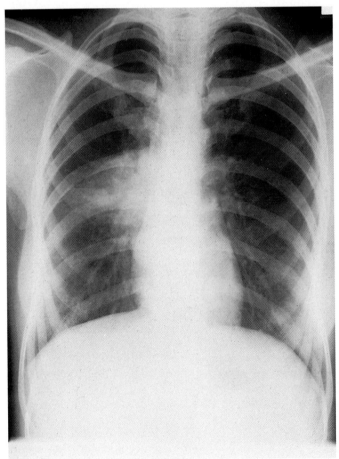

1.120

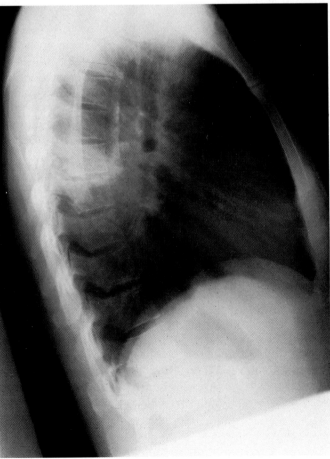

1.119, 1.120 Primary tuberculosis in the apical segment of the right lower lobe. The PA film shows the primary focus, and its position, just below the fissure, is confirmed by the lateral film. The PA film also shows slight hilar enlargement. In most cases, the primary focus heals with extensive calcification, but viable organisms remain within the healed focus. This patient was a 23-year-old Indian woman who had recently come to the UK, and the infection responded to combined anti-tuberculous chemotherapy.

granuloma continues to contain viable organisms. If host resistance is lowered in later life, TB may be re-activated, spreading locally and, via the blood stream, throughout the body and producing many possible manifestations. Major complications include:

- Miliary TB—diffuse haematogenous spread throughout the body, often visible as miliary mottling in the chest X-ray (**1.121**).
- Pulmonary TB (*see* p. 188).
- Gastrointestinal TB in the ileocaecal area (*see* p. 379).
- Genitourinary TB affecting the kidneys and other parts of the GU tract (*see* p. 298).
- Tuberculous meningitis and space-occupying tuberculomas of the brain (**1.122**, p. 492).
- Tuberculous osteomyelitis (*see* p. 158).
- Tuberculous arthritis (*see* p. 137).
- Skin manifestations including lupus vulgaris (**2.38**, **2.39**) and erythema nodosum (**1.123**, **2.40**).
- Eye involvement (**1.12**).
- Constrictive pericarditis (*see* p. 249).
- Adrenal involvement leading to Addison's disease (*see* p. 313)
- Lymph node enlargement (**1.124–1.126**).

TB in people in or from the Third World is often extra-pulmonary and investigation of any such patient with unexplained pyrexia should include chest X-ray, tuberculin skin test, culture for tuberculosis of sputum, urine and stool and, if indicated, gland or marrow biopsy. TB in the immunocompromised patient may be a primary infection or a reactivation of a previously inactive infection. By the time of diagnosis, the disease may be widely disseminated and careful investigation and management is required.

Treatment of infection with typical *M. tuberculosis* requires combination drug therapy to prevent the emergence of resistant strains of organisms. Drugs available for use include isoniazid, rifampicin, ethambutol, pyrazinamide and streptomycin.

Cell-mediated delayed hypersensitivity to TB can be demonstrated by the use of tuberculin tests, including the Mantoux, Heaf and tine skin tests (**1.127**). Patients who have latent TB infection usually react positively to these tests, but their main value is in conjunction with vaccination programmes. Those found to be 'tuberculin negative' can be immunised using BCG vaccine (**1.128**), which offers a good degree of protection against subsequent infection.

1.121

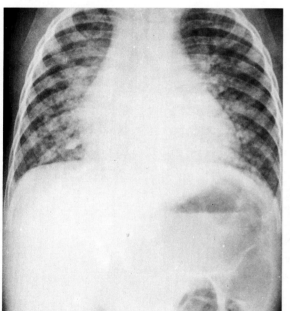

1.122

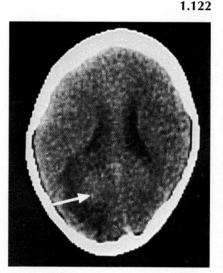

1.122 Tuberculoma of the brain is one of the many manifestations of tuberculosis. The lesion is arrowed on this CT scan.

1.123

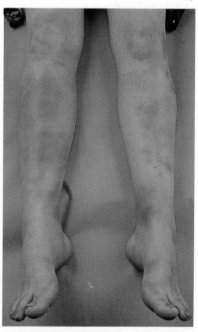

1.121 Miliary tuberculosis in a young child. The appearance of miliary mottling on the chest X-ray is characteristic, but not diagnostic, of miliary TB—similar appearances may be found in other forms of pneumonia, in sarcoidosis and in some occupational lung diseases.

1.123 Erythema nodosum is one of the skin manifestations of tuberculosis, but may also occur in a number of other conditions (*see also* **2.40**). The classic distribution is over the front of the legs, and sometimes on the extensor surface of the forearms. The appearance reflects the patchy inflammation of subcutaneous fat and small vessels, probably as the result of a type III (immune complex) allergic mechanism.

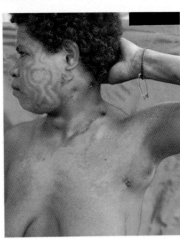

1.124 Enlarged tuberculous lymph nodes in the neck and axilla of a Fijian woman with widespread TB.

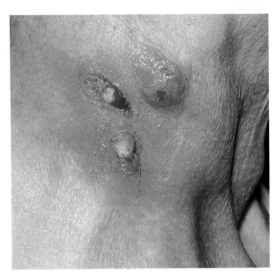

1.125 Ulcerating tuberculous lymph nodes (scrofula) in the neck of an elderly British patient.

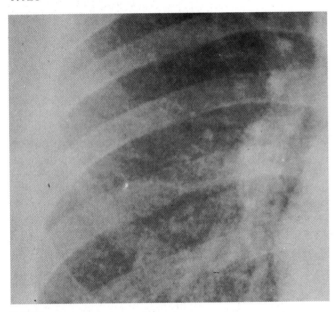

1.126 Hilar gland enlargement is a common finding in tuberculosis, usually in association with pulmonary involvement. The right hilar glands are seen to be enlarged in this close-up view.

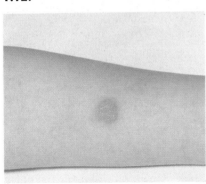

1.127 Heaf test–positive reaction. The test is carried out with purified old tuberculin, which is pricked into the skin using the Heaf applicator. In those who have no previous exposure to tuberculosis, a positive reaction appears within 48 hours, and this consists of erythema accompanied by palpable induration.

1.128 A BCG ulcer, which appeared 8 weeks after BCG vaccination. The administration of BCG is usually uncomplicated, but occasionally a severe reaction may occur, and an abscess or ulcer may be accompanied by regional lymph node enlargement.

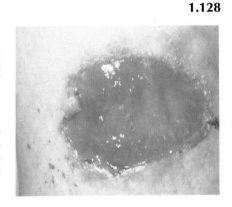

Other mycobacterial infections

A number of mycobacteria may produce tuberculosis-like disease. *Mycobacterium bovis,* formerly a common cause of tuberculosis in the West, is now a rare cause of disease in man, as a result of the careful control of the infection in cattle.

Patients with HIV infection, and other immunosuppressed patients, are not only susceptible to infection with *M. tuberculosis,* but also to infection with other mycobacteria—often termed 'atypical mycobacteria'. *M. scrofulaceum* is particularly likely to produce lymph node infections (1.124, 1.125), but other organisms such as *M. avium-intracellulare* and *M. kansasii* may produce almost any of the manifestations of typical TB. Infections with these organisms are often very difficult to treat because of multiple drug resistance.

Mycobacterium marinum may cause fish tank granulomas (1.129), which can, if necessary, be treated with antimicrobial drugs.

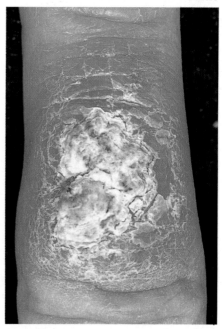

1.129 Fish tank granuloma. This middle-aged woman, who keeps tropical fish, had a 6-month history of painless nodules on the dorsum of her right index finger. The single lesion results from infection with *Mycobacterium marinium* (balnei), an organism which infects fish.

Leprosy

Leprosy, which is caused by *Mycobacterium leprae,* remains an important disease in tropical and subtropical countries. Infection is spread by droplets from infected nasal mucosa, but prolonged close contact is required. The incubation period is usually between 3 and 15 years. The spectrum of disease activity in leprosy depends upon the host's immune response to the infection.

Lepromatous leprosy develops when the response is poor. In this form, there are widespread lesions which contain enormous numbers of bacilli. There is involvement of nasal mucosa, skin (1.130, 1.131), testicular tissue and later of nerves. Marked destructive lesions of the face and palate. may result, and neurotrophic atrophy may lead to loss of the extremities (1.131–1.134).

In **tuberculoid leprosy** host immunity is good and bacilli are rarely seen in lesions. Patients present with erythematous or hypopigmented skin lesions (1.135) and with asymmetrical thickening of nerves (1.136).

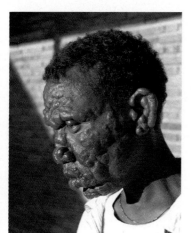

1.130 Lepromatous leprosy. There is extensive infiltration, oedema and corrugation causing 'leonine facies'. Note the depilation of the eyebrows and face, and the gross thickening of the ear.

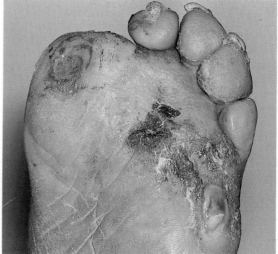

1.131 Lepromatous leprosy, showing the typical perforating ulcers resulting from neuropathy. On the lateral surface, the skin has ulcerated to expose the metatarsal head. There is associated local infection. There is also ulceration of the ball of the foot, and the great toe has been lost.

The term 'borderline leprosy' is used when there are features of both lepromatous and tuberculoid disease. This may eventually evolve into one or other form of the disease.

The diagnosis is easily made when bacilli are demonstrated in smears from nasal mucosa or skin in lepromatous disease. Biopsy of skin or affected nerve is required for diagnosis of tuberculoid disease.

Multi-drug therapy with rifampicin, dapsone and clofazimine is now recommended. Good supportive measures including surgical correction of deformities are also important. No specific vaccine is available at present. BCG vaccine has been used but doubt remains as to its efficacy.

1.132

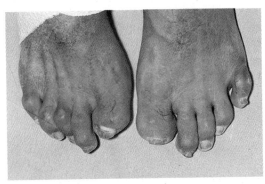

1.133

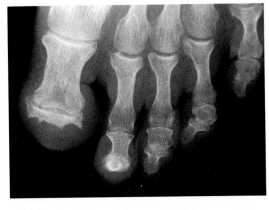

1.132, 1.133 Neurotrophic atrophy in lepromatous leprosy eventually leads to erosion of the extremities. In this patient, the terminal phalanx of each big toe showed major erosion. The other terminal phalanges were also eroded, but to a lesser extent.

1.134

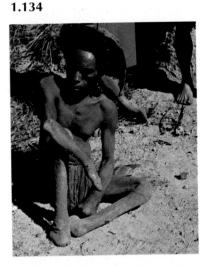

1.134 Near-total loss of the hands and feet in late-stage leprosy, as a result of long-standing neurotrophic atrophy.

1.135

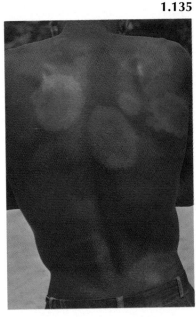

1.135 Tuberculoid leprosy. The early tuberculoid lesion is characterised by macules showing loss of sensation and hypopigmentation.

1.136

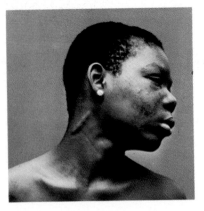

1.136 Nerve thickening in tuberculoid leprosy. Thickening of the great auricular nerve is common.

Listeriosis

The bacterium *Listeria monocytogenes* has a worldwide distribution and is found in nature in rotting vegetation, water and in 5% of human faeces. Despite this, human disease is uncommon, affecting principally pregnant women and patients who are immunocompromised. Transplacental transmission results in fetal infection which often overwhelms and kills the fetus which is aborted. Occasionally, the child is born with severe malformations. Infection acquired at term delivery usually presents with meningitis at 4–6 weeks, but these babies have disseminated disease with cardiorespiratory failure, diarrhoea and shock. The mortality in this condition is high, despite modern therapy. About half the infections occur in adults, especially in the presence of HIV infection, lympho-reticular neoplasia, treatment with steroids and cytotoxins, alcoholism, diabetes mellitus and tuberculosis. Infection presents acutely with fever, vomiting, diarrhoea and often signs of meningism. There may also be a purulent conjunctivitis which can produce corneal ulceration and the regional lymph nodes may be involved. The mortality is high, despite the use of antibiotics.

Salmonellosis

Salmonella organisms cause a range of clinical syndromes:

- Enteric fever (typhoid or paratyphoid fever).
- Focal infections (e.g. osteomyelitis).
- Enterocolitis (food poisoning) (*see* p. 379).
- Asymptomatic carrier state.

Enteric fever: the causal organisms are *Salmonella typhi* and *S. paratyphi* A, B and C. These organisms are species-specific to man, and transmission is by the faecal–oral route, either by direct contact or indirectly through contamination of water or food. Most cases diagnosed in western countries are imported.

Enteric fever is primarily a septicaemic illness which starts after an incubation period of 7–14 days, with non-specific flu-like symptoms which increase in severity during the first two weeks of the illness. The temperature rises in a step-like fashion (**1.137**), reaching its highest level in the second week, by which time there is marked toxaemia. There may be diarrhoea, but many patients remain constipated throughout the illness. Signs include furred tongue, rose spots on the trunk (**1.138**), abdominal distension and splenomegaly. During the third week, the temperature declines, but at this stage a number of potentially fatal complications may occur including intestinal haemorrhage and perforation, pneumonia, cholecystitis, meningitis and osteomyelitis. Osteomyelitis is especially common in patients who have sickle cell anaemia (**3.119, 10.45**). Death earlier in the illness is usually related to septicaemia and toxaemia. Paratyphoid is a similar but less severe illness than typhoid.

Diagnosis is by blood, stool and urine culture. The Widal test measures agglutinating antibody titres but may be difficult to interpret in immunised patients. Chloramphenicol has been widely used in treatment and is effective except in areas where there is drug resistance, in which case ciprofloxacin is used. Approximately 3% of patients will become long-term carriers, usually harbouring the organisms in the biliary tract.

Prophylaxis is by the use of killed monovalent *Salmonella typhi* vaccine.

1.137

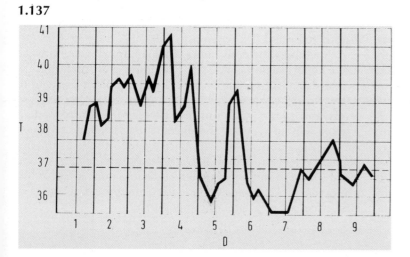

1.137 The temperature chart in a patient with typhoid shows a step-wise increase to day 4 of admission. The high fever was accompanied by confusion and severe prostration. At this point, chloramphenicol treatment was started, and the temperature showed a rapid, if occasionally incomplete, response.

1.138

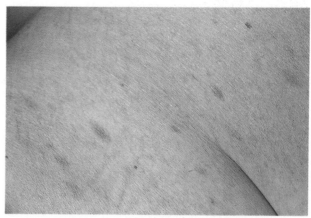

1.138 Rose spots in typhoid fever consist of pinkish macules or maculopapules, measuring 2–4 mm in diameter. The spots blanch on pressure.

Plague

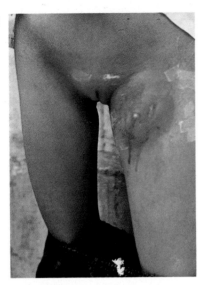

1.139 Bubonic plague. One of the most characteristic clinical features is lymphadenopathy with suppuration, especially in the inguinal and axillary regions.

Focal epidemics of plague still occur in some countries (including the USA) despite public health measures. The organism responsible is *Yersinia pestis* which is retained in a reservoir of woodland rodents (sylvatic plague) which share it with the domestic rat (murine plague). The vector from rat to man (and occasionally cats and dogs) is usually the rat flea, but cases of infection have been reported by direct transmission from an infected animal and by aerosol from infected patients.

The most common type is **bubonic plague** in which, after an incubation period of 2–4 days, the patient develops a fulminant illness with fever, headache and enlarged matted inguinal or axillary lymph nodes (buboes) (**1.139**) which may suppurate and discharge. Disseminated intravascular coagulation is common and results in bleeding from many sites, especially from the nose, and alimentary, respiratory and urinary tracts. The diagnosis can be made at this time by blood culture and by direct aspiration of the nodes. A fluorescent antibody test is also available.

When the organism is inhaled, there is rapid onset of an overwhelming pneumonia with severe toxaemia and rapid death (**pneumonic plague**). Treatment is required urgently with streptomycin, tetracycline or co-trimoxazole.

Public health measures to control the rat population in urban situations and the migration of rats are important, as there are no reasonable methods available to control the potential sylvan reservoir. Control of the flea population is possible with insecticides, but these are environmentally dangerous. Vaccination is possible in selected individuals at risk.

Cholera

Cholera is an acute diarrhoeal illness which results from colonisation of the small intestine with the organism *Vibrio cholerae*, which produces a specific exotoxin which interferes with the sodium and water homeostasis of the lining cells of the intestine. The result is massive secretion of isotonic fluid into the gut and severe extracellular fluid loss with hypovolaemic shock, potassium depletion and acid–base disturbance.

The disease is usually transmitted by the faecal–oral route, often in contaminated water (**1.4**) The incubation period may vary from a few hours to a few days before the abrupt onset of profuse watery painless diarrhoea (rice water stools—**1.140**). Muscle cramps may appear as the levels of electrolytes fall. Circulatory shock rapidly supervenes if treatment is not available—the patient has a typical appearance with extreme dehydration: sunken eyes (**1.141**), poor skin turgor, tachycardia, thready pulse and hypotension.

Acute tubular necrosis causes renal failure and this, with the severe hypovolaemic shock, is the common cause of death.

The diagnosis is made clinically and prompt replacement of water and electrolytes is the key to success. These can be given orally and monitored clinically (determination of eyeball pressure/skin turgor, or by assessment of jugular venous pressure). Biochemical control of acid–base balance and sodium and potassium levels is helpful if available. Administration of oral broad-spectrum antibiotics eradicates the infection rapidly. Public health measures to improve sanitation and provide a source of fresh water are of paramount importance.

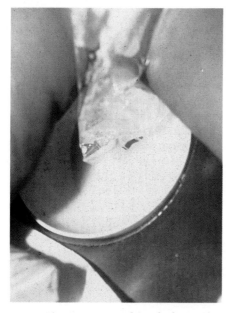

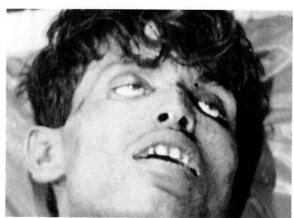

1.141 Choleraic facies. Extreme dehydration has led to the typical appearance of deeply sunken cheeks and eyes. Despite the moribund appearance of the patient with cholera, rehydration can lead to complete recovery if started before the onset of renal failure.

1.140 Rice-water stool in cholera. The large-volume, watery stool is not blood-stained, because of the non-invasive nature of the infection, but flecks of mucus and shed gut mucosal cells cause turbidity.

Legionellosis

The Legionellaceae are aerobic Gram-negative bacilli which have been found worldwide and are associated with outbreaks of pneumonia and lesser pyrexial illnessses. An increased risk of *Legionella* infection is associated with old age, male sex, cigarette smokers, alcohol excess, chronic chest disease or immuno-suppression. The airborne route of transmission has been proven in many outbreaks, usually by water aerosols from air-conditioning systems, humidifiers, shower heads and taps. Direct person-to-person transmission has not been shown, nor has infection from drinking contaminated water. The incubation period is 2–10 days.

Two distinct diseases may occur after infection with *L. pneumophila*: Pontiac fever and legionnaires' disease.

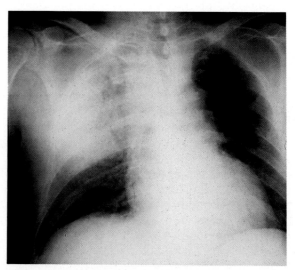

1.142 Chest X-ray in legionnaires' disease, showing extensive pneumonic shadowing in the right upper zone. The patient was severely ill, with a high fever and delirium.

- Pontiac fever, named after the city in which it was first described, is an acute pyrexial illness with fever, headache and myalgia. The disease is self-limiting over the course of a week.
- Legionnaires' disease has a spectrum of clinical severity. The features range from trivial to an acute-onset multisystem infection with pneumonia (**1.142**), encephalitis and liver and renal impairment. The dominant feature is the progressive nature of the pneumonia, which is associated with a 20% mortality (*see* p. 187). Treatment may require respiratory and renal support. Erythromycin or ciprofloxacin are the drugs of choice. Public health measures include the addition of biocides to the water used in air-conditioning cooling plants.

Bacteroides infection

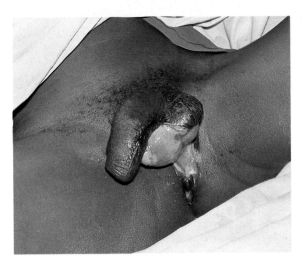

1.143 The most common and most important of the *Bacteroides* spp. is *B. fragilis*, an anaerobic Gram-negative bacillus which is a commensal of the human bowel. It may become pathogenic in the presence of tissue injury and anoxia. It is frequently found in pus from abdominal wounds, following pelvic surgery, in liver abscesses, in empyema following aspiration, and in brain abscesses. The pus is particularly foul smelling. *B. fragilis* infection is also found in spreading gangrene of skin and muscle, e.g. in Fournier's gangrene (**1.143**). Treatment is with metronidazole.

1.143 Fournier's gangrene of the scrotum, occurring in an African patient. The causative organism was *Bacteroides fragilis*. Good wound care and split skin grafting resulted in complete healing.

Brucellosis

Brucellosis in man is caused by infection with one of three species of *Brucella* organisms, depending on the animal source of infection: *B. mellitensis* (goats), *B. abortus* (cattle) or *B. suis* (pigs). The organism infects the genito-urinary tracts of animals and may be ingested in milk and milk products or meat, or directly through cuts in the skin. The disease occurs frequently in workers in contact with animals, e.g. farmers, abattoir workers, veterinary surgeons and butchers. Epidemics may occur from the ingestion of unpasteurised milk and milk products.

The incubation period is usually up to three weeks, but the first symptoms may not appear for many months and are usually low-grade 'undulant' fever (**1.11**, **1.144**), headache, myalgia, anorexia, pains in the joints and over the spine, orchitis and general debility. A more acute presentation may be high swinging fever, lymphadenopathy and tender hepatosplenomegaly. Almost every organ of the body may be involved in the acute process, which gradually subsides to be replaced by a chronic disease characterised by progressive asthenia, depression, loss of weight associated with intermittent fever, chronic bone and joint degeneration (**1.145**) and hepatosplenomegaly.

The diagnosis is made by blood culture during the acute phase or a rising titre of agglutinins. Specific immunoglobin (IgM) tests are now available. Treatment is with tetracycline or co-trimoxazole. Public health measures include testing cattle with the Brucellin skin test, certification of disease-free stock and pasteurisation of milk.

1.144

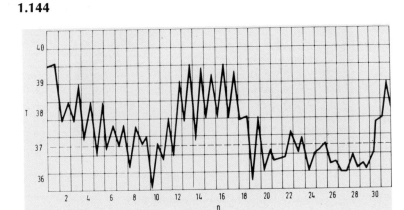

1.144 Temperature chart in brucellosis, showing typical 'undulant' fever, which is remittent and variable in character.

1.145

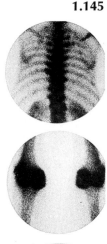

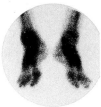

1.145 Degenerative osteoarthritis in brucellosis, as shown by a technetium-99m MDP bone scan. The patient was a Bedouin shepherd, who had suffered from fever, painful joint swellings and backache for over a year. This is a common complication of chronic brucellosis.

Pertussis

Pertussis (whooping cough) is a serious illness affecting mainly young children. The causal agent is *Bordetella pertussis,* and spread is by droplets from the respiratory tract.

Catarrhal symptoms and cough appear after an incubation period of 7–10 days. By about the tenth day of illness, the cough has usually become spasmodic and may be followed by a whoop. At the end of a spasm of coughing, mucus is expectorated and there is frequently vomiting. In severe cases there may be 20–30 spasms of coughing per day, and frequent vomiting may lead to weight loss and dehydration. The illness usually lasts about 4–6 weeks, but in some patients coughing may persist for several months.

Pneumonia and otitis media may occur as a result of bacterial superinfection. There may be mechanical complications, such as subconjunctival haemorrhage (**1.146**), epistaxis, haemoptysis or ulcers of the tongue (**1.147**). Hernias may develop and there may be rectal prolapse. Atelectasis results from mucous plugging of bronchi or bronchioles. Convulsions, either anoxic or caused by encephalopathy, can be life-threatening.

The causal organism can be identified in pernasal swabs, by culture or by immunofluorescence. The white blood count is usually raised with marked lymphocytosis.

Physiotherapy during spasms aids mucus expectoration. Small, frequent meals and attention to fluid intake prevent weight loss and dehydration. Antibiotics are of little benefit in the established case. Erythromycin given very early in the disease may have some effect and it has a place in prophylaxis in child contacts. Cough suppressants are contraindicated and sedation should be reserved for patients with convulsions.

Prophylaxis is available with combined diphtheria, pertussis and tetanus vaccine (DPT).

1.146

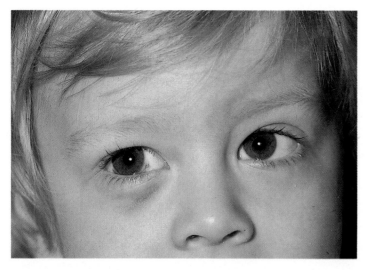

1.146 Subconjunctival haemorrhage in pertussis occurs because the intrathoracic pressure rises sharply during violent paroxysms of coughing and leads to sudden surges in capillary pressure. In this child, the subconjunctival haemorrhage is accompanied by bleeding into the lower lid—a rarer complication. No permanent harm results, and these complications resolve rapidly.

1.147

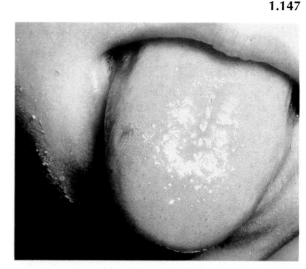

1.147 A swollen, bitten tongue is a common complication of pertussis, because of the paroxysms of coughing and choking. Ulcers of the frenum of the tongue may also occur.

Tularaemia

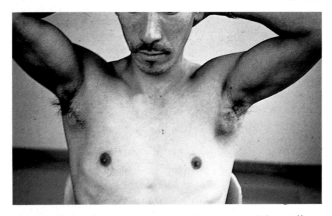

1.148 Tularaemia, causing gross enlargement of the axillary lymph nodes in a Japanese patient.

This is a zoonosis caused by the Gram-negative rod *Francisella tularensis*. It is acquired from an animal reservoir (usually a rodent) directly, by contaminated food or water, by inhalation, by handling an infected carcase or indirectly by ticks. Tularaemia occurs in most parts of the world. The clinical presentation is often with a febrile illness with a skin ulcer and enlargement of the regional lymph nodes (1.148). There may be a secondary necrotising pneumonia from the primary lesion, or inhalation of the organism may produce a primary pneumonia. Pericarditis and meningitis are rare but serious complications with a high mortality. The organisms are sensitive to streptomycin, gentamicin and tetracycline. A vaccine is available for those who are at high risk of exposure to the organism, e.g. laboratory workers, forest rangers and hunters.

Non-venereal treponematoses

For venereally transmitted treponemal disease (syphilis) *see* p. 83.

Yaws

This is a chronic infection with *Treponema pertenue* that has a worldwide tropical distribution. Children are often infected through pre-existing skin lesions when in contact with a person with infectious yaws, but congenital infection does not occur. There is an incubation period of 4–6 weeks and the primary lesion is a papule which grows and discharges ('mother yaw'). There is usually inguinal lymphadenopathy. This primary lesion heals over a period of 4–8 months. A crop of secondary lesions occurs over a period of 6 months—these often involve the skin (1.149) and long bones. Longer-term infection results in multiple destructive lesions of bones (1.150), joints and skin. Diagnosis is made by demonstration of the treponemes and by serology. Treatment of the early lesions is with penicillin. Public health measures include improvements in personal hygiene, dressing of open wounds and community prophylaxis with antibiotics.

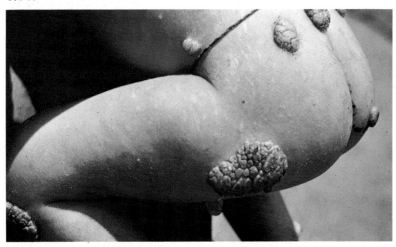

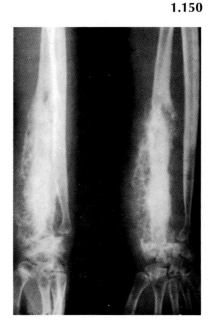

1.149 Secondary framboesiform yaws, occurring in a Papuan child. These classical lesions are often accompanied by secondary lesions at mucocutaneous junctions.

1.150 Yaws osteitis. This X-ray of the forearms shows focal cortical rarefaction and periosteal new bone formation. Similar appearances may be seen elsewhere in the body, especially in the tibia ('sabre tibia'), as in tertiary syphilis.

Pinta

Pinta is a chronic skin infection with *Treponema carateum* found in South America, which causes a generalised multicoloured rash. The lesions start slate blue and become brown and eventually white, leaving the skin mottled and blotchy (**1.151**). There is no general hazard to health and the effects are cosmetic and psychological. Penicillin controls the progress of the disease.

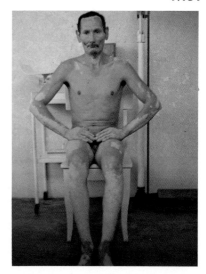

1.151 Depigmented lesions of pinta. These 'pintids' start as small papules and develop into plaques with actively growing edges which become confluent. In the late stages the 'pintids' become depigmented.

Bejel

Bejel is a chronic inflammatory disease of skin and mucous membranes caused by a non-venereal treponeme which eventually produces chronic granulomas of skin and bone. It occurs in childhood, and is found particularly in the dry regions of Africa, the Balkans and Australia. The secondary features include a maculopapular rash (**1.152**) with regional lymphadenopathy. Transmission is by direct person-to-person contact or by fomites. Widespread use of penicillin has led to a decline in incidence with eradication in some countries.

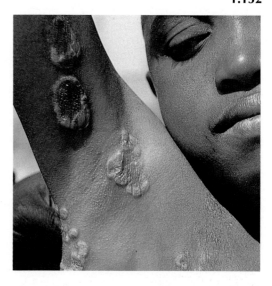

1.152 Secondary rash in bejel or 'endemic syphilis'. A florid maculopapular eruption with associated adenitis is usually the first sign of this non-venereal infection.

Cancrum oris

Cancrum oris is caused by infection with a mixed flora of anaerobic organisms including *Borrelia vincentii*. The condition is seen in malnourished, deprived children who have become immunosuppressed or who are debilitated with another disease, e.g. measles or acute leukaemia. The infection usually starts as gingivitis and rapidly spreads to involve the buccal mucosa, the cheek, the mandible and the maxilla (**1.153**). If the gangrenous areas heal, they leave major disfigurement. The mortality is very high despite antibiotic treatment.

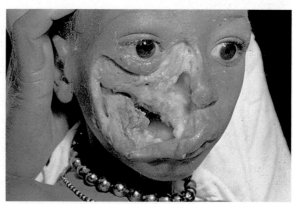

1.153 Cancrum oris in a young, malnourished African child. The infection has caused massive soft-tissue loss, followed by loss of teeth and necrosis of parts of the maxilla and mandible.

Lyme disease

Lyme disease was originally described locally in New England, USA, but has now been recognised in most countries. It is caused by a spirochaete (*Borrelia burgdorferi*) which is transmitted by bites of the animal tick (*Ixodes dammini*). Patients present with an acute febrile illness and with erythema chronicum migrans—a chronic indurated rash with a characteristic red margin and central clearing (1.154). Multiple skin lesions appear at different stages and there is associated lymphadenopathy, myalgia and arthralgia. Neurological features occur in 10–20% of cases, including meningoencephalitis, cranial nerve palsies, and peripheral neuropathy. There may also be associated myocarditis and pericarditis. Many months after these features, arthritis develops and may have a chronic relapsing course with acute exacerbations mainly affecting large joints, especially the knee. The disease is associated with erosion of cartilage and bone and may be mistaken for osteoarthritis (1.155).

The diagnosis is made by demonstrating the presence of an IgM antibody and occasionally it is possible to culture the organism from skin, joint fluid or CSF.

The acute presenting features are best treated with high-dose intravenous penicillin and the later complications with a course of tetracyline. Prevention of the disease involves the avoidance of tick bites.

1.154

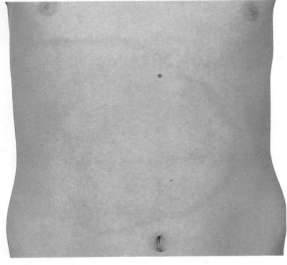

1.154 Erythema chronicum migrans. This characteristic rash should raise a strong clinical suspicion of the diagnosis of Lyme disease. Unless it is noted, the diagnosis may often be missed. Note the chronic induration, with a characteristic red margin and central clearing.

1.155

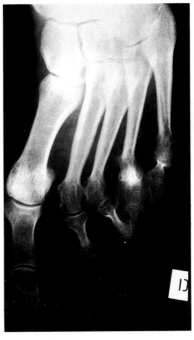

1.155 Chronic arthritis in Lyme disease. These severe arthritic changes in the foot occurred in a patient who had first noted the characteristic skin rash more than 10 years earlier.

Leptospirosis

Man acquires leptospirosis from direct or indirect contact with animals, especially rodents. Farm workers, vets, sewer workers and fish-farm workers are particularly at risk, as are people in contact with rat-infested water, e.g. canoeists and wind surfers on inland waterways. Infection gains entry through broken skin, mucous membranes or conjunctivae. The causal organisms are members of the species *Leptospira interrogans* of which there are many serotypes.

L. icterohaemorrhagiae is the serotype most often associated with classical Weil's disease which has an incubation period of 2–20 days. In the first week of illness there are influenza-like symptoms, with fever, shivering, headache, myalgia and conjunctival suffusion (1.156). If the disease progresses, the patient becomes jaundiced and haemorrhages appear on skin and mucous membranes. There are signs of meningitis and of renal failure. Death may occur in the second or third week from cardiac or renal failure. Serotypes other than *L. icterohaemorrhagiae* often cause subclinical, or less severe, anicteric illness. *L. canicola* usually presents as **aseptic meningitis.**

There is usually a polymorph leucocytosis in leptospiral infection. Early in the illness, organisms can be identified in the blood, CSF and urine by culture or dark-ground microscopy. Diagnosis is confirmed by the finding of rising titres of antibody in paired sera.

Good supportive nursing is essential. Dialysis may be required for renal failure. Antibiotics are effective only if given very early in the illness. Benzylpenicillin is the drug of choice, but tetracycline and erythromycin may also be used.

Prevention includes rodent control in farms and industrial areas and avoidance of rat-infested waters.

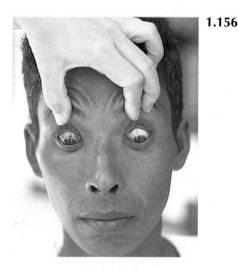

1.156 Leptospirosis causing conjunctival suffusion. This patient washed regularly in rat-infested water.

Trachoma

Trachoma is a type of chronic conjunctivitis caused by infection with *Chlamydia trachomatis,* which has a worldwide distribution. In endemic areas it is transmitted from eye to eye by hands or flies, and in non-endemic areas it may be transmitted from the genital tract to the eye, especially in the newborn. The disease presents with the features of conjunctivitis, and minute lymphoid follicles in the conjunctiva are typical of early infection (**1.157**). Chronic inflammation leads to scarring and formation of a pannus. Further scarring leads to distortion of the eyelid, with turning-in of the eyelashes (entropion) which abrade the cornea further (trichiasis). Destruction of the goblet cells leads to a 'dry eye', which in turn exacerbates the corneal injury and rapidly results in blindness (**1.158**). The diagnosis is made from the clinical picture and the therapeutic response to tetracycline. Public health measures are of paramount importance. Corneal grafting is of value in selected patients.

C. trachomatis is also a common cause of non-specific urethritis (*see* p. 86); and a strain of *C. trachomatis* is the cause of lymphogranuloma venereum (*see* p. 86).

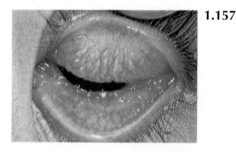

1.157 Early trachoma. Small pinhead-sized, pale follicles are present in the epithelium over the tarsal plates, as can be seen especially in the everted upper lid.

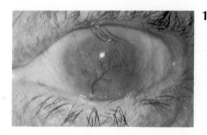

1.158 Blindness resulting from late stage corneal scarring in trachoma.

Psittacosis

This is an infection caused by *Chlamydia psittaci*, which infects parrots, parakeets, turkeys, pigeons, ducks, chickens and other birds. Infection is acquired by inhalation of dried infected bird faeces and more rarely by handling the feathers or the carcase, by a bird bite or by other close contact. The disease is found in people working with birds, such as pet shop employees, pigeon handlers and poultry workers. The incubation period is about 7–10 days followed by a mild influenza-like illness. More severe infections are associated with fever, malaise, anorexia, myalgia and headache. Chest features predominate with cough, mucoid sputum which may be blood stained and rarely pleuritic pain from pneumonia. Splenomegaly in a patient with pneumonia is an important diagnostic sign. Spontaneous recovery usually occurs over several weeks, but neurologic signs, liver or renal failure indicate a poor prognosis. The diagnosis of pneumonia is confirmed by a chest X-ray (*see* p. 186), there may be some elevation in white cell count and ESR; the diagnosis is made by isolation of the organism or, usually, by serology. Tetracyclines remain the drugs of choice.

Mycoplasma infection

Mycoplasmas are the smallest free-living organisms, which differ from other bacteria in that they lack a cell wall. The most important mycoplasmas infecting man are *Mycoplasma pneumoniae*, *M. hominis* and *Ureaplasma urealyticum*. *M. pneumoniae* is a frequent cause of respiratory infections in children and young adults, being spread by airborne droplets. The other mycoplasma organisms are associated with infections of the urogenital tract (*see* p. 86).

The spectrum of illness caused by *M. pneumoniae* ranges from mild upper respiratory infection to severe atypical pneumonia. There may also be involvement of other organs with acute myocarditis, pancreatitis, aseptic meningitis and encephalitis, ear infection (bullous) and skin involvement (erythema multiforme—*see* p. 118) and Stevens–Johnson syndrome. Patients with atypical pneumonia present with fever, lassitude, malaise and a non-productive cough. Chest pain is not usually prominent. Physical signs on examination of the chest are often less impressive than the X-ray findings which may be unilateral or bilateral (4.78). Segmental lobular consolidation is frequently seen, but there may be changes suggesting bronchopneumonia or simply a general haziness fanning out from the hilum.

Laboratory findings include a high ESR and relatively low white blood count. Cold agglutinins appear in the blood in about 50% of patients and if present may be associated with haemolytic anaemia. The diagnosis is confirmed by demonstration of rising antibody titre to *M. pneumoniae*. Mild infection usually resolves spontaneously. Moderate or severe infections should respond to a course of erythromycin or tetracycline.

Stevens–Johnson syndrome

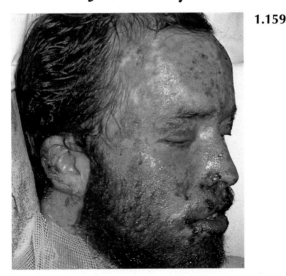

1.159

1.159 Stevens–Johnson syndrome, in its severe form, is a widespread erythema multiforme with oral, genital and conjunctival involvement, and widespread skin lesions as on this patient's face. This form of the disease is common in patients with *Mycoplasma pneumoniae* infection.

This syndrome is not strictly an infectious disease, but it may develop in response to a number of different trigger mechanisms among which are included infection with *Mycoplasma pneumoniae*, herpes simplex virus, orf and other viral agents. The ingestion of certain drugs, especially sulphonamide preparations may also precede the condition. Many cases, however, are apparently idiopathic.

Presenting features of the syndrome are fever, severe bilateral conjunctivitis, extensive inflammation of the mucosa of the mouth and genital tract and the development of an erythema multiforme-type rash, which is usually most marked on the extremities. The rash often consists of 'target'-type lesions (2.125), but there may be vesiculation with formation of larger bullae and the rash may become generalised (1.159). This occurs particularly when the syndrome develops in response to *M. pneumoniae* infection.

The disease is usually self-limiting, but progress is often slow and patients suffer a great deal of discomfort. Any underlying infection should be treated appropriately. In severe cases, systemic steroids are indicated and local application of steroid eye-drops may relieve the conjunctivitis. Intravenous fluids or nasogastric feeding with a fine-bore tube may be necessary until the patient can swallow properly. The ultimate prognosis is good.

Typhus and related infections

A range of diseases caused by the family Rickettsiaceae are harboured in the intestines of a range of arthropods (lice, fleas, ticks). They infect animals and man, often in epidemic form. Such infections are found worldwide and all have similar clinical presentations as the rickettsia invades the endothelium of blood vessels to produce vasculitis and local thrombosis followed by tissue necrosis.

The most important disease historically is typhus, which is caused by infection with *Rickettsia prowazekii*, carried by the human louse. Epidemics of infection are usually associated with disasters such as war or earthquakes. After a short incubation period (up to 7 days) there is rapid onset of fever, headache, myalgia and prostration. A rash appears soon afterwards (**1.160**), which is petechial initially before becoming confluent. Gangrene of the feet and hands (**1.161**) may then appear with areas of skin necrosis, renal failure and coma. Diagnosis is serological as culture exposes laboratory personnel to an unnecessary hazard. Tetracycline is the drug of choice and vaccination is available. Public health measures to control lice are mandatory.

Related disorders include Rocky Mountain spotted fever, murine typhus, scrub typhus and trench fever all of which are caused by different rickettsiae carried by different vectors.

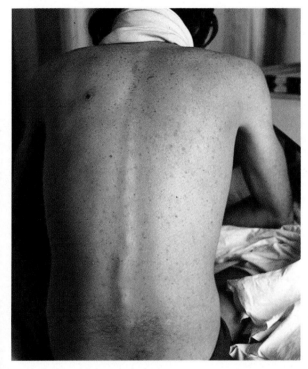

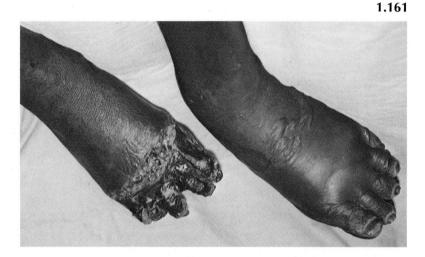

1.160 The rash in tick typhus. An 'eschar' forms at the site of the infective tick bite, and this is followed by a more generally distributed rash.

1.161 Peripheral gangrene in severe typhus. This serious complication follows the vasculitis and thrombosis associated with the disease.

Q fever

This is an acute pyrexial illness which is caused by infection by a rickettsial-like organism, *Coxiella burnetii*. Infection is usually acquired from an animal source by inhalation of dust, from infected milk, or by direct handling. The usual animal sources are cows, sheep and goats and the organism is spread by ticks. After exposure, the incubation period is about 2–3 weeks before the onset of fever, myalgia, petechial rash, headache followed by cough and pleuritic chest pain caused by pneumonia (*see* p. 187). Most patients recover rapidly, but occasionally progression occurs with hepatitis (*see* p. 397), endocarditis (*see* p. 242), uveitis and orchitis. The diagnosis is dependent on serology and treatment is with tetracycline or rifampicin.

Fungal infections

Name	Important human fungi	Relevant human disease	Page reference
Histoplasma	*H. Capsulatum* *H. duboisii*	Histoplasmosis Destructive lesions of skin and bone	62
Aspergillus	*A. fumigatus* *A. flavus* *A. niger*	Lung infections, aspergilloma, allergic bronchopulmonary aspergillosis	63
Cryptococcus	*C. neoformans*	Pneumonia, meningoencephalitis	64
Coccidioides	*Coccidioides immitis* *Paracoccidioides brasiliensis*	Pneumonia Skin lesions	64
Blastomyces	*Blastomyces dermatitidis*	Skin lesions	64
Candida	*C. albicans*	Oral, cutaneous, genital and systemic infection	65, 100
Dermatophytes	Numerous	Skin infections	100

Histoplasmosis

1.162

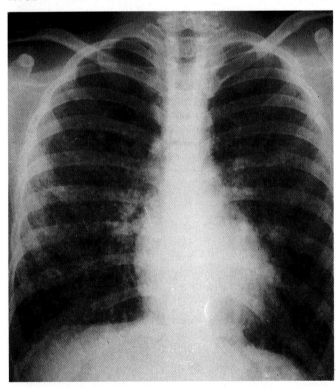

1.162 Primary pulmonary histoplasmosis may be asymptomatic, or it may result in a transient symptomatic respiratory infection. In this patient, the appearance of miliary mottling could represent miliary tuberculosis, pneumoconiosis or pulmonary metastases, and other tests are necessary to confirm the diagnosis.

Histoplasmosis occurs in many areas of the world and is particularly common in parts of the American mid-west. It is caused by a fungus, *Histoplasma capsulatum,* which is found in the soil, and transmitted by inhalation of fungal spores. The incubation period is usually 5–20 days.

In several respects, the clinical picture of histoplasmosis resembles that of tuberculosis (TB):

- **Primary pulmonary histoplasmosis**—which is often asymptomatic—is the first manifestation. It produces radiological features identical to those of the primary focus in TB (**1.119, 1.120**) and heals in a similar way. The radiological appearance may sometimes resemble miliary tuberculosis (**1.162**), and calcification may eventually occur (**1.163**). Complications at this stage may include pneumonia, pleural effusions, erythema nodosum (**1.123, 2.40**) or erythema multiforme (**2.125**).
- **Chronic pulmonary histoplasmosis** is usually clinically indistinguishable from pulmonary TB, producing a similar range of complications (*see* p. 188).
- **Disseminated histoplasmosis** may occur at any stage of the disease, leading to complications including chronic pericarditis, granulomatous hepatitis, chronic meningitis and destructive lesions of skin and bone.

Definitive diagnosis is made by culture or histology, and serology and histoplasmin skin testing are also useful. In endemic areas, over 90% of the population have serological evidence of previous infection.

Only severe histoplasmosis requires treatment with anti-fungal therapy (amphotericin B).

African histoplasmosis is caused by *Histoplasma duboisii.* It does not cause pulmonary lesions, but skin lesions (**1.164**), lymph node involvement and lytic bone lesions are common.

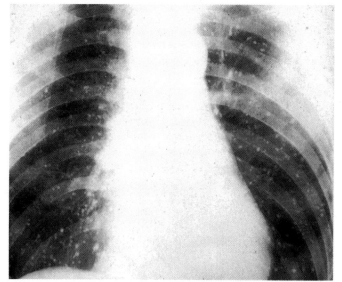

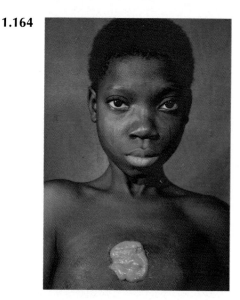

1.163 Healed pulmonary histoplasmosis. Again, the residual fibrosis and calcification are reminiscent of TB, or of healed chickenpox pneumonia.

1.164 African histoplasmosis producing a large destructive skin lesion. Similar appearances may occur in disseminated infection with *Histoplasma capsulatum*, especially in immunosuppressed patients.

Aspergillosis

Inhalation of the spores of the ubiquitous fungus, *Aspergillus fumigatus* (occasionally *A. flavus* and *A. niger*) may produce three forms of disease in the lung:

- **In normal people**, inhalation of spores may give rise to an acute pneumonia, which is usually self-limiting over several weeks. In patients who are immunosuppressed, blood-borne dissemination may take place to orbit, brain and skin.
- **In patients with pre-existing lung disease**, especially in those with bronchiectasis or cavities, *Aspergillus* can form large colonies. Balls of hyphae may reach several inches in diameter (aspergilloma) (**1.165, 4.36, 4.37**). These are usually found on routine X-ray, but may present with haemoptysis.

- **In allergic bronchopulmonary aspergillosis**, which usually occurs in previously asthmatic patients, infection is followed by intermittent episodes of asthma and pneumonia, with eosinophilia and bronchial plugging with mucus. Repeated episodes of pneumonia may produce progressive pulmonary fibrosis and/or bronchiectasis (**1.166**, *see* p. 183).

The diagnosis of aspergillosis depends on the demonstration of hyphae in the sputum, positive serology, positive skin prick test (*see* p. 90) or typical radiological appearances. Corticosteroids are of value in treating the allergic pneumonitis. Amphotericin B is used in invasive disease and surgery may be required to remove the cavity which contains the aspergilloma.

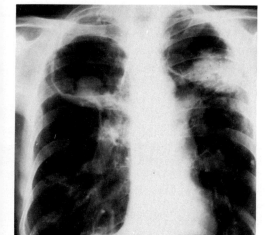

1.165 Bilateral aspergillomas, occurring in upper lobe cavities caused by old tuberculosis. If left untreated, the balls of fungus might ultimately grow to fill the cavities completely.

1.166 Allergic bronchopulmonary aspergillosis, showing widespread changes of bronchiectasis, predominantly central in distribution, with associated fibrotic scarring.

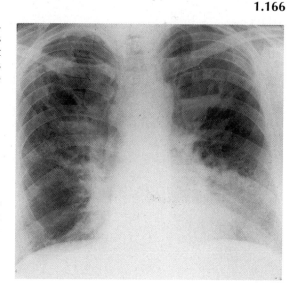

Cryptococcosis

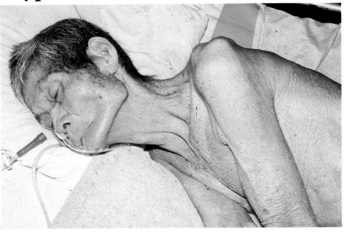

1.167 Meningoencephalitis is a potentially fatal complication of cryptococcal infection. The most common predisposing cause is now AIDS, although this patient was HIV negative.

Cryptococcus neoformans is a fungus with a worldwide distribution, which is thought to be spread in bird droppings. Inhalation of the spores of this and related fungi gives rise to a low-grade granulomatous pneumonia. This may heal spontaneously, but it is occasionally complicated by cavitation, bilateral hilar lymphadenopathy and pulmonary fibrosis.

The most serious complication is meningoencephalitis (**1.167**), a particularly common problem in patients with AIDS who have opportunistic cryptococcal infection. In addition, chronic infection of skin, bone, liver, heart and kidney may occur.

Cryptococcal infection cannot be diagnosed on clinical grounds. A CSF agglutination test is available for the diagnosis of CNS infection; in other sites, biopsy is usually necessary.

CNS infection is still potentially fatal, but treatment with amphotericin B, fluconazole or flucytosine has reduced the mortality rate.

Coccidioidomycosis

1.168

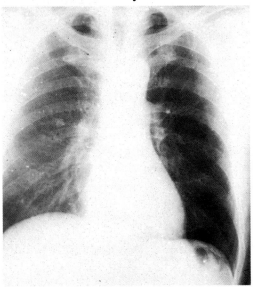

1.168 Chronic coccidioidomycosis. The nature of the coin lesion seen in the right lower zone (a coccidioidoma) was confirmed by aspiration needle biospy.

This is a common disease in South America and the Southern USA which results from the inhalation of the fungal spores of *Coccidioides immitis* which are widely disseminated in soil. Most infections are asymptomatic and the presence of the organism is detected by skin testing. In a small number of patients there is an acute pneumonia, often associated with arthralgia and erythema nodosum (**1.123, 2.40**) or erythema multiforme (**2.125**). The disease may be severe in pregnancy and in patients who are immunosuppressed. Chronic lung infection may follow (**1.168**) and there may be evidence of general dissemination to bones, joints, brain and skin. Diagnosis depends on the identification of mycelia and on serology. Treatment is with amphotericin B or ketoconazole. Surgery may be indicated for chronic pulmonary or bone lesions.

Paracoccidioidomycosis and blastomycosis are broadly similar diseases which are caused by inhalation of the fungi *Paracoccidioides brasiliensis* and *Blastomyces dermatitidis* respectively. They are found mainly in the American continent. The diseases tend to be milder than coccidioidomycosis, but skin lesions are prominent in blastomycosis and occasional dissemination of both conditions has been reported.

Candidiasis

Candidiasis results from infection by *Candida albicans*, a budding yeast-like organism which can infect the skin and the mucosa of the mouth, intestine and genital tract. Young infants, pregnant females, diabetics, people with prosthetic heart valves, patients on broad-spectrum antibiotics and people immunocompromised by drugs or disease are especially susceptible to *Candida* infections. In immunocompromised patients, dissemination of infection via the blood stream may be life-threatening. Oral or genital candidiasis is often the first opportunistic infection to appear in HIV infection.

On mucous membranes, candidiasis appears as curd-like spots or plaques ('thrush') on a red base (**1.28, 1.169, 1.170, 10.64**). Vaginal (**1.171**) or penile candidiasis is usually accompanied by irritation and itching of the region. Oesophageal candidiasis (**1.34**) causes retrosternal pain and dysphagia. Moist areas of skin are susceptible to infection (**2.50**) and the nails may be infected (**2.51**). Infants with oral candidiasis often have involvement of the skin of the groins and perineum (**1.172**). Almost any organ of the body may be involved in systemic candidiasis.

Candida organisms can easily be identified in smears made from skin or mucosal lesions and stained with methylene blue. Confirmation of infection is by culture from the local lesions or from the blood in systemic candidiasis.

Mucocutaneous candidiasis usually responds to local therapy with antifungal agents in preparations suitable for the site of infection. Oral fluconazole may be required for severe gastrointestinal or genital candidiasis. Systemic candidiasis requires intravenous therapy with fluconazole or amphotericin B alone, or combined with flucytosine. Predisposing factors such as diabetes should be sought and treated.

1.169

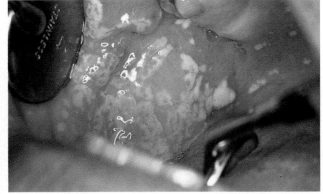

1.169 Oral thrush showing the characteristic curdy white patches of acute candida infection. In all but newborn babies this infection implies underlying disease or debility, and further investigation of the patient may be necessary. It is important not to confuse thrush with other causes of white oral mucosal lesions (e.g. lichen planus, **2.59**).

1.170

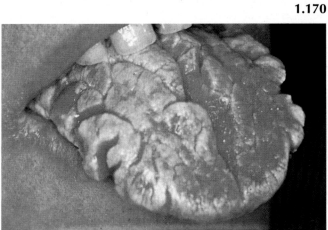

1.170 Chronic candidiasis of the mouth. The deep fissuring of the tongue is the end result of long-term candida infection (compare this appearance with the acutely infected tongue seen in **1.28**).

1.171   **1.172**

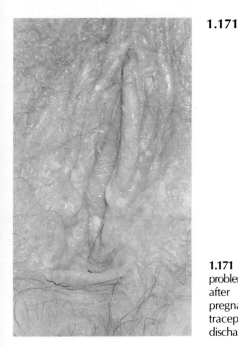

1.171 Vaginal thrush is a common problem in adult women during or after antibiotic treatment, in pregnancy and during oral contraceptive use. The curdy white discharge is chartacteristic.

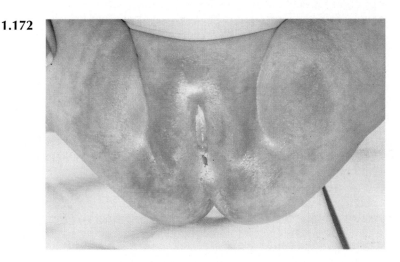

1.172 Vulvovaginitis in a baby, caused by *Candida albicans*. Infection at this age is not unusual, but in older children and adults it may suggest an underlying disorder such as diabetes.

Protozoal infections

Genus	Important human protozoa	Relevant human disease	Page reference
Intestinal and genital protozoa			
Amoeba	Entamoeba histolytica E. polecki	Dysentery, liver abscess, skin infection	66, 380, 407
Giardia	G. lamblia	Diarrhoea, malabsorption	379
Balantidium	B. coli	Diarrhoea	379
Isospora	I. belli	Diarrhoea	379
Cryptosporidium	Cryptosporidium	Diarrhoea, acute fluid loss	379
Trichomonas	Trichomonas vaginalis	Vaginitis, balinitis	86
Blood and tissue protozoa			
Toxoplasma	T. gondii	Generalised toxoplasma infection Congenital infection	67
Plasmodium	P. vivax, P. ovale, P. malariae, P. falciparum	Malaria	68
Pneumocystis	P. carinii	Pneumonia	18, 188
Leishmania	L. donovani, L. tropica, L. braziliensis	Visceral and cutaneous leishmaniasis	70
Trypanosoma	T. brucei gambiense T. brucei rhodesiense T. cruzi	African sleeping sickness American trypanosomiasis Chagas' disease	71 71

Amoebiasis

Amoebiasis is endemic in many tropical areas where sanitation is poor. Spread of infection is by the faecal–oral route, usually through ingestion of amoebic cysts in contaminated water or food. The causal agent is *Entamoeba histolytica* and the time from ingestion of cysts to the appearance of symptoms may be up to one year.

Patients infected with *Entamoeba histolytica* may present in several ways:

- With acute dysenteric symptoms: malaise, fever, abdominal pain and the passage of frequent loose stools containing blood and mucus (amoebic colitis, *see* p. 379).
- With less severe relapsing diarrhoea over a period of weeks or months.
- With symptoms mimicking those of an intestinal tumour, caused by granulomatous masses (amoebomata) in the bowel wall (**8.90**, *see also* p. 380).
- Carrier states exist without obvious clinical illness.

- Liver abscess may present without evidence of concurrent or previous bowel infection (*see* p. 407).
- Pleura, lung and pericardium may be involved in spread from the liver.
- Skin may be involved by abscess formation (**1.173**) or directly as a result of sexual contact (**1.174**).

Vegetative forms of amoebae should be sought in fresh (hot) stools or in scrapings from bowel ulcers seen at sigmoidoscopy. Suspected liver abscess is diagnosed by ultrasound, isotope scanning, CT scanning (**1.175**) or by diagnostic aspiration (**1.176, 1.177**). Antibody levels to amoebae are raised in most cases of liver abscess, but are of less value in dysenteric illness.

Both amoebic dysentery and amoebic liver abscess respond to metronidazole. Chloroquine may be used as additional therapy in liver abscess. Therapeutic aspiration of the abscess is now rarely required but progress towards healing should be monitored by ultrasound scanning. Diloxanide furoate is effective in clearing amoebic cysts from the gut in the carrier state.

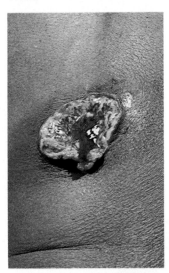

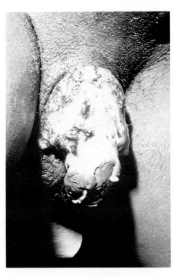

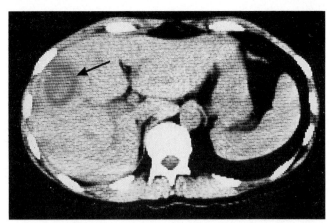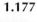

1.175 Amoebic liver abscess (arrowed) seen on a CT scan in a British woman who had returned from a vacation in Kenya two months earlier. She presented with right upper quadrant pain and fever.

1.173 Amoebiasis of the skin, resulting from direct spread from an intra-abdominal abscess.

1.174 Amoebic balanitis contracted through anal intercourse with a patient with bowel infection.

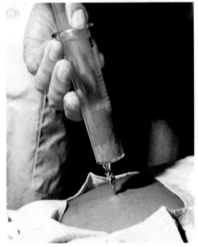

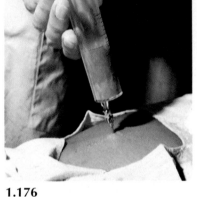

1.176 Aspiration of an amoebic liver abscess is useful for diagnostic purposes and may still have occasional therapeutic value in patients with large abscesses. Note the characteristic chocolate-coloured pus.

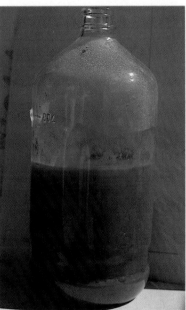

1.176

1.177 Pus from an amoebic liver abscess. Note the characteristic chocolate colour and the large volume (approximately 550 ml). All this pus was aspirated from a single abscess.

Toxoplasmosis

The causal organism is *Toxoplasma gondii,* a protozoan parasite. The organism has many vertebrate hosts but the sexual cycle occurs only in cats, which pass the infective oocysts in their faeces. Man is infected by eating meat containing tissue cysts or by the ingestion of oocytes from cat faeces.

Women infected during pregnancy may transmit the organism transplacentally to the fetus. Abortion is likely if the fetus is infected in early pregnancy. Congenital toxoplasmosis may be a severe life-threatening illness with fever, hepatosplenomegaly, rash, hydrocephalus, brain damage (**1.178, 1.179**) and choroidoretinitis (**1.180**). Infants may, however, appear normal at birth or may have only minor clinical abnormalities.

Toxoplasmosis acquired in childhood or adult life is often subclinical and can usually be diagnosed only by serology. There

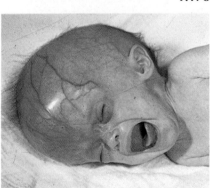

1.178 Hydrocephalus is a major complication of congenital toxoplasmosis and is usually associated with substantial cerebral damage.

may, however, be a glandular fever-like syndrome with fever, malaise and swelling of one or more glands. Occasionally the disease is more widespread with involvement of liver, spleen, heart, meninges, brain and eyes (**1.180**). Primary infection or reactivation of latent infection in immunocompromised patients is likely to cause particularly severe illness including cerebral abscesses (**1.33**).

The diagnosis is confirmed by serology. In cerebral toxoplasmosis skull X-ray and CT or MRI scanning may aid diagnosis and histology of a lymph node biopsy may also be helpful.

Acquired toxoplasmosis in immunocompetent patients usually requires no treatment. Congenital toxoplasmosis and severe illness, especially in immunocompromised people, should be treated with high-dose co-trimoxazole or pyrimethamine plus sulphonamide. Therapy may have to be prolonged and in the immunocompromised patient, maintenance therapy may be required for life. Spiramycin is advised for use in pregnancy.

Prevention includes thorough cooking of meat and meat products and the avoidance of areas such as children's sand pits likely to be contaminated with cat faeces.

1.179

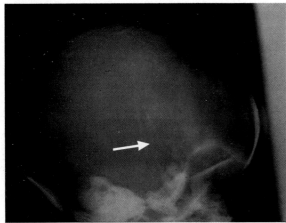

1.179 Intracranial calcification in a child with congenital toxoplasmosis. This is a common finding in congenital toxoplasmosis, but is not diagnostic of the condition. The calcification may take several forms, and is often linear, as here (arrow).

1.180

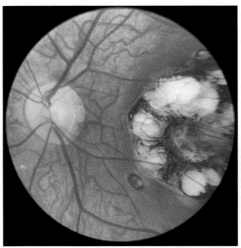

1.180 Necrotising choroidoretinitis is an invariable complication of congenital toxoplasmosis, and it also occurs in about 1% of patients with the acquired disease. Note the pigmented atrophic scar in the fundus. Ultimately, progression of the untreated disease may result in blindness.

Malaria

Malaria is the major cause of morbidity and mortality in many tropical and subtropical countries. The number of cases imported into non-endemic areas grows each year as a result of ever-increasing world travel.

Four species of the genus *Plasmodium* cause human malaria:

* *P. falciparum*—malignant tertian.
* *P. vivax*—benign tertian.
* *P. ovale*—ovale tertian.
* *P. malariae*—quartan.

The insect vector is the female *Anopheles* mosquito. Infection with *P. falciparum* causes the most severe illness. Increasing geographic spread of resistance of this organism to chloroquine and other antimalarial drugs is causing major problems in the management and control of the disease.

Presenting features of an acute malarial attack may include fever (**1.181**), rigors, sweating, headache, myalgia, gastrointestinal upset and respiratory symptoms. In severe falciparum malaria

there may be collapse, convulsions and coma (cerebral malaria, **1.182**). The presence of retinal haemorrhage in the non-comatose patient heralds the rapid onset of cerebral symptoms (**1.183**). Splenomegaly and anaemia are usual in the acute attack. Acute haemolytic crises may be associated with haemoglobinuria (Blackwater fever, **1.184**).

Chronic infection may be associated with massive splenomegaly (tropical splenomegaly syndrome (TSS)—**1.185**) or with the nephrotic syndrome (**1.186**).

The diagnosis is confirmed by examination of thick and thin blood films and the identification of parasites in red cells (**1.187**).

Chloroquine is the treatment of choice for benign tertian or quartan malaria and for falciparum malaria acquired in areas where there is no resistance of parasites to chloroquine; but chloroquine resistance is spreading and up-to-date advice is required before malaria is treated if the patient comes from an area of possible resistance. A course of primaquine should also be given to patients with benign tertian or quartan malaria to prevent recurrence.

Preventive measures include mosquito control, personal mosquito-bite avoidance measures and, often, prophylactic therapy for people entering or living in a malarious area. Advice given to travellers should take account of the relative risk of acquiring infection, the degree of resistance of parasites in the area and the potential side effects of drugs used in prophylaxis. Global control of malaria may be achieved if a reliable vaccine becomes available.

1.181

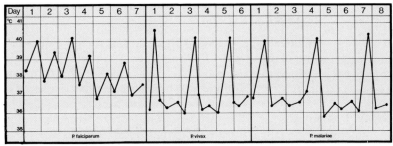

1.181 The temperature chart in malaria reflects the typical tertian and quartan fever patterns. The asexual blood stages of *P. falciparum*, *P. vivax* and *P. ovale* require 48 hours to complete their schizogony. Fever is produced when the schizonts mature, i.e. at 48-hour intervals. This gives the classical tertian periodicity of *P. vivax* and *P. ovale* infection, which is, however, uncommon in a primary attack of *P. falciparum* malaria. *P. malariae* requires 72 hours and is associated with quartan fever, i.e. 72 hours between paroxysms.

1.182 Classical decerebrate rigidity in a Thai woman with cerebral malaria.

1.182

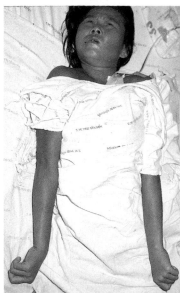

1.183

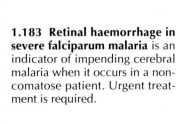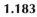

1.183 Retinal haemorrhage in severe falciparum malaria is an indicator of impending cerebral malaria when it occurs in a non-comatose patient. Urgent treatment is required.

1.184

1.184 'Blackwater' (B) compared with normal urine (A). Acute haemolytic crises resulting in haemoglobinuria occur in severe attacks of falciparum malaria (blackwater fever).

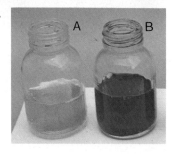

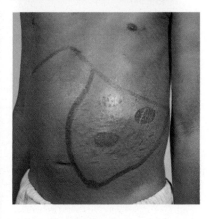

1.185 Tropical splenomegaly syndrome (TSS) is associated with chronic malaria infection and is thought to result from an abnormal immunological response. Note the outline of the massive spleen. The scars result from the local application of traditional healing techniques.

1.186

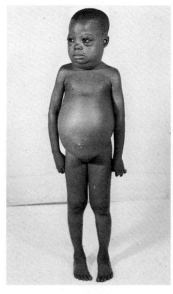

1.186 Nephrotic syndrome in a child with *P. malariae* infection. Note the gross facial and neck oedema and ascites.

1.187

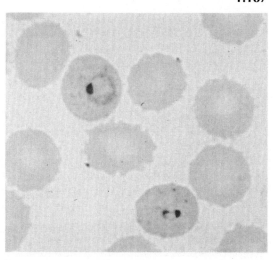

1.187 Blood film in *P. malariae* infection, showing ring form trophozoites in red cells. All blood stages in the life cycle of the parasite may be seen in films taken at different times, and blood film examination remains the cornerstone of diagnosis.

69

Leishmaniasis

This is a tropical disorder caused by infection with protozoa of the genus *Leishmania* which are transmitted to man from other humans or animals by the bite of the sandfly. The protozoa may cause either visceral or cutaneous infection.

In the visceral form, the organism (*L. donovani*) multiplies in macrophages. After an incubation period of 2–6 months there is extensive reticulo-endothelial proliferation (Kala-azar, literally 'black sickness', so called because deepening pigmentation of the skin is commonly seen). Clinically these patients present with recurrent fever, lymphadenopathy, firm, non-tender, massive splenomegaly (**1.188**) and bone marrow suppression. Leucopaenia with a relative lymphocytosis is often present. In light-skinned patients there may be hyperpigmentation of the skin, especially on the hands, feet and abdomen. The death rate in untreated patients is high from intercurrent infections, marrow suppression or bleeding. Antimony salts are still the treatment of choice. Following successful treatment of visceral leishmaniasis dermal lesions may reappear (post Kala-azar dermal leishmaniasis, PKDL, **1.189**).

The various cutaneous forms of leishmaniasis present with single or multiple chronic skin ulcers (**1.190**), and, with some species, chronic mucocutaneous lesions. They are sub-divided into 'Old World' and 'New World' cutaneous leishmaniasis and are known by a wide range of local names in different countries. Transmission occurs via sandflies or directly by contact with open lesions. The diagnosis is made by finding parasites in smears of skin adjacent to the sores or by a positive leishmanin skin test. Treatment of these local lesions is often unsatisfactory, but they may respond to direct heating to 40°C, to antimony salts or to levamisole.

1.188

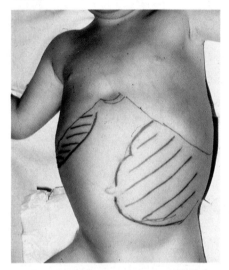

1.188 Massive splenomegaly in an 18-month-old boy with visceral leishmaniasis. For other causes of splenomegaly *see* **Table 10.6.**

1.189 Post Kala-azar dermal leishmaniasis (PKDL) in a patient who had been treated for visceral leishmaniasis two years earlier. The patient was completly cured by further chemotherapy.

1.189

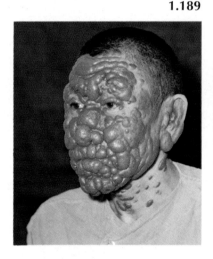

1.190

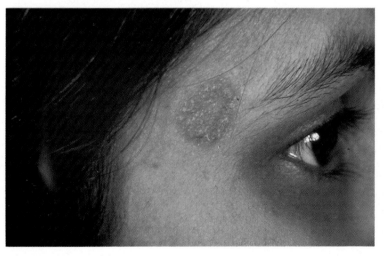

1.190 Cutaneous leishmaniasis. This lesion on the face of a woman from Western India resulted from infection with *Leishmania tropica*. This parasite often produces dry, single lesions, which represent a granulomatous response to the initial infection. The lesions may heal spontaneously, and may sometimes be treated by cryotherapy, but systemic therapy with antimony salts is often required for definitive treatment.

Trypanosomiasis

There are two major types of trypanosome infection, African trypanosomiasis, including sleeping sickness, and American Chagas' disease.

African trypanosomiasis is caused by subspecies of *T. brucei* and the natural vector is the tsetse fly. About 8–12 days after a bite by an infected tsetse fly, a trypanosomal chancre may develop at the site (**1.191**). After a period, which may vary from months to years, a systemic reaction occurs, associated with fever and lymphadenopathy (**1.192**). After an indeterminate time, the infection involves the central nervous system starting with mild behavioural changes and rapidly progressing to coma and death (**1.193**).

American trypanosomiasis (Chagas' disease) is a result of infection by *T. cruzi* and is found in Central and South America. The disease is transmitted by the faeces of blood-sucking triatomid bugs. In the acute infection, there may be a mild pyrexia and skin rash with patients occasionally developing myocarditis. The initial local skin lesion is the chagoma which is painful and swollen (**1.194**). Most patients present with chronic disease many years after the infection. The common presentations are chronic cardiomyopathy (**1.195**), and dilatation of the oesophagus (*see* p. 362) or colon. The disease may be diagnosed on blood or lymph node films, by animal culture or by serology.

1.191

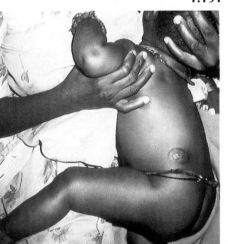

1.191 African trypanosomiasis—the trypanosomal 'chancre'. The lesion marks the site at which the tsetse fly inoculated the patient with the trypanosome. Chancres are rare in indigenous patients, but common in visitors.

1.192

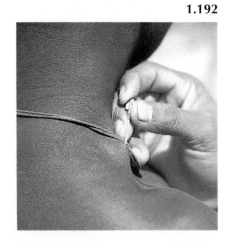

1.192 Puncture of an enlarged supraclavicular lymph node and examination of the aspirate is a valuable aid to diagnosis in African trypanosomiasis, especially in the Gambian form of the disease.

1.193

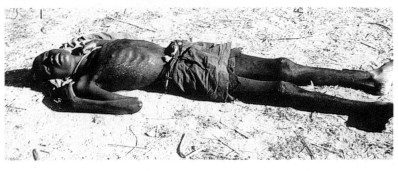

1.193 Sleeping sickness. In the Gambian form of the disease, the patient becomes more wasted and comatose, finally showing the classical picture of sleeping sickness as the CNS becomes involved. In the 'Rhodesian' form of the disease, the CNS features are usually less marked and the disease more acute.

1.194

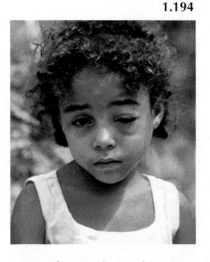

1.194 'Chagoma' in American trypanosomiasis. In this case, the inoculation occurred within the conjunctival sac, and the chagoma has caused marked local oedema with lid swelling and chemosis. This is a common site of inoculation, and this unilateral appearance is termed Romana's sign.

1.195

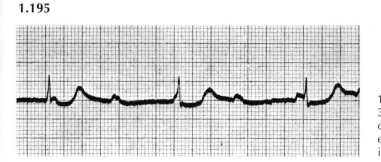

1.195 ECG in Chagas' disease, showing complete heart block (grade 3). There is no discernible relationship between P waves and QRS complexes, and the atria and ventricles are beating independently of each other. Dysrhythmias of various types and degrees are common in Chagas' disease, and death may result from Stokes–Adams attacks.

Worm infections

Class of helminth	Important human pathogen	Human disease	Page reference
Nematodes	Wuchereria bancrofti Brugia malayi Brugia timori	Filariasis—fever, lymphadenopathy, elephantiasis	72
	Loa loa	Loiasis—skin nodules (Calabar swellings) endomyocardial fibrosis	73, 246
	Onchocerca volvulus	River blindness, skin nodules	74
	Dracunculus medinensis	Dracunculosis	75
	Toxocara canis, T. cati	Visceral larva migrans—retinitis, pneumonitis, hepatitis	75
	Trichinella spiralis	Trichinosis—fever, periorbital oedema, myalgia	76
	Enterobius vermicularis	Perianal itch, granulomas of bowel	380
	Ascaris lumbricoides	Pneumonitis, allergy, asthma, intestinal obstruction, obstructive jaundice, appendicitis	380
	Trichuris trichiura	Abdominal pain and diarrhoea, prolapse of rectum	380
	Ancylostoma duodenale and Necator americanus	Diarrhoea, iron deficiency anaemia	380, 424
	Strongyloides stercoralis	Pneumonitis, asthma, encephalitis ,myocarditis (invasive in immunocompromised)	380
Trematodes	Schistosoma mansoni	Bilharziasis (Schistosomiasis)	77
	S. haematobium S. japonicum	Intestinal and urinary tract infection	77
	Paragonimus westermani	Lung cysts, haemoptysis, cerebral involvement	78
	Fasciolopsis buski	Abdominal pain and diarrhoea, allergy	381
	Fasciola hepatica	Hepatitis, obstructive jaundice	381
	Opisthorchis sinensis	Hepatitis, obstructive jaundice	381
Cestode	Echinococcus granulosus	Hydatid disease—liver, lungs, bone	78, 381
	Echinococcus multilocularis	Liver cysts	78
	Dipylidium caninum	Abdominal discomfort, pruritus ani	79
	Taenia solium, T. saginata	Usually asymptomatic. Diarrhoea occasionally. Subcutaneous nodules, Cysticerosis	381
	Diphyllobothrium latum	Usually asymptomatic. Vitamin B_{12} deficiency anaemia (rare)	

Lymphatic filariasis

The infecting nematodes, *Wuchereria bancrofti*, *Brugia malayi* and *Brugia timori* are found in the tropics worldwide and produce disease in man by lymphatic obstruction. Mosquitoes of the species *Culex*, *Anopheles* and *Aedes* transmit the larvae of *W. bancrofti*, and *Mansonia* and *Anopheles* mosquitoes transmit *B. malayi* and *B. timori*. The larvae then enter the regional lymphatics and mature. They may live in this situation for many years.

Within three months of infection, there is intermittent fever and sweats with photophobia, myalgia and lymphangitis in most areas of the body. Localised areas of swelling follow, e.g. leg oedema (**1.196**), ascites, hydrocele, pleural effusion. Local abscess formation and chronic sinuses may form. Massive chronic oedema of the legs produces elephantiasis (**1.197**). The diagnosis is made by demonstration of the parasite in blood films (**1.198**). Treatment is with diethylcarbamazine.

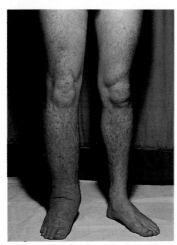

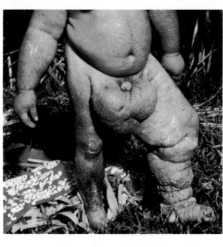

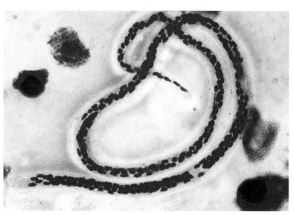

1.198 Lymphatic filariasis can be diagnosed by demonstrating the parasite (in this case *W. bancrofti*) in a blood film.

1.196 Chronic lymphatic oedema in the right leg as a result of long-standing lymphatic filariasis. The patient was a seaman who had been working in the Far East coastal trade for 15 years.

1.197 Gross elephantiasis of the leg and scrotum caused by *W. bancrofti* in a patient in Tahiti. Elephantiasis on this scale may cause incapacitating deformity and radical surgery may be required to remove surplus tissue.

Loiasis

This is filarial infection with *Loa loa* and is found in Western Central Africa. The disease is transmitted by the bite of tabanid flies of the genus *Chrysops* which live in tropical rain forests (*C. dimidiata* and *C. silacea*). Larve enter the human skin, where they mature. The adult females migrate continuously throughout the subcutaneous tissues and may pass in front of the eyes, under the conjunctivae, where they produce severe discomfort (**1.199**).

The intense subcutaneous inflammatory reaction involved in the passage of the adult worms produces skin nodules (Calabar swellings, **1.200**). In the heart, the microfilariae may cause endomyocardial fibrosis. The diagnosis may be confirmed by finding sheathed microfilariae in biopsy samples of the swellings. The migrating worms may be removed under local anaesthesia (**1.201**). Treatment is with diethylcarbamazine.

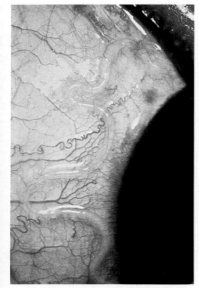

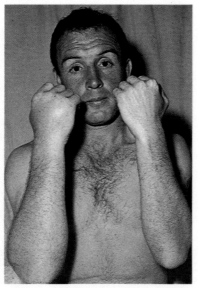

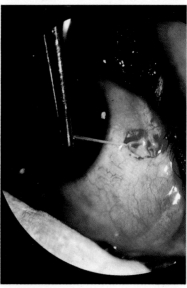

1.199 Adult *Loa loa* in the eye. The movement of the adult worm under the conjunctiva causes congestion and considerable irritation.

1.200 Calabar swelling in the right hand and arm caused by loiasis. recurrent large swellings lasting about 3 days are characteristic and are most frequently seen in the hand, wrists and forearm. They indicate the tracks of the migrating adults in the connective tissue. A marked eosinophilia (60–90%) accompanies this phase of the infection.

1.201 Extraction of *Loa loa* worm from the eye. The adult worm can be extracted with fine forceps after anaesthetising the conjunctiva.

Onchocerciasis

This is a variety of cutaneous filariasis caused by infection by the tissue-dwelling *Onchocerca volvulus*. It is found predominantly in Africa (where it is known as 'river blindness'), Yemen and South America. Larvae enter the skin following the bite of the blackfly vector of the genus *Simulium*. The larvae then migrate to the subcutaneous tissues where they mature into adults. The adult worms may then live for 10–15 years. Larvae develop from the female worms to form unsheathed microfilariae which migrate in the subcutaneous tissues and the eye. The major symptoms result from a hypersensitivity reaction to dead microfilariae. In the skin, this produces nodules which, if very large, may give an appearance called 'hanging groins' (**1.202**).

The eye lesions can be catastrophic for affected populations. They include keratitis (**1.203**) and choroiditis with eventual optic atrophy and blindness (**1.204**). The diagnosis is made by demonstrating motile microfilariae in a skin biopsy preparation (skin snip). Removal of the adult worms in the nodules by nodulectomy prevents the continued production of microfilariae. Suramin is of value in reduction of the adult worm load.

1.202

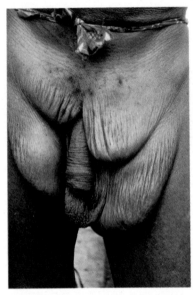

1.202 'Hanging groins' in onchocerciasis are caused by the involvement of the inguinocrural lymph nodes in a hypersensitivity reaction to dead microfilarian worms.

1.203

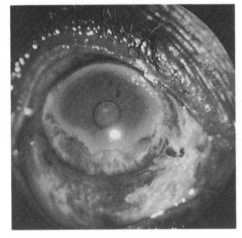

1.203 Severe keratitis in a patient with onchocerciasis.

1.204

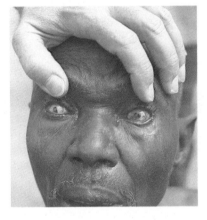

1.204 Keratitis causing blindness in onchocerciasis. This patient's disease has advanced further than the stage seen in **1.203**, and the patient is now completely blind.

Dracunculosis

Dracunculus medinensis (Guinea worm) is a nematode which migrates within the body tissues. It is widely distributed in Africa and Asia. Man is infected by drinking water containing the microcrustacean *Cyclops,* which is infected with the larval form of *D. medinensis.* The larvae are liberated in the stomach and migrate through the connective tissue planes of the body, a process that can take up to a year. Once fertilised, the female migrates to a limb where she produces a vesicle which ulcerates. This allows the female worm to protrude a loop of her uterus through the ulcerated skin. On contact with water, larvae are released and in fresh water wells the cycle continues. Patients usually present at the painful stage of vesiculation when the worms can be removed mechanically (**1.205**). If the worms die, they may be found in calcified subcutaneous nodules (**1.206**). Public health measures and education of the population are necessary for prevention. Surgery is possible for local lesions and a range of anthelmintics is available.

1.205

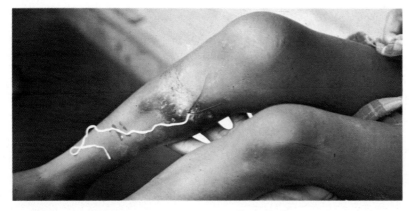

1.206

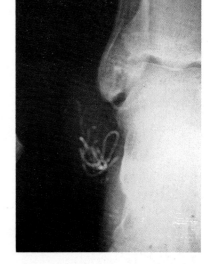

1.205 Dracunculosis in the region of the right knee joint. The infestation can cause arthritis and considerable disability, but the physical removal of some worms may be possible at this stage.

1.206 Dracunculosis. Dead, calcified worms in the region of the ankle joint, where they formed a large, palpable subcutaneous nodule.

Toxocariasis (visceral larva migrans)

The eggs of the ascarid worms, *Toxocara canis* and *T. cati,* are to be found in soil contaminated by dog and cat faeces. Infection occurs when they are accidentally ingested, usually by young children. The eggs hatch in the intestine and migrate in the blood stream to the liver and lungs but do not develop beyond the larval form. Migration of the larval worm (visceral larva migrans) may produce haemorrhage and granuloma formation. Eosinophilia is a common finding and there may also be intermittent fever, cough, asthmatic attacks, dermatitis, occasionally hepatosplenomegaly and retinitis (**1.207**). Usually, the acute attack remains undiagnosed and the healed lesions may be found coincidentally in the eye where they must be differentiated from neoplasms. The diagnosis can be confirmed serologically. Prevention is possible if pet owners de-worm their animals regularly and stop the fouling of children's play areas. Occasionally, treatment is necessary and the drug of choice is diethylcarbamazine.

1.207

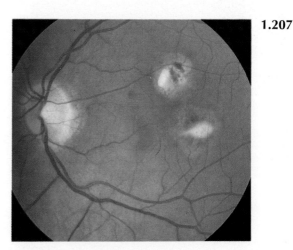

1.207 Toxocariasis. End-stage scarring of the retina in a child with otherwise subclinical toxocara infection. Sometimes the retinal appearances may suggest a melanoma or other tumour, and the eye may even be enucleated in error.

Cutaneous larva migrans

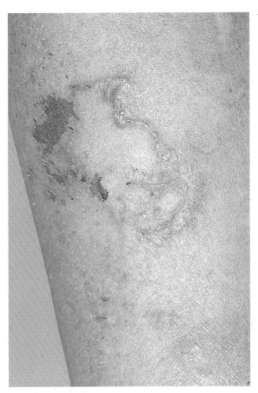

1.208

This condition is also known as 'ground itch' or 'creeping eruption' and is the result of intact skin penetration by the larvae of a range of hookworms whose normal host is non-human, e.g. *Ancylostoma braziliense, A. caninum, A. duodenale, Necator americanus* and *Strongyloides stercoralis* (*see also* p.381). The larvae cannot develop further in man, but migrate in the subcutaneous tissues where they provoke a severe erythematous and vesicular reaction, with pruritus at the point of entry (**1.208**). These lesions are often complicated by a secondary bacterial infection. The feet and lower limbs are often involved and the condition is most common in children. The diagnosis is confirmed by finding larvae in biopsy material.

1.208 Cutaneous larva migrans. The skin lesion was erythematous and itchy, and the patient had a marked eosinophilia.

Trichinosis

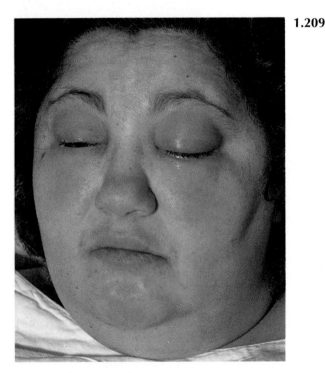

1.209

This is a worldwide disease of man which results from the ingestion of pig, bear or wolf meat containing the encysted larvae of *Trichinella spiralis*. The larvae develop into adults in the small intestine and penetrate the wall to enter the blood stream where they move to all body tissues, especially muscle and brain. Migrating larvae are associated with eosinophilia, fever, diarrhoea, myalgia and periorbital oedema (**1.209**). In severe infection, there may be evidence of meningoencephalitis, psychiatric syndromes, myocarditis and pneumonia. The disease may be suspected on clinical grounds, as it may occur as a localised outbreak, and the larvae can be found in muscle biopsies. Serology is also valuable. Thiabendazole is of value in the intestinal phase and systemic steroids may be required in severe encephalitis or myocarditis. Education in the need for thorough cooking of meat products, is important in prevention and the deep freezing of pork has significantly reduced transmission.

1.209 Gross periorbital and facial oedema are a common feature in trichinosis and are usually associated with malaise and eosinophilia.

Schistosomiasis (Bilharzia)

This is an infection with a worldwide distribution caused by three types of blood flukes of the genus *Schistosoma*—*S. mansoni*, *S. haematobium* and *S. japonicum*. Humans are infected by the cercarial stage of the parasites, released from fresh water snails, in ponds, canals, lake edges and streams. Penetration of intact skin occurs rapidly and the schistosomes migrate into the portal system to mate and then to a part of the venous system to lay eggs. *S. haematobium* is found in the bladder and pelvic organs, whereas the others are usually found in the rectal venous plexus. Eggs laid in these venous plexuses are shed into bladder or rectum and returned to the local water supply to complete the cycle through the snail population. Cercarial penetration of the skin may produce an itchy papular eruption (**1.210**) and this may be followed by myalgia, headache and abdominal pain.

In *S. mansoni* and *S. japonicum* infection, the late manifestations of the disease include abdominal pain, diarrhoea, malabsorption and, occasionally, intestinal obstruction and rectal prolapse. Cirrhosis of the liver is also frequently found with associated portal hypertension, splenomegaly (**1.211**) and oesophageal varices (**1.212**). In *S. haematobium* infection the major signs are in the urinary tract, with recurrent haematuria (**1.213**) and eventually bladder calcification, obstructive uropathy (**1.214**) and renal failure. Migration of eggs to the lungs may cause massive chronic fibrosis.

Diagnosis is by detection of the characteristic ova in the stools, urine or rectal biopsy (**1.215**) or with an ELIZA test. Public health measures may inhibit the cycle of the parasite. Treatment of the patients is with praziquantel given as a once-daily dose, depending on the patient's weight.

1.210

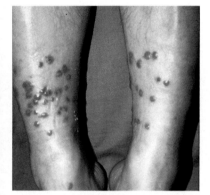

1.211

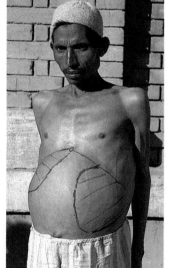

1.212

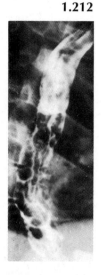

1.211 Schistosomiasis causing massive hepatosplenomegaly. The greatly enlarged spleen is accompanied by an enlarged, irregularly fibrosed liver. The appearance is typical of infection with *S. mansoni*.

1.212 Oesophageal varices are a common accompaniment of portal hypertension (*see* p. 394). Massive varices, like those outlined on this barium swallow, occur commonly in advanced schistosomiasis caused by *S. mansoni* and *S. japonicum;* they may lead to death from haematemesis.

1.210 Dermatitis resulting from the penetration of the skin by cercariae. In this case, the reaction is to avian schistosomes, which are otherwise non-pathogenic to man, but a similar, though often less marked, reaction may occur to the invasion of pathogenic schistosomes.

1.213

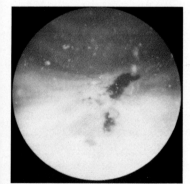

1.214

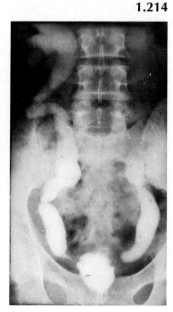

1.215

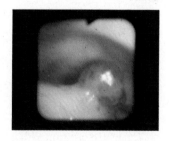

1.214 Intravenous urogram (IVU) in advanced *S. haematobium* infection, showing a severely contracted and irregular bladder, associated with severe constriction of the lower end of both ureters, and gross dilatation and tortuosity of the rest of the ureters with bilateral hydronephrosis.

1.213 Chronic deep ulceration of the bladder, seen through a cystoscope in a patient with *S. haematobium* infection. Note the bilharzial tubercles at the top of the picture, and the 'ground glass' appearance of the mucosa below.

1.215 A schistosomal polyp in the descending colon, as seen through a colonoscope. Biopsy provided diagnostic information. It is not necessary to find a polyp to achieve the diagnosis; however, 'blind' biopsy of the rectum through a proctoscope will often yield positive results.

Paragonimiasis

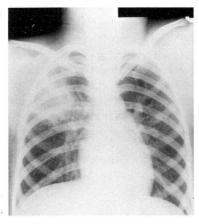

1.216 Paragonimiasis. A necrotic area is seen in the right lung field. The symptoms and signs of paragonimiasis in the lungs are often confused with those of tuberculosis.

Infection in man occurs from eating uncooked freshwater crabs and crayfish, which harbour the metacercarial form of *Paragonimus westermani* (lung fluke). The disease is found worldwide, but especially in South East Asia. The larval worm hatches in the human stomach and migrates through the gastric wall into the peritoneal cavity, and through the diaphragm into the pleural cavity and lung. The mature adult worms produce local necrosis in the lungs (**1.216**) and the patient presents with haemoptysis, cough and fever. Cavitation with massive haemoptysis, pneumonia, pleurisy and empyema are also found. Healing takes place, with eventual pulmonary fibrosis. The liver and brain may also be infected. The diagnosis can be made from sputum and faecal examination. Eosinophilia is common and should trigger a search for ova. Radiography of the chest may show infiltration, cyst formation, effusion and empyema. Public health measures include proper sanitation, and education about adequate cooking of shellfish. Drug treatment is with praziquantel or bithionol.

Hydatid disease

Human infection with *Echinococcus granulosus* is found worldwide, especially in countries with a large sheep industry. Accidental ingestion of the eggs results from contamination of food with canine faeces (usually dog). Hatching of the eggs in the intestine produces a six-hooked oncosphere which migrates through the intestinal wall and is carried to all body tissues by the circulation, especially to the liver, lungs, central nervous system and bone, where cyst formation occurs. In man that is the end of the cycle, but if the eggs were ingested by a herbivore (sheep, cattle, pig, deer) which was subsequently eaten by a canine the cysts would form adult tapeworms in the canine intestine and new egg production would be initiated.

In man, the cysts may grow to a large size and produce daughter cysts and pressure on surrounding tissues. The clinical presentation depends on the organ(s) most affected.

Cysts are contained by a definite membrane. The fluid it contains, if liberated into the body cavities, may produce anaphylactic shock and death, and it will lead to dissemination of tapeworm heads (protoscolices) which then form further cysts.

Over the course of time, cysts may become calcified.

Cysts are demonstrated by conventional X-rays (**1.217**), ultrasound and CT scanning (**1.218**). Serological diagnosis is also helpful and may be used as a screening test.

Surgery may be required to remove cysts which are causing pressure symptoms. The fluid must be aspirated and the cyst cavity filled with formalin to kill the potentially infective protoscolices and to detoxify the residual fluid. The cyst lining should then be marsupialised. Public health measures involve public education in endemic areas about transmission, personal hygiene and the prevention of feeding offal to dogs.

A more serious disease is caused by *E. multilocularis* which is found in foxes, wolves, farm dogs and cats. Man is infected in a similar fashion and the oncospheres migrate to lung, liver and brain. The developing cyst is not covered by a membrane and tends to grow progressively in size. It may be mistaken for a cancer and may embolise to other tissues. It has an untreated mortality of about 80%.

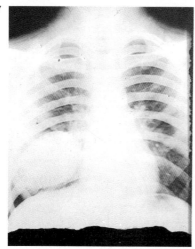

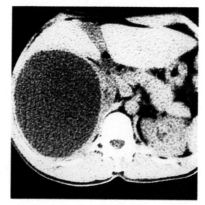

1.218 Massive hydatid cyst (*Echinococcus granulosus*) in the liver of a 14-year-old Kuwaiti boy, demonstrated by CT scanning.

1.217 Hydatid cyst in the right lung.

Dipylidiasis

This is a small tapeworm of dogs and cats (*Dipylidium caninum*), which has a normal cycle involving development of larval worms in fleas. Larvae are passed to children by the dog licking the child's face and lips. Symptoms include abdominal discomfort and anal irritation caused by active migration of the motile proglottid. The diagnosis is made by finding the distinctive eggs or proglottids in the faeces. Treatment is with niclosamide or praziquantel. Prevention involves deworming dogs, treating their fleas and not allowing them to lick young children.

Sparganosis

Infection in man is acquired by drinking water or eating raw frog or snake contaminated by copepods (crustacea) which carry a larval tapeworm (*Diphyllobothrium mansoni*). Migration of the larvae to the skin, eyes and other tissues produces an acute inflammatory reaction; e.g. in the eye, severe periorbital oedema may be found. The adult worm may be removed from its subcutaneous or conjunctival site (**1.219**). Education and public health measures are important.

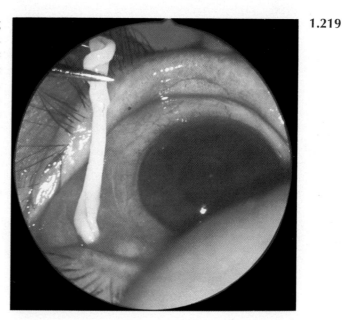

1.219 Sparganosis: removal of a mature larva from the conjunctival site to which it has migrated.

Sexually transmitted diseases

Agent	Relevant human disease	Page reference
Viruses		
Human immune deficiency virus (HIV 1 and 2)	Acquired immune deficiency syndrome (AIDS)	16
Papillomavirus	Ano-genital warts	81
Hepatitis B virus	Liver disease	398
Hepatitis C virus		
Herpes simplex virus	Cold sore, genital infection, carcinoma of the cervix	28
Bacteria		
Neisseria gonorrhoeae	Urethritis, vaginitis, cervicitis, proctitis, etc.	81
Haemophilus ducreyi	Chancroid	82
Calymmatobacterium	Granuloma inguinale	83
Treponema pallidum	Syphilis	83
Chlamydia trachomatis	Lymphogranuloma venereum	86
	Non-specific urethritis	86
	Reiter's syndrome	135
Mycoplasma hominis	Non-specific urethritis	86
Ureaplasma urealyticum		
Fungi		
Candida albicans	Vaginal discharge, balanitis	65
Protozoa		
Entamoeba histolytica	Balanitis	66
Trichomonas vaginalis	Vaginal discharge, balanitis	86
Ectoparasites		
Crab lice/pubic lice	Infestation	101

A large number of infectious diseases can be sexually transmitted, but some can also be transmitted by other routes. For example, HIV infection and hepatitis B can be transmitted by needle-sharing among drug abusers and in therapeutic blood products. Syphilis can be transmitted by unscreened blood transfusion; it is closely related to non-sexually transmitted endemic treponemal diseases (bejel, yaws and pinta—*see* p. 56–57).

In this section we cover most of those diseases which are predominantly or exclusively sexually transmitted (the STDs). HIV infection is covered on p. 16 and hepatitis B on p. 398.

Genital warts

Genital warts are sexually transmitted and are caused by DNA viruses, the human papillomaviruses (*see also* p. 98). They affect the genitalia and the perianal region and are found most commonly in men on the corona and frenum of the penis (**1.220**), and in women on the labial folds of the vulva (**1.221**), the lower third of the vagina and on the cervix. The time from sexual contact to the appearance of the lesion is about 2–3 months. The warts are usually multiple and they often grow together and spread to involve the whole perineum and anal region (condylomata acuminata—**8.8**). The rate of spread is increased in patients who are immunocompromised.

Infection with human papillomavirus is probably a causative factor in cervical neoplasia. It is strongly associated with premalignant changes in the cervical epithelium, which may progress to invasive carcinoma of the cervix. Similar epithelial changes may occur on the penis, vulva and anus, though their significance is less clear.

Spontaneous healing of warts may take place and this can sometimes be accelerated with topical applications.

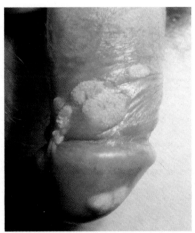

1.220

1.220 Plane warts of the prepuce and glans penis. Genital warts vary greatly in appearance. They may be sessile, filiform or hyperplastic.

1.221 Florid labial, perineal and perianal warts. Associated cervical lesions may put this patient at increased risk of carcinoma of the cervix.

1.221

Gonorrhoea

Gonorrhoea is caused by *Neisseria gonorrhoeae* (the 'gonococcus') and the disease is transmitted by sexual contact. Neonatal infection may also occur, during passage of the infant through the birth canal.

The incubation period is less than one week. In males there is purulent urethral discharge (**1.222**) and dysuria, sometimes with associated epididymitis and inflammation of regional lymph nodes. Proctitis occurs in homosexual males (**1.223**). Many females are asymptomatic, but there may be dysuria and vaginal discharge if there is cervicitis (**1.224**). Infection may spread to Bartholin's glands, the uterus, the fallopian tubes and the pelvic peritoneum, where it is one cause of chronic pelvic inflammatory disease (PID). Bloodspread may occur causing fever, skin rash and painful arthritis (**3.8**). Lesions may be seen in the mouth and pharynx following oral sex. Infants infected during birth usually develop ophthalmia neonatorum (**1.225**).

The diagnosis is by microscopy and culture of pus from the urethra, cervix, rectum, mouth or, in the case of neonates, the conjunctivae.

Single-dose therapy with procaine penicillin or amoxycillin, each given with probenecid, is usually effective. Longer treatment may be required if there is spread of infection. If the organisms are resistant to penicillin, alternative drugs include spectinomycin, the cephalosporins and ciprofloxacin. Tracing and treatment of contacts is important to prevent spread of infection.

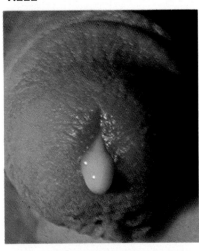

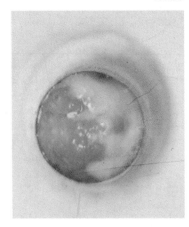

1.222 Gonorrhoea. The typical purulent urethral discharge can often be demonstrated during examination by 'milking' the urethra. The patient also has associated meatitis.

1.223 Gonococcal proctitis as seen through a proctoscope. Note the erythematous mucosa and the profuse purulent exudate.

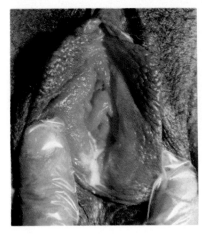

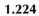

1.224 Gonorrhoea in a symptomatic woman. Note the purulent discharge, which usually indicates the presence of cervicitis.

1.225 Ophthalmia neonatorum. Purulent conjunctivitis follows 2–5 days after birth in the infected infant, and may be associated with septicaemia.

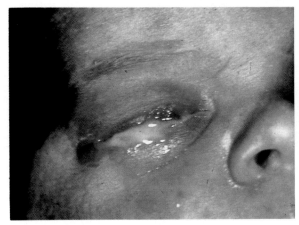

Chancroid

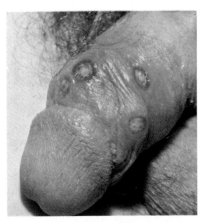

1.226

1.226 Chancroid of the prepuce, showing typical multiple ulcerating lesions.

This STD is characterised by painful genital ulceration followed by tender inguinal lymphadenopathy. The organism responsible is *Haemophilus ducreyi,* a Gram-negative bacterium with a worldwide distribution (though infection in developed countries is now rare). It is most common in men, but this suggests significant underdiagnosis in women. The incubation period is usually 2–5 days. The first lesion is a tender, painful macule which becomes pustular and, on bursting forms a painful ulcer which has a necrotic grey membrane. Lesions are usually found on the glans or shaft of the penis (**1.226**) or around the anus. In women, they may appear on the cervix, vagina, vulva or perianal region. They may also be found occasionally on other skin surfaces and in the mouth. Regional lymphadenopathy (buboes) is invariable and may occasionally suppurate and leave chronic fistulae.

The diagnosis can be made in most cases by microscopy of exudate or pus; treatment is with co-trimoxazole or tetracycline. Sexual partners should be identified and screened if possible.

Granuloma inguinale

This is an infectious diease resulting from *Calymmatobacterium granulomatis,* a Gram-negative bacterium. It is usually transmitted sexually and is found predominantly in the Far East but some cases have been reported in homosexuals in the USA and Europe. The clinical signs develop 1–10 weeks after exposure. An indurated papule usually forms on the penis, labia or anal margin but extragenital lesions are common on the face, lips and neck.

These primary lesions may be tender and produce a foul-smelling discharge. Regional lymphadenopathy is usual (**1.227**) and suppuration and secondary infection are common. Extensive scarring may be found in the healing phase (**1.228**). Diagnosis is by finding the typical 'Donovan' bodies in Gram-stained exudate. Exclusion of the other venereal infections is essential.

1.227

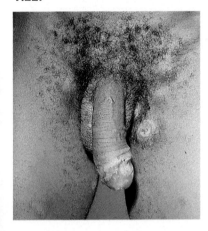

1.228

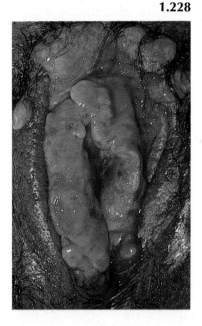

1.227 Granuloma inguinale, showing a typical ulcer on the inner thigh. The ulcerated lesion is deep and its floor is covered by a thick, offensive, purulent exudate. Bilateral inguinal lymphadenopathy is present.

1.228 Granuloma inguinale of the vulva. The disease often runs a chronic course and is associated with mutilating ulceration, chronic swelling and ultimately extensive scarring.

Syphilis

This is a sexually transmitted disease characterised by an initial illness followed by a long latent period before late manifestations of the disease appear. The causative organism is the spirochaete, *Treponema pallidum.* Congenital syphilis results from transplacental infection of the fetus.

Three stages of the disease are recognised:

- **Primary stage.** After an incubation period of about 3 weeks, a painless ulcerated lesion (chancre) develops at the site of inoculation. In the male, the lesion is usually on the penis (**1.229**) or anus (in homosexuals). In females the lesion may be on the vulva (**1.230**), but if it is in the vagina or on the cervix it may be missed. Chancres are highly infective, but are self-limiting and heal in about 4–6 weeks.
- **Secondary stage.** This represents systemic spread of infection and follows about 2 months after the primary lesion. Features of this stage include fever, widespread macular rash (**1.231**), wart-like lesions (condylomata lata) in the genital area (**1.232**), snail-track ulcers on the buccal mucosa (**1.233**), generalised lymphadenopathy and occasionally aseptic meningitis. This stage is also self-limiting and is followed by a latent period of from 2–20 years, before symptoms of the tertiary stage appear.
- **Tertiary stage.** Features of this stage include the development of chronic granulomatous lesions (gummata) in skin (**1.234**), mucosa and bone, vascular lesions (aortic aneurysm—**1.235**) and lesions of the central nervous sytem (meningo-vascular syphilis (**11.8**), general paralysis of the insane, tabes dorsalis) which may also lead to destructive joint disease (**1.236, 1.237**). Adequate therapy in the early stages of syphilis should prevent the tertiary stage developing.
- **Congenital syphilis** may result in abortion or stillbirth. Infants may be severely affected at birth or may appear normal and develop manifestations of disease in later childhood (**1.238, 1.239**).

The diagnosis is confirmed by finding spirochaetes in the primary lesion or in exudates during the secondary stage. Serological tests include non-specific antigen tests (e.g. VDRL) or specific antitreponemal tests (TPI, TPHA, FTA). CSF examination should be carried out if neurosyphilis is suspected.

Penicillin is the drug of choice. Treatment usually involves a 14-day course of long-acting penicillin given parenterally. Steroid cover should be used in the first few days of therapy to prevent a Jarisch–Herxheimer reaction (caused by toxins released by the dying spirochaetes). Alternative drugs for patients with penicillin allergy include erythromycin and tetracycline.

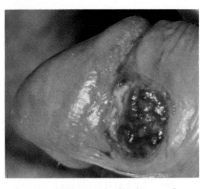

1.229 Syphilis—typical primary chancre in the coronal sulcus. A small red macule enlarges and develops through a papular stage, becoming eroded to form a typical round, painless ulcer. If untreated, the ulcer usually heals after 4–8 weeks.

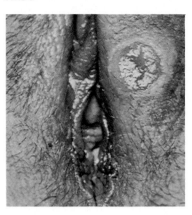

1.230 Syphilis—typical chancre of the labium majus.

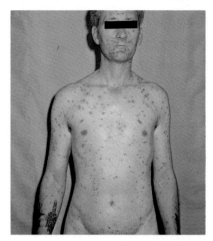

1.231 Secondary syphilis. This patient has a very typical papulosquamous rash (syphilide). Note the facial lesions, the colour and the symmetrical distribution of the rash.

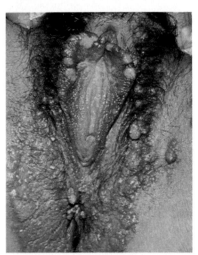

1.232 Secondary syphilis. Gross condylomata lata of the vulva and anus. Note the resemblance to warts (condylomata acuminata).

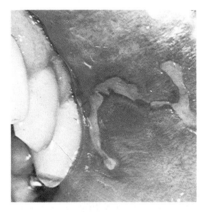

1.233 Secondary syphilis—classic 'snail-track' ulcer of the buccal mucosa. Other mucosal lesions at this stage may be round or oval in shape.

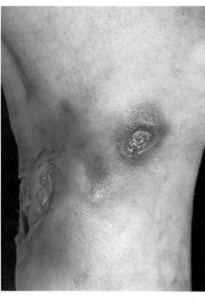

1.234 Tertiary syphilis—gummata of the skin. The lesions start as subcutaneous masses, which increase in size before breaking down to form typical gummatous ulcers. The ulcers are painless, and have sharply defined 'punched out' edges and an indurated base that is occupied at this stage by a slough of necrotic tissue. In contrast to the ulcerating lesions in primary and secondary syphilis, *T. pallidum* organisms cannot be found.

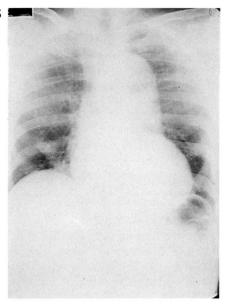

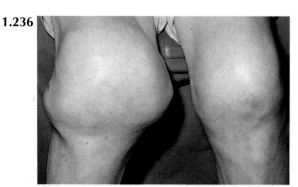

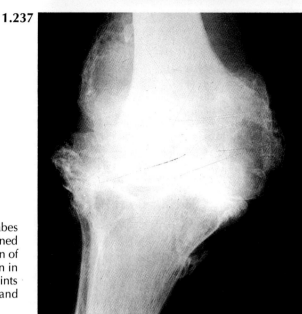

1.235 Tertiary syphilis—a large aortic aneurysm on chest X-ray. The aneurysm results from vasculitis affecting the vasa vasorum of the aorta.

1.236, 1.237 Tertiary syphilis—Charcot joints. In tabes dorsalis, impared pain and position sensation, combined with muscular hypotonia, often lead to the destruction of joints and inappropriate new bone formation, as seen in these clinical and radiological examples. Charcot joints may also occur in patients with diabetes, leprosy and syringomyelia.

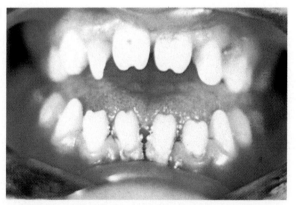

1.238 Congenital syphilis (Hutchinson's teeth). The incisors have a typical appearance with a 'peg' or 'screwdriver' shape and marginal notching.

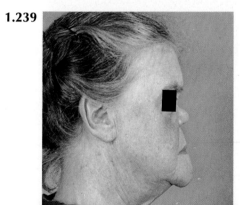

1.239 Congenital syphilis. Treponemal infection of bone leads to epiphysitis, retardation of bone formation and separation of the epiphyses, with resulting interference with growth. In the nasal bones, the infection results in destruction of the nasal septum and the classic 'saddle nose', giving the characteristic facies of congenital syphilis.

Lymphogranuloma venereum

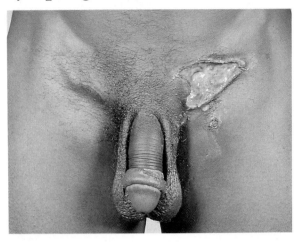

1.240

1.240 Lymphogranuloma venereum showing superficial penile and scrotal ulceration, enlarged lymph nodes (buboes) in the right inguinal region, and an ulcerated inguinal bubo in the left groin.

This is a sexually transmitted disease caused by a strain of *Chlamydia trachomatis* which is found in many tropical countries. The primary lesion appears, within a few days of sexual contact, on the genitalia, in the anus or in the mouth as a small indurated papule, and heals rapidly without leaving a scar. Lymph node enlargement develops in 2–8 weeks and the nodes undergo suppuration and may discharge though the skin (**1.240**). There may be systemic upset with fever, arthralgia, splenomegaly, generalised lymphadenopathy and meningism. Healing may be associated with extensive scarring and local oedema resulting from lymphatic obstruction; strictures of the vagina, urethra or rectum may form.

The diagnosis is made by finding the organism in the local lesions or by serology. Treatment is with tetracycline, and suppurating lymph nodes should be aspirated via normal skin to prevent fistulae forming.

Non-specific urethritis (NSU)

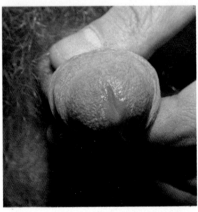

1.241

1.241 Typical non-specific urethritis, with mucopurulent discharge. Although the discharge is often more watery than that in gonorrhoea (**1.222**), gonorrhoea must always be excluded by Gram stain and culture.

Chlamydia trachomatis is one of the most common causes of sexually transmitted non-specific (or non-gonococcal) urethritis. The incubation period is short (5–10 days) and is usually followed by a urethral (**1.241**) or vaginal discharge and severe dysuria. A variety of complications may occur including cervicitis, salpingitis and urethral stricture.

Mycoplasma hominis and *Ureaplasma urealyticum* are other recognised causes of non-specific urethritis.

Diagnosis is usually made by the finding of a leucocytic urethral exudate and excluding gonorrhoea, as culture may be difficult and serology unreliable.

Treatment is with tetracycline for the patient and sexual partners.

Trichomoniasis

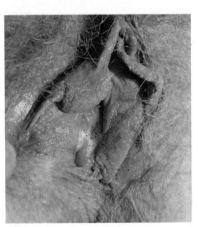

1.242

1.242 Trichomoniasis. Typical vulvovaginitis, with profuse, foul-smelling purulent frothy discharge.

This is a sexually transmitted disease caused by the protozoan *Trichomonas vaginalis*. In the female, it presents as an acute or recurring vaginitis characterised by an extremely irritant, foul-smelling vaginal discharge which is often frothy and yellow (**1.242**). The symptoms may subside, but the patient continues to carry the trichomonads and is infectious to her sexual partners. In the male, the organism may cause recurrent urethritis and prostatitis. The diagnosis is made by the finding of numerous motile organisms in a wet mount of vaginal, prostatic or urethral secretions or a spun sample of urine.

Treatment of all sexual partners with metronidazole is important.

2. Skin Diseases

History and examination

As in most areas of medicine, a careful history and full examination of the dermatological patient is essential. The duration and evolution of a rash, its colour, morphology and distribution will often provide more information than most investigations.

Investigative techniques

Skin biopsy

Histology of a lesion will establish, confirm or refute the clinical diagnosis in most cases. The biopsy should be well planned: early lesions are more informative as secondary infection or excoriation mask underlying changes. A representative lesion should be selected, with attention to local anatomy, healing and potential scar formation. While a punch biopsy is adequate for some conditions, an ellipse of skin, including normal and abnormal skin is preferable (2.1) The size and depth of biopsy depend on the nature of the lesion and on the investigations required. Tissue should be sent fresh for culture or immunofluorescence staining (3.78), or fixed in formalin for routine histology. Special stains, e.g. for fungal elements, should be requested (2.2).

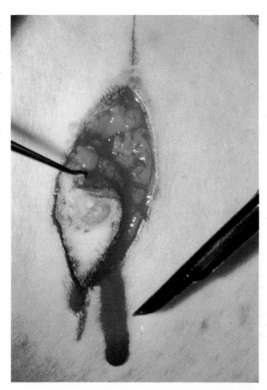

2.1

2.1 Excision biopsy of a lesion on the leg. The ellipse for excision is placed in the direction of the skin-crease line, and a small margin of normal skin is removed with the lesion.

Samples for microbiological investigation

Swabs can be taken from lesions with exudate or pus; blister fluid can be aspirated for culture or microscopy of bacterial or viral lesions. Interpreting results requires some knowledge of commensal organisms and potential pathogens (Table 2.1).

Blood samples may be needed for culture, ASO titres, fluorescent treponema antibody-absorption (FTA-ABS) tests, paired samples for viral titres or serology for other infections such as hepatitis or HIV infection. Fungal elements are found in keratin from nail clippings, hairs and skin scrapings: the skin should be scraped firmly, using a scalpel blade held at 45° to the skin surface. Scrapings are collected in a fold of paper or on microscope slides. Examination under Wood's light may be useful in diagnosis, and in identifying areas from which scrapings or biopsies should be taken (2.3, 2.4).

Direct miscroscopy reveals fungal hyphae and spores (2.2) and culture allows identification of the dermatophyte species. Scabies infestation may be confirmed by looking for adult mites in skin scrapings (2.5).

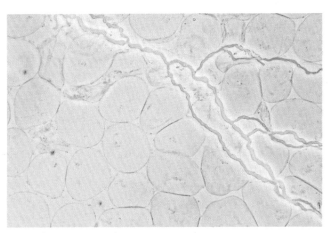

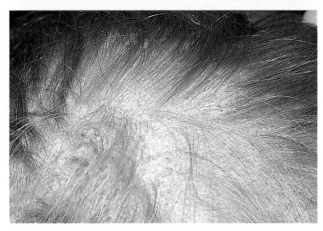

2.2 Fungal hyphae in a skin biopsy. Biopsy was carried out in this case because of diagnostic uncertainty. Often, with superficial lesions, microscopic examination of skin scrapings yields similar results.

2.4

2.3, 2.4 Wood's light is a long-wave ultraviolet light (UVA), which is useful in evaluating a range of skin conditions. In this patient, a superficial fungal infection of the scalp fluoresces blue-green (**2.3**). The appearance of the scalp of the same patient in normal light is shown in **2.4**. The patient has ringworm (*see* p. 100).

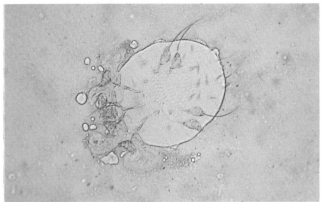

2.5 Scabies mite. The discovery of even a single mite or egg seen microscopically in skin scrapings confirms the diagnosis.

Table 2.1 Skin commensals and common pathogens.

Commensals

Corynebacterium	'Diphtheroids' (Gram-positive rods) aerobic or anaerobic, e.g. *C. acnes*
Micrococcaceae	Gram-positive cocci, e.g. *Staphylococcus albus* (*S. aureus* in 10%)
Gram-negative bacilli	e.g. *Proteus* 5–15%
Pityrosporum ovale	Yeast in sebaceous glands or scalp
Candida	Varying species, including *C. albicans*
Demodex folliculorum hominis	A mite on face or scalp

Pathogens

Corynebacterium	*C. minutissimum* (erythrasma) *C. acnes* (acne vulgaris)
Micrococcaceae	*Staphylococcus aureus*
Streptococci	Beta haemolytic Group A (C, D and G may be pathogens)
Gram-negative bacilli	*Pseudomonas, Klebsiella, E. coli*
Yeasts	*Candida albicans* (opportunistic) *Pityrosporum orbiculare* (pityriasis versicolor)
Fungi	Dermatophytes: *Trichophyton, Epidermophyton* and *Microsporum*

Patch testing

This investigation reproduces a delayed hypersensitivity reaction to suspect allergens applied to the skin surface under a special chamber (**2.6**, **2.7**). After 72 hours, a positive test shows erythema and blistering at the contact site (**2.8**). A vast range of potential allergens exists: choosing the correct 'battery' of test substances depends on the history, nature of the rash and knowledge of potential sensitisers (**Table 2.2**).

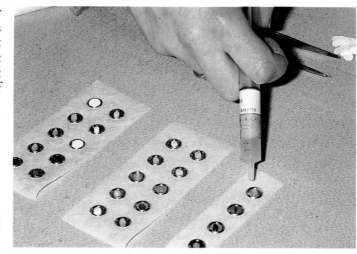

2.6

2.6 Preparation for patch testing. Common sensitisers are dissolved in water or soft paraffin ointment and applied in sequence to special aluminium chambers (Finn chambers).

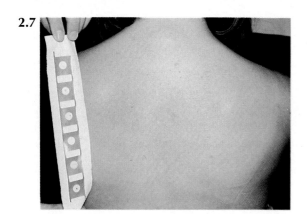

2.7

2.7 Patch testing. The aluminium chambers are mounted on hypo-allergenic tape and applied to the back.

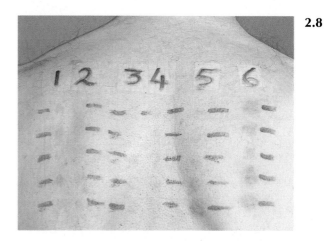

2.8

2.8 Positive patch test results in a gardener who became sensitised to chrysanthemums and other plants and developed contact dermatitis.

Table 2.2 Common causes of contact dermatitis.

Allergen	Component of:
Nickel	Coins, buckles, jewellery
Formaldehyde Ethylene diamine Parabens Wool alcohols Chlorocresol	Preservatives, stabilisers or bases for creams or ointments
Chinoform	Topical antiseptics
Neomycin	Topical antibiotic
Paraphenylenediamine (PPD)	Hair and textile dye
Thiuram mix Mercapto-mix Carba-mix PPD-mix	Rubber additives

Prick tests

Prick tests with allergen extracts result in immediate (type I) skin reactions (**2.9, 2.10**). In atopic dermatitis, frequent false positives occur.

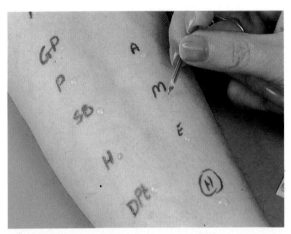

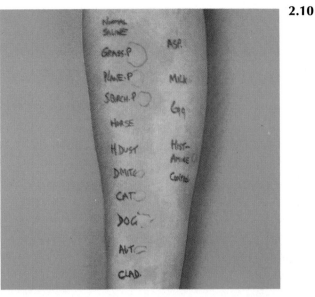

2.9 Skin-prick testing may be useful in urticaria, asthma, rhinitis, allergic conjunctivitis and other allergic conditions, though false positive results are common in atopic eczema. The skin is cleaned, prick sites are marked and a small drop of each allergen solution is placed on the skin. A lance is introduced through the drop to a depth of about 1mm into the skin, and pulled out, raising the skin in the process. The skin should not bleed. The site is blotted dry, and the maximum reaction is assessed after 15–20 minutes.

2.10 A multiple positive prick-test result. This patient had mild chronic eczema, and symptoms of hayfever from April to August, which correlates with the positive reactions to grass, plane and silver birch pollens. He also developed nasal and eye symptoms on contact with cats; but, despite the positive skin test, dogs did not cause obvious symptoms. There was nothing to suggest that *Alternaria* contributed to his rhinitis. The other allergens gave negative results—the flare reactions should be regarded as non-specific, and there was no measurable weal.

IgE and RAST tests

IgE is often but not always raised in atopic dermatitis, but does not reflect severity of rash or response to treatment. Radio-allergo-sorbent tests (RAST) record levels of specific IgE, indicating potential sensitisers such as animal dander or house dust mites.

Other tests

Haematological and biochemical tests are frequently used in both primary skin disorders and dermatological manifestations of systemic disease, and to monitor drug therapy with, for example, methotrexate, retinoids or dapsone.

Immunological investigations including ANA, immune complexes, complement levels or auto-antibodies may be required. Underlying medical or surgical problems should be investigated.

Psoriasis

Psoriasis is a common disorder affecting around 2% of the population. Onset may be at any age, with peaks around 20 and 60 years. Males and females are affected equally. A positive family history is found in 30% of patients: those developing the disease at an earlier age have an increased association with HLA CW6.

Psoriasis is characterised by variability and unpredictability. The rash may be intermittent, undergo spontaneous remission or be lifelong. In general a chronic condition, it may flare acutely and, rarely, be life-threatening. Patients generally feel well but they can experience considerable emotional distress and social isolation. There is an association between psoriasis and high alcohol intake.

The most common presentation is chronic plaque psoriasis, generally affecting extensor surfaces in a symmetrical pattern (2.11, 2.12, 3.46). Lesions are clearly demarcated erythematous plaques covered with coarse scales which may be removed by gentle scraping (2.13).

Flexural involvement (2.14) is also common, but not usually scaly, often leading to misdiagnosis. Perineal lesions may be present. The scalp may be involved alone or with other lesions: psoriasis in the scalp may be 'felt' and seen. The hairline (2.15) and behind the ears are common sites. A resistant plaque in the sacral area is also very common.

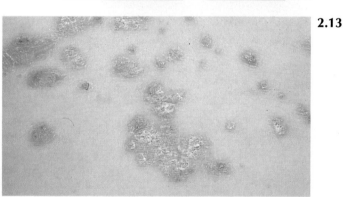

2.11 Psoriasis affecting the extensor surfaces of the arms. Other plaques are visible on the trunk.

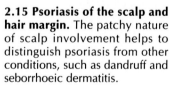

2.12 Psoriasis on the extensor surfaces of the knees and legs in an elderly patient.

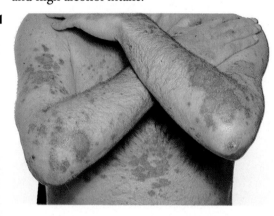

2.13 Psoriasis. Typical small plaques, showing typical silvery scales. These can be removed by gentle scraping with a spatula or fingernail.

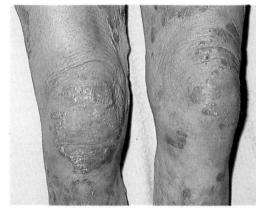

2.15 Psoriasis of the scalp and hair margin. The patchy nature of scalp involvement helps to distinguish psoriasis from other conditions, such as dandruff and seborrhoeic dermatitis.

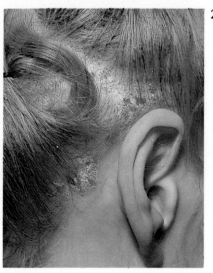

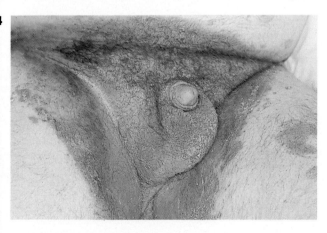

2.14 Perineal psoriasis caused severe pruritus in this man. The discoloration of the lesions results largely from tar therapy.

Involvement of nails may occur as a coarse 'pitting' as on a thimble (3.5) or as onycholysis (2.16) or gross thickening of the nail with underlying hyperkeratosis.

Guttate psoriasis is an abrupt onset of psoriasis with 'droplet' shaped erythematous scaly lesions scattered widely over trunk and limbs with no predilection for extensor surfaces (2.17). It may be triggered by a preceding streptococcal throat infection, and is more common in children and young adults. It usually clears completely but classic psoriasis may appear in later life.

Erythrodermic psoriasis (2.18) can be a life-threatening condition. The rash starts as common psoriasis but spreads to become confluent and often indistinguishable from other forms of erythroderma.

Arthropathy occurs in 10–15% of psoriatic patients. Classically, distal interphalangeal joints (3.47) and large joints such as the ankles and knees are involved and the rheumatoid factor is negative. The arthritis can be severe, producing an 'arthritis mutilans' of the hands and feet with resultant severe disablility (3.48, 3.49).

Localised chronic pustular psoriasis may occur without other evidence of psoriasis (2.19, 3.50). Generalised pustular psoriasis is a rare presentation which may be fatal. It may be precipitated by topical or systemic steroid use, drug reactions or infections. Crops of sterile pustules occur, with fever and systemic upset.

The diagnosis of psoriasis is usually made on clinical features but histology is diagnostic. The aetiology of the condition remains obscure despite much research. It is a chronic hyperproliferative inflammatory disorder, with a combination of increased epidermal turnover and inflammation, involving both lymphocytes and polymorphonuclear leucocytes with an associated vasodilatation of superficial dermal vessels.

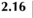
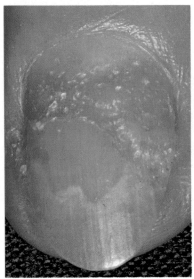

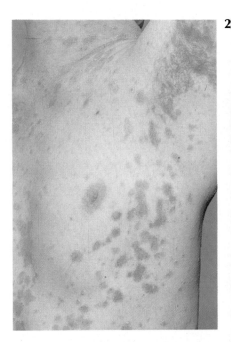

2.16 Psoriasis affecting the nail, causing pitting, onycholysis, discoloration and thickening.

2.17 Guttate psoriasis in a 17 year old. The condition resolved completely within a few months.

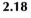
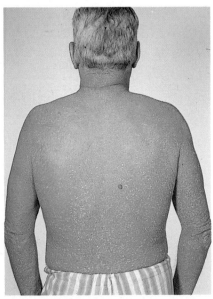

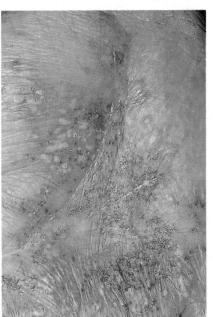

2.18 Erythrodermic psoriasis is potentially life-threatening, and it closely resembles other forms of erythroderma in which the whole skin surface is involved. The management of patients with severe erythroderma is as urgent as that of a patient with severe burns.

2.19 Pustular psoriasis of the palms. The palms and soles are the most common areas for this localised form of psoriasis. The pus is usually sterile, and the hands are not tender or oedematous.

Dermatitis

'Dermatitis' and 'eczema' are synonymous, but 'eczema' is usually restricted in clinical use to atopic dermatitis. Dermatitis may be exogenous (contact, irritant, infective or photodermatitis) or endogenous (e.g. atopic, seborrhoeic, discoid). Often the diagnosis is made on the pattern of rash. A detailed history is most important.

Dermatitis means inflammation in the skin. This may be acute with weeping, crusting and vesicle formation; subacute; or chronic with dryness, scaling and fissuring and lichenification (in atopics). The rash is almost always itchy and secondary infection is common.

Atopic dermatitis usually begins in childhood, between 2–6 months of age, affecting around 2% of the population. A family history of atopy occurs in 70% of cases. Hayfever and/or asthma may develop as the child gets older. Over 90% of children are clear by the age of 12, but predicting this for an individual child is difficult. In infants the face, neck and trunk are involved (**2.20**), with sparing of the napkin area. Flexural involvement appears later, behind knees, elbows, wrists and ankles and in the groins (**2.21**). Secondary infection is common (**2.22**). Itch can be severe and causes much distress to patients and families. Food allergy, especially to eggs, fish and dairy products may be relevant, but few patients benefit from exclusion diets.

Neurodermatitis or lichen simplex is chronic dermatitis perpetuated by the itch-scratch cycle. Common sites include the arms (**2.23**), the neck and the lower leg.

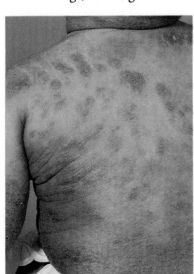

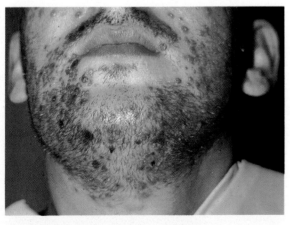

2.22 Secondary infection in eczema. Patients with atopic dermatitis have defective cell-mediated immunity, and are more susceptible to bacterial, viral and fungal infections. This man has a herpes simplex infection (eczema herpeticum), which has prevented him from shaving (*see* p. 28).

2.20 Infantile eczema in a dark-skinned child, affecting the face, neck and trunk. In a light-skinned child, the lesions are pinkish rather than bluish in colour.

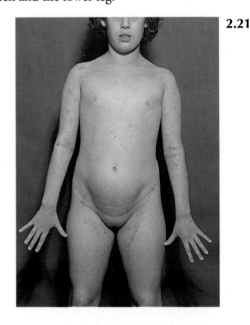

2.21 Flexural atopic dermatitis. This girl shows the typical childhood distribution. As the lesions are itchy, they are usually scratched repeatedly and become excoriated. In the long term, lichenification results (*see* **2.23**). Even non-flexural skin is dry and may be itchy.

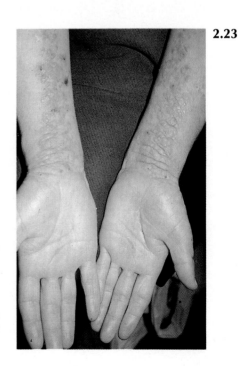

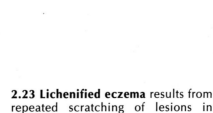

2.23 Lichenified eczema results from repeated scratching of lesions in eczematous patients.

Discoid dermatitis is characterised by discrete patches of dermatitis, in a symmetrical pattern, often on extensor surfaces, of unknown cause (**2.24**).

Contact dermatitis is allergy (type IV) to a substance on the skin surface. The relevant factor may be immediately obvious, e.g. nickel, perfume, or shoe rubber (**2.25–2.27**). A wide range of potential allergens exists in domestic and industrial life: a careful history and patch tests should establish the diagnosis. The rash can be chronic, patchy and some distance from the allergen, e.g.nail varnish allergy may present with dermatitis on the face or neck.

Stasis dermatitis is associated with venous insufficiency. It is often complicated by oedema, infection and contact dermatitis to topical medicaments (**2.28**). A secondary, widespread symmetrical dermatitis may develop.

Seborrhoeic dermatitis presents in infancy as cradle cap, with scattered erythematous patches on the head and neck (**2.29**) and an associated napkin rash. In adults scaling in the scalp, blepharitis, red scaly patches in naso-labial folds (**2.30, 2.31**), around the ears and on the presternal area are characteristic; intertrigo may occur.

In **irritant dermatitis** the rash is caused by physical or chemical irritation of the skin: allergy is not involved. Soaps, detergents, foods and DIY materials can all produce this pattern. Hand dermatitis is the most common form (**2.32**).

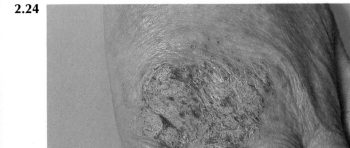

2.24 Discoid dermatitis. Round plaques of eczema develop, usually on the extensor surfaces of the limbs. The condition often occurs in patients who have no previous history of atopic dermatitis. In this patient the lesions are 'weeping' serous fluid.

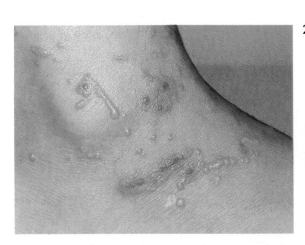

2.25 Contact dermatitis to poison ivy is a common problem in North America. This 15-year-old boy presented with linear eczematous lesions on his ankle.

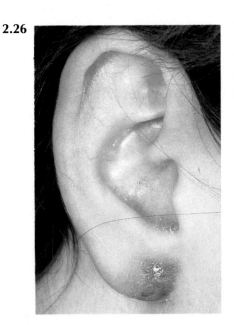

2.26 Contact dermatitis to nickel affects 10% of European women. Nickel is a common component of jewellery such as rings, necklaces and ear-rings. Nickel in ear-rings gave rise to ear-lobe eczema in this young woman.

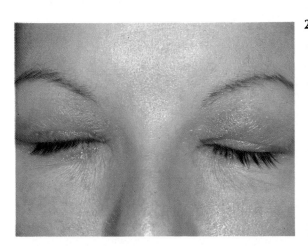

2.27 Contact blepharitis. Characterised by redness and swelling of the eyelid margins, this can result from contact dermatitis caused by eye make-up, as in this 22-year-old woman.

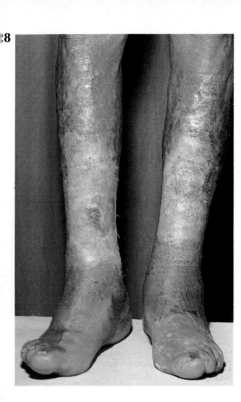

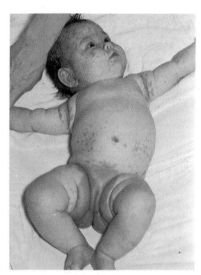

2.28 Stasis eczema is commonly seen in elderly women, in association with venous insufficiency or frank ulceration. Often, as here, there is also marked pigmentation as a result of haemosiderin deposition.

2.29 Seborrhoeic dermatitis in infancy. Napkin rash is associated with scattered erythematous patches on the abdomen, trunk and head and neck, but the extremities are spared.

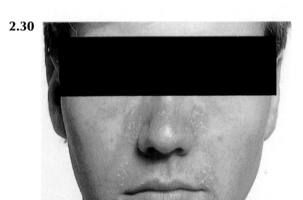

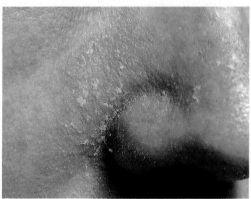

2.30, 2.31 Florid seborrhoeic dermatitis—in close-up in **2.31**, showing typical red, scaly lesions. This patient was HIV positive at the ARC stage (*see* p. 17); but although this is a common problem in patients with HIV infection, most patients with seborrhoeic dermatitis do not have HIV infection.

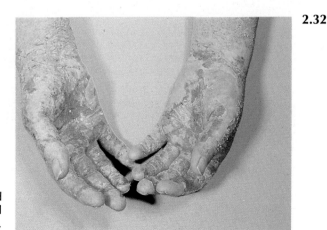

2.32 Irritant dermatitis, presenting as hand dermatitis in a 39-year-old man. It resulted from exposure to irritant chemicals at work.

Urticaria

Urticaria is common, and usually presents as acute, transient but recurrent, pruritic, erythematous cutaneous swellings caused by fluid transfer from the vasculature to the dermis (**2.33**). It often produces only minor weals, and some patients may exhibit dermographism (**2.34**). Rarely urticaria is part of a severe and life-threatening reaction—severe angioedema (**2.35**, **2.36**), in which the patient is at risk of asphyxiation from laryngeal involvement—and similar reactions can occur in other organs including the gastrointestinal tract, joints and bronchi.

The aetiology of urticaria is usually unknown, though both immunological and non-immunological factors may be involved. Most patients will require treatment on a symptomatic basis with antihistamines, but in some cases an exclusion diet may be helpful.

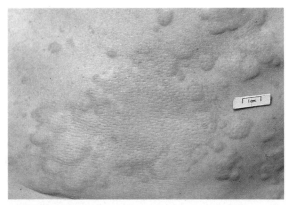

2.33

2.33 Urticaria in close up, showing characteristic small, punctate weals, surrounded by an erythematous flare.

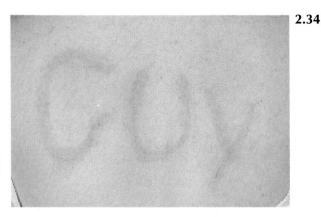

2.34

2.34 Dermographism is a form of urticaria in which the patient responds to anything more than a very light touch with a weal and flare reaction. This can be simply tested with firm finger pressure, as shown in this patient from a well-known London teaching hospital.

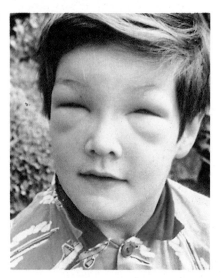

2.35

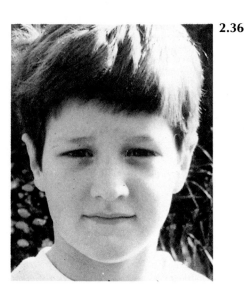

2.36

2.35, 2.36 Severe angioedema in a 9-year-old boy following a bee sting. The patient required immediate treatment with adrenalin to overcome a generalised anaphylactic response, and showed gross facial swelling. **2.36** shows the same patient without angioedema.

Infections and infestations

Bacterial infections

Surface commensals include diphtheroids and micrococci—mainly *Staphylococcus epidermidis*. A minority of people carry *Staphylococcus aureus* in the nares, perineum or axillae (**Table 2.1**). Damaged epidermis predisposes to secondary infection.

Staphylococcal infections include impetigo (**1.103**) which is highly contagious (it can also be caused by *Streptococcus pyogenes*). Furuncules (**2.37**) are boils which may occur singly or in crops: multiple or large lesions (carbuncles) suggest underlying diabetes mellitus (**1.92**). Staphylococci may cause toxic epidermal necrolysis in children (**1.94**).

Erysipelas (**1.100**) is a **streptococcal infection**, usually associated with systemic upset. Recurrent attacks may occur, leading to chronic lymphoedema.

Syphilis should be remembered as a cause of skin rashes (*see* p. 83). The primary chancre is typically a painless ulcer. Secondary syphilis (**1.231**) must be distinguished from pityriasis rosea, measles, drug eruptions, guttate psoriasis and lichen planus. Tertiary syphilis (**1.234**) resembles granulomatous conditions such as sarcoid.

Tuberculosis (*see* p. 46) may present as lupus vulgaris, a chronic nodular, scarring rash (**2.38**, **2.39**). Warty tuberculosis or scrofuloderma occur less commonly. **Erythema nodosum** (**1.123**, **2.40**) or induratum may be associated with tuberculosis.

Skin lesions in **leprosy** reflect the patient's immune response (*see* p. 49).

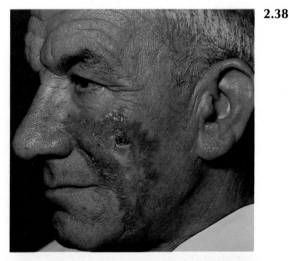

2.38

2.38 Lupus vulgaris on the cheek. This is a rare presentation of tuberculosis in the Western world, but it still occurs in developing countries and in immunosuppressed patients. The slowly extending lesion is hyperpigmented at its margin, and depigmented in the healing central zone. Ulceration has also occurred. This patient is generally pigmented as a result of Addison's disease, following tuberculous infection of the adrenals (*see* p. 313).

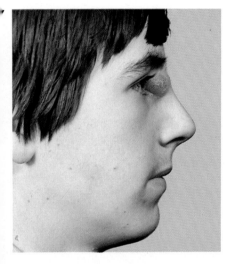

2.37 A boil (furuncle) is caused by a staphylococcal infection of a hair follicle with the accumulation of pus. This results in severe pain, and is usually followed by the spontaneous discharge of yellow pus. A boil in this location carries the risk of septicaemia and cavernous sinus thrombosis (*see* p. 501).

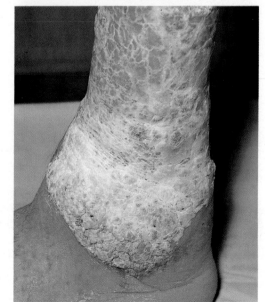

2.39

2.39 Extensive, chronic lupus vulgaris leads to ulceration, desquamation and fibrosis. Disease of this severity is now rarely seen because of the efficacy of modern chemotherapy.

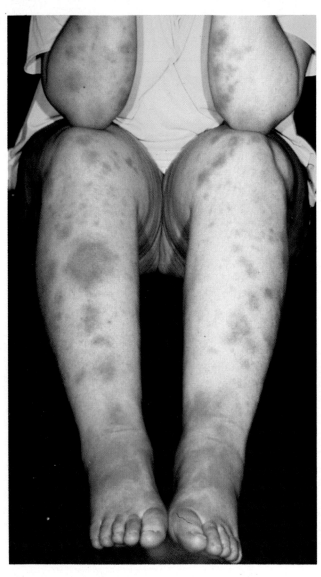

2.40 Erythema nodosum. occurring in a classic distribution over the front of the legs and forearms. The appearance reflects the patchy inflammation of subcutaneous fat and small vessels, probably as the result of a Type III (immune complex) allergic mechanism. Erythema nodosum has many causes, of which the commonest in the Western world is now drug therapy—especially with sulphonamides. This patient also had arthralgia and a mild fever, and further investigation revealed an underlying diagnosis of sarcoidosis.

Viral infections

Viral warts are caused by the human papilloma virus (more than 50 subtypes exist). Warts are common; their morphology varies with anatomical site and viral subtype. Spontaneous resolution occurs (30% in 6 months), but painful or multiple lesions may need treatment (**2.41, 2.42,** *see* p. 81).

Herpes simplex types I and II cause primary (sometimes asymptomatic) and recurrent infections, usually on extragenital and genital sites respectively. Recurrent lesions are preceded by tingling or pain, they usually appear in the same place and are triggered by various factors. Grouped vesicles on an erythematous base persist for a few days (*see* p. 28). Secondary bacterial infection may occur. Infection may complicate atopic dermatitis (Kaposi's varicelliform eruption).

Herpes zoster (shingles) is caused by the varicella zoster virus, reactivated in a sensory nerve root (where it persists following chickenpox). Pain in the affected dermatome precedes the rash of scattered blisters and erythema (**2.43**) (*see* pp. 17, 30). Haemorrhagic lesions and scattered lesions elsewhere on the body suggest underlying neoplasia or immunosuppression. Corneal ulcers and scarring may follow involvement of the ophthalmic branch of the trigeminal nerve. Post herpetic pain is common (*see also* p. 30)

Molluscum contagiosum is caused by a pox virus. The umbilicated pearly lesions (**2.44**), often multiple, are more common in childhood and resolve spontaneously after becoming inflamed. Residual marks may persist for some months.

Pityriasis rosea occurs in children and young adults (a viral aetiology is suspected but unproven). A herald patch (**2.45**) precedes subsequent lesions which tend to be distributed along the rib lines (**2.46**). The lesions are usually asymptomatic but may be itchy. They persist for 4–6 weeks.

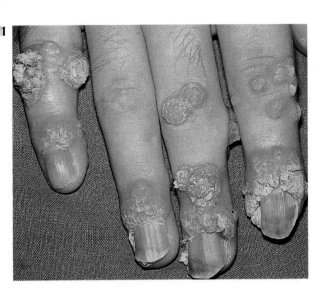

2.41 Multiple viral warts on the fingers. A florid collection of warts like this should raise the suspicion of a possible underlying impairment in cell-mediated immunity.

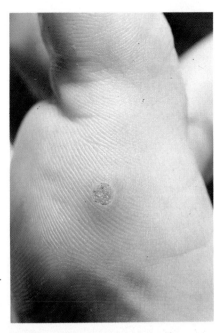

2.42 A plantar viral wart, popularly known as a 'verruca' Single and multiple plantar warts are common, especially in school-children who may acquire them from swimming-bath floors. They are characteristically flat with a callus on the surface, but may extend subcutaneously. They are often painful, and should be treated—to relieve symptoms and prevent transmission to others.

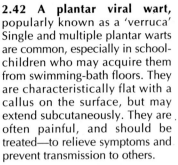

2.43 Shingles in the L3 dermatome, showing the characteristic type of distribution and appearance of the rash. This patient had AIDS.

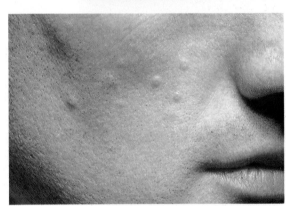

2.44 Molluscum contagiosum lesions on the face. Note the umbilicated, pearly lesions. The condition occurs in otherwise normal patients but it is particularly common in patients with HIV infection.

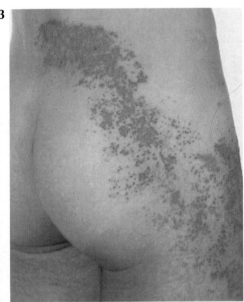

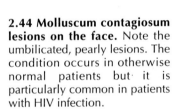

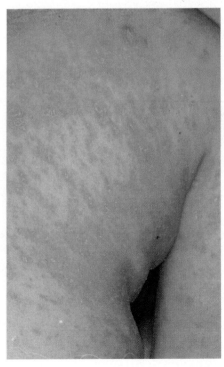

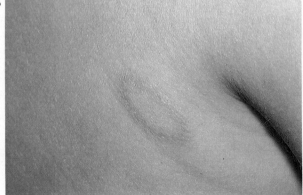

2.45 The herald patch in pityriasis rosea commonly precedes the later multiple lesions by several days. It is usually oval, and has a surrounding collar of fine white scales.

2.46 Pityriasis rosea. The herald patch can still be seen, but there is now a widespread itchy skin eruption, largely following the lines of the ribs.

Fungal and yeast infections

Dermatophyte fungi (genera *Trichophyton, Microsporum* and *Epidermophyton*) live on keratin and evoke a variable amount of inflammation. Clinical lesions are termed tinea or ringworm. Presentation depends on body site, but it is usually plaques of scaling erythema, with variable itch (**1.3, 2.2–2.4, 2.47, 2.48**). Nail involvement causes onycholysis and dystrophy, and scalp infection causes patchy hair loss (**2.49**).

Candida infections caused by *Candida albicans* yeast commonly occur in moist, flexural sites (**2.50**). Predisposing factors include diabetes mellitus, pregnancy, broad-spectrum antibiotics or obesity (*see also* p. 65). Chronic paronychia may be complicated by additional bacterial infection; wet work or poor circulation are predisposing factors, and the fingernails may be infected (**2.51**).

Pityriasis versicolor is caused by yeasts (*Pityrosporum orbiculare*) producing widespread scaly lesions on the upper trunk and back (**2.52**), pale in dark skins and darker in fair skins. Recurrent attacks are common.

2.47

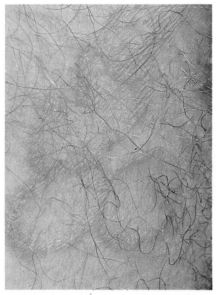

2.47 Tinea corporis. These annular lesions ('ringworm') are on the thigh. Note the scaly margins, which can be scraped and examined for fungal hyphae and spores (**2.3–2.5**).

2.48

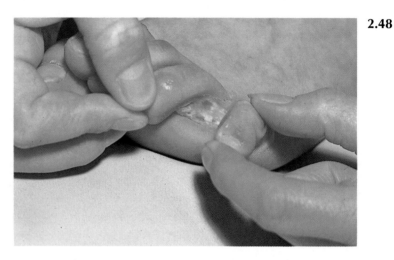

2.48 Tinea pedis ('athlete's foot') is a very common infection, especially in those who wear tight or poorly ventilated footwear.

2.49

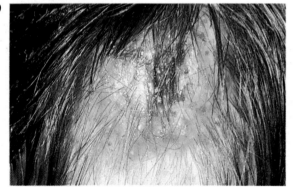

2.49 Fungal infection of the scalp, which has resulted in severe pustular inflammation and hair loss.

2.50

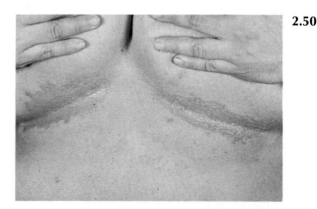

2.50 Candidiasis of the skin (intertriginous candidiasis) below both breasts in an obese diabetic.

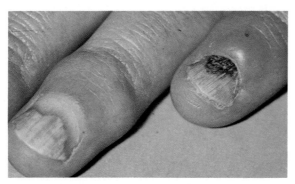

2.51 Moniliasis of the fingernails in a diabetic patient.

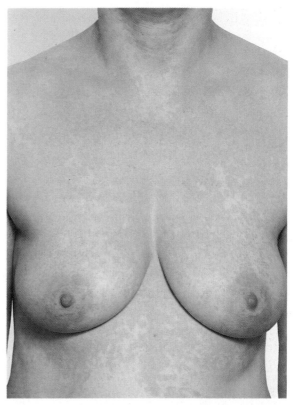

2.52 Pityriasis versicolor. Typical lesions in a 28-year-old woman.

Infestations

These result from invasion of the body by arthropods, including insects, mites and ticks.

Insect bites are reactions to injected antigens, causing weals, persisting papules and sometimes blisters (2.53). Papular urticaria describes lesions occurring in recurrent crops, often secondarily infected.

Scabies is caused by the mite *Sarcoptes scabiei* var. *hominis* (2.5). Transmission occurs through close body contact. The adult mite lays eggs in burrows in the skin (2.54). Sensitisation to the mites results in a widespread secondary eczema (2.55) and severe pruritus, worse at night. Household contacts must be treated to prevent recurrences.

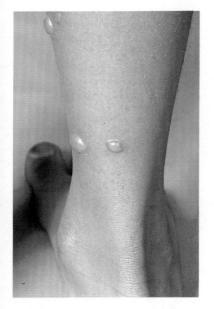

2.53 Insect bites producing a bullous reaction in an 8-year-old child.

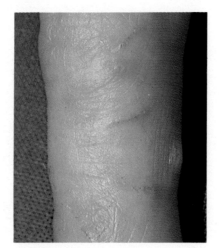

2.54 Scabies. Typical burrows on the finger.

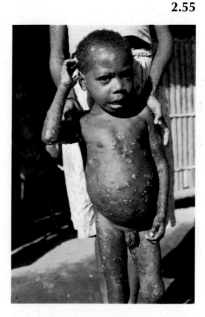

2.55 Scabies with secondary infected eczema in a boy from Papua.

2.56

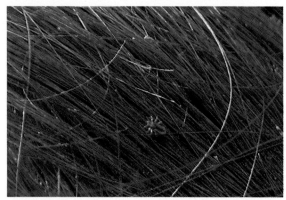

Lice infestations are caused by *Pediculus humanus* (var. *capitis* and *corporis*) and *Phthirus pubis.* The lice suck blood, causing pruritus, scratching and secondary infection. Their eggs, known as nits, are attached to hairs (or clothing with body lice) (**2.56**). Head lice occur irrespective of cleanliness, whereas body lice are found on the vagrant or unhygienic. Pubic lice (crab lice) are commonly sexually transmitted.

2.56 Head louse infestation (pediculosis capitis). This close-up picture shows a single louse clearly enough to count its six legs, and a number of egg capsules (nits) attached to the hairs.

Lichen planus

Lichen planus accounts for 1–2% of new dermatology referrals. It affects both sexes equally, usually in the 30–60 year age group.

The classic presentation is easy to diagnose with 'purple, pruritic, polygonal papules'. These commonly occur on the wrists, low back, ankles and feet (**2.57**), but the lesions may be widespread. If severe, lesions may blister. Koebner's phenomenon may be seen (**2.58**).

Mucosal lesions are common and may present before or without other affected sites. Mouth lesions are diagnostic, with lacy white striae on the buccal mucosa (**2.59**). Ulceration may occur. Genital lesions affect the vulva or the glans and shaft of the penis.

Hair loss may occur, sometimes with irreversible scarring alopecia (**2.60**). Nail changes include irregular coarse pits or linear streaks, or adhesions between the skin and the nail plate,

causing pterygium formation.

The histology is characteristic and should confirm the diagnosis if required.

Most cases settle within 1–2 years, but the rash may recur or become chronic. Post-inflammatory hyperpigmentation may persist. Topical or systemic steroid treatment may be required in severe cases.

The aetiology remains unknown. An association with primary biliary cirrhosis and other auto-immune diseases has been reported.

Lichenoid reactions, mimicking lichen planus, may occur with drugs such as gold, chloroquine, methyldopa, thiazide diuretics or following contact with colour photograph developer.

2.57

2.58

2.57 Lichen planus. The polygonal papules on the dorsum of the foot are typical of the chronic form of the disorder, and the lesions are commonly itchy. Dystrophic nail changes are common in lichen planus.

2.58 Koebner's phenomenon in lichen planus. Typical lesions may occur in a scratch when the disease is active, as here along the lines of bramble scratches.

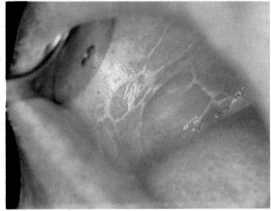

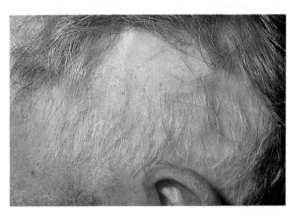

2.59 Oral lesions are relatively common in lichen planus. The classic appearance is of white reticulations on the buccal mucosa, as here, but the disease may also take an erosive form and similar lesions may occur on the tongue. Biopsy is usually advisable to confirm the diagnosis.

2.60 Lichen planus in the scalp of a 68-year-old man. There is depigmentation and scarring caused by biopsy-proven lichen planus that was active for over 30 years.

Bullous disorders

Blisters develop when fluid collects between layers of the skin, as a result of inflammation (external or internal) or shearing forces. They are a feature of many conditions, some covered elsewhere in this book, e.g. dermatitis, (p. 93), herpes simplex (p. 28) and insect bites (p. 101). Immunofluorescent staining characteristics are important to distinguish the bullous disorders listed below.

In **dermatitis herpetiformis**, groups of itchy blisters appear on elbows (2.61), shoulders, buttocks (2.62) and knees. There may be an associated gluten enteropathy (*see* p. 369). Blisters are subepidermal in site and immunofluorescence shows granular IgA deposits in dermal papillae.

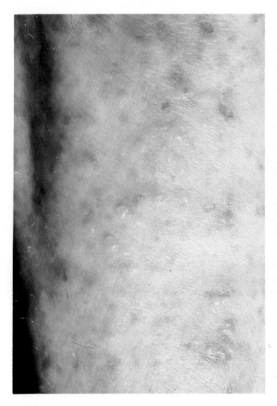

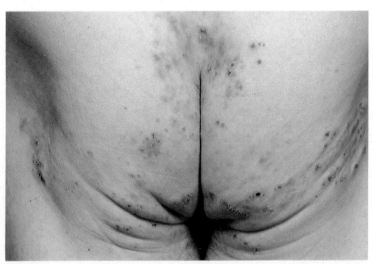

2.61 Dermatitis herpetiformis on the elbow. This 65-year-old man had a history of a recurrent eruption of vesicles and crusts on his elbows, head, neck and lower back. The lesions are intensely itchy, and the vesicles are easily ruptured by scratching.

2.62 Dermatitis herpetiformis in the sacral and buttock areas. The vesicles have been ruptured by scratching, and are healing, leaving pigmented scars.

In **bullous pemphigoid**, large tense blisters on any body site (2.63) occur, predominantly affecting elderly patients. Blisters are subepidermal and immunofluorescence shows linear IgG at the dermo-epidermal junction. Oral lesions are uncommon.

Pemphigus gestationis (herpes gestationis) is a rare dermatosis of pregnancy resembling pemphigoid. It remits *post partum*, but tends to recur with subsequent pregnancies.

In **pemphigus vulgaris**, erosions are the predominant lesion, as the blisters are flaccid and easily ruptured (2.64, 2.65). All body sites are affected; oral lesions are common and may be the presenting site. Blisters form within the epidermis;

immunofluorescence shows diffuse staining of intercellular cement substance between epidermal cells, with IgG and C3. The course is prolonged, often with serious complications despite therapy.

Blisters are a feature of most of the **cutaneous porphyrias**, due to skin fragility and light sensitivity.

Epidermolysis bullosa comprises a group of blistering disorders of varying inheritance patterns and presentation. Blisters form within the dermo-epidermal junction as the skin responds abnormally to shearing forces (2.66).

2.63

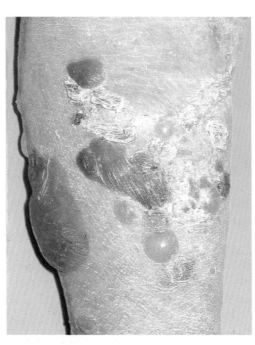

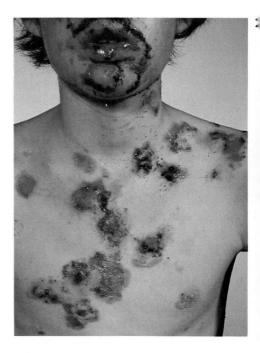

2.63 Pemphigoid. Some of the blisters have become haemorrhagic, as often occurs.

2.64 Pemphigus vulgaris in a 13-year-old boy. The blisters rupture easily, and are often associated with similar lesions on mucous membranes, especially in the mouth.

2.65

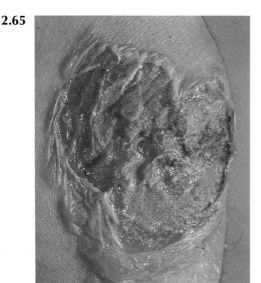

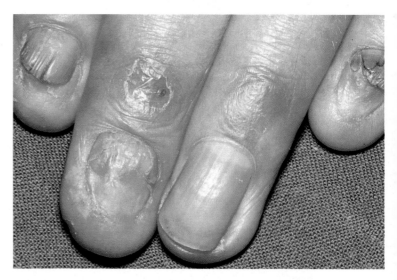

2.65 Pemphigus vulgaris blisters are thin and painful, with an intraepidermal split. They often become secondarily infected.

2.66 Epidermolysis bullosa (dominant dystrophic form). From early childhood, minor trauma has caused blistering in this patient. The blisters heal with scarring, as shown here. Note also the dystrophic nail changes.

Acne vulgaris

Acne is a very common disorder of the pilosebaceous unit. It occurs in adolescence, tends to present earlier in females and may persist for some years (though infantile acne may also occur rarely). It results from a combination of factors. There is increased sebum production, although this alone does not cause acne. Infection and inflammation caused by *Propionibacterium acnes* occurs within the sebaceous glands, where breakdown of fatty acids triggers inflammation. Increased end-organ sensitivity within the sebaceous gland to normal levels of androgen hormones accounts for hormonal influences. Duct abnormalities and obstruction in the pilosebaceous unit also have a role.

The face (2.67), back (2.68) and chest are affected, with a range of lesions from small papules and pustules, to comedones and deeper, painful cysts and a background of seborrhoea. Subsequent scars may be hypertrophic or depressed (2.69).

Drug-induced acne may follow treatment with corticosteroids, androgenic hormones, oral contraceptives, anticonvulsant drugs, bromides or iodides.

Acne rosacea occurs in an older age group than acne vulgaris and has a vascular component to it. Flushing, often precipitated by hot foods, warm environment or sunlight occurs in association with small papules and pustules over the forehead, cheeks and chin in a symmetrical pattern (2.70). Seborrhoea is not necessarily present and skin microflora are often normal. An association with the mite *Demodex folliculorum* has been suggested. Rosacea lymphoedema may be persistent, keratitis may occur and rhinophyma (2.71) may develop. The rash is exacerbated by topical steroids and sometimes by sunlight.

2.67

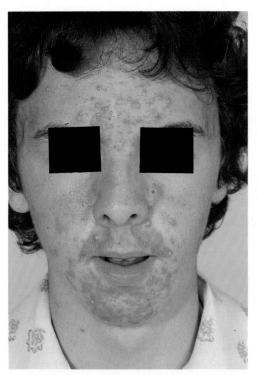

2.67 Acne vulgaris usually involves the face. This 17 year old shows the typical features of moderately severe acne. He has many papular and pustular lesions at different stages of evolution, and the older lesions are healing with scarring.

2.68

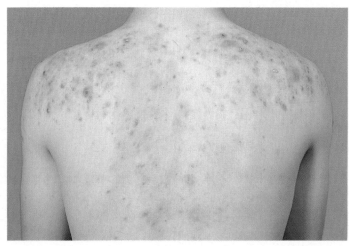

2.68 Acne vulgaris on the shoulders and back—another common site. Again, a wide range of lesions are seen, including some large pustules, and scarring is occurring on healing.

2.69

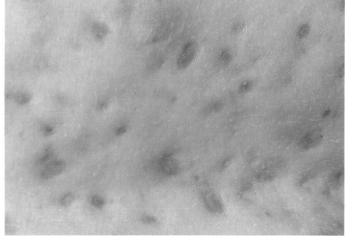

2.69 Acne scars—a close-up view. In this patient, the scars are depressed, but hypertrophic scars may also occur

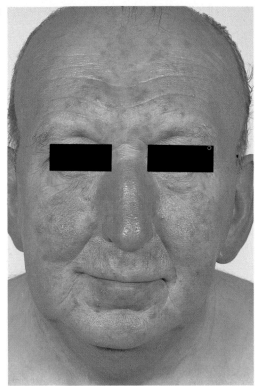

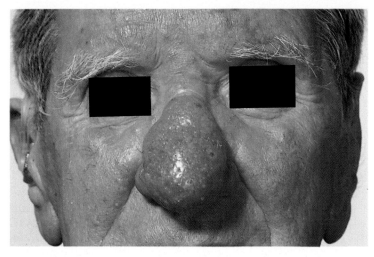

2.70 Acne rosacea. This patient shows typical papules and pustules, superimposed on a generally erythematous facial skin. His eyes are normal, but keratitis may occur.

2.71 Rhinophyma usually occurs as a long-term complication of acne rosacea. In this elderly man, the nose is characteristically red and bulbous. The 'strawberry' appearance results from hyperplasia of the sebaceous glands and connective tissue. The follicle openings become prominent.

Disorders of pigmentation

The dominant pigmentation of the skin is melanin and most disorders result from excess or insufficiency of this. Other pigments include haemosiderin, bilirubin and carotene.

Congenital disorders of pigmentation include freckles, simple lentigenes and café-au-lait patches in neurofibromatosis (2.72). Less common conditions include oculocutaneous albinism (defective melanin production which affects hair, eyes and skin, 2.73). Incontinentia pigmentii (initial blisters leave whorled pigmentary lesions in adult life) and lentigenes round the mouth in Peutz–Jeghers syndrome (2.74). Xeroderma pigmentosum patients show excessive freckling in light-exposed areas. Urticaria pigmentosa presents in childhood as scattered brownish-pink macules that urticate on rubbing.

Vitiligo (2.75) develops in 1% of the population. The white patches show total loss of melanocytes. A personal or family history of other autoimmune disorders may be present.

Hyperpigmentation may be a sign of underlying endocrine disease, such as Addison's disease, acromegaly, Cushing's syndrome and hyperthyroidism. Patchy facial pigmentation (cholasma) is common in pregnancy and in women taking oral contraceptives. Tumours may cause diffuse pigmentation through ectopic ACTH production or localised pigment changes such as acanthosis nigricans (2.76).

Hyperpigmentation is seen in cirrhosis, renal failure, haemochromatosis (slate-grey colour) and porphyria.

Connective-tissue disorders such as SLE, dermatomyositis or morphoea may cause local or diffuse pigment changes.

Drugs causing pigmentation include antimalarials, phenothiazines, hydantoin, minocycline, busulphan, cyclophosphamide, bleomycin and arsenic. Psoralens used for photochemotherapy produce a deep tan.

Exogenous causes of pigmentation include carotene (carotenaemia) and compounds containing silver (argyria). Tattoos are a common form of exogenous pigmentation.

Post-inflammatory hypo- or hyperpigmentation may result from inflammatory conditions such as lichen planus, dermatitis (2.77), or discoid lupus erythematosus, especially in dark-skinned subjects.

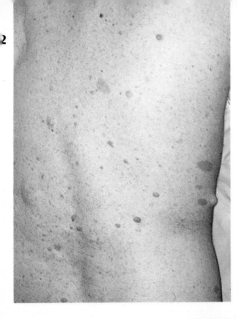

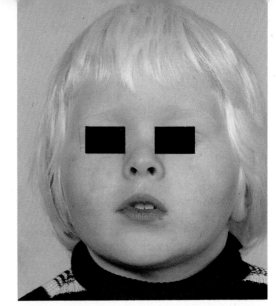

2.72 Neurofibromatosis (Type I, *see* p. 517) (von Recklinghausen's disease). Note the subcutaneous nodular tumours arising in the sheaths of peripheral nerves, the pigmented pedunculated tumours on the skin surface and the brown (café-au-lait) patches.

2.73 Albinism. This child has typical white skin and hair. His eyes were also affected; he had pink irises and photophobia.

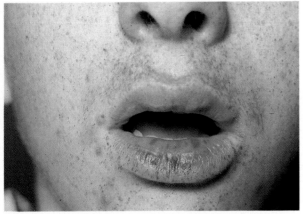

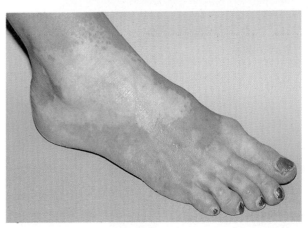

2.74 Peutz–Jeghers syndrome. Dark brown pigmentation is found particularly on the lips and around the mouth, but also on the hard and soft palate, buccal mucosa and, occasionally, on the feet and hands. There is an association with multiple intestinal polyps, some of which undergo malignant transformation.

2.75 Vitiligo is often first noticed in the hands, but may be found throughout the body. It is characterised by multiple, well-demarcated areas of hypopigmentation which progressively enlarge. It is often associated with other autoimmune disorders, and—in about one-third of cases—there is a family history.

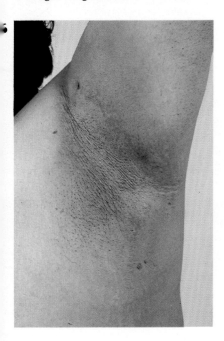

2.76 Acanthosis nigricans in an Asian patient. Patchy velvety brown hyperpigmentation and thickening of flexures develops. In older patients, this is often a marker of underlying malignant disease but the condition may occur in diabetes and other endocrine disorders and as an isolated abnormality.

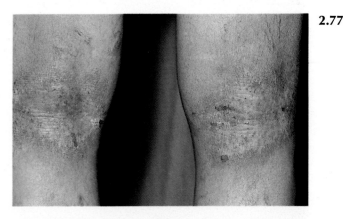

2.77 Hyperpigmentation and lichenification are common complications of chronic atopic dermatitis. Note the thinning of the skin around the gross lesions, which results from inappropriate use of topical corticosteroid therapy.

Disorders of keratinisation

Abnormalities of keratin maturation may present as scaling with or without inflammation. Scaling is also a feature of conditions such as psoriasis and dermatitis.

Ichthyosis vulgaris is a common (1:300), autosomal dominant condition which appears in early childhood. The scales are small, spare the flexural areas and the condition improves with age. There is an association with keratosis pilaris. X-linked ichthyosis presents in early infancy, with larger, darker scales (**2.78**) and flexural involvement, and persists in adult life. Acquired ichthyosis is usually associated with underlying conditions such as Hodgkin's disease, other lymphomata, sarcoid or malabsorption.

Keratosis pilaris is a common abnormality of keratinisation at the hair follicle ducts which presents in childhood as roughened areas on upper outer arms and legs (**2.79**). The face and eyebrows may be affected.

Darier's disease (keratosis follicularis) is a rare autosomal dominant condition which appears in the mid-teens as small scaly reddish-brown papules on chest, back, scalp or flexures (**2.80**). Histology is diagnostic. Nail abnormalities include linear streaks and notching. Punctate lesions may be seen on hands or feet.

Keratoderma of palms and soles may be inherited or acquired. Various patternings such as punctate, striate or diffuse thickening occur. Rarely, diffuse keratoderma (tylosis) has been associated in some families with underlying neoplasia (**2.81**).

2.78

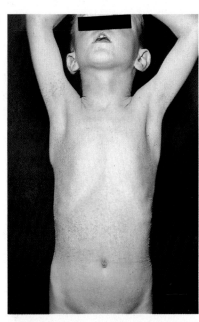

2.78 Ichthyosis vulgaris, is a dominant condition that causes scaly skin from early childhood onwards. Its name reflects the resemblance of the skin to scaly fish skin.

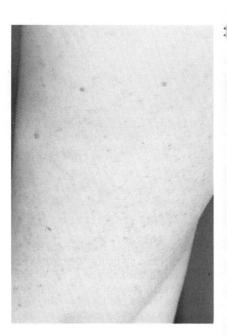

2.79 Keratosis pilaris on the leg. In this common disorder, the hair follicles are plugged with keratin, giving the skin a rough texture. The disorder is only of cosmetic importance.

2.80

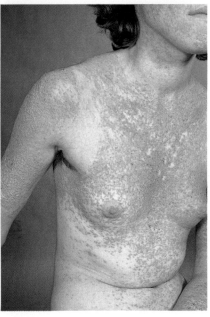

2.80 Darier's disease. In this dominant familial disorder there are large numbers of hard reddish papules, which may coalesce.

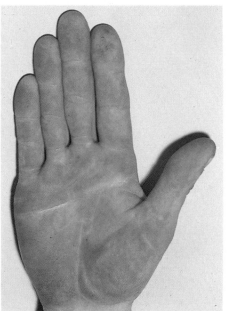

2.81 Keratoderma of the palm in a 5-year-old girl with familial tylosis.

Hair disorders

Hair loss (alopecia)

Alopecia areata is a common cause of focal hair loss (**2.82**). Regrowth usually occurs within weeks or months. Alopecia totalis (**2.83**) with loss of all body hair (alopecia universalis) can occur, and fine pitting of the nails may be seen. A family or personal history of autoimmune disorders may be present.

Fungal infection of the scalp causes patchy hair loss (**2.49**). If significantly inflamed, the lesion is called a kerion. Permanent scarring may result.

Traction alopecia results from repeated tension on the hairs, as in some Afro-Asian hair styles (**2.84**).

Trichotillomania is patchy hair loss caused by rubbing or pulling, commonly in childhood; hairs are broken off close to the surface.

Scarring alopecia may result from inflammatory dermatoses, such as lichen planus (**2.60**), discoid lupus erythematosus or scleroderma, or from trauma, burns or irradiation.

Diffuse hair loss following pregnancy, severe febrile illnesses or operations, is termed telogen effluvium (loss in telogen growth phase). Cyclophosphamide causes anagen effluvium. Iron-deficiency anaemia, hypo- or hyperthyroidism, SLE and drugs such as heparin, vitamin A derivatives (retinoids) and oral contraceptives may cause hair loss.

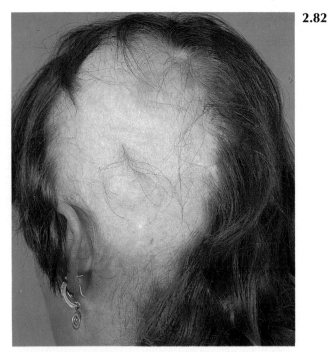

2.82 Alopecia areata in a 24-year-old woman. There are no features to suggest infection of the scalp.

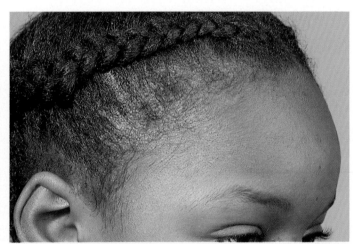

2.83 Alopecia totalis developed from severe alopecia areata in this patient. a similar appearance may result from the use of some cytotoxic chemotherapy for malignant disease.

2.84 Traction alopecia has resulted from the combing involved in maintaining an 'Afro' hairstyle in this patient.

Excessive hair

Hirsutism is male-pattern hair growth in women (**2.85**, **2.86**, **7.55**). Mild facial hirsutism is common, increasing after the menopause. In younger women, especially with menstrual irregularity or with other signs of virilisation, investigations to exclude conditions such as polycystic ovaries, ovarian tumours, virilising adrenal tumours or Cushing's syndrome should be considered.

Hypertrichosis, an overall increase in hair, may be drug induced, such as by minoxidil, or associated with anorexia nervosa or porphyria.

2.85

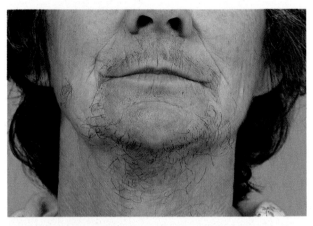

2.86

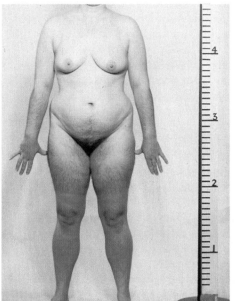

2.85 Hirsutism was the presenting symptom in this woman who was found to have an arrhenoblastoma.

2.86 Hirsutism with male-pattern pubic and body hair. Note the extensive hair on her forearms and thigh, and the evidence of shaving of the lower thighs and legs.

Nail disorders

Nail abnormalities are present in some genodermatoses, such as nail–patella syndrome, pachyonychia congenita and ectodermal dysplasias. Scarring of nails occurs in some forms of epidermolysis bullosa (**2.66**). Subungual exostoses cause overlying nail dystrophy.

Acute or chronic trauma may cause subungual splinter haemorrhages (**3.27**, **3.28**) or haematomas, gross thickening of the nail (onychogryphosis) or onycholysis of individual nails. Habit tic nail dystrophy of thumb-nails and bitten nails, with damaged cuticles are common.

Yellow nails (**2.87**) are seen with chronic lymphoedema and some chronic lung diseases. Other colour changes include leukonychia in liver disease (**2.88**), half-and-half nails in renal disease, and changes with some drugs such as antimalarials or tetracyclines.

Koilonychia (**2.89**) is seen in iron-deficiency anaemia.

Clubbing of nails (**2.90**, **2.91**, **4.3**, **4.67**, **4.108**, **5.3**, **11.104**) is associated with cyanotic heart disease and some chronic lung and gut diseases or it may be congenital.

Beau's lines are horizontal grooves that appear on all nails following severe illness.

Splinter haemorrhages may be seen in vasculitis, in association with connective tissue diseases (**3.28**) or in bacterial endocarditis.

Onycholysis (**2.16**) may be drug induced or associated with hyperthyroidism. Median nail dystrophy occurs without skin changes and the cause is unknown. Peripheral vascular disease predisposes to chronic paronychia. Dystrophic changes may occur in many dermatological conditions.

Tumours may develop under or around the nail base, including malignant melanoma (**2.92**), glomus tumours and myxoid cysts. Viral warts are common in the periungual site and vigorous treatment may damage nail growth.

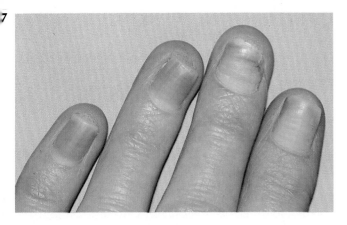

2.87 Yellow nail syndrome is a disorder in which there is progressive yellowing and thickening of the nails with absence of the lunula and a degree of onycholysis. There is often an association with a number of lung conditions and peripheral lymphoedema.

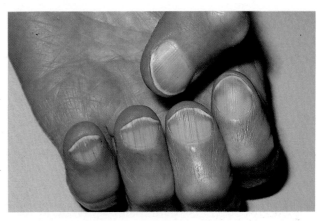

2.88 Leukonychia (opaque white nails) are a marker of chronic liver disease and of other conditions in which the serum albumin is low, such as nephrotic syndrome. In this patient, marked ridging of the nails is also present.

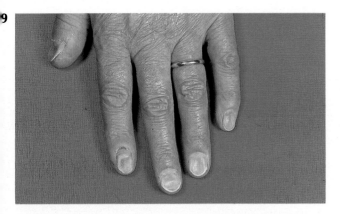

2.89 Koilonychia is usually a marker of underlying iron deficiency. The nails are brittle and spoon-shaped, as is particularly evident here in the thumb and index finger. This middle-aged woman had long-standing menorrhagia.

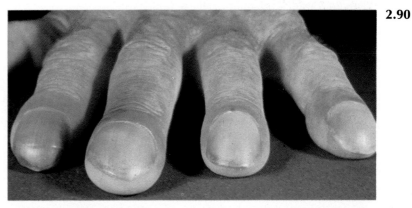

2.90 Gross clubbing of the nail in a 72-year-old man with carcinoma of the bronchus. Note the so-called 'nicotine sign'—staining of the index and middle finger by tar from his heavy cigarette smoking.

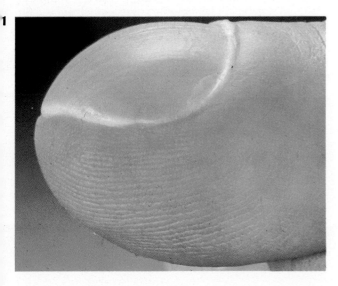

2.91 Gross clubbing of the nail. Note the filling-in of the nail fold, the increased curvature of the nail in both directions, giving a 'beaked' appearance, and the increased volume of the finger pulp.

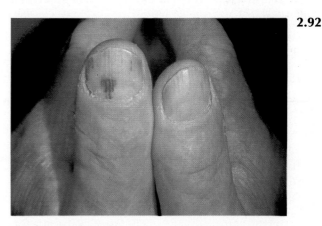

2.92 Subungual melanoma. A persistent dark lesion below a nail should be biopsied, as this is a common site for malignant melanoma.

Skin tumours

Skin tumours are common and may originate from the epidermis, melanocytes or any of the dermal components. Early detection of malignant tumours is vital.

Common benign tumours

Seborrhoeic keratoses or **basal cell papillomas** occur in the middle years, mainly on the trunk and face, with a roughened warty, greasy surface and a superficial, stuck-on appearance (2.93). Lesions may be multiple, sometimes heavily pigmented, and they can be traumatised. They are commonly misdiagnosed as malignant melanomas.

Skin tags are simple papillomas which occur round the neck and in body folds (2.94).

Milia are common on the face or at the site of healed blisters (2.95). They are superficial cysts of sweat ducts.

Keratoacanthoma (2.96) is a rapidly growing ulcerating tumour, more common in middle-aged or elderly subjects. It should resolve spontaneously within 9 months. Clinical distinction from a squamous cell carcinoma can be impossible.

If the history is uncertain, biopsy is essential.

Cavernous haemangiomata (2.97) appear at or soon after birth. Single or multiple lesions, of varying size occur at any site. Ulceration and trauma with haemorrhage can occur, but lesions are best left to regress spontaneously.

Capillary haemangiomata (port-wine stains), are present from birth and do not fade with age. Cosmetic camouflage may be needed, and unilateral facial haemangioma may be associated with cerebral haemangiomata in the Sturge–Weber syndrome (11.112).

Dermatofibromas (2.98) are more common in women, often pigmented, may be multiple and generally occur on limbs.

Keloids are persisting areas of exuberant scar tissue.

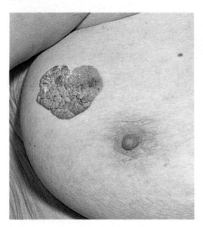

2.93

2.93 Seborrhoeic keratosis (seborrhoeic wart). These benign lesions are increasingly common with age, and they appear predominantly on unexposed Caucasian skin.

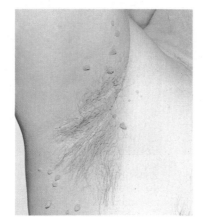

2.94

2.94 Skin tags in the axilla. These are small benign papillomas.

2.95

2.95 Milia on the eyelid. These are harmless, superficial, keratin-filled cysts, which are usually found on the face. In this location, it is important not to confuse these with xanthelasmas (*see* p. 339).

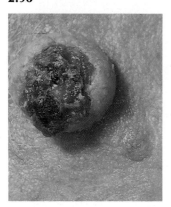

2.96

2.96 Keratoacanthoma on the neck. This ulcerating tumour, with a central keratin plug, grows rapidly but resolves spontaneously. Biopsy may be necessary to exclude a malignant lesion.

2.97 Cavernous haemangioma. 'Strawberry naevi' appear early in life and enlarge progressively. Parents can be reassured that most will resolve spontaneously before puberty.

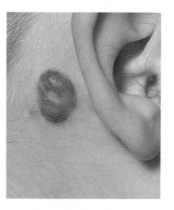

2.97

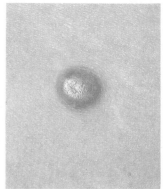

2.98

2.98 Dermatofibroma on the thigh. The lesion is raised, pink and firm, and is surrounded by a halo of hyperpigmentation. These benign lesions are often multiple on the legs and thighs in middle-aged women.

Melanocytic tumours

Congenital melanocytic naevi (moles) appear during the first few years of life. Most people have 20–30. Some have many more. The common mole should be uniformly pigmented, with a regular margin (2.99–2.101). Occasionally, congenital moles are large (greater than 1 cm) (2.102), multiple or confluent (bathing trunk pattern). These lesions carry a risk of malignant transformation. Moles deeper in the dermis appear blue in colour (2.103). Moles tend to regress in old age.

If moles change in size, become irregular in shape and pigmentation, itch or bleed they should be regarded as unstable and potentially malignant. Sunburn can irritate and activate moles. During pregnancy, moles tend to increase in size and darken.

Malignant melanomas (2.92, 2.104, 2.105) arise *de novo* or from pre-existing moles. The incidence of this tumour is increasing, especially in fair-skinned people with high sun exposure. The prognosis is much better if tumours are detected early. Melanoma may develop after some years in a lentigo (2.106). Amelanotic melanomas may be missed, especially in periungual sites.

2.99

2.100

2.101

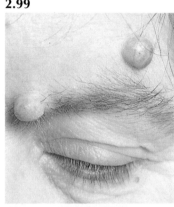

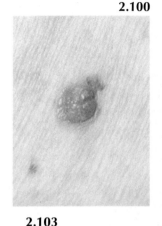

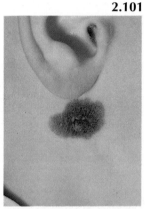

2.99–2.101 Benign melanocytic naevi (moles), showing a range of normal appearances. Pigmentation is even, but may vary from pale (2.99) to dark brown (2.101). There is no hint of malignant change in 2.99. The irregular margin in the lesion seen in 2.100 aroused sufficient suspicion for the lesion to be biopsied (2.1). Despite the slightly irregular margin, the mole in 2.101 is almost certainly benign; but, if it were to change in shape, pigmentation or size, or if it were to bleed, biopsy would be necessary.

2.102

2.103

2.104

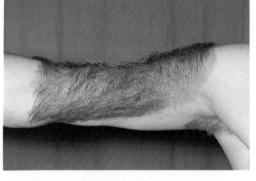

2.102 A large congenital pigmented melanocytic naevus. Note that hairs can grow in melanomas. Large lesions like this should be carefully observed for malignant change.

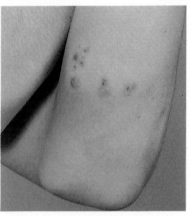

2.103 A group of blue naevi on the arm. These lesion are usually benign.

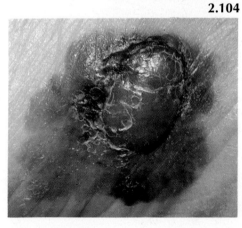

2.104 Malignant melanoma. Note the superficial spread in the skin and the varying level of pigmentation. The lesion had also bled. Prognosis depends on the depth of invasion of the tumour in the skin.

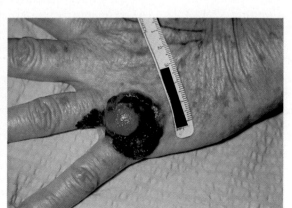

2.105

2.106

2.105 Malignant melanoma on the hand. The centre of the tumour is now amelanotic, but the local invasion remains pigmented and the patient has widespread secondary deposits.

2.106 Malignant lentigo. Lentigo is a flat, dark brown lesion on the cheek of an elderly person. It should be regarded as a melonoma-in-situ, and may become frankly malignant, as here.

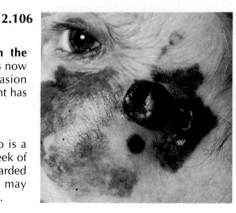

Non-epithelial malignant tumours

Secondary tumour deposits may occur in the skin (2.107). Common tumours that metastasise to the skin include breast, stomach, bronchus and kidney. Hodgkin's disease and B-cell lymphomas may have skin lesions.

Mycosis fungoides is a cutaneous T-cell lymphoma. It commonly presents as a patchy superficial dermatitis (2.108) that evolves slowly into plaques and tumours.

Kaposi's sarcoma is another important skin tumour. Formerly rare outside Africa, it has now become a common complication of AIDS, especially in male homosexuals (*see* p. 19).

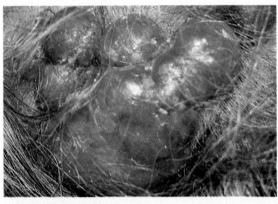

2.107

2.107 Skin secondaries, in this case in the scalp from a primary carcinoma of the bronchus. Such lesions are relatively uncommon.

2.108

2.108 Mycosis fungoides—an advanced case. The individual lesions grow slowly over a period of years. They are red, thickened plaques, often with fine scales, which are itchy, and may ulcerate.

Pre-malignant and malignant epithelial tumours

Solar keratoses (2.109, 2.110) occur on sun-exposed sites as patches of erythema and scale which gradually thicken. The adjacent skin shows signs of sun damage with wrinkling and loss of elasticity. Common sites are the face, ears and backs of hands. Malignant change occurs in a minority of lesions. Lesions on ears must be distinguished from chondrodermatitis nodularis helicis chronica: these lesions are characteristically painful.

Bowen's disease (2.111) appears as persistent erythematous, slightly scaly patches, which gradually enlarge. The surface is usually flattened and occasionally ulcerates. Patches may be multiple and occur on any body site.

Leukoplakia (2.112) presents as persistent white patches on mucous membranes, in the mouth or vulva, and may be an indication of underlying dysplasia.

Basal cell carcinomas are slow-growing, locally invasive malignant tumours (2.113, 2.114). The pearly margin, telangiectatic vessels and central ulceration are classic, but variations occur, multifocal and morphoeic lesions being less characteristic.

Squamous cell carcinomas occur on sun-exposed sites (2.115), often in areas of chronic scarring or inflammation, implicating a role for environmental carcinogens in their evolution.

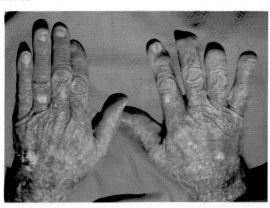

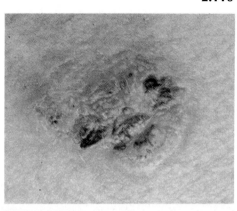

2.109 Solar keratoses—small, firm and scaly plaques—are commonly found on the extensor aspects of the hands and other exposed areas of skin in elderly people.

2.110 Solar keratosis. These lesions occur after long exposure to sunlight and are potentially malignant, with a latent period of at least 10 years.

2.111 **2.112**

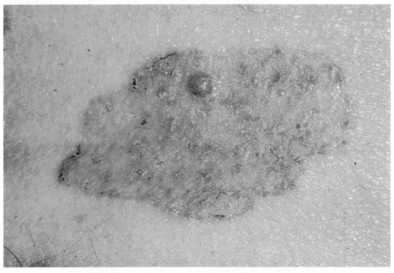

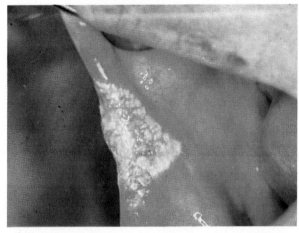

2.111 Bowen's disease—a persistent brownish patch which slowly enlarges and may become malignant. A carcinoma may develop under the crust or as a nodule, as here.

2.112 Leukoplakia may take several forms, all involving white patches on mucous membranes. In speckled leukoplakia, white areas alternate with areas of atrophic red epithelium. The risk of malignant transformation is high.

2.113 **2.114** **2.115**

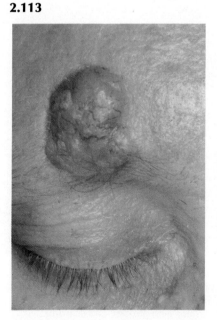

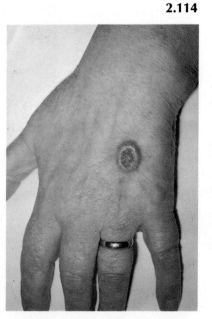

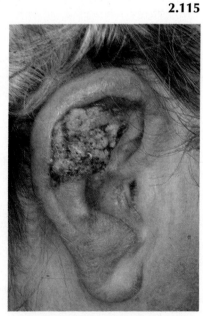

2.113 Basal cell carcinoma (rodent ulcer) begins as a slowly enlarging nodule.

2.114 Basal cell carcinoma ulcerates at a later stage, usually with a shallow ulcer, with a very narrow indurated edge and a smooth shallow base.

2.115 Squamous cell carcinoma begins as a small nodule, but slowly grows to produce the typical lesion seen here. The ulcer has thick edges and an irregular granular base; and it usually produces a serous discharge.

Vasculitis and connective tissue disorders

Vasculitis implies the presence of inflammation within blood vessel walls, with resultant vessel damage, haemorrhage or infarction. The clinical expression of this process depends on the size of the vessel involved, from capillaries to small muscular or larger arteries. Circulating factors may initiate the inflammation (immune complexes, cryoglobulins); the vessel damage ranges from endothelial cell swelling to fibrinoid necrosis of the vessel wall or a granulomatous response. Skin lesions of vasculitis tend to be purpuric and palpable, they may ulcerate and are painful.

Conditions where vasculitis is the predominant feature include Henoch–Schönlein purpura (2.116) (small vessel vasculitis, with purpura, arthritis, and glomerulonephritis—*see also* pp. 284, 458), polyarteritis nodosa (*see* pp. 148, 287).

Vasculitis may be a feature of drug reactions and of other diseases such as connective tissue disorders, drug reactions, malignant disease or infections.

Discoid lupus erythematosus (DLE) presents as chronic plaques, commonly on face, scalp or ears (2.117), with erythema, scaling and follicular plugging. Lesions persist, with scarring and depigmentation, but other features of LE are absent.

Systemic lupus erythematosus (SLE) may present with an acute facial rash of butterfly distribution (3.72, 3.73). The other features of SLE are described on p. 142.

Rheumatoid arthritis may be associated with vasculitis and subcutaneous nodules (3.26–3.28). It may also be accompanied by pyoderma gangrenosum, a destructive necrotic ulceration which may destroy large areas of skin (2.118). Pyoderma gangrenosum may also complicate other diseases, especially ulcerative colitis and Crohn's disease.

Systemic sclerosis has several skin manifestations (*see* p. 144).

Morphoea is a condition without systemic features. Scarring occurs in the skin (2.119) and may affect adjacent bone, but the condition usually resolves spontaneously.

Dermatomyositis commonly presents with skin features (3.85–3.87), as may other connective tissue disorders, including **relapsing polychondritis** (3.91).

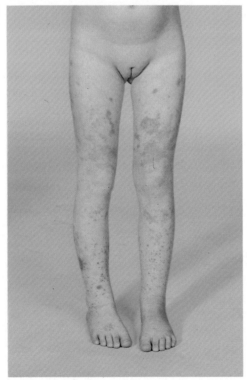

2.116 Henoch–Schönlein purpura, associated with swelling of the left knee and renal involvement in a child aged 4 years.

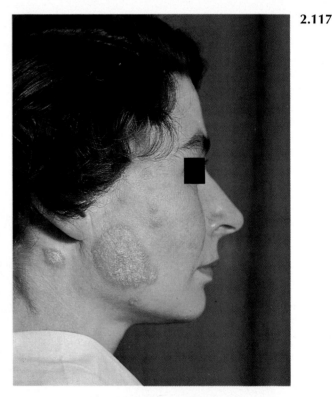

2.117 Discoid lupus erythematosus. Slowly enlarging recalcitrant pink scaly plaques are seen on the face, ears and scalp. The lesions are aggravated by sunlight, and they clear centrally with atrophy and scarring.

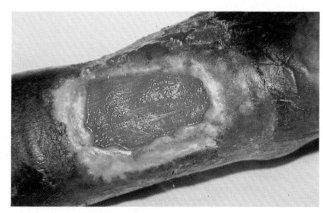

2.118 Pyoderma gangrenosum. This West Indian man developed a pustule over the lower leg which progressed to a tender, superficial necrotic ulcer. Note the typical purple undermined edge. The lesion persisted for months and partially responded to topical corticosteroids and minocycline. Eventually, it responded to systemic corticosteroids. No underlying disease was identified.

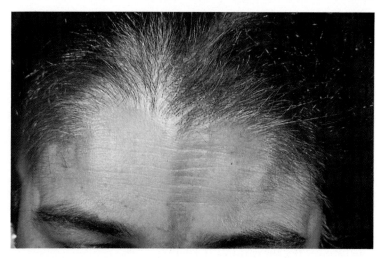

2.119 Morphoea 'en coup de sabre' (resembling the scar from a sabre cut). This form of localised morphoea can involve subcutaneous tissues and even bone. It is a variant of linear morphoea and, if the scalp is involved, can be associated with scarring and subsequent hair loss. Despite the severe local involvement, systemic sclerosis is not seen in this condition.

The skin in other multisystem disorders

A number of mutisystem disorders have cutaneous manifestations or complications. Many have already been mentioned, but others are also of importance.

Many **systemic infections** have skin manifestations (*see* Chapter 1), and a broad range of skin complications has been noted in HIV infection and AIDS (**Table 1.2**).

Diabetes may be associated with a number of skin conditions, including acanthosis nigricans (**2.76**), staphylococcal (**1.92, 2.37**) and candidal infection (**2.50, 2.51**), gangrene (**7.93**), and trophic changes, especially in the skin of the legs. Two specific, and probably related, conditions are seen most commonly in diabetics, though they may also occur in non-diabetic patients:

- **Granuloma annulare** presents as groups of flesh-coloured papules in rings or crescents, most commonly on the extensor surfaces of the hands and fingers (**2.120**).
- **Necrobiosis lipoidica** presents as erythematous plaques over the shins (**2.121**). These gradually develop a waxy appearance and a brown pigmentation. Care is needed to prevent skin breakdown and ulceration.

2.120 Granuloma annulare on the finger. Note the ring of flesh-coloured papules.

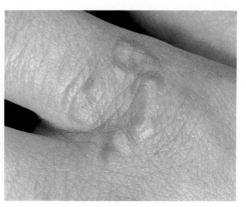

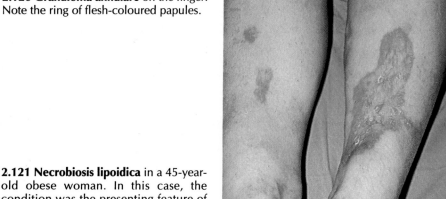

2.121 Necrobiosis lipoidica in a 45-year-old obese woman. In this case, the condition was the presenting feature of her diabetes. Note the surface scaling, scarring and some ulceration.

Drug reactions in the skin

Skin rashes are the most common sign of adverse reactions to drug therapy, although any organ system may be involved. Many drug reactions are not truly allergic in their nature, and it is important to distinguish between the characteristics of non-allergic and allergic reactions (**Table 2.3**). Drugs which have been frequently implicated in allergic reactions are listed in **Table 2.4**.

Drug therapy may lead to a wide range of skin pathology. The classic 'drug rash' is exemplified by the common reaction to penicillins (**2.122**), but its origin is not always truly or simply allergic. Patients with EB virus infection (glandular fever) are far more likely than others to develop a rash when given ampicillin, for example (**1.87**).

Morbilliform eruptions are common (**2.123**), and they may sometimes develop into severe **erythroderma** (exfoliative dermatitis), clinically indistinguishable from that found in other conditons such as psoriasis (**2.18**).

True immediate-type hypersensitivity to penicillin and many other drugs may lead to **urticaria** (**2.33**), **angioedema** (**2.35**) and life-threatening **anaphylaxis**. Similar reactions may sometimes occur through idiosyncratic direct release of mediators by non-allergic mechanisms.

Fixed drug eruptions are rashes or individual lesions which recur in the same site each time the causative drug is given (**2.124**). Sulphonamides, barbiturates and the laxative phenolphthalein are common causes.

Erythema multiforme is a rash composed of a symmetrical eruption of iris-like ('target') lesions, which may blister, affecting principally the hands and feet, but spreading proximally (**2.125**). The term is a misnomer, as the lesions are often surprisingly uniform. Erythema multiforme may be provoked by drug therapy, but it may also be the result of infections, malignancies or radiotherapy. It is a component of, and may develop into, the life-threatening **Stevens–Johnson syndrome** (*see* p. 60).

Another major drug reaction is **toxic epidermal necrolysis**, the 'scalded skin syndrome' (**2.126**). Drug allergy is the most common cause of this syndrome in adults. In other respects this resembles the childhood conditon, which is more commonly provoked by infection (**1.94**).

Erythema nodosum (**1.123**, **2.40**) may be provoked by drug therapy; so too may **vasculitic and purpuric reactions** (**2.116**, **10.8**, pp. 148, 455). Sometimes it may be difficult to determine whether these reactions result from the patient's underlying condition or the drugs used in its treatment.

Some drugs are used despite a known high incidence of rashes. Gold therapy may be used for its powerful effect in severe rheumatoid arthritis, for example, but it often provokes a psoriasis-like eruption, which may persist despite withdrawal of the drug (**2.127**).

A number of drugs may produce **phototoxic or photoallergic reactions,** in which only light-exposed skin devolps an abnormality (**2.128**). It is important to distinguish these patients from those with photosensitivity resulting from conditons such as SLE or porphyria.

Table 2.3 Differences between non-allergic and allergic drug reactions.

Difference	Non-allergic	Allergic
Quantities required to provoke reaction	Large	Minute
Cumulative effect	Often necessary	Usually none
Relationship between allergic effect and pharmacological action	Often present	No connection
Same effect reproduced by pharmacologically different chemicals	Rare	Common
Clinical picture	Uniform	Varied

Table 2.4 Drugs frequently implicated in allergic drug reactions.

- Aspirin
- NSAIDs
- Penicillins
- Sulphonamides
- Antituberculous drugs
- Nitrofurans
- Antimalarials
- Griseofulvin
- Hypnotics
- Anticonvulsants
- Anaesthetic agents

- Muscle relaxants
- Tranquillisers
- Antihypertensives
- Antiarrhythmics
- Iodinated contrast media
- Antisera and vaccines
- Organ extracts, e.g. insulin, ACTH
- Heavy metals
- Allopurinol
- Penicillamine
- Antithyroid drugs

2.122

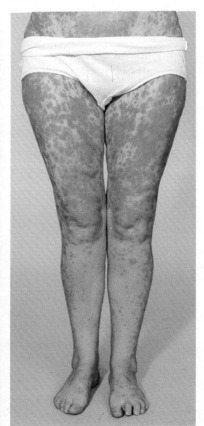

2.122 Ampicillin rash often presents as a symmetrical erythematous maculo-papular eruption. This patient had a history of previous penicillin rashes, which had not been taken into account when the ampicillin was prescribed.

2.123 A morbilliform eruption in a patient treated with co-trimoxazole. The offending agent here is usually the sulphonamide component, and similar rashes may occur when other sulphonamides are administered.

2.123

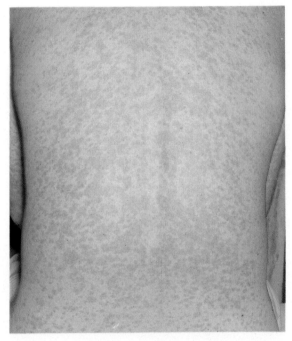

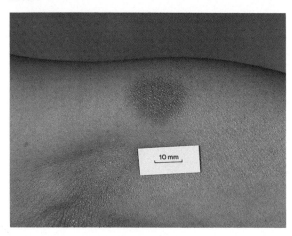

2.124 Fixed drug eruption, so-called because the lesion recurs at the same site after each administration of the causative drug. A common cause, as here, is phenolphthalein, found in various proprietary laxative preparations. The lesion is intensely itchy.

2.125

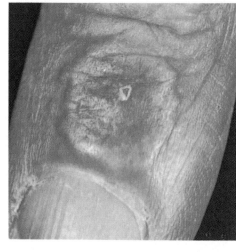

2.125 Erythema multiforme in a patient on sulphonamide treatment. This single. 'target' lesion was accompanied by others elsewhere on the hand and body, some of which showed central blistering.

2.126

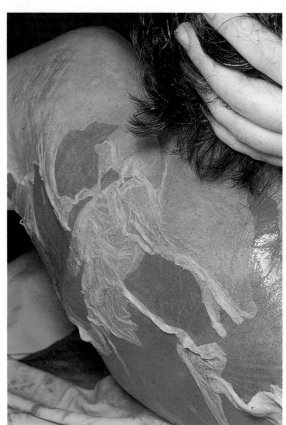

2.126 Toxic epidermal necrolysis, the 'scalded skin syndrome' in an adult. The most common cause is drug allergy.

2.127

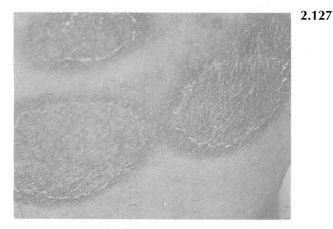

2.127 Gold sensitivity is most commonly manifest as a psoriasiform eruption. Gold rashes are not uncommon in rheumatoid patients, and they may persist despite withdrawal of gold therapy.

2.128

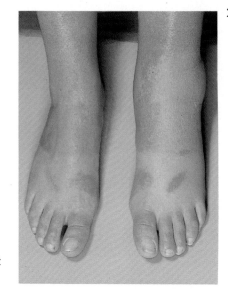

2.128 A phototoxic drug eruption, occurring in exposed skin not covered by footwear. This woman had been treated with doxycycline.

3. Diseases of joints and bones

History and examination

In a patient with joint disease, a detailed clinical history and examination is essential to determine the severity of the disease and the nature and extent of subsequent investigations.

The most common symptoms are pain and stiffness. In inflammatory arthritis, these are worse in the morning and are relieved by movement of the joint(s); and there is redness, swelling and an increase in skin temperature over the joint. These features are uncommon in mechanical joint diseases and pain is worse on use of the joint and towards the end of the day. It is relieved by rest.

Information regarding the number and the distribution of joints affected is important. For example:

- Gouty and septic arthritis tend to present as a monoarthritis (one joint) (**3.1**).
- Ankylosing spondylitis and enteropathic arthritis are oligoarticular (four or fewer joints).
- Rheumatoid arthritis (RA) and systemic lupus erythematosus (SLE) are polyarticular (five or more joints) (**3.2**).
- A proximal and symmetrical distribution is suggestive of RA.
- An asymmetrical presentation favours seronegative arthritis.
- In seronegative arthritis, there may also be axial joint involvement with spinal and lower back pain.

The variation of the symptomatology over time also provides useful diagnostic information. For example:

- RA tends to be relapsing and remitting.
- Osteoarthritis (OA) is usually persistent and insidiously progressive.
- Gouty arthritis is usually episodic.

Although most forms of arthritis are spontaneous in their onset, in some patients specific factors of aetiological importance can be identified. For example, trauma may precipitate an attack of gout and aggravate OA and an infection may cause non-specific polyarthralgia (rubella), Reiter's syndrome (genital or intestinal infection) or a septic arthritis (gonorrhoea).

Extra-articular features are also important:

- Skin psoriasis suggests psoriatic arthritis.
- Nodules occur in RA and gouty arthritis.
- Ocular symptoms may occur in most forms of arthritis, but their manifestations are different, e.g. RA patients may complain of dryness of the eyes, and seronegative spondyl-arthritis patients may have a history of transient conjunctivitis and/or iritis.
- The seronegative arthropathies are also often complicated by mucocutaneous lesions.

Joint function can be assessed by asking patients simple questions about difficulty in dressing and washing unaided, working in the kitchen, climbing up and down stairs, getting in and out of a car, etc.

Simple general observation will provide much information. The patient may have difficulty sitting on, or rising from, a chair, have an abnormal gait and show reluctance to shake hands in fear of pain. Distribution of joint involvement should be noted. On inspection of the individual joints look for erythema, swelling, deformity and muscular atrophy resulting from disuse (**3.3**):

- Deformities are classified as either fixed or reducible, and in accordance with their deviation from the normal anatomical position (e.g. valgus, varus, ulnar, radial, flexion, etc.).
- The range of active movement should be assessed, so that limitation of joint movement is noted before palpation.
- On palpation, joint tenderness should be noted. An increase in skin temperature indicates active inflammation. The type of swelling may be appreciated (thickened synovium has a boggy feeling; osteophytes feel hard and irregular).
- Joint effusion may be demonstrated (**3.4**) and crepitation can be felt (fine crepitation caused by bone and cartilage irregularities).
- Grip strength can be assessed either by asking the patient to squeeze the examiner's second and third digits or with a modified sphygmomanometer.

A comprehensive and systematic examination should also be carried out to reveal extra-articular features such as episcleritis, nodules (**3.26**) and vasculitis in RA; skin psoriasis and nail lesions in psoriatic arthropathy (**2.16**, **3.5**); iritis (**3.43**), mucocutaneous lesions and cardiac complications in ankylosing spondylitis; conjunctivitis (**3.6**) and urethritis in Reiter's syndrome; tophus deposition in gouty arthritis (**3.7**); and septic vesicular lesions in gonococcal arthritis (**3.8**).

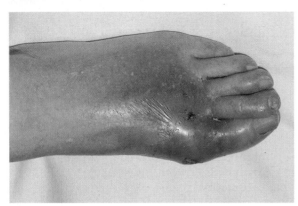

3.1 Monoarthritis. The acute onset of a hot, red, very tender metacarpo-phalangeal joint of the great toe is a classical presentation of gout (*see* p. 140).

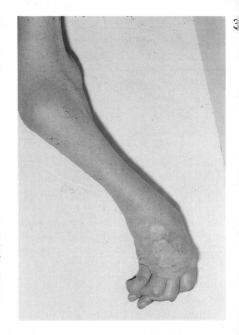

3.2 Polyarthritis in chronic rheumatoid arthritis. The finger joints are not acutely inflamed, but there is major residual deformity of the hand. The elbow joint is also severely disorganised. The end result is major impairment of hand and arm movement.

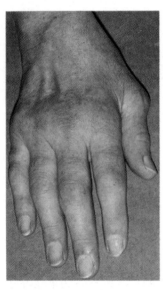

3.3 Rheumatoid arthritis. There is swelling of the metacarpophalangeal and the proximal interphalangeal joints, subluxation with ulnar deformity, and a fixed flexion deformity in the first metacarpophalangeal joint. Note also the disuse atrophy of the intrinsic muscles of the hands.

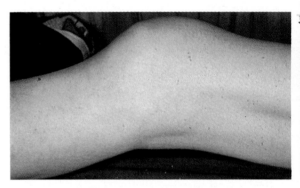

3.4 Knee effusion in rheumatoid arthritis. The knee is swollen, tender to touch, warm on palpation and is held in flexion. A patellar tap can be demonstrated, and the effusion can be confirmed by aspiration.

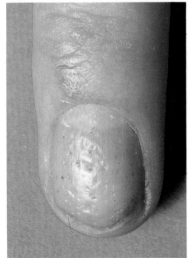

3.5 Pitting of the nails may be a clue to the diagnosis of psoriatic arthropathy. This patient also has a small psoriatic plaque on the finger. More severe nail changes may occur (*see* **2.16**).

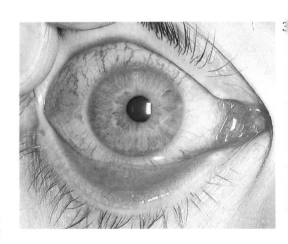

3.6 Conjunctivitis is a frequent extra-articular feature in many rheumatic disorders.

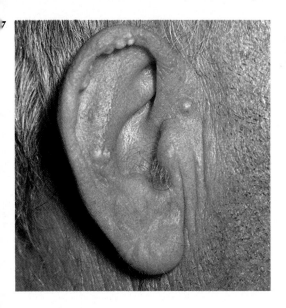

3.7 Tophaceous deposits in the ear are often a feature of chronic gout. They may discharge a thick toothpaste-like material, which can be shown on polarised light microscopy to be uric acid (*see* **3.12**).

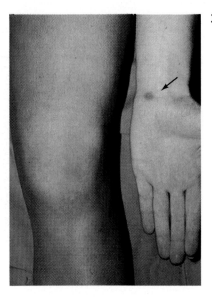

3.8 Gonococcal arthritis of the knee. The association of extra-articular skin lesions, such as the vesicular lesion seen here on the volar surface of the wrist (arrowed), with the arthritis points to a systemic infection.

Investigations

An investigative programme for the rheumatological patient may include: haematology, immunopathology, blood biochemistry, joint fluid analysis, and radiography.

Haematology

Full blood count

- Leucocytosis and thrombocytosis suggest an inflammatory process.
- A normochromic, normocytic anaemia may indicate a chronic disease such as RA.
- A microcytic anaemia (**3.9**) may indicate chronic gastrointestinal blood loss caused by the use of non-steroidal anti-inflammatory drugs (NSAIDs).

Erythrocyte sedimentation rate (ESR)

- A raised ESR or plasma viscosity suggests an inflammatory condition.

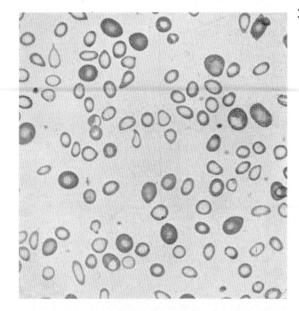

3.9 Microcytic anaemia in a patient with chronic rheumatoid arthritis. Most red cells have a central pallor (hypochromia) and a small diameter (microcytosis). The anaemia resulted from long-term gastrointestinal blood loss as a side-effect of non-steroidal anti-inflammatory drug use.

Immunopathology

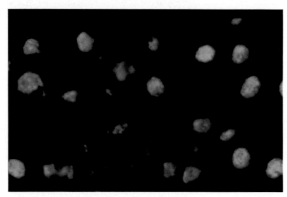

3.10 Antinuclear antibody as revealed by indirect immunofluorescence. The test serum came from a patient with systemic lupus erythematosus (*see* p. 142).

Rheumatoid factor

- Positive in 80% of patients with RA; high titres indicate aggressive disease.
- May also be found in other connective tissue disorders such as Sjögren's syndrome, SLE and systemic sclerosis.

Anti-nuclear factor (ANF) (3.10)

- Common in connective tissue disorders, but relatively non-specific.

Other subclasses of ANF

- e.g. anti-DNA antibodies in SLE, anti-RNP in mixed connective tissue disorder.

Blood biochemistry

Renal and liver function

- Abnormal function may indicate extra-articular complications and provide guidance to treatment.

Uric acid level

- High level may suggest gouty arthritis.

Calcium level

- Hypercalcaemia in sarcoidosis (uncommon) and in some cases of chondrocalcinosis.

Joint fluid analysis

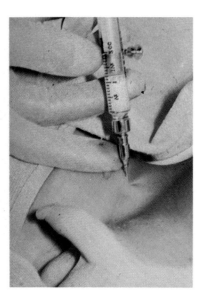

Naked eye appearance on aspiration (3.11)

- Colour, viscosity and turbidity; active synovial inflammation gives a thin turbid appearance.

Microscopy

- White cell count with differential—polymorphonuclear cells predominant in RA, gouty arthritis and septic arthritis; mononuclear cells predominant in OA.
- Under polarised light—urate crystals are negatively birefringent (**3.12**); calcium pyrophosphate dihydrate crystals are weakly positively birefringent (**3.13**).

3.11 Joint aspiration may yield valuable information. In this case, pus containing *Staphylococcus pyogenes* was aspirated from the hip joint of an infant.

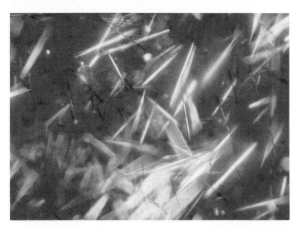

3.12 Polarised light microscopy reveals strongly negative birefringence in the needle-shaped urate crystals found in a joint aspirate from a patient with acute gout.

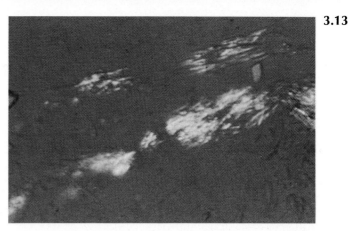

3.13 Polarised light microscopy reveals weakly positive birefringence in the rhomboidal crystals of calcium pyrophosphate dihydrate ingested by leucocytes, which are found in joint aspirates from patients with pseudo-gout.

Radiography

Plain radiographs
- Useful in assessing soft-tissue swelling, joint space loss, erosions, sclerosis, calcification, etc. (**3.14**, **3.15**).

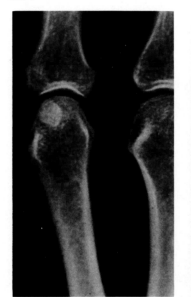

3.14, 3.15 Radiographs of the proximal interphalangeal joint showing progressive changes of rheumatoid arthritis from normality (**3.14**) to severe erosion (**3.15**). Note the loss of the joint space, the formation of exostoses, the irregularity of the articular surfaces (and the subluxation of an interphalangeal joint).

Other investigations

These are less often requested and include:

- Arthrography.
- CT scanning.
- MRI scanning.
- Arthroscopy and synovial tissue biopsy (**3.16**).
- HLA-B27 tissue typing.
- Scintigraphy.
- Thermography.

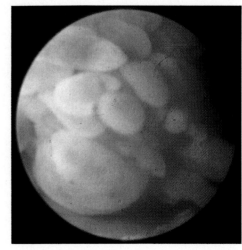

3.16 Arthroscopy can be easily performed in many joints. The procedure may give a visual diagnosis, allow confirmation biopsy and may also allow corrective surgery. Arthroscopy of the knee in this patient with rheumatoid arthritis revealed multiple synovial villi.

The Arthropathies

Rheumatoid Arthritis (RA)

RA is a common condition with a worldwide distribution, more prevalent in the temperate climates. In Western communities the prevalence is approximately 3%, with women more commonly affected than men (**3.1**), and the peak age of onset is 30–50 years.

The aetiology is unknown, but is most probably multifactorial. The high risk conferred by HLA-D4 and common family history suggest a genetic component. Environmental factors such as viral infections have been suggested. The initial pathology is synovitis with oedema, vascular dilatation and polymorphonuclear cell infiltrate. This is followed by lymphocyte and plasma cell infiltration and proliferation of the synovial lining cells. As the disease progresses, the synovial tissue becomes fibrosed and granulation tissue (pannus) develops and erodes the cartilage (**3.17**).

Over 70% of patients present with a bilateral and symmetrical polyarthritis (**3.18**), usually of insidious onset. All synovial joints may be affected, but certain joints are more commonly affected (**3.19**). Patients complain of joint pain, stiffness and swelling which are worse in the early morning. There may also be constitutional symptoms with general malaise and anorexia. The clinical course is that of relapse and remission.

Later, characteristic **deformities** of the joints develop:

- In the hands, there is subluxation and ulnar deviation (**3.18**) at the metacarpophalangeal joints. Swan-neck (**3.20**) and boutonnière (**3.21**) deformities occur at the interphalangeal joints. Dorsal subluxation of the ulnar styloid at the wrist is common, and may contribute to rupture of the fourth and fifth extensor tendons when there is also inflammation within the extensor tendon sheaths (**3.22**).
- In the forefoot, the metatarsophalangeal joints become dislocated. There is clawing of the toes and patients complain of a painful sensation like 'walking on pebbles' (**3.23**).
- Varus and fixed flexion deformities of the knees (**3.4**) are common and popliteal (Baker's) cysts are sometimes felt. Rupture of these cysts causes sudden calf pain with swelling which can mimic deep vein thrombosis (**3.24**, **3.25**).
- The disease also commonly affects the elbows and in more advanced cases the hips and neck.

3.17

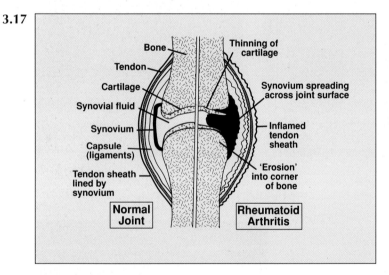

3.17 A diagramatic cross-section of a normal synovial joint (left) and a joint affected by rheumatoid arthritis (right).

3.18

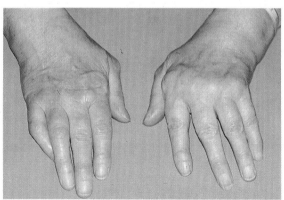

3.18 Advanced rheumatoid arthritis affecting the metacarpophalangeal and proximal interphalangeal joints of the hands. There is also wasting of the small muscles of the hands. Ulnar deviation and other deformities have occurred as a result of subluxation.

126

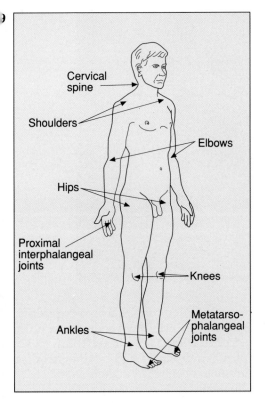

3.19 Joints commonly affected by rheumatoid arthritis.

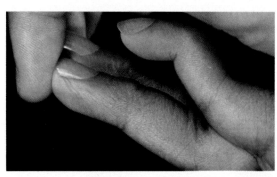

3.20 Swan-neck deformity is common in advanced rheumatoid arthritis. It is brought about by disruption of the volar plate of the proximal interphalangeal joint, sometimes with associated rupture of the insertion of flexor sublimis.

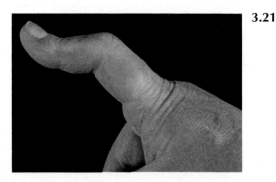

3.21

3.21 Boutonnière deformity. This common deformity in advanced rheumatoid arthritis results from the rupture of the central slip of the extensor tendon over the proximal interphalangeal joint. The lateral slips of the extensor tendon mechanism are displaced to the sides and maintain the deformity.

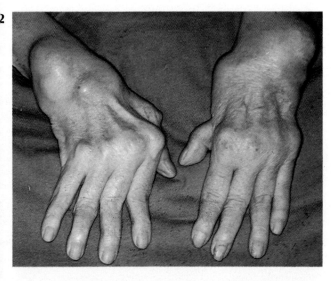

3.22 Severe advanced rheumatoid arthritis of the hands. There is massive tendon swelling over the dorsal surfaces of both wrists, severe muscle wasting, ulnar deviation of the metacarpophalangeal joints and swan-neck deformity of the fingers.

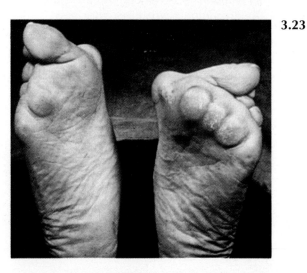

3.23

3.23 Rheumatoid arthritis of the feet. Gross destructive changes with multiple subluxations cause painful deformity which severely limits mobility.

127

3.24

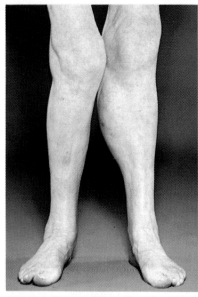

3.24 Advanced rheumatoid arthritis has resulted in a valgus deformity of the right knee and swelling of the left calf caused by the rupture of a Baker's cyst.

3.25

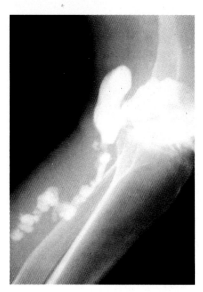

3.25 Arthrogram showing a ruptured Baker's cyst. Contrast has leaked from the Baker's cyst producing the clinical picture shown in **3.24**.

Patients may present with extra-articular features. These patients tend to have a poorer prognosis:

- Skin manifestations include subcutaneous nodules found over any bony prominence that is subject to external pressure, e.g. extensor surface of the elbow (**3.26**). Vasculitic skin rashes and nail fold and finger pulp infarcts are not uncommon (**3.27, 3.28**). Patients may also complain of Raynaud's phenomenon—a condition characterised by finger blanching (vasospasm), usually precipitated by cold or emotion (**3.29**, p. 255).
- Keratoconjunctivitis sicca (dry eyes) and episcleritis are common ocular manifestations (**3.30**). Scleritis and scleromalacia are rare but serious, as they can lead to eyeball perforation (**3.31**).
- Cardiac and pulmonary complications are usually limited to pericardial and pleural involvement (**3.32**). Rare cardiac complications may include constrictive pericarditis, myocarditis and endocarditis. Rheumatoid nodules may occur in the lung (**3.33, 4.103**). Diffuse fibrosing alveolitis (**3.32, 3.33, 4.120**), Caplan's syndrome (**4.115**) and obliterative bronchiolitis are uncommon pulmonary complications.
- Neurological manifestations include mononeuritis, which is a true extra-articular complication, and the carpal tunnel syndrome and cervical myelopathy, which are compression neuropathies secondary to the arthritis process. Involvement of the cervical spine can result in cord transection and sudden death if the neck is manipulated inadvertently, for example under an anaesthetic.
- In the kidneys there may be amyloid deposition, but clinical manifestations are usually limited to mild proteinuria with only very few patients developing nephrotic syndrome or renal failure.

3.26

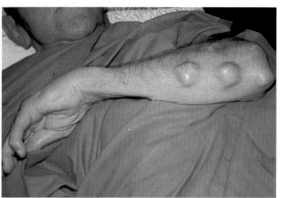

3.26 Rheumatoid nodules. The upper forearm and elbow are the most common sites for skin nodules in rheumatoid arthritis. These nodules result from vasculitis, and they may ulcerate or become necrotic.

3.27

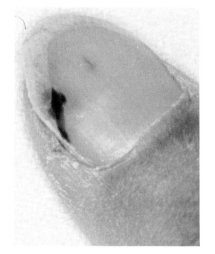

3.27 Nail bed infarction caused by vasculitis may occur in rheumatoid arthritis.

3.28

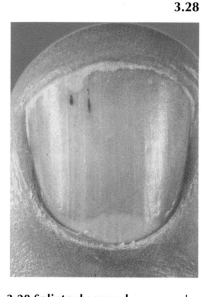

3.28 Splinter haemorrhages may be another result of vasculitis in rheumatoid arthritis, but they are a rather non-specific sign; they may be caused simply by trauma, and have little value in diagnosis.

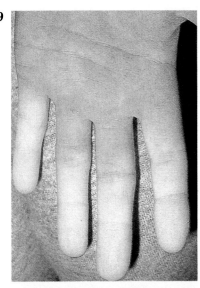

3.29 Raynaud's phenomenon, in which there is uncomfortable blanching of the fingers as a result of vasospasm, may occur in patients with rheumatoid arthritis and other connective tissue disorders.

3.30 Rheumatoid episcleritis may present acutely as a localised painful area of inflammation. It is the most common ocular complication of rheumatoid arthritis and indicates a poor prognosis.

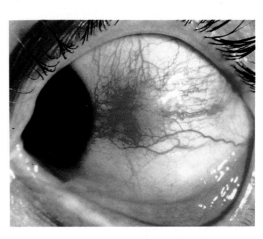

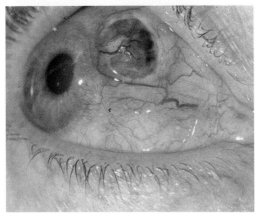

3.31 Scleromalacia perforans in rheumatoid arthritis. Long-standing inflammation of the sclera has resulted in thinning, which exposes the underlying choroid to secondary infection and the risk of eyeball perforation.

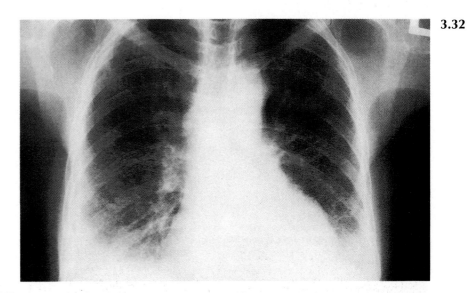

3.32 Pleural effusion is a common complication of rheumatoid arthritis, and it may precede joint symptoms. In this patient it occurred later in the disease, and was accompanied by some reticular nodular shadowing, representing early fibrosing alveolitis, in both lower zones.

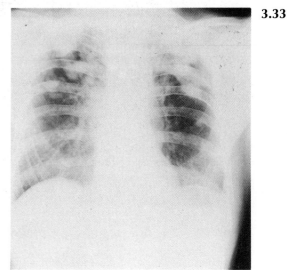

3.33 Multiple rheumatoid nodules in the lung. These nodules are more common in men. They may cavitate; and they may require further investigation to exclude the possibility of malignancy. This film also demonstrates some fibrotic changes in both lungs.

Immunological investigations show a positive rheumatoid factor (a circulating immunoglobulin of the IgM type) in about 80% of patients. The most common **haematological manifestation** is a normochromic, normocytic anaemia (*see* p. 426), but hypochromic anaemia may occur, especially where NSAID therapy has caused GI blood loss (**3.9**, **8.34**, **8.35**, p.425). The platelet and white cell count may be high and the ESR may be raised. Some patients may develop Felty's syndrome which is an association of splenomegaly and neutropenia with RA.

There may not be any radiological changes in the early stages, but later there is soft-tissue swelling and periarticular osteoporosis followed by joint space narrowing and periarticular erosions (**3.14**, **3.15**). In long-standing cases subluxation, secondary OA and bony ankylosis are seen (**3.34**).

The principles in the **management** of all forms of arthritis are similar. The main object is to reduce pain and enable the patient to maintain as near normal a life as possible. Physiotherapists can recommend appropriate exercises to maintain full joint movement and strengthen weak muscles. Wax bath, ice packs, ultrasound and weak electrical current stimulation (interferential therapy) may also alleviate some of the joint symptoms. Occupational therapists can advise on joint protection and can provide aids and appliances which allow sufferers to be independent.

The two main types of **drug treatment** used in RA are the non-steroidal anti-inflammatory agents (NSAIDs) and the so-called 'disease modifying anti-rheumatoid drugs' (DMARDs):

- NSAIDs are the mainstay of treatment but may produce upper gastrointestinal side-effects.
- DMARDs include gold in oral and injectable forms, penicillamine, sulphasalazine and hydroxychloroquine. They induce remission of the arthritis, but gold and penicillamine are particularly associated with high side-effect profiles such as bone marrow suppression, nephrotoxicity and hepatotoxicity. DMARDs should therefore be used only when first-line treatment fails or when patients develop extra-articular complications.

In advanced cases, immunosuppressive drugs such as low-dose methotrexate and azathioprine may be used. Corticosteroids have potent anti-inflammatory effects and may be useful in the treatment of an acute flare, although long-term use should be actively discouraged. Intra-articular injections of steroids are also useful in these cases, as is bed rest.

Surgery may have an important role, especially in the more advanced stages of RA. Useful operations range from the removal of local areas of diseased synovial tissue (**3.35**), to the removal of subluxed metatarsal heads, and the total replacement of hip, knee, shoulder and elbow joints or the small joints of the hands (**3.36**).

3.34

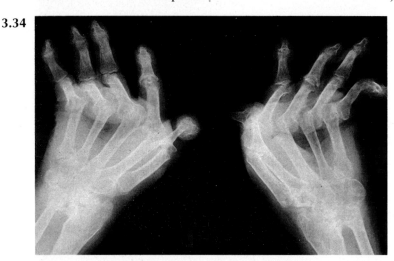

3.34 Radiographic appearance of severe rheumatoid arthritis in the hands. The bones are severely osteoporotic, and there are extensive destructive changes with subluxation of many of the finger joints. This radiograph corresponds with the degree of clinical change seen in **3.22**.

3.35

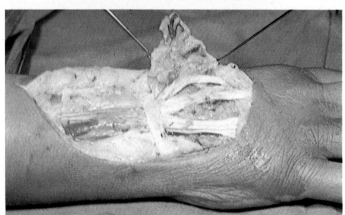

3.35 Surgical removal of diseased synovial tissue in a patient with rheumatoid arthritis.

3.36

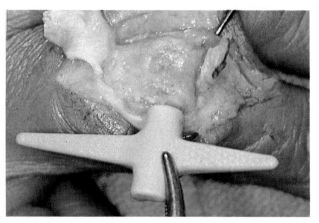

3.36 Proximal interphalangeal joint replacement. A prosthesis is assessed for size.

Juvenile chronic arthritis (JCA; Still's disease)

Arthritis is uncommon before the age of 16 years (incidence 0.7–1 per 1,000) although arthralgia is a common problem. The essential criterion for JCA is persistent synovitis in one or more joints for at least 3 months.

There are five main types of JCA:

- Systemic Still's disease has an equal sex incidence and is most common in 2–3 year olds. It is characterised mainly by systemic features including a high spiking fever, morbiliform rash, lymphadenopathy, hepatosplenomegaly and pleuropericarditis. Arthritis is usually a minor feature.
- Polyarticular Still's disease which is seronegative for rheumatoid factor (3.37). The features include micrognathia (secondary to temporomandibular joint involvement with abnormal mandibular growth) (3.38), loss of neck extension (cervical spine involvement, 3.39), unequal limb lengths (premature closure or overgrowth of the epiphyses) and fixed flexion deformities of the lower limbs.

- Pauciarticular (four or fewer joints) Still's disease which usually affects the large joints of 2–5-year-old girls. ANAs are usually positive and chronic iritis (3.40) may lead to blindness. Regular slit-lamp examination is necessary.
- Seropositive polyarthritis which resembles adult RA.
- Juvenile ankylosing spondylitis which is more common in HLA-B27-positive males of 10–15 years of age. The clinical features resemble those of the adult form, although back pain is not prominent.

Treatment is with NSAIDs. DMARDs may be effective in the polyarticular type JCA but are associated with a high incidence of side-effects. Corticosteroids should be avoided because of their retarding effect on growth. Physiotherapy and joint protection are important. Long periods of rest may sometimes be necessary.

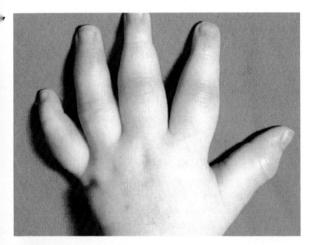

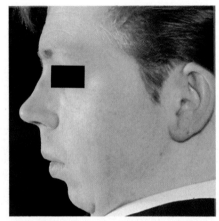
3.38

3.37 The hands in juvenile chronic arthritis. There is marked swelling of the proximal interphalangeal joints.

3.38 Micrognathia in a young adult who had juvenile chronic arthritis. The condition was associated with polyarticular Still's disease, and with cervical spine involvement (3.39).

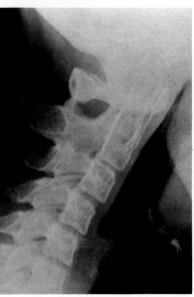

3.39 Cervical spine involvement in Still's disease. Ankylosis of the upper cervical spine is shown on this radiograph.

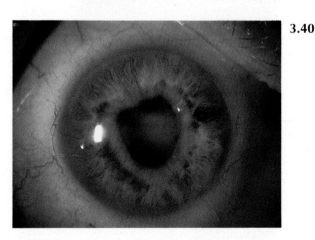
3.40

3.40 Iridocyclitis in pauciarticular Still's disease. Distortion of the pupil is caused by adhesion of the iris to the lens (posterior synechiae).

Seronegative spondarthritis

This term describes a group of conditions with a number of common characteristics. These include the absence of rheumatoid factor and other auto-antibodies in the blood, involvement of the spine, a peripheral inflammatory arthritis, similar extra-articular features (predominantly mucocutaneous) and a high incidence of the tissue antigen HLA-B27.

Ankylosing spondylitis

Ankylosing (fusion) spondylitis (spinal vertebral joint inflammation) primarily affects young males (9 males: 1 female); although cases in females are being increasingly recognised, they tend to have milder disease. The aetiology is unknown but there appears to be a strong genetic component. A family history is common and over 90% of patients possess the HLA-B27 tissue antigen. However, 7% of the population are HLA-B27-positive and the prevalence of ankylosing spondylitis is 1%. Thus environmental factor(s) are also likely to be important.

Low back pain with morning stiffness occurs as a result of sacro-iliac joint involvement. The pain is worse at rest and is often felt in the buttocks, especially when seated. It may radiate to the back of the thighs mimicking sciatica, although the latter is usually unilateral and relieved by rest. As the disease progresses upwards, pain is experienced at higher spinal levels. Thoracic spine involvement may present with pleuritic chest pain, but unlike true pleurisy it is usually bilateral. On examination, there is loss of lumbar lordosis and a fixed kyphosis usually compensated for by extension of the cervical spine, eventually producing the stooped 'question mark' posture (3.41). Sacro-iliac joints are tender on percussion and springing of the pelvis. Movements of the spine at various levels are restricted (3.42) and so is chest expansion. Changes in the peripheral joints, usually the larger ones, are similar to those seen in RA and show signs of inflammation. Extra-articular manifestions include iritis (30%) which may sometimes precede spinal involvement (3.43). About 4% of patients develop aortitis with signs of a collapsing pulse and the early diastolic murmur of aortic incompetence. Cardiac conduction defects occur in 10% of patients. Pulmonary restriction resulting from chest wall involvement and lung fibrosis (1.5%) may also be apparent.

Blood tests are often not very helpful. ESR may be raised but rheumatoid factor is not present in the blood. HLA-B27 tissue typing is not of diagnostic value and may be useful only in the difficult case. Radiological changes of sacro-iliitis include widening of joint space and juxtarticular erosion and sclerosis (3.44). In the spine there is squaring of the vertebrae caused by erosion of their corners. Syndesmophytes (bony deposition) form at the margin of the vertebrae. These may join together and produce the classic appearance of a 'bamboo spine' (3.45). There may also be radiological evidence of enthesopathy (calcification and new bone formation in the soft tissues) with erosions, sclerosis and soft-tissue calcification around the ischial tuberosities, iliac crests, greater trochanters, patellae and calcanea.

Physiotherapy is most important, and appropriate back exercises should be done daily in order to avoid spinal deformities. Hydrotherapy is also valuable. Pain control can usually be achieved by NSAIDs. Sulphasalazine, though not fully proven to be effective, may sometimes be used in advanced cases. Iritis may be recurrent, leading to severe ocular damage, and should be treated vigorously with topical steroids. Spinal irradiation, which was popular in the 1950s, is not used now because of risks of the later development of malignancy.

3.41

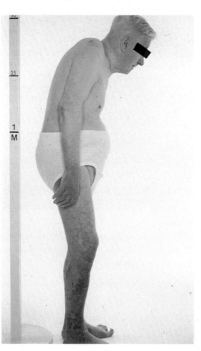

3.41 Advanced ankylosing spondylitis. Eventually, the trunk may become fixed in a fully bent position, so that the patient cannot see directly ahead—the classic 'question mark' posture.

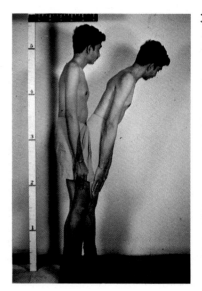

3.42 Ankylosing spondylitis. At an earlier stage the deformity is much less marked, but these superimposed pictures show gross loss of forward flexion on attempted toe-touching as a result of severe spinal involvement.

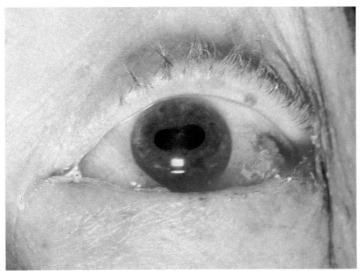

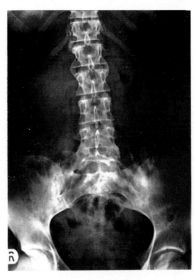

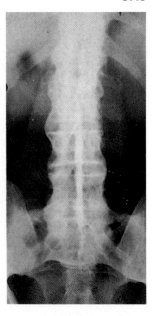

3.43 Acute iritis may be an early problem in ankylosing spondylitis. Note the irregular pupil and the haziness in the anterior chamber of the eye.

3.44 Sacro-iliac joint involvement in ankylosing spondylitis is often the earliest objective evidence of the disease. Initially there is blurring and later obliteration of the sacro-iliac joints. This radiograph also shows a relatively early stage of syndesmophyte formation with ankylosis between lumbar vertebrae.

3.45 'Bamboo spine'. This AP X-ray of the lumbar spine in advanced ankylosing spondylitis shows rigid ankylosis resulting from calcification of the spinal ligaments. The anterior spinal ligament is particularly obvious. The sacro-iliac joints are ankylosed.

Psoriatic arthropathy

This occurs in 7–8% of patients with psoriasis. There is a strong genetic influence and a family history is common. Skin psoriasis usually precedes the onset of the arthritis, but the reverse may happen occasionally. Skin lesions may be found on the scalp, behind the ears, in the umbilicus and the natal cleft, as well as in the common places such as the extensor aspect of the elbows and knees and the trunk (**3.46** and *see* p.91).

There are five forms of psoriatic arthropathy:

- The distal phalangeal type (**3.47**) is more common in males and is usually accompanied by nail lesions such as pitting (**3.5**), ridging, onycholysis (lifting of the nail—**2.16**) and hyperkeratosis.
- The polyarthritic form may be indistinguishable from RA but it is persistently seronegative.
- Oligoarthritis usually affects the knees or the other large joints with an asymmetrical distribution.
- A spondylitic form resembles ankylosing spondylitis and 60–70% of these patients are HLA-B27-positive.
- Arthritis mutilans (5%) is rare but severe (**3.48**) and is usually associated with extensive skin psoriasis.

The pathology is similar to RA but there is more fibrosis of the joint tissues resulting in ankylosis, and bony changes with periosteal inflammation producing the classical sausage-shaped digits (dactylitis) (**3.47**). Extra-articular features are rare. Features in the blood are similar to those seen in ankylosing spondylitis. There are no specific radiological features, but the distribution of the arthritis can provide an important guide to the diagnosis. Periosteal new bone formation reflects periostitis. The 'pencil-in-cup' appearance of the hand radiograph is caused by periarticular bone dissolution with cupping of the proximal ends of the phalanges and whittling of the distal bone ends (**3.49**).

Most patients have mild arthritis and respond to standard NSAID treatment. In more advanced cases, corticosteroids and immunosuppressive agents such as methotrexate or azathioprine may be required. Unlike RA, patients do not respond to penicillamine.

3.46

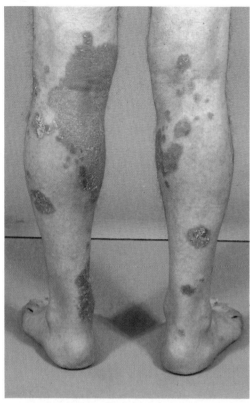

3.47

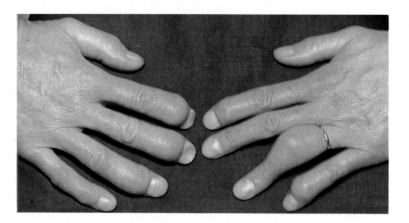

3.47 Psoriatic arthritis involving mainly the distal interphalangeal joints. There is also deformity and swelling of the left fourth proximal interphalangeal joint (dactylitis).

3.46 Typical psoriatic skin lesions on the legs. Not all patients with psoriatic arthropathy have such obvious skin lesions.

3.48

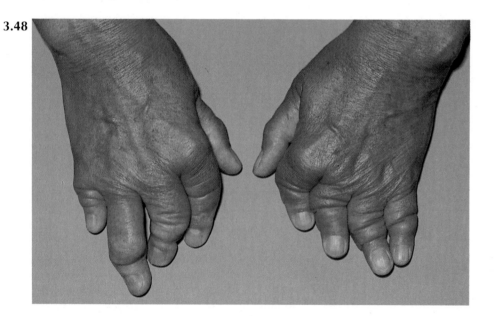

3.48 Severe psoriatic arthritis (arthritis mutilans). There is a gross destructive arthropathy, involving all joints of the hands and wrists. The phalanges have 'telescoped' (*see* 3.49), resulting in shortening of the fingers and gross impairment of function.

3.4

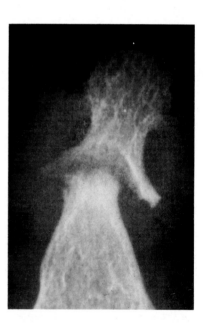

3.49 Pencil-in-cup deformity of the distal phalanx in psoriatic arthropathy. There is loss of the head and splaying of the base of the distal phalanx.

Reiter's Syndrome

This condition has a high male to female ratio (20:1) and up to 90% of patients possess the HLA-B27 antigen. It is likely to be a generalised reaction to an infection, either urogenital or intestinal, and is sometimes called 'reactive arthritis'. *Chlamydia trachomatis* has been shown to be the infective organism of the genital type, while the dysenteric form may follow infections by *Shigella flexneri*, *Shigella dysenteriae*, *Yersinia enterocolitica* and occasionally *Salmonella* species.

The classical symptom triad comprises **urethritis**, **conjunctivitis** (3.6) and **arthritis**, although all three may not be evident. The arthritis usually affects the large joints in the lower limbs and some patients (especially HLA-B27-positive) develop spondylitis. Extra-articular complications are common and involve the skin (keratoderma blenorrhagicum, 3.50) and mucocutaneous surface—mouth ulcers (3.51), circinate balanitis (3.52) and cervicitis.

The acute episode may take a month or longer to settle and patients often respond to conservative treatment such as NSAIDs. Iritis, if severe, should be treated with topical steroids. Later there may be exacerbations with remissions and up to 80% of patients may develop chronic joint disease, visual problems or urethral strictures. The urethritis can be treated by erythromycin or tetracycline, but neither alters the course of the arthritis.

3.50

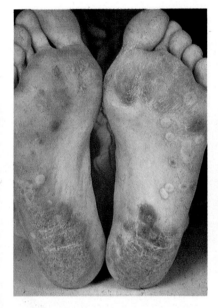

3.51

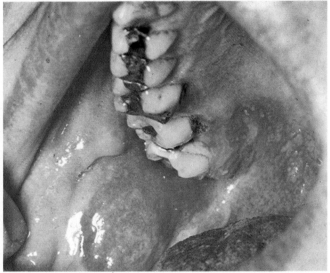

3.52

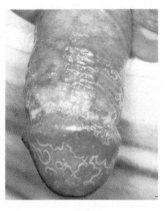

3.52 Circinate balanitis in Reiter's syndrome. Small, discrete, round or oval red macules or erosions often become confluent.

3.51 Reiter's disease, with vesicular lesions and erythema of the hard palate and lesions on the cheek.

3.50 Keratoderma blenorrhagicum in Reiter's syndrome. Pustular psoriasis may produce the same clinical and histological features (*see* p. 92).

Behçet's syndrome

This is a syndrome of unknown aetiology in which small blood vessels, especially small venules, become acutely inflamed. This results in areas of recurrent ulceration in many organs of the body, especially in the mouth and genitalia, inflammation in the eyes, acute inflammatory joint disease and central nervous system and gastrointestinal involvement. The disease has a worldwide distribution with a high incidence in Japan and the Middle East and this is associated strongly with HLA-B5.

Males are affected more often than females (1:2) and the common clinical manifestations are painful oral aphthous ulcers (3.53) which are recurrent and often heal without scarring. These are accompanied by genital ulceration (3.54, 3.55) and ocular symptoms caused by uveitis (3.56). The presence of uveitis and other central nervous system involvement carries a poor prognosis with a high incidence of blindness and death. Joint involvement is usually asymmetrical, acutely affecting the large joints of the lower limb which are not permanently damaged.

There is no specific therapy for the disease. Corticosteroids are of value in the management of acute uveitis.

135

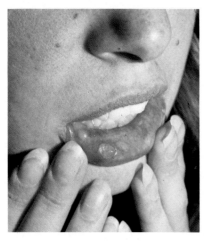

3.53 Behçet's syndrome. Acute ulceration of the lip, accompanied by scarring from previous episodes.

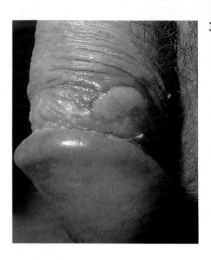

3.54 Behçet's syndrome. A typical penile ulcer, with an erythematous margin.

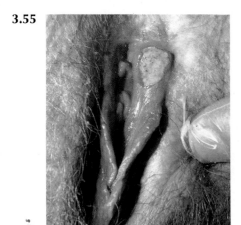

3.55 Behçet's syndrome. Ulceration of the labium minus in the same patient as in **3.53**.

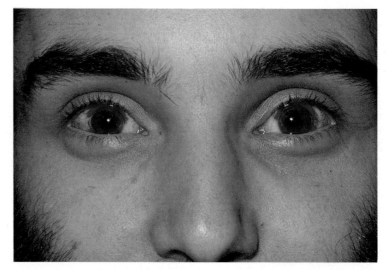

3.56 Uveitis in Behçet's syndrome is most common in patients who have HLA-B5. In this patient, there are severe changes with scleral haemorrhage.

Other seronegative spondarthritis

These include arthritides associated with inflammatory bowel disease (Crohn's disease and ulcerative colitis) and Whipple's disease, a rare malabsorption condition. Treatment of the bowel conditions often leads to remission of the arthropathy.

Infective arthritis

Infective arthritis may be caused by bacteria, viruses or fungi which usually are blood borne to the joint. A primary focus may be identified elsewhere, e.g. a boil on the skin or otitis media, etc. The common infecting organisms are shown in **Table 3.1**. Arthritis may be acute or chronic. Acute septic arthritis often involves joints that have been previously damaged by rheumatoid/osteoarthritis, or occurs in patients who are immunocompromised. The patient usually presents with fever and rigors; the affected joint is swollen, tender to touch and has an effusion (**3.8**).

There may be other clinical clues, e.g. purpura (*see* p. 455) and the joint may be held protected in flexion. In patients with pre-existing joint disease, there is often difficulty in deciding if the changes are caused by a flare-up of the basic disease or infection, in which case the diagnosis is made by joint aspiration of a purulent aspirate (**3.11**); there is usually systemic leucocytosis and blood culture may be positive.

Treatment with appropriate antibiotics is mandatory to stop cartilage erosion and repeated aspiration of the effusion or surgical drainage of the joint may be required.

Chronic infective arthritis may be caused by organisms such as *Mycobacterium tuberculosis, Borrelia burgdorferi* (*see* p.58) and a range of fungi. Tuberculous arthritis remains a problem in the elderly, in alcoholics, diabetics and those who are immunocompromised. In developing countries, TB remains a major public health problem associated with poverty, overcrowding and malnutrition. In areas of the world where AIDS is epidemic there has been a dramatic rise in the incidence of TB.

Tuberculous arthritis is usually caused by dissemination of the disease from lung or kidney. It usually involves a single joint—most commonly the hip, knee (**3.57**), sacro-iliac joints or intervertebral joints of the spine (**3.58**). The onset is insidious with systemic upset, malaise, anorexia, weight loss and night sweats followed by discomfort and swelling of the affected joint. There may be features of tuberculosis elsewhere in the patient, especially in the lung and kidney.

Diagnosis may be made by joint aspiration or synovial biopsy. Radiology is unhelpful initially, showing only soft-tissue changes, but with time there is progressive cartilage and bone erosion. Treatment is to immobilise the joint in the acute phase and give the appropriate antibiotic.

Table 3.1 Organisms commonly associated with infective arthritis.

Bacteria	*Staphylococcus*
	Streptococcus pyogenes
	Neisseria meningitidis
	Neisseria gonorrhoeae
	Salmonella spp.
	Pneumococcus
	Pseudomonas aeruginosa
	Borrelia burgdorferi
	Mycobacterium tuberculosis
Viruses	Hepatitis B
	Rubella
	Mumps

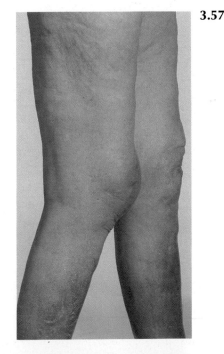

3.57 Tuberculous effusion of the right knee. In this patient, arthritis followed untreated pulmonary tuberculosis. The knee joint was destroyed, and arthrodesis was required. Note the signs of weight loss in the legs.

3.57

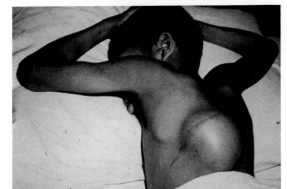

3.58

3.58 A 'cold' abscess may be the presenting feature of tuberculosis of the spine, as in this child who presented with a painless loin swelling. Such abscesses may be associated with tuberculosis of the intervertebral joints or with osteomyelitis of the spine (**3.120**).

Osteoarthritis (OA)

This common degenerative disease of the joints affects approximately 10% of all adults (men and women) and the prevalence increases with age.

The aetiology is multifactorial, although a polygenic inheritance pattern is recognised in the generalised 'nodal' form affecting middle-aged females. Mechanical factors include previous limb trauma, abnormal joint congruity, joint hypermobility, congenital dislocation of the hip and certain occupations—'wicket keeper's thumb', 'Zulu dancer's hip', etc. OA may also be secondary to metabolic disorders such as ochronosis, acromegaly and gout or to other inflammatory arthropathies, e.g. RA.

OA most commonly affects the weight-bearing joints, in particular the knees and the interphalangeal joints of the hands (3.59). The wrists, shoulders and ankles are less often involved. Not all patients with joint symptoms have radiographic changes; and not all radiographic changes are associated with symptoms. Pain can be severe and incapacitating and is worse on use of the joint and at the end of the day. Morning stiffness is not common, though stiffness after prolonged inactivity may occur. Clinical signs in advanced cases include crepitus, limitation of movement and joint deformities. The hands are often functionally affected (3.60). Heberden's nodes are found at the distal interphalangeal joints (3.61) and Bouchard's nodes at the proximal interphalangeal joints (3.62) of the hands. There may be valgus (knock knees) and varus (bow knees, 3.63), deformities of the knees and fixed flexion of the hip.

Blood tests are usually unhelpful, but they may sometimes reveal underlying metabolic disorders. X-rays (3.64, 3.65) may show loss of joint space resulting from cartilage damage. Osteophytosis (formation of new bone), altered bone contour, subchondral sclerosis (increased bone density) and cystic formation result from bony remodelling. There may also be soft-tissue swelling and periarticular calcification (calcium phosphate crystal deposition).

Treatment primarily involves pain relief, initially with simple analgesics. NSAIDs may be added if these are required, though the use of these drugs in the elderly population should be minimised. Intra-articular steroid injections are useful when there are signs of inflammation. Obese patients should lose weight. Appropriate exercises should be taught to strengthen the various muscle groups acting on the affected joint. Surgery may be considered when pain becomes intractable and severe limitation of mobility is present. Secondary causes should be sought and treated.

3.59

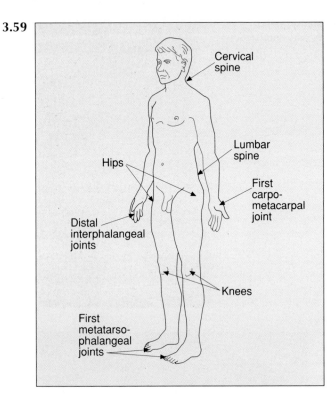

3.59 Joints commonly affected by osteoarthritis.

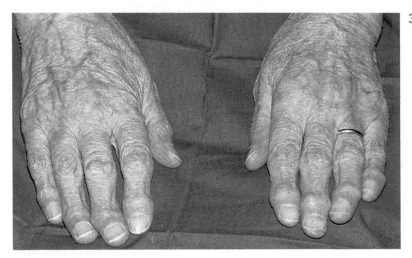

3.60 Osteoarthritis of the hands showing Herberden's nodes at the distal interphalangeal joints and Bouchard's nodes at the proximal interphalangeal joints.

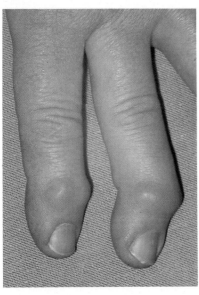

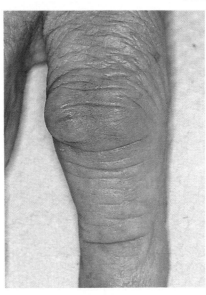

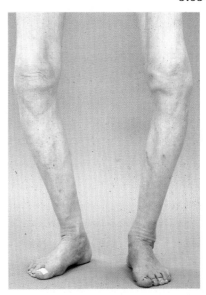

3.61 Herberden's nodes in OA are bony protuberances from the base of the terminal phalanx. They are usually painless, but may occasionally ache.

3.62 Bouchard's nodes in OA occur at the proximal interphalangeal joint.

3.63 Varus deformity of the knees may result from OA.

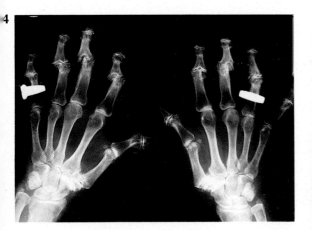

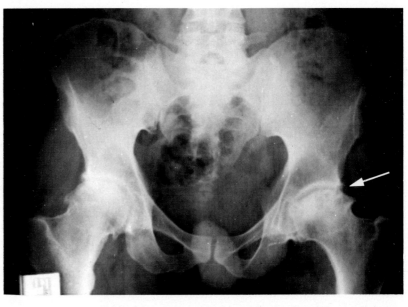

3.64 Osteoarthritis of the hands. This radiograph shows a moderately advanced case, with typical changes in the distal and proximal interphalangeal joints: loss of joint space, subchondral sclerosis, osteophytosis and subarticular cysts.

3.65 Advanced bilateral OA of the hips. Both hips show cartilage thinning and osteophytes around the femoral head. The left hip shows partial collapse of the femoral head (arrow). Hip replacement surgery may be necessary to relieve symptoms.

Osteochondritis

This is a rare disease of unknown aetiology, in which non-traumatic necrosis of bone and cartilage occurs, usually involving the fragmentation and separation of sections of the epiphyses. Most commonly involved are the tibial tuberosity, calcaneal apophysis, vertebral epiphysis and the femoral epiphysis (**3.66**). Treatment is by immobilisation of the part to encourage spontaneous healing.

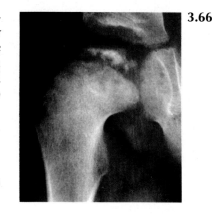

3.66

3.66 Osteochondritis of the femoral head of a young boy. In this age group and joint, the condition is also known as Perthes' disease.

Crystal arthropathy

Gout

This disease is most common in males and post-menopausal females. The classic history is of an abrupt onset of pain and swelling (usually at night) in the big toe with red, shiny skin overlying it (**3.1**, **3.67**), but any joint or joints may be affected (**3.68**). The serum uric acid level is high and joint aspiration reveals needle-shaped crystals (monosodium urate monohydrate) which appear negatively birefringent under a polarised light microscope (**3.12**). The acute episode subsides with desquamation of skin.

Uric acid is the breakdown product of the purine residues of nucleic acid. Two-thirds of it is excreted via the kidney and the rest via the gut. Most patients have primary gout, but possible secondary causes include:

- Increased dietary intake of purines, e.g. sweetmeats, offal.
- Over-production, as in the myelo- and lympho-proliferative disorders, carcinomatosis and the rare specific enzyme defects in purine biosynthesis and degradation, e.g. Lesch–Nyhan syndrome, a condition characterised by mental retardation and self mutilation.
- Decreased renal excretion in renal failure and with inhibition of the renal tubular excretion pathway, e.g. the use of thiazide diuretics, lead poisoning and in conditions causing acidaemia (diabetic ketoacidosis, starvation and excessive alcohol ingestion).

Not all patients with hyperuricaemia have gout. However, the likelihood of crystal formation increases as the uric acid level increases, more so at low temperatures, and this explains the peripheral distribution of gout. As well as the first metatarsophalangeal joint (70%), the small joints in the hands, wrists, ankles and knees are also often involved. During the acute phase, there may be a leucocytosis and the ESR is usually raised. Radiography of the joints shows soft-tissue swelling. In chronic cases, there are additional features such as joint space narrowing, subarticular (compared with RA which is periarticular) 'punched-out' cystic lesions and secondary osteoarthritic changes (**3.69**).

NSAIDs are useful during acute attacks. Intra-articular steroids are also useful. Colchicine is rarely used because of its side-effects. Chronic tophaceous gout, which is characterised by the deposition of urate (chalky, toothpaste-like appearance) in the periarticular and subcutaneous tissues (**3.68**, **3.70**), is now rare, as hyperuricaemia can be adequately controlled by allopurinol. The first metatarsophalangeal joint, other finger joints (**3.68**), the ear lobe (**3.7**), elbow and Achilles tendon are the most common sites involved. Allopurinol may aggravate gout during an acute attack.

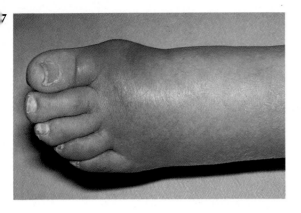

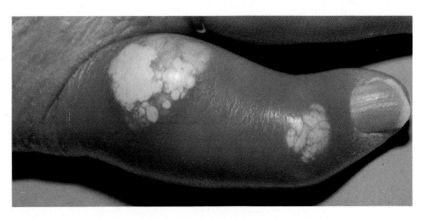

3.67 Gout. A classic attack of acute gout affects the big toe (*see also* **3.1**).

3.68 'Acute on chronic' gout in the little finger. The tophi helped to confirm the diagnosis. On aspiration, they were found to contain uric acid crystals (*see* **3.12**).

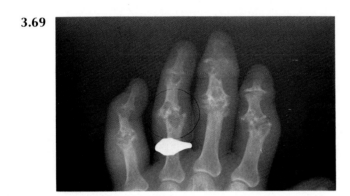

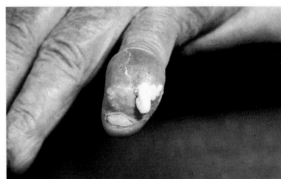

3.69 Gout. This radiograph of the hand shows destructive changes in the proximal and distal interphalangeal joints with multiple punched-out areas caused by urate deposition.

3.70 Chronic gout with a discharging tophus in the finger.

Pseudo-gout

This condition is characterised by the deposition of calcium pyrophosphate dihydrate crystals in the cartilage and synovium (**3.71**). There is no evidence of an underlying disease in most patients, but a metabolic disorder, e.g. hyperparathyroidism, hypothyroidism and haemochromatosis, may be found in some patients. Calcium pyrophosphate dihydrate crystals are rhomboid and weakly positively birefringent (**3.13**). The clinical features are similar to those seen in gout, although the onset is slower and the course milder. Conservative treatments such as NSAIDs and intra-articular steroid injections are usually effective.

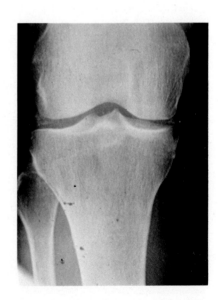

3.71 Chondrocalcinosis of the right knee. The radiograph shows calcification in both menisci.

Connective tissue diseases

The term 'connective tissue diseases' is synonymous with 'collagen vascular diseases'. Both describe a group of conditions characterised by the occurrence of vasculitis, multisystem involvement, arthritis or arthralgia and abnormal immunological features, e.g. autoantibodies and immune complex deposition.

Systemic lupus erythematosus (SLE)

This autoimmune disorder is uncommon in Caucasians (prevalence 0.1%), although it is being increasingly diagnosed with the development of more sensitive diagnostic tests. It is more common in other races, with a prevalence of up to 1 in 250 amongst black women. The peak age of onset is 20–40 years and females are more often affected (**3.72**).

The aetiology is unknown, but there is a slight increase in incidence in the families of patients with SLE and in subjects with the histocompatibility markers DR2 and DR3. The aetiological role of environmental factors, such as exposure to sunlight and certain viral infections, is being investigated but is not yet clear. Some drugs may produce a lupus-like syndrome (**Table 3.2**). Almost all patients possess an anti-nuclear antibody (ANA) against nuclear antigens (**3.10**). This is, however, a non-specific marker and may be found in other connective tissue disorders. The antibody to double stranded DNA (anti-dsDNA) is more specific and occurs in 60–70% of patients. The primary pathology is that of a multisystem inflammatory process, probably secondary to antigen-antibody reactions.

Patients may present with constitutional symptoms, such as anorexia, tiredness, fever and weight loss, and many organ systems may be involved:

- **Skin involvement** is most common (90%). Rashes may be local or generalised. The classic 'butterfly rash' on the face may occur in isolation (**3.72, 3.73**), but a more generalised rash may also occur—usually in sun-exposed areas (**3.74**). The inflammatory process may manifest itself as a vasculitis, with periungual infarcts (**3.75**), erythematous nodules, palpable purpura, livedo reticularis (**3.93**) and Raynaud's phenomenon (**3.29**) being common findings. Alopecia, localised or generalised, may occur (*see* p. 109).
- **Lung involvement** (40%) results in pleurisy and pulmonary infarcts.
- **Cardiac involvement** (50%) results in pericarditis, myocarditis and endocarditis (**3.76**).
- **Nephritis** occurs in 40–75% of patients and is often associated with a poor prognosis. The most common histological lesion is a diffuse proliferative glomerulonephritis (*see* p. 289).
- **Neurological complications** (30–35%) include epilepsy, focal neurological signs such as hemiparesis, aseptic meningitis, cranial and peripheral neuropathies (**3.77**) and psychiatric disturbances (**11.30**).
- **Blood involvement** may give rise to leucopenia, thrombocytopenia, lymphadenopathy and a thrombotic tendency which is more marked in those patients with positive anti-cardiolipin or anti-phospholipid antibodies.
- **Joint involvement** may resemble RA, but there is usually no evidence of erosive changes on radiographs.

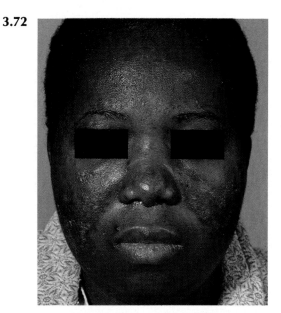

3.72 Systemic lupus erythematosus is most common in black women of child-bearing age, such as this 33-year-old West Indian woman who presented with a rash over her cheeks.

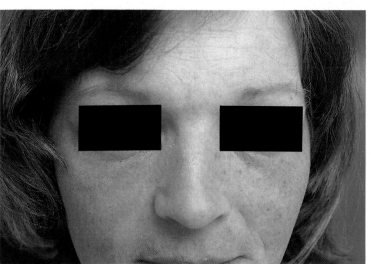

3.73 Systemic lupus erythematosus. The classic bat or butterfly wing rash in a white patient, who presented after a holiday in Majorca. The rash was fairly mild, but accompanied by severe polyarthropathy.

Investigations may show a raised ESR in addition to the above. ANA is present in over 90% of patients. Anti-dsDNA may also be present, as may other subclasses of ANF such as the anti-Ro and anti-Sm antibodies. The immunoglobulin levels may also be increased. The lupus band test on a skin biopsy may be of value (3.78). Radiography is usually unhelpful. Advances in diagnostic techniques and monitoring systems have improved both the morbidity and mortality (there is now a 95% 5-year survival rate in SLE from diagnosis). Patients should be advised to avoid excessive sunlight exosure. Sun-blocking creams can be very useful. Mild disease usually requires only symptomatic drug treatment, e.g. chloroquine is useful when there are troublesome skin lesions and for suppressing moderate joint disease. When the condition becomes active, systemic steroids and immunosuppressive agents, e.g. azathioprine and cyclophosphamide are the mainstay of treatment. Pregnancy is not a contraindication, but there is an increased rate of fetal loss and complications during pregnancy. SLE may flare during the post-partum period.

Table 3.2 Drugs which may induce a systemic lupus erythematosus-like syndrome.

Frequently	Rarely
Hydrallazine	L-dopa
Procainamide	d-Penicillamine
Isoniazid	Phenylbutazone
Phenothiazine	Reserpine
Oral contraceptives*	Quinidine
	Co-trimoxazole*
	Penicillin*

*May also exacerbate existing SLE.

Features of drug-induced SLE:
(1) renal and central nervous systems are rarely involved;
(2) the syndrome resolves on withdrawal of the offending drug.

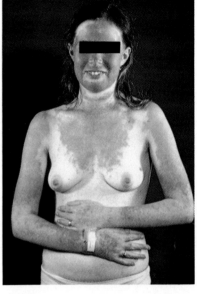

3.74

3.74 Systemic lupus erythematosus. A persistent erythematous rash may occur in sun-exposed areas.

3.75

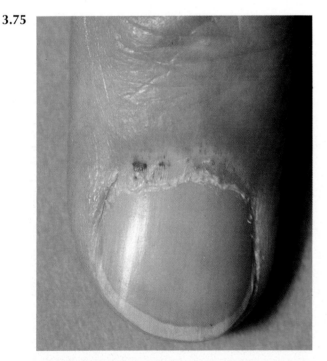

3.75 Erythema, telangiectasia and a small periungual infarct, together with ragged cuticles. These appearances are often seen in SLE, but also in other non-organ-specific autoimmune disorders such as dermatomyositis.

3.76

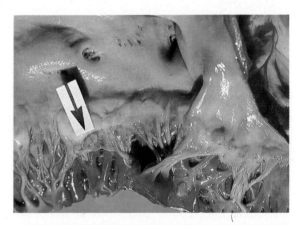

3.76 Cardiac involvement in SLE includes immune complex deposition and (arrowed) thickening of the heart valves (Libman–Sacks endocarditis). It can simulate rheumatic heart disease.

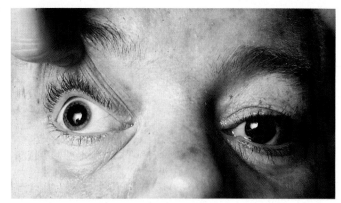

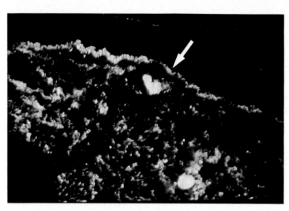

3.77 Third nerve palsy. The right eye faces 'down and out', the pupil is fixed and dilated and the patient has a unilateral ptosis (the upper lid is lifted here to reveal the other signs). Cranial neuropathy is a frequent neural manifestation of SLE.

3.78 The lupus band test demonstrates the deposition of complement and immunoglobulin in the skin at the dermoepidermal junction, shown here as a continuous band of IgM (arrow) by direct immunofluorescence (the background fluorescence in the dermis is not significant in this context). Non-lesional, light-exposed skin should be used for this test.

Systemic sclerosis (SSc)

This is an uncommon idiopathic multisystem disease, also known as scleroderma, which predominantly affects the skin and blood vessels. There is a female preponderance (female:male = 3:1). Progressive fibrosis and atrophy are the main pathological features.

There are two types of SSc:

- The **diffuse type** is characterised by skin and vascular changes and visceral involvement is common. The skin is thickened and tight and this sometimes results in contractures (**3.79**). Telangiectasia are a common feature (**3.80**), and Raynaud's phenomenon occurs in over 95% of patients (**3.29, 5.133**). It may be accompanied by calcinosis (**3.81**) and may lead to ulceration and autoamputation of the digits. Involvement of the locomotor system may present as myositis and polyarthritis. Involvement of the gastrointestinal tract may present as dysphagia (**3.82**), bowel distension, diarrhoea and weight loss resulting from malabsorption. Basal pulmonary fibrosis (*see* p. 194) develops in 45% of patients. Cardiac involvement may result in a restrictive cardiomyopathy or conduction defects. Renal involvement is associated with a high mortality, and patients usually present with proteinuria and hypertension, which may be malignant (*see* p. 294).

- The **limited type**, which has a better prognosis, is also known as the CRST or CREST syndrome and is characterised by calcinosis (**3.83, 3.84**), Raynaud's phenomenon, oesophageal involvement, sclerodactyly and telangiectasia (**3.80**).

There are no specific diagnostic tests. The ESR may be slightly raised and the full blood count may show an anaemia of chronic disorder. Both RA latex and ANA may be positive. The anti-scl 70 and anti-centromere antibodies are more specific autoantibodies and have been shown to be present in some but not all patients with the diffuse and limited types of SSc, respectively.

Treatment is symptomatic. Raynaud's phenomenon may be controlled by simple measures such as stopping smoking and using warm gloves. In more severe cases, vasodilator drugs such as nifedipine can be used. Antacids and/or H$_2$-antagonists are useful for patients with dyspeptic symptoms. Oesophageal dilatation may be useful in patients who have developed a stricture. Hypertension should be treated. Specific treatment for SSc has been disappointing. Penicillamine has been tried, but it probably has only a limited use in patients with rapid skin progression.

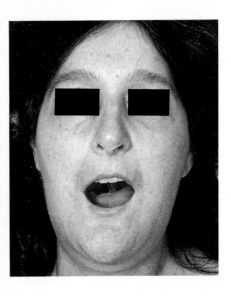

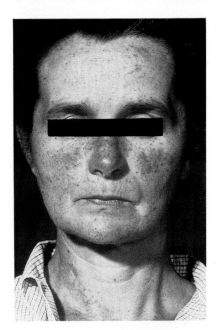

3.79 Systemic sclerosis. The skin around the mouth is tight, and the patient has opened her mouth as far as possible. Her skin is generally waxy and shiny.

3.80 Systemic sclerosis. Some puckering of the perioral skin is seen and multiple telangiectasia are visible on the face and neck.

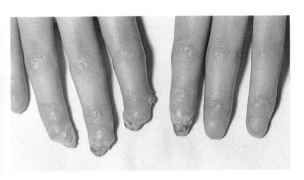

3.81 Calcinosis and sclerodactyly occur in digits with severe Raynaud's phenomenon, and the condition may sometimes progress to gangrene.

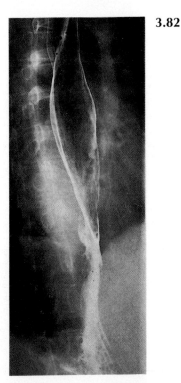

3.82 Systemic sclerosis affecting the oesophagus. The oesophagus is rigidly dilated, and there is loss of peristaltic movement.

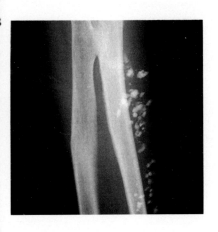

3.83 Calcinosis in the forearm of a patient with advanced systemic sclerosis.

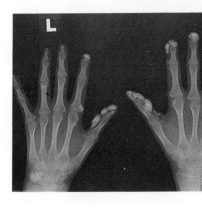

3.84 Calcinosis in the soft tissue of the fingertips in a patient with systemic sclerosis.

Polymyositis and dermatomyositis

These conditions are closely related to each other and are uncommon. The incidence is not known, but is probably comparable to that of SSc. There are five types:

- Primary dermatomyositis.
- Primary polymyositis.
- Secondary dermatomyositis/polymyositis (90% of cases have an underlying malignant condition).
- Childhood dermatomyositis/polymyositis.
- Dermatomyositis/polymyositis associated with a collagen vascular disease.

The cause is unclear, but a viral aetiology has been suggested, such as rubella, influenza and Coxsackie infections.

The proximal (shoulder and pelvic girdle) muscle groups are commonly affected and patients may have difficulty lifting their arms and getting up and down stairs. Involvement of the skin gives rise to a heliotrope rash on the eyelids with periorbital oedema (**3.85**, **3.86**). This rash may spread to the shoulders, chest, arms and hands. In the hands, Goddron's patches may be found: these are scaly, erythematous lesions on the dorsum of the hands, knuckles and extensor surfaces of the other small joints (**3.87**). Nail fold infarcts are common. Other features include dysphagia, arthralgia, calcification of the subcutaneous tissues and muscles (**3.83**), Raynaud's phenomenon (**3.29**), and myocarditis. Pulmonary involvement, in the form of fibrosing alveolitis or aspiration pneumonia, is accompanied by a high mortality.

Laboratory investigations reveal raised muscle enzyme levels, abnormalities in the electromyograph and inflammatory cell infiltration in muscle biopsy. Treatment is with high-dose steroids and/or immunosuppressive drugs such as azathioprine, cyclophosphamide and methotrexate. Bed rest is imperative in the acute phases. A search for an underlying malignancy is mandatory in all adult cases.

3.85

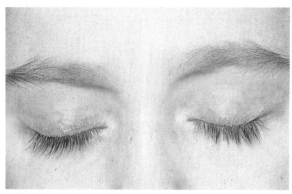

3.85 Dermatomyositis. Slight oedema of the eyelids with a red-mauve discoloration and some telangiectasia.

3.86

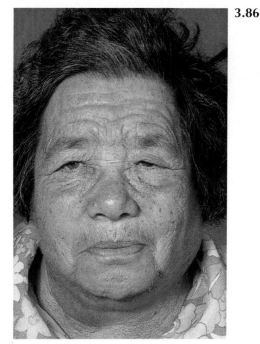

3.86 Dermatomyositis. This elderly lady has characteristic erythemia and oedema of the face. She also complained of proximal muscle weakness. Investigation revealed that she had an underlying carcinoma of the bronchus.

3.87

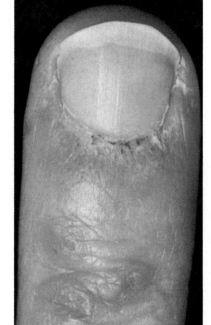

3.87 Dermatomyositis. Nail-fold erythema and telangiectasia with ragged cuticles are useful physical signs of non-bullous, non-specific autoimmune disorders, and are commonly seen in dermatomyositis and in SLE. Violaceous plaques and papules may also occur on the knuckles, knees, and elbows in dermatomyositis.

Sjögren's syndrome

This condition is characterised by dryness of the eyes (sicca syndrome) and mouth (xerostomia), caused by chronic dysfunction of the exocrine glands. Females (age 40–60 years) are more often affected (female : male = 9:1). It may occur alone or in association with RA or other connective tissue disorders.

Patients complain of burning and itchy sensation in the eyes and there is impaired tear production. Involvement of the salivary glands results in xerostomia (3.88) with difficulty in speaking and swallowing, and a high incidence of dental caries. The parotid glands may be enlarged. Any mucous membrane covered areas may also be affected, e.g. nose, throat, larynx, bronchi and vagina. Other features include pancreatitis, pleuritis, vasculitis, renal tubular acidosis and chronic interstitial nephritis. There is an increased incidence of malignant lymphomas.

Rheumatoid factor (70%) and other autoantibodies (anti-Ro and anti-La antibodies) may be present. Schirmer's tear test, a simple bedside test, can be performed to detect the diminished tear production (3.89). Staining with rose bengal solution may also be diagnostic as the superficial ulcers take up the stain (3.90).

No specific treatment is available, but artificial tears can be used to lubricate the eyes with good effect though artificial saliva is less effective. Attention should be paid to oral hygiene.

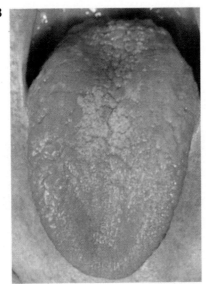

3.88

3.88 A bone-dry tongue—xerostomia —in Sjögren's syndrome. Xerostomia results from the involvement of the salivary glands.

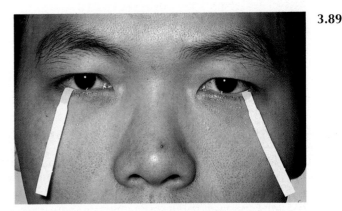

3.89

3.89 Schirmer's test for dry eyes. A strip of sterile filter paper of standard pore size is placed over the lower lid. The patient is asked to close the eyes gently, and after 5 minutes the length of the wet area is measured. Diminished tear production is present if it is less than 15mm.

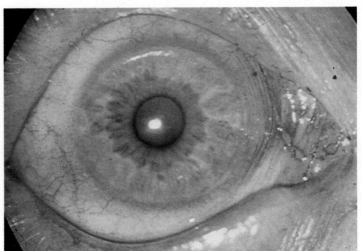

3.90

3.90 Rose bengal staining of the eye of a patient with Sjögren's syndrome. Tiny superficial ulcers have taken up the pink stain and are seen on the nasal side.

Relapsing polychondritis

3.91

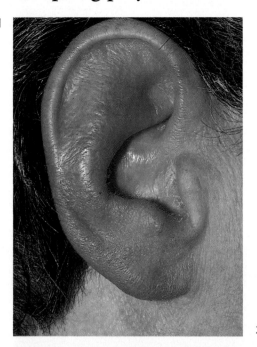

Relapsing polychondritis is a rare condition in which there is softening and collapse of cartilaginous structures. It often presents with painful swollen ears (**3.91**) and may also involve cartilage in the nose, respiratory tract and joints, and the fibrous tissue in the globe of the eye. Steroid therapy may control symptoms.

3.91 Relapsing polychondritis causing painful ears in a 58-year-old man.

Overlap syndromes and mixed connective tissue disease (MCTD)

Occasionally, patients may present with a constellation of clinical and laboratory abnormalities which fit into more than one disease profile. These patients are said to have an overlap syndrome and most common amongst these are disorders with features of RA combined with those of SLE, or of SSc associated with those of SLE and of polymyositis. In the latter group, antibodies to the n-ribose nucleoprotein (nRNP) may be found. These cases are often referred to as MCTD. This condition has a more favourable prognosis than that of SLE or SSc alone and often responds to small doses of prednisolone.

The Vasculitides

This is a mixed group of conditions characterised by inflammatory infiltration of the blood vessels. It may be localised or systemic and the pathology may range from simple inflammation to necrotising arteritis or granuloma formation. Blood vessels of all sizes may be affected, so there is a wide spectrum of presentation. Most cases are idiopathic, but some complicate other conditions as in the case of rheumatoid vasculitis, SLE and dermatomyositis/polymyositis.

Polyarteritis Nodosa

This rare condition primarily affects young males (age 20–50 years). Any small or medium-sized arteries may be affected. There is fibrinoid necrosis and polymorphonuclear-cell (in some cases eosinophil) infiltration with narrowing of the lumen and thrombosis. Local ischaemia and healing by fibrosis leads to the formation of small aneurysms (nodosa). The aetiology is unknown, but 20–40% of patients possess the hepatitis B antigen (*see* p. 398).

Clinical features include general malaise, weight loss and arthralgia. A purpuric vasculitic skin rash is common (**3.92**). Vasculitic digital infarcts are common (**3.27, 3.28, 3.75**). Patients may also present with livedo reticularis (**3.93**). Cardiac involvement may present as pericarditis, myocardial infarction or a persistent tachycardia. Pulmonary infiltration may occur (**4.101**). In the gastrointestinal tract there may be small bowel infarcts, haemorrhage and intussusception. Infarction of the gall bladder and pancreatitis may also occur. Neurological complications include mononeuritis multiplex, polyneuritis and occasionally subarachnoid haemorrhage. Half of these patients are hypertensive, which may be related to renal involvement, which is associated with a poor prognosis (*see* p. 287).

Investigations reveal an elevated ESR and a high white cell count, anaemia, hyperimmunoglobulinaemia and sometimes hepatitis B antigen. Anti-neutrophil cytoplasmic antibodies (ANCA), though not specific, may also be present. Biopsy of muscle or kidney shows fibrinoid necrosis of the wall of medium-sized arteries and arterioles with cellular infiltrates. Visceral angiography may reveal characteristic aneurysms (**6.62**).

Treatment is with high-dose corticosteroids, usually in combination with an immunosuppressive agent, e.g. azathioprine. The prognosis is variable. Although spontaneous remission may occur, death usually occurs in months to years as a result of renal complications.

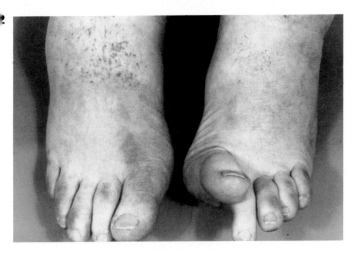

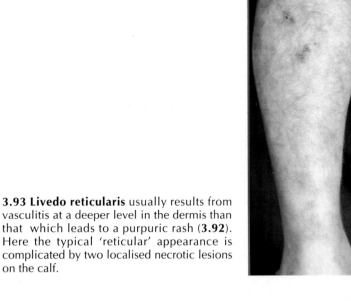

3.92. Polyarteritis nodosa. A vasculitic purpuric rash has developed over the dorsum of both feet and the patient has developed a mononeuritis—he is unable to dorsiflex his right toe.

3.93 Livedo reticularis usually results from vasculitis at a deeper level in the dermis than that which leads to a purpuric rash (**3.92**). Here the typical 'reticular' appearance is complicated by two localised necrotic lesions on the calf.

Wegener's granulomatosis

This is another uncommon condition of unknown aetiology. Small to medium arteries are affected and the pathology is that of necrotising granuloma formation. Wegener's granulomatosis consists of the clinical triad of upper respiratory tract granuloma, fleeting lung shadows and necrotising glomerulonephritis. Initial presentation may be rhinorrhoea and nasal mucosal ulceration followed by collapse of the nasal septum (**3.94**). There is later involvement of the lungs (*see* p. 193) and kidneys (*see* p. 288).

Corticosteroid therapy and cyclophosphamide may be of benefit but the prognosis is poor.

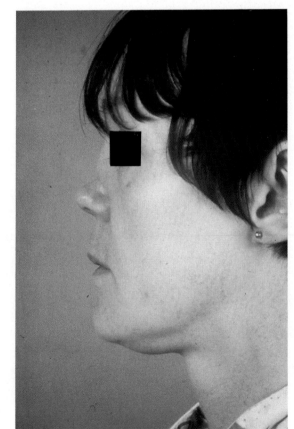

3.94 Wegener's granulomatosis. The classic appearance following collapse of the nasal septum resulting from granulomatous infiltration.

Churg–Strauss syndrome

This condition is like polyarteritis nodosa but less generalised. The small arteries and veins are predominantly involved and there may be extravascular granuloma formation. Patients present with hypereosinophilia and asthma, and chest radiographs show pneumonic-like shadows (*see* p.193). There may also be peripheral nerve involvement but renal complications are less common. Bronchospasm responds well to steroids.

Polymyalgia rheumatica (PMR) and temporal arteritis (TA)

PMR is a disorder which affects middle-aged or older patients. It is often of abrupt onset and presents with fever, malaise, weight loss and pain and stiffness in the proximal (shoulder–pelvic girdle) muscles. Patients have difficulty getting out of bed and walking up and down the stairs. Full blood count reveals a normochromic, normocytic anaemia and the ESR is almost always elevated. The course of treated PMR is usually limited to 1–2 years.

PMR and TA are described together as they often coexist. TA is a synonym for giant-cell arteritis, which affects mainly the large arteries, most frequently the temporal artery, with inflammatory cell infiltration and giant-cell formation in all layers of the vessels. Involvement of the ophthalmic artery in TA may lead to blindness. Additional symptoms which may be present include: headache, which is usually unilateral and throbbing; visual disturbance; scalp tenderness; and jaw claudication. The temporal artery may appear thickened, tender and non-pulsatile (**3.95**). The ESR is characteristically over 100 mm in the first hour. Temporal artery biopsy may show giant-cell lesions (**3.96**), but these are patchy and a negative biopsy does not rule out the diagnosis.

If TA is suspected, treatment with high-dose corticosteroids (e.g. prednisolone 60 mg/day) should be started immediately, before any biopsy results are available, in order to prevent irreversible blindness. The dose should be continued for several weeks before tapering down. Lower doses of steroid (e.g. prednisolone 10–15 mg/day) may be used with good response if there is polymyalgia without cranial symptoms. The steroid dose should be very slowly reduced over the course of 1–2 years, using the ESR and clinical symptoms as guides to disease activity.

3.95

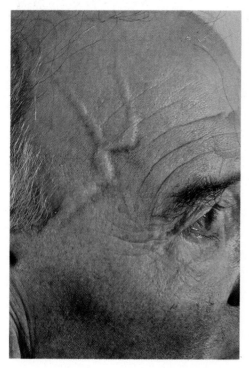

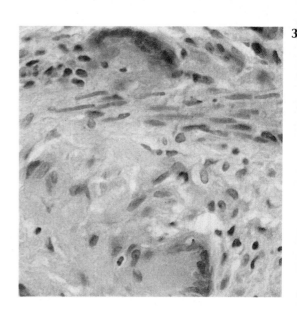

3.95 Temporal arteritis. The right temporal artery is dilated in this 74-year-old man who had severe headache, burning and tenderness over the artery and visual disturbance. Biopsy was diagnostic of temporal arteritis.

3.96 Temporal arteritis. The histological appearance of a temporal artery biopsy is diagnostic. All layers of the vessel are involved with inflammatory cell infiltration and this high-power view shows two characteristic giant cells.

Ehlers–Danlos syndrome

The Ehlers–Danlos syndrome is a group of rare inherited disorders of connective tissue in which patients have hyperextensible skin, hypermobile joints, fragile tissues and a bleeding diathesis associated with poor wound healing. There are many subtypes associated with a range of collagen defects; the common ones are transmitted as autosomal dominant traits. Type 1 has been widely described clinically and has the most severe manifestations. The extremely hyperextensible skin (**3.97**) and the hypermobile joints (**3.98**) were often features found in side shows (India-rubber man). With time, the skin becomes redundant and sags, particularly over joints. It is liable to bleed and wound healing is defective: this results in large pigmented scars especially over the knees and elbows. As all tissues are involved, a wide range of signs may be found, including retinal detachment, blue sclerae, dislocated lens, mitral valve prolapse, conduction defects, and aneurysm formation caused by defects in large arteries. No specific treatment is available to correct the defects, but advice should be given for skin and joint protection.

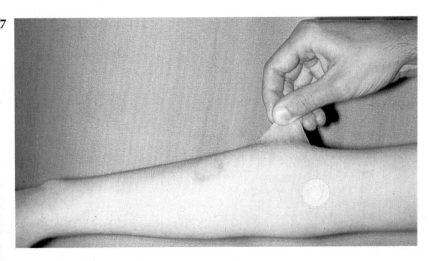

3.97 Ehlers–Danlos syndrome showing hyperelasticity of the skin.

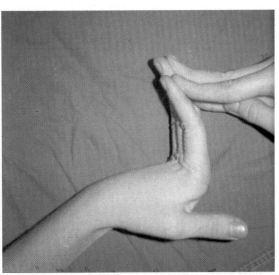

3.98 Ehlers–Danlos syndrome showing extreme extensibility of the fingers.

Diseases of bone

Bone is a collagen-based matrix with mineral laid upon it, and its strength depends on both components. The mineral phase is composed mainly of calcium, magnesium and phosphorus. Vitamin D, parathormone and calcitonin are important factors in bone mineralisation. New bone is deposited by osteoblasts and old bone resorbed by osteoclasts. Bone is a living and dynamic tissue, constantly remodelling itself throughout life.

Osteoporosis

Osteoporosis is the most common metabolic bone disease. Its frequency increases with age, and women are more commonly affected than men. The weakened bone fractures easily and accounts for much morbidity and indirect mortality in the elderly. There is an absolute decrease in bone mass (mineral and non-mineral) resulting from an increased bone resorption rate. However, the rate of bone formation and the quality and architecture of the bone are normal. The aetiology of most cases remains unclear, but the effects of ageing, failure of oestrogen secretion at the time of menopause, lack of physical activity, inappropriate secretion of parathormone or calcitonin, or some combination of these factors, may contribute. In other cases, direct causes may be found and these include Cushing's syndrome, diabetes, thyrotoxicosis, hypogonadism, RA (local osteoporosis), chronic renal failure and drugs such as glucocorticoids and long-term heparin.

Asymptomatic osteoporosis is common. In patients who are symptomatic, backache is a common complaint. There may be episodes of severe pain caused by fractures of the weakend bones. Collapse of vertebrae may result in loss of height (**3.99**). The lumbar and thoracic vertebrae, the upper end of the humerus (**3.100**), the lower end of the radius and the neck of the femur are the most common sites of fracture (**3.101**). The bone radiographs show loss of bone density, reduction in the number and size of trabeculae and thinning of the cortex. The lumbar and thoracic vertebral bodies become biconcave in shape, with anterior wedging caused by compression or collapse (**3.102**) Blood levels of calcium, phosphate and alkaline phosphatase are normal.

Treatment is unsatisfactory once the condition is established and prophylaxis is preferable. Any primary factor such as endocrine disease or the use of long-term corticosteroids should be corrected if possible. Hormone replacement therapy in the post-menopausal female is helpful if started early. Other prophylactic measures include regular exercises against gravity and adequate intake of vitamin D and calcium.

3.99

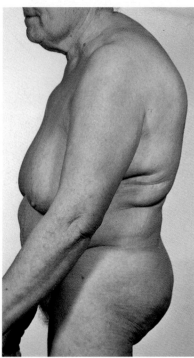

3.100

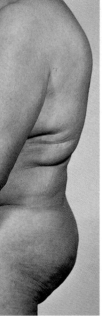

3.99 Osteoporosis results in loss of height, and vertebral collapse is associated with chronic backache, bouts of severe back pain and kyphosis (Dowager's hump). Creases often appear in the skin, and the ribs may rub on the iliac crest.

3.100 Osteoporosis has caused a loss of cortical thickness and an opening up of the trabecular pattern in this radiograph of the humerus.

3.102

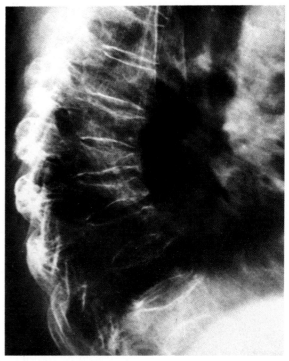

3.101

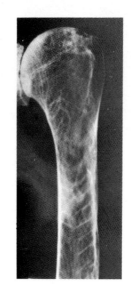

3.101 Osteoporosis is the usual underlying disorder in fracture of the neck of the femur in the elderly. This patient has a subcapital fracture, which may lead to ischaemic necrosis of the femoral head.

3.102 Osteoporosis leads to vertebral collapse. This radiograph shows wedge-shaped flattening of the vertebral bodies in the mid-thoracic region.

Vitamin D deficiency — osteomalacia and rickets

Deficiency of vitamin D in adults (osteomalacia) and children (rickets) is now fairly uncommon in the Western world although it may occur in Asian immigrants and the elderly, as a result of a combination of dietary insufficiency and lack of exposure to sunlight. It may also be caused by malabsorption of any cause, including previous gastric surgery, coeliac disease and deficient bile salt production. Other less common causes include chronic use of long-term anticonvulsants, liver and renal failure and familial conditions such as vitamin D-resistant rickets and X-linked hypophosphataemia.

The main function of vitamin D is to ensure an adequate concentration of calcium for the formation of calcium salts in bone. Deficiency results in poor bone mineralisation and a reduction in tensile strength.

Childhood rickets usually presents with bony deformity or failure of adequate growth. Signs include bossing of the frontal and parietal skull bones (**3.103**), delayed closure of the anterior fontanelle, rickety rosary (enlargement of the epiphyses at the costochondral junctions of the ribs), pigeon deformity of the chest and bowing or other deformities of the legs (**3.104**).

In the adult, osteomalacia may produce skeletal pain and tenderness and spontaneous bony fractures. Muscle weakness is often present and there may be a marked proximal myopathy.

In both conditions, tetany may be manifest by carpopedal spasm and facial twitching. Investigations show low or low-normal plasma calcium, low serum phosphate and increased alkaline phosphatase. Radiographs show rarefaction of bone (defective mineralisation) and translucent bands (pseudo-fractures, Looser's zones), especially in the pelvis, ribs and long bones (**3.105**). In children, there may be additional changes in the epiphyseal zone which becomes broadened (**3.106**). Bone biopsy may sometimes be required for diagnosis in adult cases.

Prevention is better than cure. Education and living standards should be improved in the susceptible populations. Free access to and adequate dietary intake of Vitamin D should be ensured. Supplements should be given to epileptic patients on long-term anticonvulsants. High replacement doses are required in patients with renal disease and those with vitamin-D resistance.

3.104

3.103

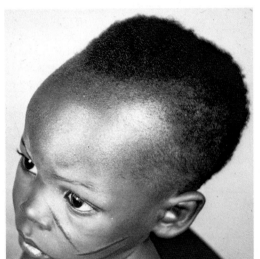

3.103 The skull in rickets. In infancy, the frontal bones are prominent and bossed. There is delayed closure of the fontanelles. The entire skull is soft to the touch and it can be distorted in a way which resembles a table tennis ball to which pressure has been applied.

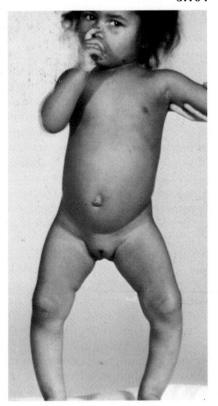

3.104 Rickets. Weight-bearing bones in the arms and legs show lateral and forward bowing.

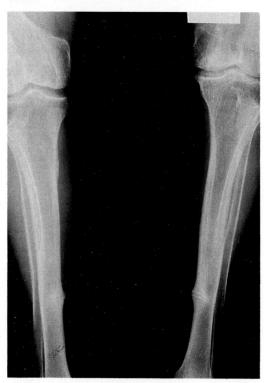

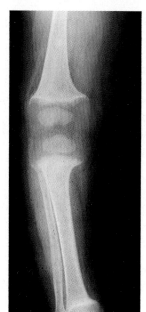

3.105 Pseudo-fractures (Looser's zones) at the lower end of both tibias in osteomalacia.

3.106 Rickets. In this radiograph of the right leg of a child, there is widening and cupping (a champagne glass appearance) of the ends of the long bones, increased space between diaphysis and epiphysis and poor mineralisation of the bones.

Hyperparathyroidism

Parathormone (PTH), from the parathyroid glands, controls the concentration of calcium and inorganic phosphorus in the blood. It raises the plasma calcium by enhancing the removal of mineral from the skeleton, increasing absorption from the bowel and reducing tubular reabsorption in the kidneys. It also increases the synthesis of vitamin D and lowers the serum phosphate by enhancing its excretion. Under normal physiological conditions, parathormone levels rise as the plasma calcium falls. Abnormally raised parathormone levels may result from a parathyroid adenoma (primary hyperparathyroidism) and conditions which cause a tendency to hypocalcaemia, e.g. chronic renal failure (secondary hyperparathyroidism). If secondary hyperparathyroidism becomes long-standing, the glands may become autonomous and continue to secrete excess parathormone (tertiary hyperparathyroidism).

Patients with mild hyperparathyroidism may be asymptomatic. Clinical features in the more severe cases are related to hypercalcaemia and patients complain of malaise, anorexia, nausea and vomiting, drowsiness or confusion. Peptic ulceration and acute pancreatitis may be the presenting features. Kidney involvement may present with renal colic from stones, haematuria or polyuria/nocturia from tubular damage. Bone pain suggests involvement of the bones and backache is common. Pseudogout may occur (*see* p. 141).

The plasma calcium may be high and the phosphate level low. Alkaline phosphatase is raised, reflecting increased osteoblastic activity in response to bone resorption. Radiological changes in the early stages include demineralisation or subperiosteal erosions in the phalanges (**3.107**). Cystic changes (**3.108**) are rare. A lateral skull radiograph may reveal a typical 'ground glass' appearance (**3.109**). Other radiological features include nephrocalcinosis (*see* p. 301) and soft-tissue calcification elsewhere. Calcification may sometimes be seen in the eye (**3.110**).

It is important to exclude other causes of hypercalcaemia such as malignancy (particularly multiple myeloma p. 465), sarcoid and drugs, including excess vitamin D. Detection of PTH by radioimmunoassay in the presence of hypercalcaemia is diagnostic of hyperparathyroidism and the second stage is the localisation of the tumour or tumours. The best approach is surgical exploration of the neck, which in experienced hands has a 90% success rate in locating and removing the adenoma. Other methods involve CT scanning, radionuclide scanning and selective venous sampling for PTH. Definitive treatment is surgical resection.

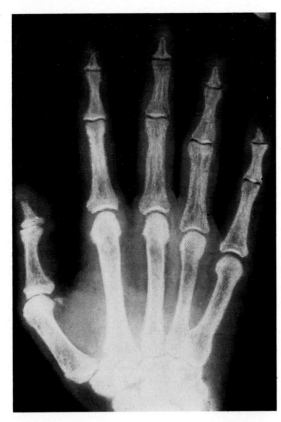

3.107 Hyperparathyroidism. There are subperiosteal erosions along the cortical surfaces of the middle and distal phalanges especially obvious in the index finger, and gross resorption of the distal phalanges.

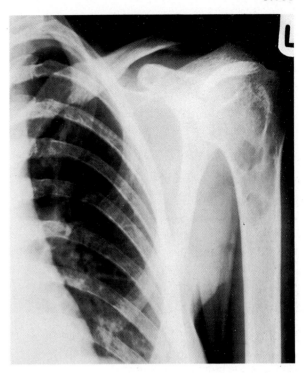

3.108 Hyperparathyroidism. A solitary bone cyst in the upper humerus. It is important to remember hyperparathyroidism in the differentiated diagnosis of bone cysts and tumours.

3.109

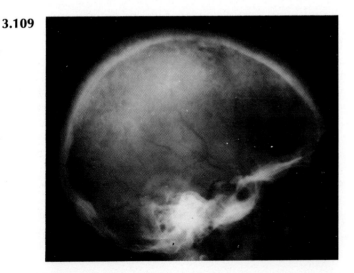

3.109 X-ray of the skull in hyperparathyroidism showing the typical granular or mottled (ground glass) appearance. Some cystic areas are also present—the so-called pepper-pot skull.

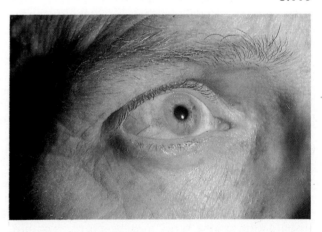

3.110 Ectopic calcification in the lateral and nasal margins of the right eye (band keratopathy) in a patient with primary hyperparathyroidism.

Renal Osteodystrophy

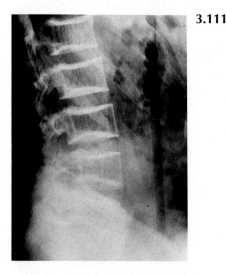

3.111

3.111 'Rugger-jersey spine' in secondary hyperparathyroidism caused by the demineralisation of the vertebral bodies, with simultaneous new bone formation at the subchondral plates.

Patients with chronic renal failure may develop various forms of bone disease. These include osteomalacia, hyperparathyroidism (secondary and tertiary) and osteosclerosis. Osteomalacia is caused by failure of the damaged kidneys to produce the metabolically active 1,25-dihyroxycholecalciferol. Poor absorption of dietary calcium and retention of phosphate lowers the serum calcium. This leads to the development of secondary hyperparathyroidism and, if this becomes long-standing, tertiary hyperparathyroidism. Clinical features and radiological appearances are as those described in the previous related sections. The cause of osteosclerosis, the third type of bone lesion, is less clearly understood, although it may be a direct result of excess parathormone. It produces the characteristic 'rugger-jersey spine', a radiographic appearance caused by the formation of alternate bands of sclerotic and porotic bone in the vertebrae (**3.111**).

Renal osteodystrophy can be partially prevented and treated. Aluminium hydroxide gel given by mouth binds phosphate and lowers its concentration, and vitamin D resistance can be overcome by giving the newer biologically active derivatives. Resection of the parathyroid glands is now rarely indicated.

Paget's Disease of the Bone

This condition, also known as osteitis deformans, is common in the elderly (up to 10%). The aetiology is unknown, but there is a weak familial tendency. Geographical clustering of this condition, e.g. in North Lancashire in England, emphasises the importance of environmental factors. There is an increase in osteoclastic activity, compensated for by an increase in osteoblastic activity which results in disorganisation of the normal bone architecture and an increase in bone vascularity. Any bone can be affected, but the legs and the axial skeleton (including the skull) are most commonly involved (**3.112**).

Patients are often asymptomatic and Paget's disease of the bone is commonly an incidental finding. Those who are symptomatic complain of constant and localised bone pain, unrelieved by posture or rest. There may be bone deformities such as frontal bossing (**3.113**), distorted facial features and bowing of the tibia (**3.114**). The affected bone may feel warm on palpation and a bruit may be heard. Complications include: blindness caused by nerve compression; deafness secondary to ossicular involvement or to nerve compression by the enlarging bone; secondary OA; and pathological fractures (**3.115**). High-output cardiac failure and osteosarcoma are rare but serious complications.

Investigations show raised alkaline phosphatase, reflecting the compensatory increase in osteoblastic activity, but normal calcium and phosphate levels. There is also an increase in urine excretion of hydroxyproline. Radiographs show lucency zones, caused by bone resorption and osteolysis, and areas of increased bone density (**3.115, 3.116**).

Drug treatment is indicated only when patients become symptomatic or develop complications. In such cases, calcitonin and diphosphonates may be used. Conservative measures, such as the use of simple analgesics, physiotherapy and correction of inequality of leg length, are also required.

3.112

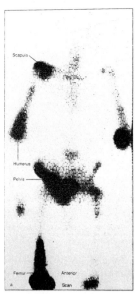

3.112 Paget's disease. In this isotope bone scan, the dark areas indicate bone which is affected by Paget's disease.

3.113

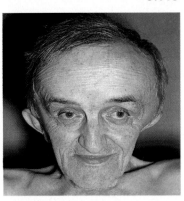

3.113 Paget's disease. Frontal bossing of the skull leads to a distorted facial appearance. This patient has gross changes and he presented with deafness secondary to ossicular involvement.

3.114

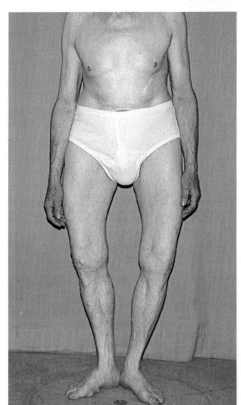

3.114 Paget's disease. Bone deformity has led to bowing of the legs and compression of the trunk, giving the appearance of relatively long arms.

3.115

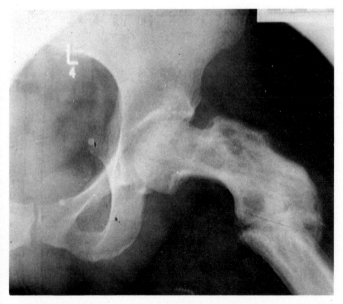

3.115 Paget's disease, with a pathological fracture of the upper femoral shaft. Lucency zones and areas of increased bone density are seen.

3.116

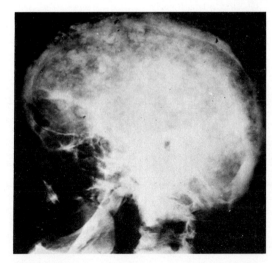

3.116 Skull X-ray in Paget's disease. Areas of lucency and increased bone density are seen. There is frontal bossing and new bone accretion on the cortex.

Osteomyelitis

Infection in bone may result from blood-borne or direct spread of a number of micro-organisms (Table 3.3) and various conditions predispose to bone infection (Table 3.4). Direct spread of infection to the bones occurs most commonly in diabetics with neuropathic foot ulcers (3.117, 3.118) and in patients with penetrating bed sores.

Acute osteomyelitis is usually caused by *Staphylococcus aureus*. It often presents with fever, pain and tenderness over the affected bone, but the presentation may be more non-specific without initial localising features. Blood culture or needle biopsy are usually required for definitive diagnosis, but treatment can sometimes be started on clinical grounds alone.

Chronic osteomyelitis results from undiagnosed or inadequately treated acute osteomyelitis. Within two weeks of onset of acute osteomyelitis, radiographic changes can often be seen, and these progress to include periosteal elevation, bone erosion, areas of sclerosis and areas of cystic degeneration (3.118). Avascular necrosis of the bone leads to the development of a bony sequestrum (3.119). Intermittent episodes of acute flare-up of the disease may occur over many years, with fever, local pain and sinus formation.

Treatment of chronic osteomyelitis often involves a combination of surgery and antibiotic therapy. Patients with sickle cell disease should receive long-term penicillin prophylaxis to prevent *Salmonella* osteomyelitis (3.119).

Chronic tuberculous osteomyelitis results from blood or lymphatic spread. The long bones and vertebral bodies are most commonly involved. Tracking of pus produces a 'cold' abscess (3.58) and destruction and subsequent collapse of the vertebrae leads to gross kyphosis (Pott's disease of the spine, 3.120). Surgery and anti-tuberculous therapy are commonly required.

Table 3.3 Organisms which may cause acute osteomyelitis.

Staphylococcus aureus

Pseudomonas aeruginosa

Salmonella sp.

Gram-negative bacilli

Neisseria gonorrhoeae

Pasteurella multocida

Mixed aerobic and anaerobic organisms

Streptococci

Brucella sp.

Candida sp.

Table 3.4 Osteomyelitis: predisposing conditions.

Acute osteomyelitis

Blood-borne
Skin sepsis and ulcers (especially in diabetes)
Intravenous drug abuse
Sickle cell disease
Chronic urinary tract infection
Chronic diverticulitis
Gonorrhoea
Malnutrition
Immunodeficiency

Direct spread
Open fractures
Penetrating trauma, e.g. animal bite
Prosthetic joints
Penetrating ulcer, e.g. in diabetic neuropathy
Finger pricks for blood sampling in diabetes

Chronic osteomyelitis

Inadequately treated acute disease
Tuberculosis

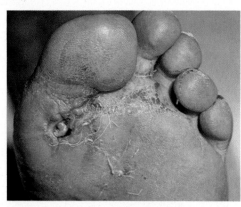

3.117 A purulent discharging ulcer at the base of the big toe in a diabetic patient. The ulcer is associated with osteomyelitis of the first metatarsal head (see **3.118**).

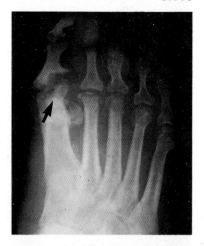

3.118 Osteomyelitis at the base of the ulcer seen in **3.117**, associated with X-ray changes including bone erosion and sequestrum formation.

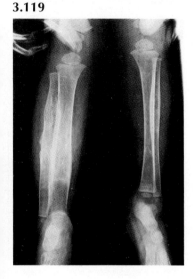

3.119 Salmonella osteomyelitis is a common complication of sickle-cell disease. In this child, extensive unilateral osteomyelitis has caused long bone sequestrum formation and a 'bone within a bone' appearance.

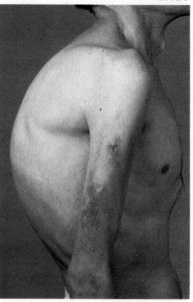

3.120 Pott's disease of the spine. Chronic tuberculous osteomyelitis of the lower thoracic vertebrae has caused a typical angular kyphosis.

Tumours of bone

Primary tumours of bone are rare and occur mainly in the young (**3.121**).

Secondary metastases in bone are common, especially from malignant tumours of the bronchus, breast, prostate, thyroid and kidney. Most metastases are osteolytic (**3.122**), but secondaries from carcinoma of the prostate are often sclerotic in character (**3.123**). Multiple metastases are common

(**3.124**), and lytic bone lesions are also a feature of multiple myeloma (*see* p. 465).

Bone secondaries are often painful and may cause hypercalcaemia. Symptomatic treatment is usually necessary, and specific hormone treatment or chemotherapy may be helpful in some cases.

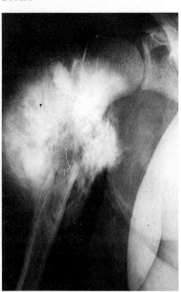

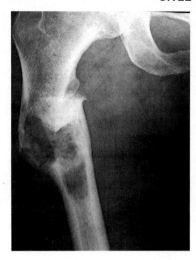

3.121 Osteosarcoma of the humerus in a 15-year-old boy. The radiograph shows lytic defects within the bone, periosteal new bone formation and a characteristic 'sunray' spiculation in the soft tissues.

3.122 An isolated lytic secondary in the femur. The deposit is the site of a pathological fracture, but has otherwise stimulated little bone reaction. The primary tumour was in the thyroid gland.

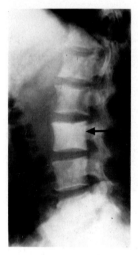

3.123 A sclerotic secondary deposit (arrowed) occupying the body of the third lumbar vertebra. The primary tumour is carcinoma of the prostate.

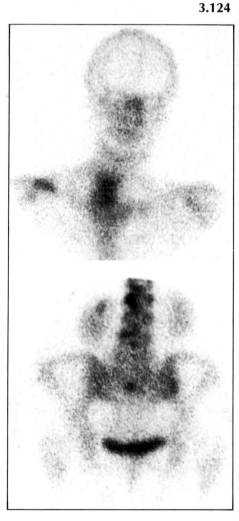

3.124 Multiple bone metastases are seen in this 99m Tc-MDP bone scintigram of a 60-year-old woman with breast cancer. A similar appearance may occur with other metastases, e.g. from renal tumours.

4. Respiratory Disorders

History and examination

A full medical history is important in any patient with respiratory symptoms or signs. Specific questions should always be asked about:

- Cough.
- Sputum—production, volume and colour.
- Breathlessness—onset, duration and positional variations.
- Wheezing.
- Fever.
- Chest pain.
- Nasal or upper respiratory tract symptoms.
- Weight loss.
- Smoking history.
- Occupation.

On general examination, there may be clues to the underlying disease:

- Cachexia (4.1) may occur in malignant disease, and in severe chronic lung diseases including fibrosis, infection and emphysema.
- Impaired growth in a child or young adult may be the result of chronic asthma or of its treatment by systemic steroids (4.2).
- 'Nicotine' stained fingers occur in heavy smokers (4.3), and typical pigmented scars may occur in coal miners (4.4); in association with finger clubbing (2.90, 2.91, 4.3, 4.67, 4.108, 11.104) both signs have an ominous significance, suggesting underlying bronchial carcinoma, pulmonary fibrosis, bronchiectasis or chronic sepsis.

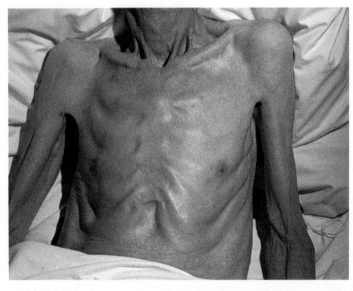

4.1 Cachexia may occur in a number of severe disorders including malignant disease and chronic lung diseases such as pulmonary fibrosis, tuberculosis and emphysema. Note the obvious signs of weight loss, with widespread muscle and soft-tissue wasting.

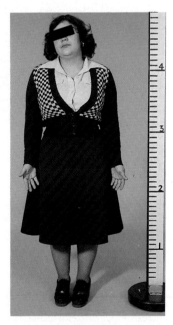

4.2 Growth retardation in a 19-year-old asthmatic. As the scale shows, she is 4' 10" (1.47m) tall. Asthma itself causes growth retardation, but here—as so often—chronic systemic steroid treatment has compounded the problem. Note the characteristic steroid facies. Inhaled steroids do not have the same growth-retarding effect as systemic steroids, but systemic treatment is still required in some patients. Whenever possible, systemic steroid treatment should be administered in short-term 'pulses' or on an alternate-day basis, as these manoeuvres may help to prevent unwanted side-effects.

4.2

- Cyanosis—best seen in the lips (4.64), tongue (4.5) and fingers (4.67)—indicates significant desaturation of circulating haemoglobin.
- A plethoric appearance may result from polycythaemia (4.6) most commonly secondary to chronic hypoxia in lung disease.

On examination of the chest:

- Distortion of the thoracic cage suggests chronic disease and may take many forms. Look for:
  —Barrel-shaped chest in obstructive airways disease (4.7).
  —Flattening of the chest wall overlying lung damage or collapse.
  —Kyphoscoliosis may be a primary abnormality (4.8), or secondary to other disease (3.41, 3.99).
  —Scars from previous thoracic surgery.

- The respiratory rate and depth may be raised or lowered:
  —Is there hypoventilation or hyperventilation?
  —Are the accessory muscles of respiration in use (4.9)?
  —Is the patient fatigued?
  —Does the patient breathe out through pursed lips (4.10)?
- Respiratory movements may be asymmetrical.
- Cervical lymph nodes may be visible (4.11) or palpable.
- Look and palpate for a goitre.
- Feel in the suprasternal notch for tracheal deviation.
- Examine a sputum sample if possible.
- Key findings in the main groups of lung disease on palpation, percussion and auscultation are summarised in **Table 4.1**.

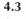 4.3

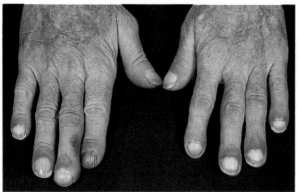

4.4 Impregnation of coal dust is commonly found in the hands of coal miners, and may give a clue to the presence of occupational lung disease (pneumoconiosis).

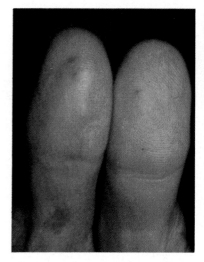

4.3 'Nicotine' stained fingers—a misnomer, because it is the tar from cigarettes which causes the staining. This patient smoked 40 cigarettes per day, but staining is more dependent on the action of smoking cigarettes right to the stub than on the total number smoked. This patient also has acute, recent onset clubbing (note the reddening and swelling of the nailfolds). He had lung cancer.

4.5

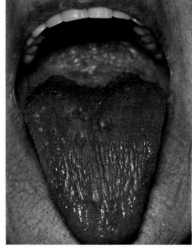 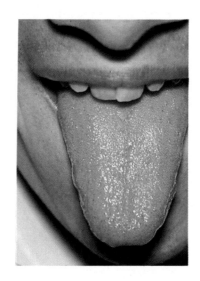

4.5 Central cyanosis is seen in the tongue, lips and earlobes. It is due to the presence of high levels of deoxygenated haemoglobin (>5g/dl). Here, the cyanotic patient's tongue (left) is compared with a normal individual (right). The blue appearance is characteristic, and may occur in severe respiratory or cardiovascular disease.

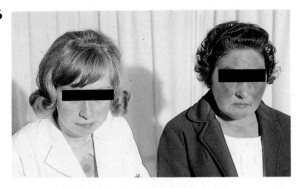

4.6 Secondary polycythaemia has developed in the patient on the right as a consequence of chronic hypoxic lung disease. Compare her appearance with the normal woman on the left.

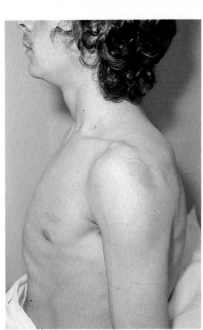

4.7 Barrel-shaped chest in a patient with asthma. This picture was taken during an acute attack. The hyperinflation results from air-trapping associated with inflammatory changes, hypersecretion of viscid mucus and smooth muscle contraction in the small airways. Note the associated indrawing of the intercostal muscles. Similar changes are seen in patients with chronic bronchitis and emphysema.

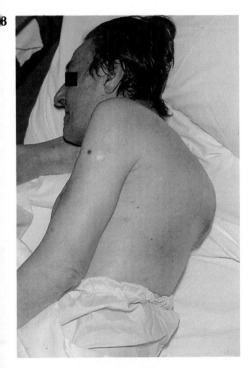

4.8 Severe kyphoscoliosis of unknown aetiology. Flexion (kyphosis) and lateral deviation (scoliosis) of the spine have the combined effect of reducing chest volume (see **4.33**). This compromises respiratory function, so that otherwise minor chest infections may precipitate respiratory failure.

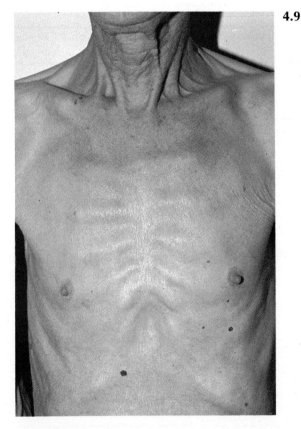

4.9 Dyspnoea in a patient with severe asthma. Note the contraction of the accessory muscles of respiration.

4.10

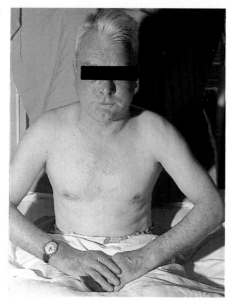

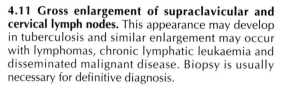

4.10 Pursed lip expiration is a common manoeuvre adopted by patients with severe chronic bronchitis and emphysema. The patient starts to breathe out against closed or nearly closed lips to keep the intra-bronchial pressure high and prevent collapse of the bronchial wall and expiratory obstruction. Later in expiration the lips are blown forwards and open, often with a grunt ('Fish-mouth breathing').

4.11 Gross enlargement of supraclavicular and cervical lymph nodes. This appearance may develop in tuberculosis and similar enlargement may occur with lymphomas, chronic lymphatic leukaemia and disseminated malignant disease. Biopsy is usually necessary for definitive diagnosis.

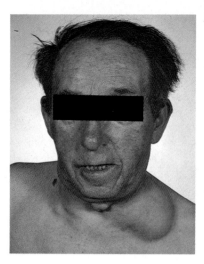

Table 4.1 Physical signs in respiratory disease.

Lung pathology	Chest expansion	Mediastinal shift	Percussion note	Breath sounds	Voice sounds	Added sounds
Asthma	Reduced on both sides	Nil	Normal	Vesicular with prolonged expiration	Normal	Expiratory wheeze
Chronic bronchitis	Reduced on both sides	Nil	Normal	Vesicular with prolonged expiration	Normal	Expiratory wheeze and crackles
Consolidation (lobar pneumonia)	Reduced on affected side	Nil	Impaired	Bronchial	Increased	Crackles
Lung or lobar collapse	Reduced on affected side	Towards affected side	Impaired	Diminished vesicular	Reduced	Nil
Localised fibrosis	Reduced on affected side	Towards affected side	Impaired	Bronchial	Increased	Crackles
Pneumothorax	Reduced on affected side	To opposite side	Hyper-resonant	Diminished vesicular	Reduced	Nil
Pleural effusion	Reduced on affected side	To opposite side	Stony dull	Diminished vesicular, occasionally bronchial at air fluid margin	Reduced	Rarely a pleural rub

Investigations

Sputum

Naked-eye examination of the sputum can give vital clinical information:

- Consistently large volumes suggest bronchiectasis.
- Rupture of an abscess, empyema or cyst into a bronchus may produce a sudden increase in volume.
- Infected sputum is usually yellow or green because of the large number of polymorphs it contains.
- Blood in the sputum produces a pink tinge in the typical frothy sputum of left ventricular failure, deep red flecks in bronchial carcinoma and pulmonary embolism, and a rusty colour in pneumococcal pneumonia (4.12).
- Black sputum may be found in workers in a dusty environment or following smoke inhalation .
- Thick viscid sputum, sometimes taking the form of bronchial casts, is often seen in asthma (4.13).
- Rupture of a hepatic amoebic abscess into the lung gives an 'anchovy sauce' appearance to sputum.
- Rupture of a hepatic hydatid cyst into a right lower lobe bronchus produces bile-stained sputum.

Microscopic examination of sputum may show asbestos fibres (4.14), Charcot–Leyden crystals derived from eosinophils, fungal spores or clumps of pathogenic bacteria (4.15).

Sputum culture is of value in identifying bacteria and fungi and in testing for drug sensitivity. Culture normally takes 24–48 hours for pyogenic bacteria (up to eight weeks for mycobacteria). Therapy should often be started without waiting for the results of culture.

For sputum cytology, as much sputum as possible should be sent fresh to the laboratory. The results are excellent with central tumours (80–90% positive, 4.16), but much less successful with peripheral tumours.

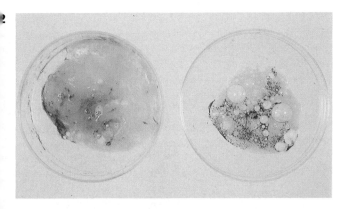

4.12 Rusty red sputum (left) compared with fresh haemoptysis (right) in two sputum samples. The rusty red sputum comes from a patient with pneumococcal pneumonia, while the haemoptysis occurred in a patient with small cell lung cancer.

4.13 Asthmatics commonly cough up thick rubbery mucus plugs, and occasionally these can teased be out to reveal bronchial casts, as here.

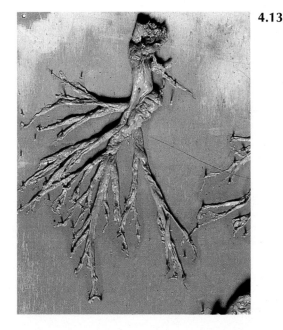
4.13

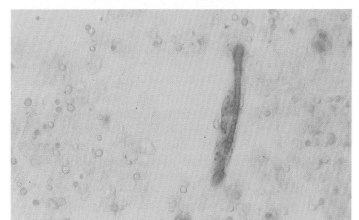
4.14

4.14 Asbestos body in sputum. The typical drumstick appearance represents an asbestos fibre surrounded by a ferroprotein complex. It is indicative of asbestos exposure with associated increased risks of bronchial malignancy and (with blue asbestos) mesothelioma.

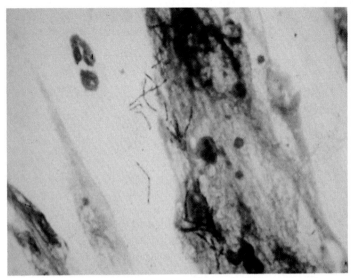

4.15 Ziehl-Neelsen staining of sputum showed many red-staining tubercle bacilli in this patient with pulmonary tuberculosis.

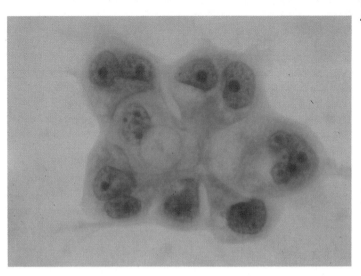

4.16 Adenocarcinoma cells in a sputum smear. The assessment of the appearances on sputum cytology is a very specialised field, and an expert opinion is essential for the definitive diagnosis of malignancy.

Skin tests

Skin-prick testing may be useful in establishing the patient's sensitivity to common allergens (*see* p. 90). Multiple positive skin tests are common in asthmatic patients (**4.17**). Radioallergosorbent tests (RASTs) on venous blood are an alternative method of identifying specific IgE antibodies.

Tuberculin tests (**1.127**) are of little value in diagnosing tuberculosis in individual patients, but have a role in screening contacts and in pre-BCG assessment.

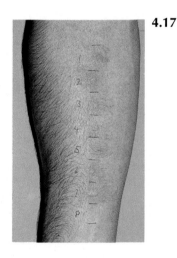

4.17 Multiple positive skin tests—a common finding in asthmatic patients. Note the negative control (8) which rules out dermographism as the cause of the positive results (*see also* **2.9**, **2.10**).

Blood tests

Venous blood samples taken for automated blood counts may provide major clues or confirmation of a suspected respiratory disease. A high haemoglobin concentration may be a reflection of polycythaemia, either primary or secondary (**4.6**) and a low haemoglobin may cause breathlessness. The total white cell count may be elevated in a range of acute bacterial infections and its subsequent fall is a reflection of successful therapy. Normal or low white cell counts are found in mycoplasma or viral infections. Eosinophilia (**1.17**) suggests an allergic component or parasitic infection.

A range of serologic tests which depend on agglutination, precipitation and complement fixation provide evidence of the presence in the patient's serum of specific antibodies against viral, bacterial, fungal, protozoal and helminth infections. Samples of blood should be tested on admission and repeated after 10–14 days to detect a rising titre.

Blood gases

The presence of respiratory failure may be suspected by the signs of central cyanosis. It is important to define the type and extent of failure of oxygenation and this is best done by measurement of arterial blood gas tensions (PaO_2 and $PaCO_2$), oxygen saturation (SaO_2) and pH (**4.18**). The response to drugs and the therapeutic response to oxygen can then be monitored easily. Haemoglobin saturation reflects oxygen carriage by the blood and thus the adequacy of tissue oxygenation (if perfusion is satisfactory) and the requirement for oxygen therapy. The arterial partial pressure of carbon dioxide ($PaCO_2$) is a good indication of ventilation, low values indicating hyperventilation and vice versa; it is often more important than the PaO_2 in assessing the need for assisted ventilation.

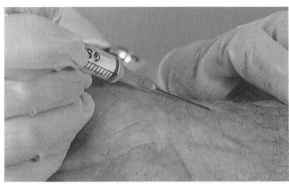

4.18

4.18 Arterial blood sampling can be carried out from the femoral, brachial or radial arteries, but the most common site is the radial artery in the patient's non-dominant arm. Firm pressure should be applied after withdrawal of the needle to prevent local haematoma formation.

Pulmonary function tests

Simple pulmonary function tests may easily be done at home or at the bedside using a peak flow meter or gauge (**4.19**). This gives reasonably reliable and repeatable results and can be used to monitor therapy in asthma and chronic obstructive airways disease.

By use of a spirometer (**4.20**) and other equipment, a number of volume and flow rates can be estimated:

- The **forced vital capacity** (FVC) is the total volume of gas expired.
- The **forced expiratory volume in one second** (FEV_1) is the volume of gas expired in the first second of expiration.

- The **peak expiratory flow** (PEF) is the fastest flow rate recorded during expiration.
- After a full expiration, some gas remains in the lung, the **residual volume**. In order to measure this it is necessary to measure the volume of gas in the lungs at full inspiration (**total lung capacity**, TLC) and obtain the residual volume by subtracting the vital capacity. TLC is usually measured by helium dilution; a subject rebreathes a known volume and concentration of helium which is diluted in the lung so that the TLC can be calculated by measuring how much the helium has been diluted.

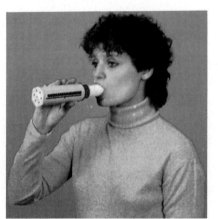

4.19 Mini peak flow meter in use. The patient takes in a deep breath, and then makes a maximal expiratory effort through the instrument. The procedure is repeated three times and the highest peak expiratory flow (PEF) is recorded. This can be compared with a nomogram which shows the patient's sex, age and weight, and plotted on a chart to show the progress or response to treatment.

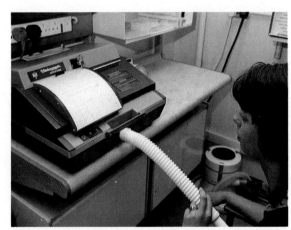

4.20

4.20 A spirometer provides a simple means of assessing air flow obstruction. The patient takes a maximal inspiration and then exhales as fast as possible for as long as possible. The volume expired against time is measured, and the forced expiratory volume in one second (FEV_1) and the forced vital capacity (FVC) can be simply calculated from the graph produced (**4.22**).

167

- **Airways resistance** can be measured by body plethysmography (**4.21**).
- There are methodological difficulties in measuring oxygen transfer from lung to blood, so **carbon monoxide transfer factor** is commonly measured. The transfer of carbon monoxide depends on how much haemoglobin can be 'seen' by the inspired gas; therefore transfer is low when the pulmonary capillary bed is damaged or obscured by inequalities of ventilation or perfusion. It is also low in anaemia and can be increased with polycythaemia or if haemorrhage into the lungs has occurred.

The results of simple spirometry provide much useful information (**4.22**) and even simple lung function tests are of great value in following the course of disease and response to treatment.

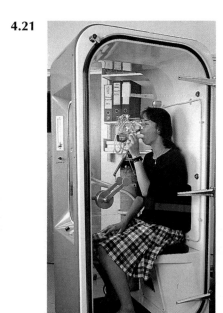

4.21 Body plethysmography allows the simultaneous measurement of thoracic gas volume and airways resistance. Such techniques are not available in every centre, but may provide valuable additional information, especially in relation to the assessment of the effects of drug therapy.

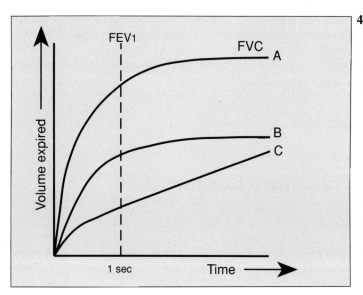

4.22 Typical results of spirometry in a normal patient (A), a patient with a restrictive defect (B) and a patient with an obstructive defect (C). In a restrictive defect (B), the FEV_1/FVC ratio is preserved at the normal level, but both absolute values are reduced. In an obstructive defect (C), both absolute values are again reduced, but the FEV_1/FVC ratio is considerably reduced, as the forced expiratory time required to reach the FVC is greatly prolonged.

Imaging

A posteroanterior (PA) chest X-ray will often provide valuable diagnostic information about the nature and location of respiratory disease (**4.23–4.30**).

A lateral chest X-ray is helpful in identifying the position of abnormalities seen on the PA film (**4.31–4.35**) and may occasionally show significant abnormalities not seen on the standard film.

Tomography allows a radiograph of a specific slice of the chest; it is particularly useful for demonstrating lung cavities (**4.36, 4.37**), the lumen of the trachea and major bronchi, and the position and nature of abnormal shadows noted on the plain radiograph.

Computerised axial tomography (CT) of the lung is most commonly used for the assessment of the extent of lung cancer but is being increasingly used in diffuse lung disease (**4.38**) and has replaced bronchography as the first-line investigation of suspected bronchiectasis.

Magnetic resonance imaging shows cardiovascular structures in the chest. Its role in pulmonary disease is still developing.

Pulmonary and aortic angiography may be used to define the anatomy of the arterial tree (**5.155**).

Radionuclide scans of lung (V/Q scan) are particularly useful in suspected pulmonary embolism (**5.154**). In this technique, xenon gas is inhaled and a gamma-camera image is produced of the alveolar distribution of the radioactivity (**4.39**). Then an intravenous injection of macroaggregates of human albumin (each 100μ) labelled with 99mTc is injected. These microspheres embolise harmlessly in the lung vessels and the distribution of the radioactivity is a reflection of the pulmonary blood supply (**4.40**).

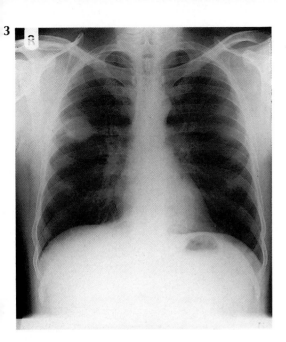

4.23 An early peripheral bronchial carcinoma in the right mid-zone, found by chance on a chest X-ray. The hilum appears normal, and this was confirmed at tomography. This patient underwent a successful and probably curative lobectomy.

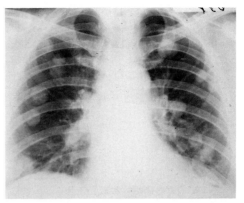
4.24

4.24 Cannonball metastases in both lung fields. Single or multiple round, discrete shadows resulting from secondary deposits occur with a number of tumours, including those of the kidney, ovary, breast, pancreas and testicle, and they are also seen in malignant melanoma.

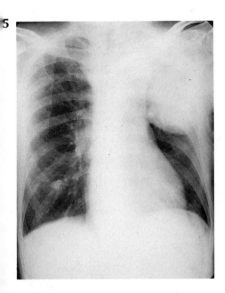

4.25 Left upper-lobe opacity. The patient presented with pain in the chest and haemoptysis (**4.12**), and the underlying diagnosis proved to be small cell carcinoma of the bronchus. Much of the shadowing is the result of infection and collapse of the lung distal to the point at which the tumour causes bronchial obstruction. Note the extensive calcification in the right hilum and lower zone–the result of healed tuberculosis.

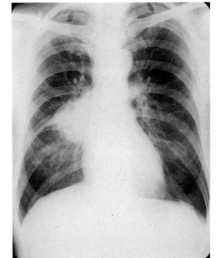
4.26

4.26 Carcinoma of the bronchus involving the right hilum and mediastinum. Bronchoscopy showed widening of the carina, which suggested lymph node involvement in the mediastinum and a friable, bleeding tumour in the right main bronchus. CT scan confirmed involvement of the great vessels. The tumour was thus inoperable.

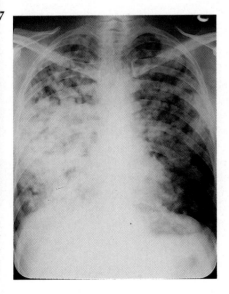

4.27 'Snowstorm' miliary mottling in both lung fields. In this case, the underlying diagnosis was testicular seminoma, with disseminated haematogenous metastases. Such an extreme picture is usually the result of malignant disease, but the chest X-ray may look similar in a number of infectious conditions, especially miliary tuberculosis (*see* **1.121**), and in dust diseases.

4.28 The chest X-ray is a poor guide to the severity of asthma. Although this 4-year-old girl had acute severe asthma requiring urgent treatment, her chest X-ray showed nothing more than mild hyperinflation.

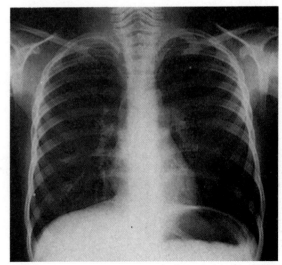
4.28

4.29

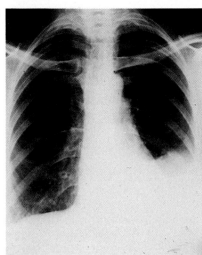

4.29 Left pleural effusion, which developed during an influenza-like illness in a young woman, and was associated with fever and pleuritic pain.

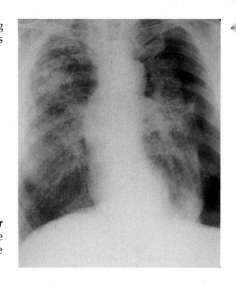

4.30 Left pneumothorax developed in this former coalminer with known pneumoconiosis. Note the obvious lung edge in the left chest and the diffuse miliary mottling of pneumoconiosis in both lungs.

4.31

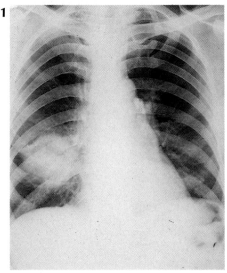

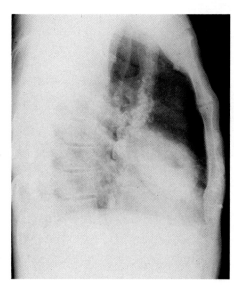

4.31, 4.32 Staphylococcal lung abscess in the right lung of an intravenous drug abuser. The abscess is in the lower zone on the PA film, and the lateral film shows that it is above the oblique fissure—i.e. in the middle lobe of the lung. Note that there is also extensive calcification of the left hilum, which results from healed tuberculosis.

4.33

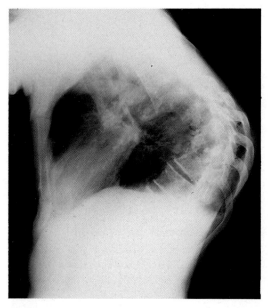

4.33 Kyphoscoliosis resulting from tuberculosis involving the thoracic vertebral bodies (T6-8). The significant reduction of lung volume is obvious (see **4.8**).

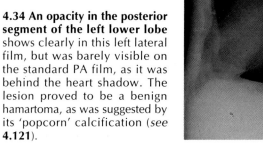

4.34 An opacity in the posterior segment of the left lower lobe shows clearly in this left lateral film, but was barely visible on the standard PA film, as it was behind the heart shadow. The lesion proved to be a benign hamartoma, as was suggested by its 'popcorn' calcification (*see* **4.121**).

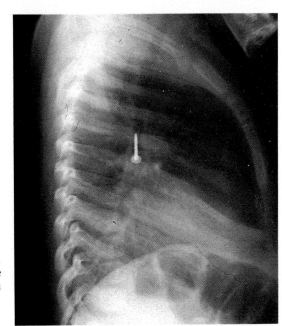

4.35

4.35 An inhaled foreign body—a nail—impacted in the right lower lobe bronchus. This young patient presented with a persistent cough and wheeze, but did not realise that he had inhaled a nail. Foreign bodies should always be borne in mind as a differential diagnosis of wheezing, especially in children.

4.36 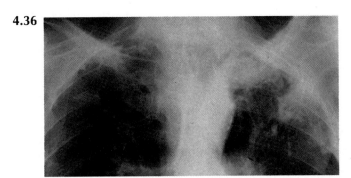 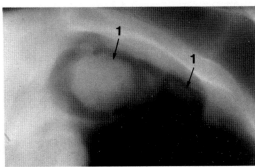 **4.37**

4.36, 4.37 Tuberculous cavities containing aspergillomas at the left apex. This patient's left apical shadowing was further investigated by tomography, which clearly demonstrates the round mycetomas or fungus balls (1) within the chronic tuberculous cavities.

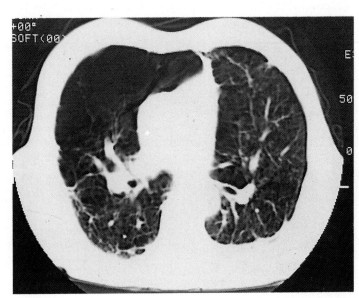

4.38

4.38 CT scan at upper hilar level demonstrating bullous emphysema. A very large bullus is present anteriorly in the right lung, together with numerous smaller bullae in both lungs.

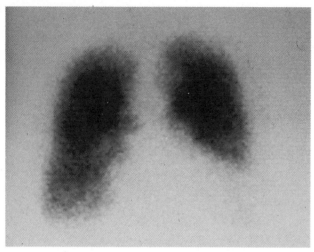
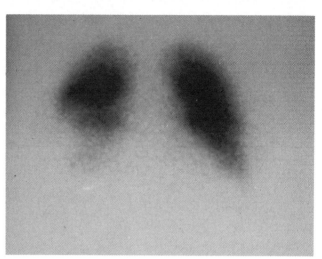

4.39, 4.40 Radionuclide ventilation (4.39) and perfusion (4.40) scans. 4.39 shows a normal distribution of xenon during ventilation, while **4.40** shows multiple perfusion defects in the right lung field when technetium ^{99}M albumin microspheres were injected. This 'unmatched' perfusion defect is typical of multiple pulmonary emboli.

Bronchoscopy

The flexible fibreoptic bronchoscope (4.41) has made bronchoscopy easier, quicker, safer and less traumatic than before. Excellent views can be easily obtained of all major and segmental bronchi (4.42) and samples of mucus collected via the aspiration channel. In addition brush biopsies, suction catheters and biopsy forceps can be passed through this channel. Samples suitable for culture, cytology and histology can be easily obtained.

Bronchoscopy is the investigation of choice for mass lesions on the central and mid-zones, especially if carcinoma is thought to be obstructing bronchi (4.43). In those who are very frail, however, sputum cytology may be the investigation of choice. The use of bronchoscopy to obtain good specimens for microbiology and lung histology has reduced the requirement for open lung biopsy in patients with pulmonary infiltrates. Broncoscopy can be useful therapeutically in the removal of secretions or foreign bodies causing airways obstruction, and some central tumours are amenable to laser resection via the bronchoscope. Lung biopsy is possible by advancing the biopsy catheter through the lung parenchyma under fluoroscopic control (4.44). This avoids the need for an open lung biopsy in many patients.

4.41

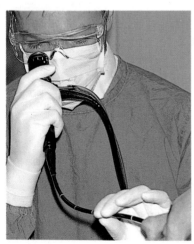

4.41 Fibreoptic bronchoscopy is a simple technique which can be performed on the conscious patient. The bronchoscope is usually passed through the nose. This picture demonstrates the gown, mask, gloves and eye protection which are required if the patient is HIV positive. These patients often require bronchoscopy for the diagnosis of opportunistic lung infections.

4.42 Tracing the source of haemoptysis is often possible using the fibreoptic broncho-scope. Here it has been traced to a sub-division of the right upper lobe bronchus labelled B³b.

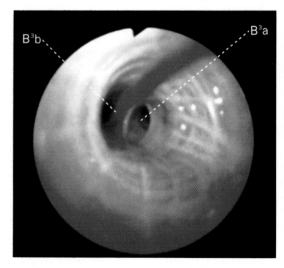

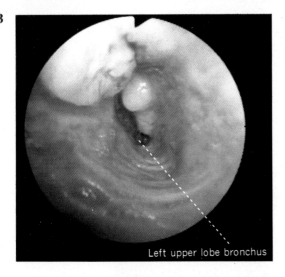

Left upper lobe bronchus

4.43 Squamous cell carcinoma seen through the fibreoptic bronchoscope at the opening of the left upper lobe bronchus. The white tumour has a relatively smooth surface. Biopsy through the bronchoscope is simple.

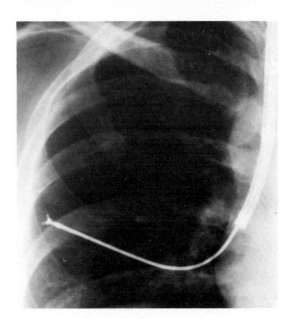

4.44 Biopsy of a peripheral lesion through the fibreoptic bronchoscope. Direct vision is not possible, but the forceps have been positioned under radiographic control and a biopsy should be obtained when their jaws are closed.

Pleural aspiration and biopsy

Aspiration of pleural fluid is of major value for both diagnostic and therapeutic reasons. Naked-eye inspection may suggest the presence of pus, the effusion may be blood stained suggesting carcinoma or pulmonary embolism, or milky white (chylous) as a result of obstruction of the thoracic duct, usually by tumour.

- Pleural transudates are associated with generalised oedema and are pale in colour with a specific gravity of less than 1015, total protein less than 2.5 g per 100 ml.
- Pleural exudates represent inflammation and are usually darker in colour with a specific gravity above 1018 and a total protein greater than 3 g per 100 ml.
- The glucose level is often decreased in the presence of infection, in contradistinction to rheumatoid pleural effusion.
- Total white cell count and cell type are of value.

Polymorphs indicate bacterial infection and lymphocytes suggest tuberculosis. Culture of the fluid may show the organism responsible and cytology the diagnosis of tumour.

At the time of pleural aspiration, it is often convenient to carry out a pleural biopsy with a side-cutting needle. This is 'blind', but relatively atraumatic. Pleuroscopy and mediastinoscopy can be used to provide direct vision for biopsy. If the diagnosis is already made, then an opportunity to instil antibiotics, cytotoxics or sclerosants may be taken.

Pleural aspiration and biopsy are not always harmless procedures. They may result in damage to the lung or abdominal organs, pneumothorax or haemothorax (4.45). In the longer term, biopsy of a mesothelioma may result in spread of the tumour (4.46).

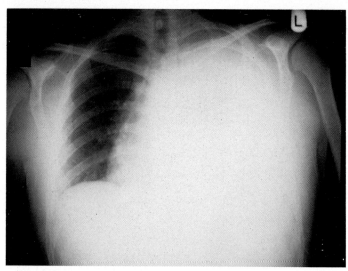

4.45 Haemothorax following pleural aspiration and biopsy. Before biopsy, the patient had only a small pleural effusion, but now there is a massive haemothorax resulting from arterial bleeding, which has caused a shift to the right of the mediastinum.

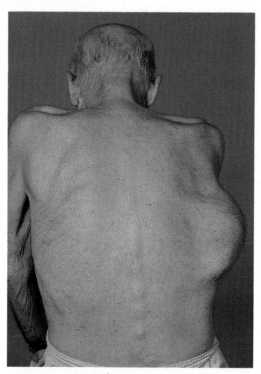

4.46 Mesothelioma has invaded down the needle track of a previous pleural biopsy into the subcutaneous tissues of this patient with an asbestos-linked pleural plaque (*see* **4.119**).

Lymph-node biopsy

Biopsy of a palpable node, usually in the neck, may provide a rapid histological diagnosis. When no nodes are felt, removal of the scalene node may provide diagnostic information.

Upper respiratory tract disorders

The common cold is discussed on p. 20, and rhinitis, sinusitis, tonsillitis, pharyngitis and laryngitis may also occur as part of a number of the childhood exanthemata such as measles (p. 24), and in infectious mononucleosis (p. 32) and streptococcal infection (p. 38).

Other medical disorders of the upper airway include allergic and non-allergic rhinitis. Allergic rhinitis (4.47) may be seasonal—most commonly caused by allergy to grass or other pollens (hay fever)—or perennial—most commonly cauded by allergy to the faeces of the house-dust mite. Skin-prick testing is often helpful in diagnosis (*see* p. 90 and 166).

Non-allergic or vasomotor rhinitis produces similar symptoms, but the cause is usually obscure.

Allergic rhinitis is often associated with other atopic disorders including conjunctivitis, asthma, urticaria and eczema. It usually responds to topical corticosteroid or sodium cromoglycate therapy. Unlike asthma, however, most of the symptoms of allergic rhinitis often respond to oral antihistamines.

Chronic rhinitis may be associated with the formation of nasal polyps (4.48), especially in a group of patients who also have asthma and are sensitive to aspirin and dietary salicylates. Surgical removal of polyps may be needed to control obstructive symptoms.

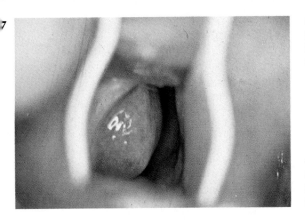

4.47 Allergic rhinitis produces a greyish appearance in the nasal mucous membrane, especially when chronic.

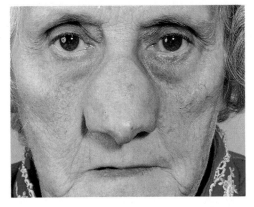

4.48 Nasal polyps produced near-total nasal obstruction and anosmia in this patient. Her nose was obviously enlarged.

Inhalation of foreign bodies

Foreign bodies may be inhaled and lodge at any level in the respiratory system (e.g. **4.35**). Large objects may cause potentially fatal obstruction at the level of the larynx. In a conscious patient, such obstruction may often be dislodged by sharp blows to the back or by use of Heimlich's manoeuvre (**4.49**).

If these techniques fail, emergency cricothyrotomy using an intravenous cannula (**4.50**) or even a sharp knife and the empty shaft of a ball-point pen may re-establish an airway.

At lower levels in the respiratory tract, inhaled foreign bodies are not usually immediately life-threatening (**4.35**); but failure to diagnose and remove foreign bodies may lead to traumatic damage to the lungs or to the collapse of segments of the lung distal to the obstruction with subsequent lobar pneumonia.

Chest X-ray is diagnostic for radio-opaque objects and bronchoscopy often allows removal of the foreign body.

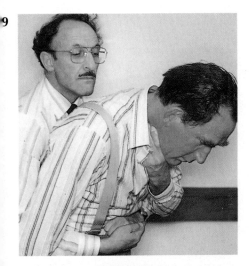

4.49 The Heimlich manoeuvre can be used in an attempt to dislodge an inhaled foreign body. One fist is clenched and positioned in the epigastrium and the other hand is placed on top. The patient is squeezed suddenly so that the fist moves backwards and upwards, causing a violent expulsion of air from the lungs.

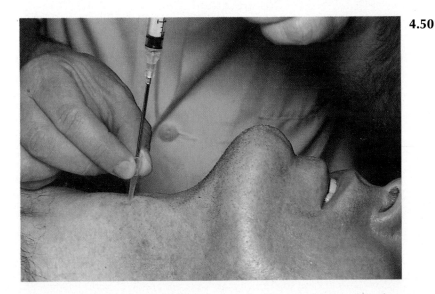

4.50 Cricothyrotomy is indicated as a last resort in obstructive asphyxia, when endotracheal intubation is impossible because of a foreign body, oedema or the absence of equipment. The surface marking for insertion of the needle is the space between the thyroid and cricoid cartilages. The syringe is aspirated to ensure that the needle and cannula are in the tracheal lumen, and the syringe and needle are then withdrawn, leaving the cannula in place.

Asthma

Asthma is commonly defined as: 'a disorder of function characterised by dyspnoea caused by widespread narrowing of peripheral airways in the lungs, varying in severity over short periods of time either spontaneously or with treatment'.

Asthma is a common disorder. Its prevalence is highest in the second decade of life, when it may affect 10–15% of the population in developed countries such as the UK, the USA and New Zealand. It is much less common in most Asian countries. Occupational asthma is a common problem in those exposed to sensitising substances in industry.

In non-occupational asthma the allergens involved are similar to those causing allergic rhinitis and conjunctivitis, though pollen (4.51) is a less common cause of asthma (perhaps because of the relatively large size of pollen grains) and dust mite faecal particles are probably the most common cause of allergic asthma worldwide (4.52).

Asthma is accompanied by bronchial hyper-reactivity—an increased responsiveness of the airways to non-specific stimuli. Although the degree of hyper-reactivity may be influenced by allergic mechanisms, its pathogenesis is unclear, and non-allergic factors are also involved. It is now clear that asthma is a fundamentally inflammatory condition.

Asthma is often divided into two sub groups:

- Extrinsic asthma—a definite external cause is implied.
- Intrinsic asthma—no causative agent can be identified.

Those with extrinsic asthma are typically atopic individuals who show positive skin-prick reactions to common inhaled allergens, whereas those with intrinsic asthma are not. Ninety per cent of asthmatic children have positive skin tests to one or more substances in a standard battery (*see* p. 90), whereas only 50% of adults do.

The extrinsic/intrinsic classification is of little practical value. Non-atopic patients may develop asthma in middle age from extrinsic causes such as sensitisation to occupational agents, intolerance to aspirin, or the use of beta-blockers for the treatment of hypertension or angina. Extrinsic causes should thus be considered in all cases of asthma and avoided whenever possible. Other treatment for the two sub-groups is similar.

4.51

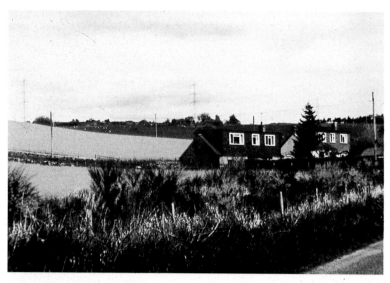

4.52

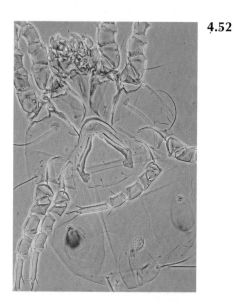

4.51 Pollen from the oil-seed rape is one of a number of pollens which may provoke asthma in susceptible subjects. It is important to remember environmental and occupational trigger factors in the assessment and management of patients with asthma.

4.52 The house-dust mite, *Dermatophagoides pteronyssinus*. The faecal particles of this and related mite species are the most common cause of allergic asthma worldwide. The faecal particles are about 20 μm in diameter—small enough to be inhaled into the smaller, peripheral airways in the lung. Dust mites are most common in moist, temperate environments. They feed on shed scales of human and animal skin, and thus commonly infest mattresses, pillows, carpets and soft furnishings. They are about 0.5 mm in length and invisible to the naked eye. Dust mite allergy also plays a major role in perennial rhinitis and possibly in eczema.

Well over 200 different causes of occupational asthma have been recognised, and some are of major importance in industry (Table 4.2). Some occupational materials produce asthma by a classic Type I mechanism, and specific IgE antibody can be found in the serum. In other cases, the precise mechanism has still to be determined.

The spectrum of clinical presentation of asthma ranges from very mild symptoms (4.53) to an acute life-threatening illness (4.54).

Physical signs in asthma are dependent upon the stage at which the disease presents (Table 4.3), but it is important to realise that the severe asthmatic may show few signs. In particular, wheezing may disappear at severe levels of airway obstruction. Even in severe asthma, the chest X-ray may appear normal or show no more than the signs of hyperinflation (4.28), though it may show complicating conditions such as pneumonia or pneumothorax (4.135).

Simple respiratory function tests are very helpful in the diagnosis and management of asthma, but it is usually important that they are repeated. Even repeated measurement at the same time of day may mask regular variations in PEF (4.55), so several measurements per day are needed. Measurement following simple provocation tests, e.g. exercise, may be very useful in patient assessment (4.56, 4.57). Some patients, especially children, may exist at low levels of PEF without complaint, but if this is recognised and treated there may be major quality-of-life benefits (4.58).

The treatment of severe acute asthma usually requires hospital admission for oxygen therapy, nebulised bronchodilators and systemic corticosteroids (4.59). The mainstay of treatment for chronic asthma is regular inhaled corticosteroid therapy (4.60), supplemented by inhaled β_2 agonists for occasional symptomatic relief. Inhaled sodium cromoglycate, oral theophylline and oral β_2 agonist therapy are sometimes of value. Oral steroid therapy is effective, but its long-term use should be avoided because of the risk of side-effects (4.2).

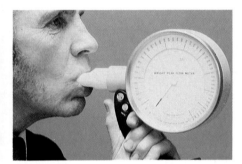

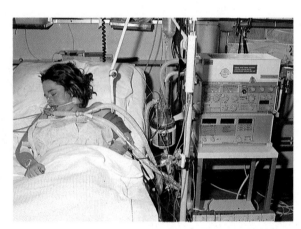

4.54

4.53, 4.54 The range of presentation of asthma. The patient in **4.53** was found to have a degree of reversible airways obstruction incidentally during a medical examination for other reasons. He had never been aware of symptoms. The patient in **4.54**, by comparison, presented as a medical emergency with acute severe breathlessness and required immediate intensive care including intermittent positive-pressure ventilation.

4.55

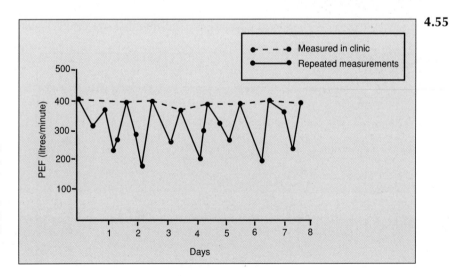

4.55 Diurnal variation in PEF. Even daily measurements of airflow obstruction in a hospital or general practice setting may not show any evidence of airflow obstruction, because the typical morning 'dip' in PEF usually occurs between 4.00 a.m. and 7.00 a.m., with spontaneous improvement in peak flow over the next few hours. In these circumstances only home monitoring of PEF reveals the extent of the patient's asthma.

Table 4.2 Some important causes of occupational asthma.

IgE related

Allergens from animals (including insects)	Laboratories
Allergens from flour and grain	Farmers, millers, grain handlers
Proteolytic enzymes	Manufacture of 'biological' washing powders (but not their use)
Complex salts of platinum	Metal refining
Acid anhydrides and polyamine hardening agents	Industrial coatings

Non-IgE related

Isocyanates	Polyurethane varnishes, industrial coatings
Colophony fumes	Soldering, electronics industry

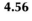 4.56

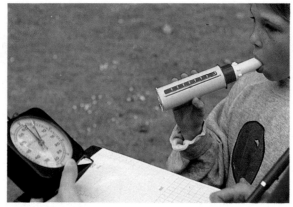

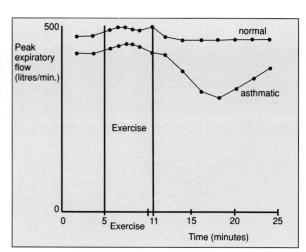 4.57

4.56, 4.57 PEF responses to an exercise test. In normal and asthmatic patients there is a small degree of bronchodilatation during exercise, but in asthmatic patients this initial bronchodilatation is followed by bronchoconstriction, reaching its maximum 5–10 minutes after the end of exercise. A 15% drop from baseline levels of PEF is considered a positive test, and the fall in PEF can be rapidly reversed with an inhaled bronchodilator.

4.58

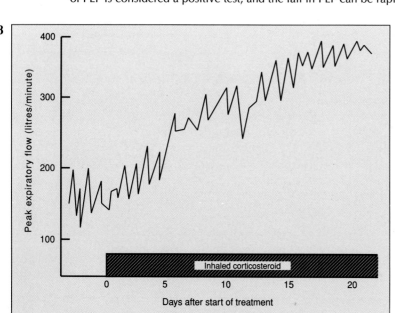

4.58 The importance of adequate control in asthma. An apparently asymptomatic 8-year-old boy had been monitored for four weeks and found to have a PEF which varied between 120 and 200 litres per minute. He reported no bronchodilator usage. Nevertheless, when inhaled steroid therapy was started, his peak flow rate showed progressive improvement over the next three weeks and remained at the new level when treatment was continued. At the new peak flow rate he found that he felt much more 'well' than before, and both his school work and his performance in games improved.

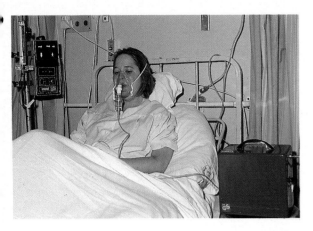

4.59 An acute asthmatic patient in hospital, receiving oxygen, nebulised β₂ agonist and intravenous hydro-cortisone. Careful monitoring of therapy is required.

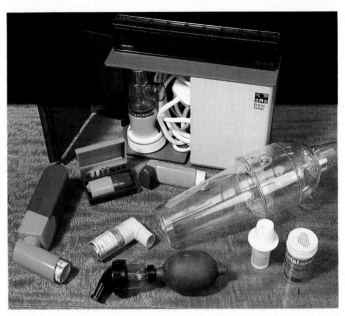

4.60 A range of asthma drug-administration devices produced by one patient in response to the question: 'What treatment are you receiving?'. In asthma, as in most other conditions, it is essential for doctor and patient to have an agreed treatment plan which minimises the number of drugs required and avoids confusion.

Table 4.3 Physical signs in asthma.

In the acute attack
- Tachypnoea
- Hyperinflated chest, with symmetrically reduced chest wall movement
- Prolonged expiration with vesicular breath sounds
- Expiratory wheeze
- Cough—especially in children
- Thick yellow-green sputum—does not necessarily indicate infection
- No mediastinal displacement
- Normal percussion
- Normal vocal resonance

In the severe acute attack
- Tachycardia
- The wheeze may disappear as a result of reduced air-flow
- Variable jugular venous pressure (high during expiration)
- Pulsus paradoxus (an exaggerated fall in systolic BP on inspiration)
- Rapid progress to life-threatening respiratory distress with cyanosis

In chronic or recurrent episodic asthma
- Signs of other allergic disorder may be present
- Pigeon chest—if asthma started in childhood
- Growth retardation—if asthma started in childhood
- Cushingoid features if long-term systemic steroid treatment used

Respiratory infections

Acute bronchitis

Viral infections of the upper respiratory tract often lead to secondary bacterial infection of the lower respiratory tract, especially in patients with pre-existing respiratory disorders. These infections may damage bronchial epithelium, leading to exacerbations of asthma or obstructive airways disease and to bronchitis and pneumonia, most commonly with *S. pneumoniae* or *H. influenzae* (*see* p. 186).

Chronic bronchitis and emphysema

Chronic bronchitis is a clinical syndrome in which there is excess mucus secretion by bronchial goblet cells. This stimulates the cough reflex so that sputum is produced daily for at least 3 months of the year. There are often episodes of superimposed viral or bacterial infection in which the sputum may be yellow or green and often contains a fleck of blood. Many patients also have an intermittent wheeze with objective evidence of airways obstruction on pulmonary function tests and some may have acute severe bronchoconstriction in response to respiratory infections or to irritants or allergens (asthmatic bronchitis).

Emphysema is a pathological or radiological rather than a clinical diagnosis and is commonly associated with chronic bronchitis. Destruction of the alveolar septae results in the formation of large bullae in the lungs, with hyperinflation of the chest (4.61, 4.62) and impaired respiratory function.

The common combination of chronic bronchitis and emphysema has also been termed chronic obstructive airways disease (COAD) or chronic obstructive pulmonary disease (COPD). Up to 20% of adult males worldwide have the disease, and this proportion is higher in heavily industrialised countries. Chronic bronchitis occurs in the majority of heavy smokers, but significant airways obstruction and/or emphysema occurs in only a minority.

The characteristic clinical features of chronic bronchitis and emphysema are cough, productive of thick yellow-green sputum, wheeze and progressive breathlessness. The symptoms are usually worse in winter and exacerbated by atmospheric pollution, dry air, intercurrent infections and industrial exposure to irritant gases or dusts.

4.61

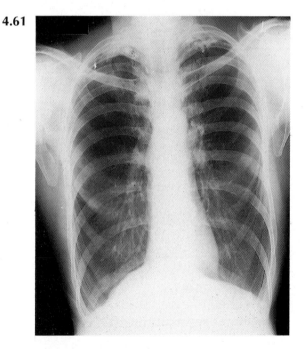

4.61 Emphysema. The PA chest X-ray shows hyperinflation of both lung fields, producing depression of both diaphragms and a characteristic long, thin mediastinum. There is some 'tenting' of both diaphragms as a result of previous infections. There are also calcified lesions and some scarring at both apices and both hila as a result of old, healed tuberculosis.

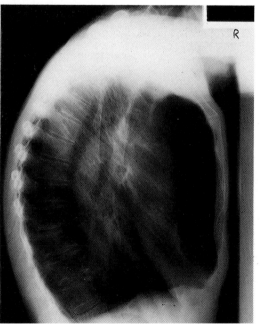

4.62

4.62 Emphysema. The right lateral chest X-ray shows a marked increase in the PA diameter of the chest, and confirms the diaphragmatic depression. In this patient the hilar calcification resulting from old, healed tuberculosis is also well seen in the lateral view. He also has marked osteophytes and degenerative changes in the discs (Schmorl's nodules) of the spine.

Two common presentations occur:

- The 'pink puffer' (**4.63**) usually has significant emphysema with a barrel-shaped chest, but is thin and maintains a normal $PaCO_2$ by increasing his respiratory rate.
- The 'blue bloater' (**4.64**) tends to be fatter, polycythaemic, centrally cyanosed and to show signs of pulmonary hypertension (**4.65**, **4.66**, **5.98**, *see* p. 241). As the disease progresses, the $PaCO_2$ rises and leads to a compensated respiratory acidosis (**4.67**, **4.68**).

The most important step in management is to persuade the patient to stop smoking, though this may be difficult. Bronchodilators may achieve some reversal of airways

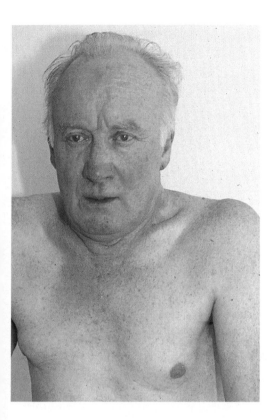

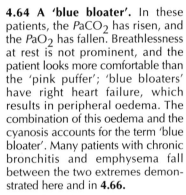

4.63 A 'pink puffer'. Some patients with severe long-standing chronic bronchitis and emphysema are breathless and have a hyperinflated chest, but a well maintained PaO_2 and a low $PaCO_2$. These patients are not cyanosed but are breathless, hence the term 'pink puffer'.

4.64 A 'blue bloater'. In these patients, the $PaCO_2$ has risen, and the PaO_2 has fallen. Breathlessness at rest is not prominent, and the patient looks more comfortable than the 'pink puffer'; 'blue bloaters' have right heart failure, which results in peripheral oedema. The combination of this oedema and the cyanosis accounts for the term 'blue bloater'. Many patients with chronic bronchitis and emphysema fall between the two extremes demonstrated here and in **4.66**.

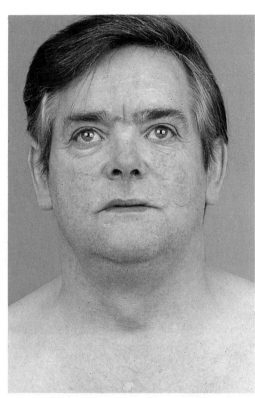

4.64

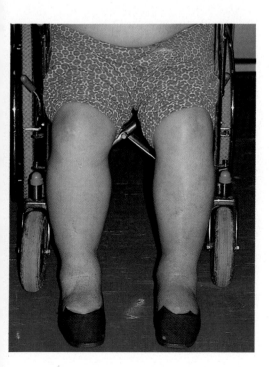

4.65 Chronic bronchitis with right heart failure causing gross peripheral oedema. The patient was a typical 'blue bloater' and he was not unduly breathless.

4.66 Cor pulmonale in a patient with emphysema. The bronchovascular markings at both hila are enlarged, reflecting pulmonary artery dilatation resulting from hypertension. The heart is generally enlarged.

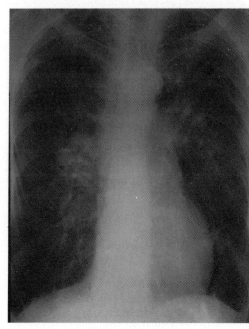

4.66

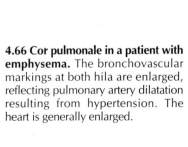

obstruction, and corticosteroids have a role in some patients. Complications such as right heart failure and polycythaemia (4.6) may require treatment. Long-term oxygen therapy for more than 15 hours daily has been shown to improve mortality and morbidity in some severely affected patients (4.69).

Infections are frequent, and it is important to educate patients in the early recognition of symptoms and signs, e.g. change of sputum colour and quality, fever or increasing wheeze. Many patients should be given a supply of antibiotics to keep at home for self-medication. There is little evidence that long-term antibiotic prophylaxis is of value, but influenza vaccination each winter may be worthwhile.

Chronic bronchitis and emphysema are very rare in non-smokers. Airways obstruction in a non- or light-smoker is usually caused by asthma, rarer causes being emphysema in alpha-1-antitrypsin deficiency, obliterative bronchiolitis or industrial lung disease, e.g. byssinosis.

4.67

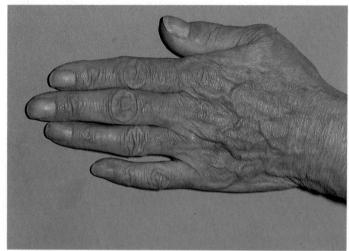

4.67 Respiratory acidosis produces peripheral vasodilatation, giving hands which are warm and dry, cyanosed and show features of a hyperkinetic circulation: a bounding pulse and tachycardia, with dilatation of the peripheral veins. A flapping tremor of the hands may also develop. This patient also has early finger clubbing, which is an indication for further investigation.

4.68

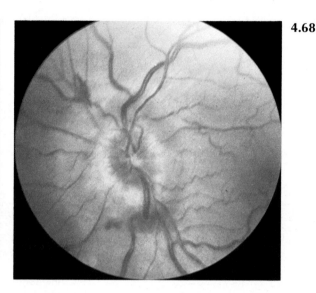

4.68 Papilloedema occurs in respiratory failure as a result of the increased cerebral and retinal blood flow caused by CO_2 retention. This papilloedema is similar to that seen in raised intracranial pressure of other causes.

4.69

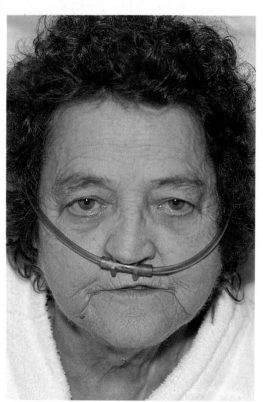

4.69 Long-term oxygen therapy from cylinders or an oxygen concentrator may be of value in patients with chronic stable respiratory failure. The flow rate and concentration are adjusted to relieve arterial hypoxaemia while avoiding carbon dioxide narcosis.

Sleep apnoea syndrome

With the aid of sleep laboratories, in which patients can be observed (and videoed) while having recordings of EEG, ECG and ear oximetry, a variety of disturbances in sleep patterns have now been recorded. The most common is the sleep apnoea syndrome which occurs as a result of intermittent pharyngeal obstruction during REM sleep. It is most common in grossly obese chronic bronchitics who have nasal obstruction and abuse alcohol or take hypnotics. The clinical presentation is often from the spouse who complains of explosive episodes of snoring or snorting; general poor sleep-quality and recurrent daytime tiredness are the patient's complaints. Investigation often shows alarming falls in ear-oxygen saturation during apnoeic episodes (4.70).

Management consists of control of preventable factors such as obesity, abstinence from alcohol and drugs, and treatment of local nasal factors. Continuous oxygen by catheter may be of value and a variety of prosthetic devices are being evaluated.

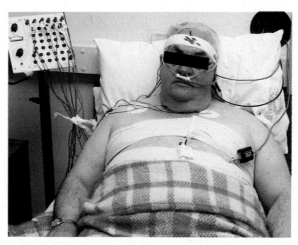

4.70

4.70 Sleep apnoea under investigation in a sleep laboratory. The syndrome should always be considered in patients with chronic respiratory disease who complain of daytime somnolence, or whose partners complain about the patient's snoring or apnoeic episodes at night. Alarming falls in arterial oxygen saturation may be found during sleep apnoea, and the syndrome is a cause of sudden death at night.

Bronchiectasis

Damage to the elastic and muscle fibres in the bronchial wall may lead to bronchiectasis—the abnormal dilatation of a bronchus (or bronchi). The pathological process by which the damage is initiated is often not clear, but a number of conditions are associated with subsequent development. These include:

- Impairment of mucociliary function as seen in Kartagener's syndrome and in cystic fibrosis.
- Impairment of immunity as in hypogammaglobulinaemia, which predisposes to recurrent infection.
- Acute suppurative or necrotising pneumonia resulting from viral or bacterial infections including tuberculosis.
- Persistent infection with Aspergillus, as in asthmatics.
- Bronchial obstruction by lymph nodes or by a foreign body.
- Inhalation of corrosive materials, e.g. gastric contents or industrial hydrocarbons.
- In some races there may be a hereditary element of bronchiectasis.

The end result of all these processes is a vicious circle of events in which there is alteration of normal drainage and mucus production, recurrent bacterial superinfection and acceleration of the lung damage.

The onset is usually insidious and the symptoms and signs are progressive. The first features include a chronic cough productive of increasing volumes of sputum which is intermittently infected (yellow or green) and often tinged with blood. Basal bronchiectasis may be associated with sudden coughing up of large volumes of sputum on changing posture. Episodes of superinfection may be associated with fever, signs of pneumonia, lung abscess, empyema and septicaemia. Copious foul-smelling sputum may be produced and occasionally major haemoptysis may lead to exsanguination. In the quiescent phase residual signs often persist, especially showers of coarse crepitations associated with areas of bronchial breathing. Finger clubbing (2.90, 2.91) is usual and may be progressive.

The clinical course is often progressive, with gradual loss of respiratory function and cor pulmonale is found in the late stages of the disease. Chronic disease may rarely be associated with secondary amyloid which presents with peripheral oedema and proteinuria (see p.290).

Diagnosis is made on history and examination, and the disease localised by plain X-ray (4.73), tomogram, bronchogram (4.71) or CT scanning (4.72). Monitoring of respiratory function tests, blood gases and renal function is important. The white cell count and ESR are raised in acute exacerbations.

Treatment consists of intensive physiotherapy and postural drainage. Antibiotics may be given for acute exacerbations or for prolonged periods as prophylaxis. Bronchodilators are of value when indicated by pulmonary function tests, and surgery should be considered for localised disease if the rest of the lung tissue is reasonably normal. Vaccination against influenza is probably of value as many acute exacerbations are precipitated by virus infections.

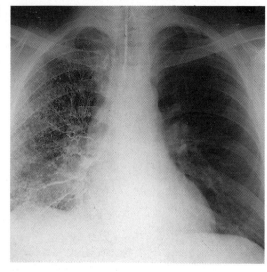

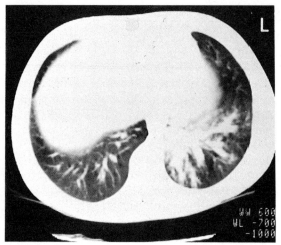

4.71 Bronchiectasis. This bronchogram shows diffuse bronchiectasis in the right lung, with dilatation of many of the proximal bronchi, and pooling of the contrast medium in the lower bronchi.

4.72 Bronchiectasis in the left lower lobe in a CT scan. Note the typical thickened bronchial walls, cystic changes and occluded tube-like branching bronchi. A CT scan is a good screening test for bronchiectasis, and is much less unpleasant for the patient than a bronchogram.

Cystic fibrosis

Cystic fibrosis is the most common fatal inherited disease in European populations; with a carrier frequency of 1:20 it affects 1:2,000 children. Recently, the abnormal gene was located on chromosome 7 and the structure of an abnormal protein has been identified. Prenatal diagnosis can now be made precisely and population screening for heterozygotes is theoretically possible.

The disease is characterised by production of mucus of high viscosity and a severe biochemical derangement of the sweat glands, which secrete an excess of sodium and chloride (3–5 times greater than normal). A major clinical feature of the disease is bronchiectasis (4.73 and *see* p. 183); and the majority of patients have pancreatic malabsorption (and thus require oral pancreatic enzyme preparations with food) (4.74). Other complications include meconium ileus, presenting at birth (4.75) pneumothorax, haemoptysis, cor pulmonale and diabetes mellitus.

In the past, most patients died in childhood from severe respiratory involvement, but the life expectancy of patients has increased with early diagnosis and prophylactic treatment. This has highlighted additional problems such as stunting of normal growth (resulting from malabsorption), infertility, because of lack of ciliary movement in the vas deferens, enhanced formation of gall stones and eventually cirrhosis of the liver.

Treatment of bronchiectasis and attention to nutrition are the mainstays of therapy; some patients are fortunate and receive a successful heart–lung transplant, but the majority still die early from respiratory failure (4.76). In affected families, genetic counselling is important and prenatal diagnosis should be offered.

184

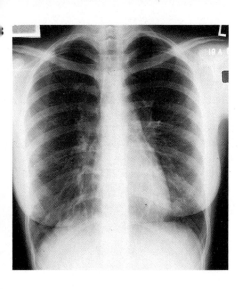

4.73 Bronchiectasis in cystic fibrosis. This chest X-ray of an 18-year-old shows hyperinflation, bronchial wall thickening and 'tramline' shadows in the areas affected by bronchiectasis.

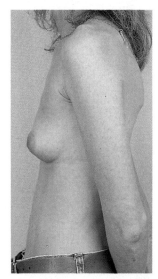

4.74

4.74 Cystic fibrosis presenting at the age of 18 years (the same patient as in **4.73**). This girl had previously been diagnosed as asthmatic, but she presented with weight loss (note the loose trousers and belt), and a sweat test confirmed the diagnosis. Her malabsorption was corrected by pancreatic enzyme supplements.

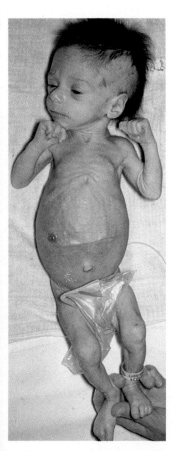

4.75 Cystic fibrosis presenting in the neonate. Note the emaciated appearance and distended abdomen, which follow surgery for meconium ileus. The meconium in cystic fibrosis is abnormally sticky, and this may result in intestinal blockage and peritonitis.

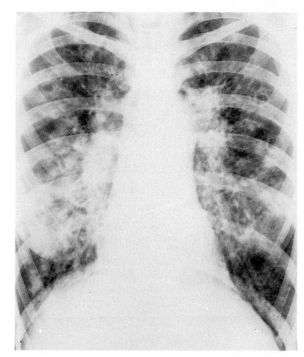

4.76

4.76 Terminal cystic fibrosis in a 16-year-old girl. There is hyperinflation, and gross lung destruction with 'tramlines' and large pulmonary vascular markings. The patient had severe pulmonary hypertension and she died two days after this X-ray was performed.

Pneumonia

Pneumonia is an inflammation of the lung, usually caused by bacteria, viruses or protozoa. If the infection is localised to one or two lobes of a lung it is referred to as 'lobar pneumonia' and if the infection is more generalised and involves primarily the bronchi it is known as 'bronchopneumonia'. A wide range of infecting organisms has been implicated (**Table 4.4**). In up to 30% of patients no organism is identified, usually because of prior antibiotic administration. In many patients there is a preceding history of an upper respiratory virus infection. Most community acquired pneumonia can be managed at home, and has a low mortality; studies of such patients admitted to hospital have shown a mortality of 6–24% depending on the population studied and the presence or absence of such risk factors as old age and underlying disease.

The usual clinical presentation in pneumonia caused by *Strep. pneumoniae* is acute, with the abrupt onset of malaise, fever, rigors, cough, pleuritic pain, tachycardia and tachypnoea, often accompanied by confusion, especially in the elderly. The signs include a high temperature, consolidation and pleural rubs, and herpetic lesions may appear on the lips. There may also be signs of pre-existing disease, especially chronic bronchitis and emphysema or heart failure in the elderly. The sputum becomes rust coloured over the following 24 hours (**4.12**). The diagnosis is made on clinical grounds and confirmed by chest X-ray (**4.77**). The white cell count and ESR are usually elevated. Blood should be sent for culture before antibiotic therapy is given and a baseline blood sample taken for serology. Sputum should be sent for culture. Direct Gram-staining of a fresh sputum sample may show the organism. Pneumococcal antigen can be identified in sputum, urine or serum. Antibiotic therapy should not be delayed whilst awaiting sputum culture results.

The symptoms usually resolve rapidly over 7–10 days and the signs over a slightly longer period. Radiological resolution should be complete by 12 weeks. Persistence of changes in the

Table 4.4 Pneumonia: infecting organisms in descending order of frequency.

	Per cent *
Community acquired	
Streptococcus pneumoniae	34
Mycoplasma pneumoniae	18
Influenza virus A	7
Haemophilus influenzae	6
Legionella pneumophila	2
Staphylococcus aureus	1
Coxiella burneti	(Rare—may be epidemic)
Chlamydia psittaci	
Hospital acquired	
Gram-negative bacilli	50
Staph. aureus	
Strep. pneumoniae	
L. pneumophila	30–40 (depending on the local situation)
H. influenzae	
Pseudomonas spp.	
Immunocompromised patients	
Pneumocystis carinii	85
Cytomegalovirus	
Mycobacterium avium-intracellulare	
Mycobacterium tuberculosis	
Strep. pneumoniae	
H. influenzae	
L. pneumophila	
Actinomyces israelii	
Aspergillus fumigatus	
Nocardia asteroides	

* Data from British Thoracic Society Survey, 1991.

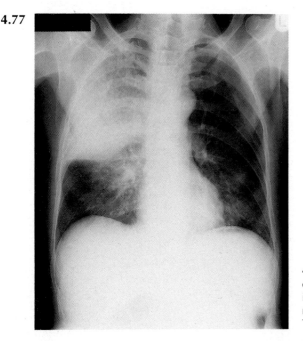

4.77

4.77 Pneumonia in the right upper lobe caused by *Streptococcus pneumoniae*. The consolidation involves the whole of the right upper lobe, and a small amount of fluid is present in the horizontal fissure. There are also some areas of consolidation in the right and left lower zones, probably as the result of transbronchial spread of infection. This patient produced typical rusty red sputum (**4.12**).

X-ray after this, or recurrence of pneumonia, suggests some other pathological process and should trigger a search for underlying carcinoma. Careful examination should be made at presentation for clinical features of AIDS (*see* p. 16).

Mycoplasma pneumoniae (p. 60) is the most common cause of the 'atypical' pneumonias. Infection usually occurs in older children and young adults, who present with pharyngitis and bronchitis; pneumonia occurs in the minority and is rarely severe (**4.78**). Psittacosis (p. 60) is acquired from birds and Q fever (p. 61) from animals, commonly farm livestock; they also cause 'atypical pneumonia', although the Q-fever organism, *Coxiella burnetii,* may also cause endocarditis. The diagnosis of the 'atypical' pneumonias is usually made by serology.

Staphylococcal pneumonia typically occurs as a complication of influenza, especially in the elderly and, although uncommon, is important because of the attendant high mortality. It is a destructive pneumonia, which frequently leads to the formation of cavities within the lung (**1.64**, **1.93**, **4.31**, **4.32**). Such cavitating pneumonia was most frequently caused by tuberculosis in the past but now *Staphylococci, Klebsiella* and anaerobic organisms are the most common causes.

Legionnaires' disease is pneumonia caused by *Legionella pneumophila* (*see* p. 53 and **1.142**). Infection is most common in debilitated or immunocompromised patients. Most cases occur sporadically, but outbreaks from contaminated water droplet sources occur. The disease may present with a wide spectrum of additional symptoms, such as headache, cerebellar ataxia, renal failure or hepatic involvement. Special medium is necessary for the culture of the organism and the diagnosis is usually made by serology.

Aspiration pneumonia results from the aspiration of gastric contents into the lung and is associated with impaired consciousness (e.g. anaesthesia—**4.79**, epilepsy, alcoholism) or dysphagia. Multiple organisms may be isolated.

Nosocomial pneumonia occurs when infection takes place in hospital; patients may be debilitated, immunocompromised or have just undergone a major operation. The causative organism(s) are often Gram-negative or the Gram-positive coccus, *S. aureus*. The high mortality is usually related to the severity of the underlying disease. Lung abscess and/or empyema (a collection of pus within the thoracic cavity) may be caused by specific organisms or may complicate any aspiration pneumonia. Septic pulmonary emboli can lead to multiple lung abscesses, pulmonary infarcts may become infected cavities and abscesses can develop distal to lesions obstructing a bronchus.

Treatment of all pneumonias should be started immediately and the antibiotic chosen should be the 'best guess' (decided on by the origin of the pneumonia and its clinical severity). If community acquired, then high-dose parenteral penicillin (or erythromycin) will usually be effective. If legionnaires' disease is suspected on epidemiological grounds, rifampicin should be given with erythromycin. If staphylococcal pneumonia is suspected, because of preceding influenza, flucloxacillin should be added to the regime. In hospital-acquired pneumonia, combination therapy is required to cover the range of possible pathogenic organisms (especially Gram-negative bacilli). Combinations such as gentamicin with piperacillin or a cephalosporin may be used. In aspiration pneumonia, where anaerobes may be present, metronidazole should be added to these combinations. Supportive measures should include oxygen, intravenous fluids, inotropic agents where necessary, bronchial suction and assisted ventilation. Physiotherapy and bronchodilators are of value in pneumonia complicating chronic bronchitis and emphysema.

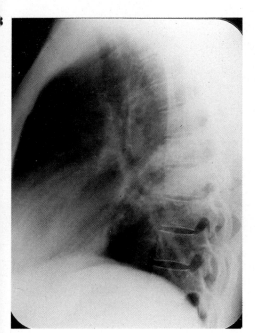

4.78 Pneumonia caused by mycoplasma pneumoniae. This patient presented with fever and left lower posterior pleuritic chest pain. There is patchy consolidation in the upper part of the left lower lobe, as seen in this left lateral film.

4.79 Postoperative pneumonia is common following abdominal surgery. This patient underwent urgent surgery for a perforated duodenal ulcer. Note the gas shadows below both diaphragms. He has a right basal consolidation, which results from a combination of aspiration and poor chest movement postoperatively.

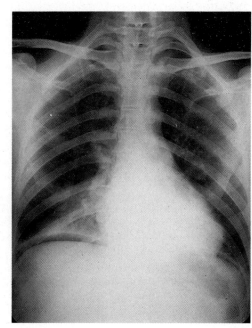

4.79

Infection in the immunocompromised host

There has been a steady increase in the number of patients whose immune system has been damaged by malignancy, organ failure, drugs or the HIV virus. In such immunocompromised patients, infections of the lung are common and may be caused by organisms which are not usually pathogenic in the normal host. Invasive fungal infections tend to occur in neutropenic patients, whereas T-cell defects often lead to infection with viruses, mycobacteria and protozoa such as *Pneumocystis carinii*. The tempo of infection in the immunocompromised patient can be extremely rapid; it is important to take steps to identify the pathogen and to start therapy as soon as possible.

Pneumocystis carinii

Pneumocystis carinii is the most important cause of fatal pneumonia in immunosuppressed patients. It is believed that the infection is acquired in early childhood, and that reactivation occurs when the immune system becomes damaged. The incubation period is approximately 1–2 months before the insidious appearance of a low-grade progressive pneumonia, which presents as severe dyspnoea with, at first, only minimal chest signs and X-ray changes (**4.80**). The pneumonia progresses rapidly, and within a few days gross pneumonic changes may be seen on the chest X-ray (**1.32**). Diagnosis depends on demonstrating the organism in sputum, bronchial lavage or lung tissue, which may require a lung biopsy (**4.44**). Treatment is with sulphonamide or pentamidine; both of these may be used in prophylaxis. Mortality remains high despite treatment.

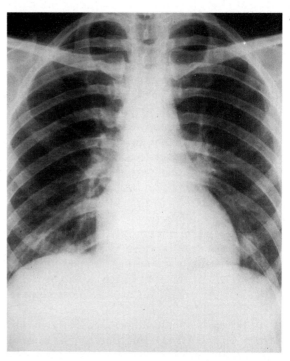

4.80

4.80 *Pneumocystis carinii* **pneumonia** on presentation in a patient with AIDS. The changes on X-ray are very minor, but the patient was markedly hypoxic and a transbronchial biopsy revealed *Pneumocystis carinii*. Unless the infection is treated promptly, gross pneumonic changes follow (*see* **1.32**).

Pulmonary tuberculosis

Tuberculosis may infect many parts of the body (see p. 46), but pulmonary infection is its most common manifestation.

Primary infection usually involves the lungs (**1.119, 1.120**). Within months, further pulmonary complications may occur, including lobar collapse, bronchiectasis, miliary tuberculosis (**1.121**) or the development of a pleural effusion (**4.81**).

More commonly, the 'primary complex' in the lung heals and calcifies. The patient remains well, often for many years or even for life. If host resistance is lowered later in life, by malignant disease or its treatment, by diabetes mellitus, by malnutrition or by HIV infection, however, or if reinfection with large numbers of organisms occurs, the patient may develop active adult pulmonary tuberculosis.

Pulmonary tuberculosis is characterised by fever, tiredness, malaise, anorexia and weight loss, associated with an increasingly productive cough. There may be few or no signs on examination, but X-ray changes are always present, and may include patchy or nodular pneumonic shadowing in the upper zones (**4.82**), cavitation (**4.82–4.84**), calcification (**4.85**), fibrosis (**4.86**) and· lymph node enlargement (**1.124–1.126, 4.11**). Pleural effusion (**4.81**) and calcification may also be seen.

The diagnosis may be strongly suggested by the X-ray appearances. However, microbiological confirmation is necessary to exclude chronic necrotising pulmonary

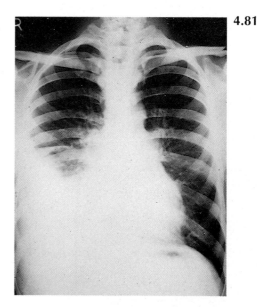

4.81

4.81 Tuberculous pleural effusion. This patient presented with a 6 month history of malaise and weight-loss, but no symptoms directly referable to the chest. The large right pleural effusion is accompanied by fluid in the horizontal fissure. Aspiration and culture confirmed the diagnosis.

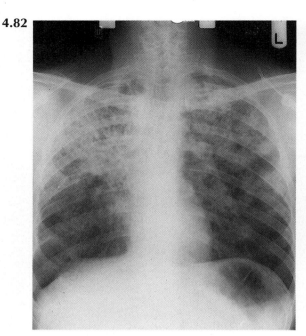

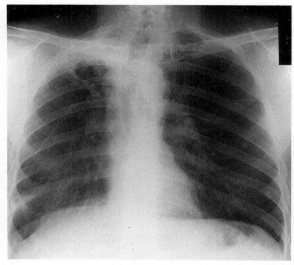

4.82, 4.83 Active tuberculosis in a Greek immigrant to the UK (**4.82**), who presented with weight-loss, low-grade fever and fresh haemoptysis. He gave a family history of tuberculosis. This film shows multiple areas of shadowing, especially in the upper lobes, and several lesions have started to cavitate. Despite the extensive nature of the disease, chemotherapy resulted in dramatic healing of the lesions as seen in a film taken 3 years later (**4.83**), which shows only minimal residual scarring at both apices.

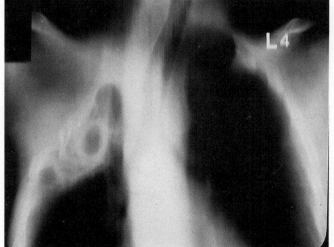

4.84 Cavitating right apical tuberculosis revealed on tomography. This 'slice' shows 3 separate cavities, surrounded by dense inflammation and fibrosis, with pulling of the trachea to the right. The chest wall has been surgically collapsed (thoracoplasty). This obsolete technique was used before effective chemotherapy became available in an attempt to accelerate the healing of the cavities.

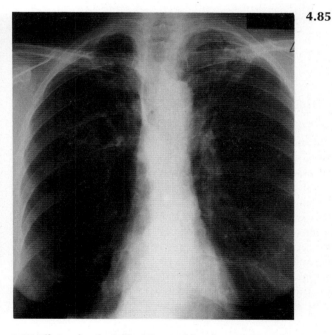

4.85 Bilateral apical fibrosis resulting from pulmonary tuberculosis. The hila are elevated, and streaky linear shadows extend from the hila to the apices. Scattered calcified upper zone nodules are also present bilaterally.

aspergillosis, which produces a similar picture, histoplasmosis (p. 62) and coccidioidomycosis (p. 64)—especially in those living in or who have visited an endemic area for these diseases, and cryptococcosis in immunocompromised patients. Similar appearances may also occur with atypical mycobacterial infections in normal and immunocompromised patients (*see* p. 49).

Pulmonary tuberculosis requires treatment with antituberculous chemotherapy for a period of 6–9 months. Investigation and immunisation of contacts is necessary (p. 46). Patients with signs of previous tuberculosis (as in **4.82**, **4.87**), who are about to undergo immunosuppressive drug treatment or manoeuvres such as haemodialysis for renal failure, should be given prophylactic antituberculous therapy.

4.86

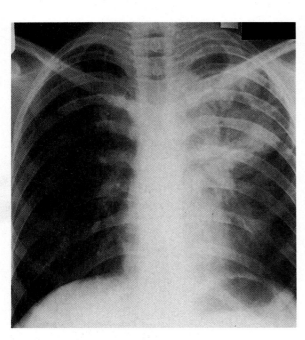

4.86 Tuberculous left upper zone pneumonia, confirmed by sputum examination. The presence of an air bronchogram in the left upper zone confirms that the underlying pathology is consolidation rather than collapse.

4.87 Tuberculoma. This solid, calcified lesion in the right lower lobe (as confirmed by a lateral film) represents the healed stage of tuberculosis. There is associated bilateral hilar lymph node calcification. It is important to exclude the possibility of lung cancer whenever solitary lesions are seen.

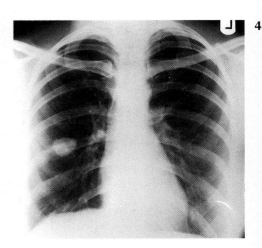

Pulmonary infiltrations

Sarcoidosis

This multisystem disorder is most often found in the lung parenchyma and related lymph nodes, but it can involve the skin, eyes, peripheral lymph nodes, gut, liver, bone and central nervous system. The pathological process is a granulomatous reaction of the type seen with insoluble antigens, but as yet no single factor has been positively identified. It is not contagious, but there is a slightly increased incidence within families and in women. In the USA it is much more common in black patients.

The most common clinical presentation of sarcoidosis is respiratory. It is often found on chest X-rays in patients with non-specific features such as tiredness, weight loss or recurrent fever. The characteristic lesions are:

- Bilateral hilar lymphadenopathy (**4.88**), usually asymptomatic, which will subside without treatment in about 80–90% of patients.
- Pulmonary infiltration with bilateral hilar lymphadenopathy (**4.89**, **4.90**), which may cause symptoms including dyspnoea, cough and fever, but which subsides in 40% of patients.
- Pulmonary fibrosis following diffuse infiltration, ultimately leading to bullae formation and/or fibrosis (**4.91**, **4.92**), associated with symptoms and a restrictive defect on respiratory function testing.

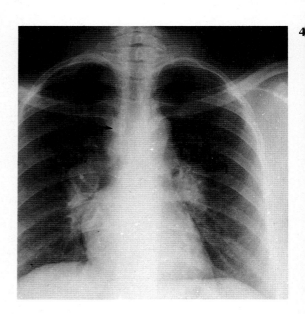

4.88 Bilateral hilar lymphadenopathy (1) in a patient with sarcoidosis. Note that there is increased right paratracheal shadowing (2) and shadowing in the aortico-pulmonary window (3). These shadows indicate more widespread lymph node enlargement, but the prognosis at this stage is good, even without treatment.

Evidence of the disease should be sought in the skin, eye and peripheral lymph nodes.

The most common skin lesion in sarcoidosis is erythema nodosum (1.123, 2.40). However, this is a non-specific sign, the most common cause of which is a reaction to sulphonamides. Sarcoid nodules may be found in the skin in about 5% of cases particularly on the face, especially the nose (lupus pernio) (4.93, 4.94), in scars and elsewhere (4.95).

Eye involvement may present acutely with a painful eye and acute impairment of vision (4.96). More often there is progressive visual impairment from posterior uveitis (4.97). There may also be involvement of the lacrimal glands (producing dry eyes) and of both parotids (uveoparotid fever) producing a dry mouth. The seventh cranial nerve may be involved by this process or by more proximal involvement. Localised involvement of bones may give tender swellings (4.98) and X-rays may show localised bone cysts. Involvement of heart, gut and liver are rare.

Hypercalcaemia is often found in established disease as a result of additional α-hydroxylation occurring in the sarcoid lesions in the lung. This may result in metastatic calcification or stone formation in the urinary tract (*see* p. 301).

The diagnosis is made by biopsy of lymph nodes, skin or lung. Lung function tests often show a restrictive defect and the Mantoux test is often negative. The Kveim test is now of largely historical interest; the theoretical possibility of HIV transmission limits its use.

Treatment of sarcoidosis depends on the extent of the disease and the tissues involved. Parenchymal lung disease, acute eye involvement and central nervous system or heart signs require a prolonged course of steroids. Minor skin or lymph node involvement can be watched over a period of months for spontaneous resolution. The level of angiotensin-converting enzyme is often raised and may be used to follow the course of disease activity, but this is not a specific diagnostic test.

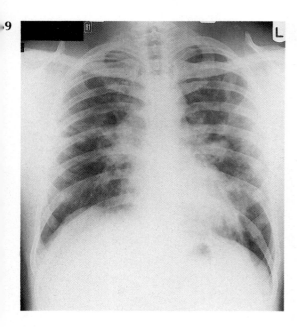

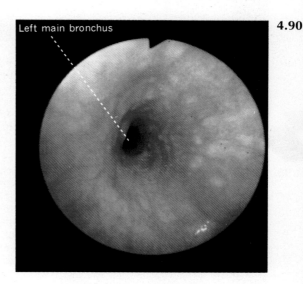

4.89 Pulmonary infiltration with bilateral hilar lymphadenopathy in a patient with sarcoidosis. Note the nodular pattern in both lung fields with relative sparing of the apices in this patient. In this young man, the important differential diagnosis included secondary deposits, especially as a cystic testicular swelling was found; but in this case the diagnosis of sarcoidosis was confirmed by lung biopsy, and the swelling was a simple hydrocoele.

Left main bronchus

4.90 Bronchoscopic findings in a patient with infiltrative sarcoidosis. The lumen of the left main bronchus is so narrowed that a fibreoptic bronchoscope can hardly pass through it. There are dilated mucosal vessels, and multiple sarcoid nodules in the mucosa.

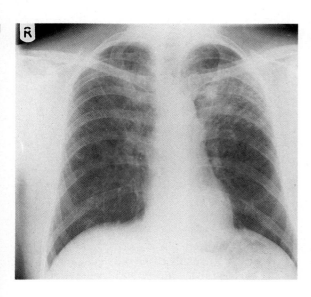

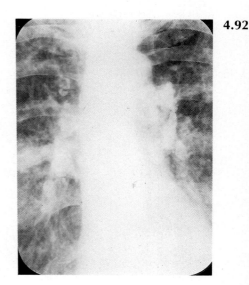

4.91 Extensive chronic fibrotic sarcoidosis. This degree of fibrosis results in severe irreversible impairment of respiratory function.

4.92 'Eggshell' calcification is often seen in chronic sarcoidosis, as in the left hilar nodes in this patient.

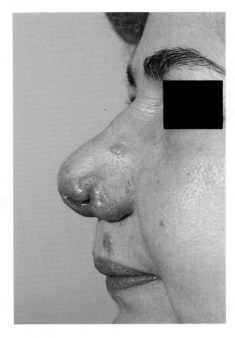

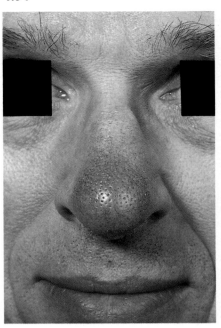

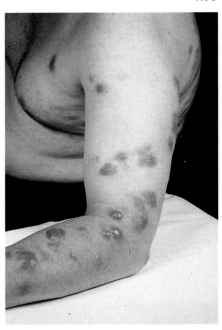

4.93 Skin infiltration has resulted in destructive lesions of the nose in this patient with sarcoidosis. Note the presence of a separate lesion on the upper lip.

4.94 Lupus pernio is the term used to describe a dusky purple infiltration of the skin of the nose in chronic sarcoidosis. It is important to distinguish this appearance from rhinophyma and acne rosacea.

4.95 Sarcoid lesions may occur in the skin at any site, and they may take noular, papular or plaque forms. Biopsy is usually necessary for diagnosis.

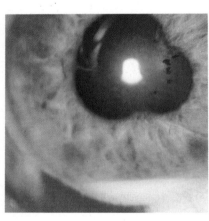

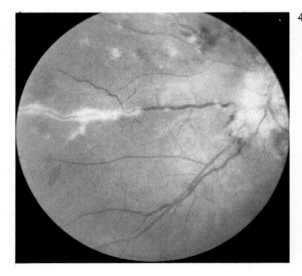

4.96 Acute anterior uveitis in sarcoidosis. Note the fluid level of pus in the anterior chamber (hypopyon) and the distortion of the pupil caused by the development of posterior synechiae. A cataract may form if this eye involvement does not receive prompt treatment.

4.97 Posterior uveitis is a relatively common complication in sarcoidosis, and may cause choroiditis and retinitis. In this patient, a focal retinal periphlebitis alternates with stretches of unaffected vein.

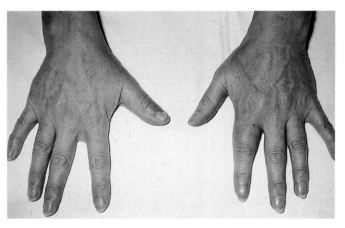

4.98 Dactylitis in sarcoidosis. The left index finger shows obvious signs of inflammation and swelling, particularly of the proximal phalanx and interphalangeal joint, and the other digits are also involved.

Histiocytosis X

This is a disease of unknown aetiology, which is associated with the presence of granulomas that are rich in eosinophils. There are two forms found in young children (Letterer–Siwe and Hand–Schüller–Christian disease) and one in adults (eosinophilic granuloma). The granulomas may be found in bones and in the lung parenchyma where they produce progressive restrictive lung disease and may produce pneumothorax (4.99). Hypothalamic/pituitary axis involvement may lead to diabetes insipidus, panhypopituitarism or obesity.

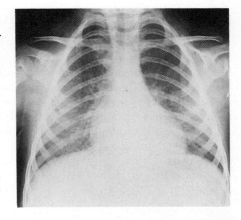

4.99 Histiocytosis X in a child. Granuloma formation has produced generalised miliary mottling.

Vasculitis

The vasculitic diseases most commonly affecting the lung are Wegener's granulomatosis and the Churg–Strauss syndrome. Classical polyarteritis nodosa rarely affects the upper and lower respiratory tracts; renal involvement (*see* p. 287) is much more common.

Wegener's granulomatosis

Wegener's granulomatosis consists of the clinical triad of upper respiratory tract granulomas (3.94), fleeting lung shadows and necrotising glomerulonephritis (*see* p. 149).

Chest X-rays show nodular masses and pneumonic infiltrates (4.100). Cavitation may also occur. In the early stages, the chest X-ray changes are 'fleeting': lesions clear from one area as new lesions appear elsewhere. Immunosuppressive therapy may help to reverse the lung changes, but renal involvement usually requires complex therapy (*see* p. 288).

Churg–Strauss syndrome

The Churg–Strauss syndrome (*see* p. 150) usually occurs in subjects with asthma, and is characterised by a high blood eosinophil count, pulmonary infiltrates and involvement of the locomotor system, skin, gut and nervous system but rarely the kidneys.

Polyarteritis nodosa

Polyarteritis nodosa is a multisystem disorder characterised by widespread vasculitis (*see* p. 148). Pulmonary involvement may rarely occur, presenting with cough, haemoptysis, fever or asthmatic symptoms. Chest X-ray may show pneumonic infiltration (4.101) and biopsy of lung or other tissue may be required for definitive diagnosis.

4.100

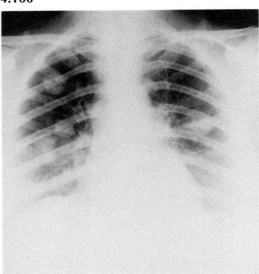

4.101

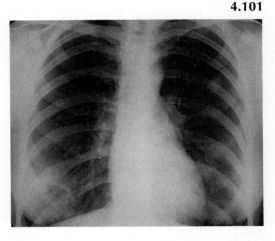

4.100 Wegener's granulomatosis, showing multiple bilateral nodular lesions and pneumonic infiltration in both lower zones.

4.101 Polyarteritis nodosa with pulmonary infiltration in the both lower zones. The appearance is not diagnostic, and the diagnosis must be based on the clinical picture and confirmed by angiography and/or biopsy.

Pulmonary complications of the connective tissue diseases

Fibrosing alveolitis, indistinguishable from the cryptogenic variety (4.102) (*see* p. 196), may occur in any collagen disease, but is most commonly seen in rheumatoid arthritis. There is an excess mortality from respiratory infection in rheumatoid arthritis. Other pulmonary complications also occur, including bronchitis; obliterative bronchiolitis and bronchiectasis; multiple (3.33) or single (4.103) pulmonary nodules, which may cavitate; and pleural effusions (3.32), which occur predominantly in men. In Caplan's syndrome, pulmonary lesions occur in a patient with rheumatoid arthritis who has been exposed to dust as a coal miner or in an industrial setting; they may progress to massive pulmonary fibrosis (4.115). Complications seen in other connective tissue diseases include: pleurisy, pleural effusions and lung atelectasis in systemic lupus erythematosus; pulmonary hypertension and basal fibrosis (4.102) in systemic sclerosis; and upper zone fibrosis in ankylosing spondylitis.

4.102

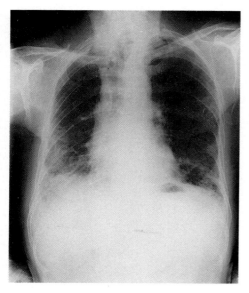

4.103

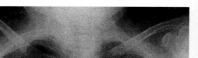
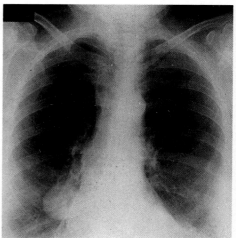

4.102 Fibrosing alveolitis causing diffuse lower zone shadowing in a patient with rheumatoid arthritis. The appearance is indistinguishable from that seen in patients with cryptogenic fibrosing alveolitis, and similar appearances may occur in other connective tissue disorders including systemic sclerosis. The apparent mediastinal shift in this film results largely from rotation of the patient, whose arthritis prevented accurate positioning.

4.103 A single rheumatoid nodule in the right lower zone in a 55-year-old woman with rheumatoid arthritis. Note the rheumatoid changes in the left shoulder. Rheumatoid nodules are more common in men, and solitary nodules often require biopsy to exclude malignancy.

Pulmonary infiltration with eosinophilia

The association of blood eosinophilia and pulmonary shadowing may occur in a number of situations, many of which are imperfectly characterised.

Simple pulmonary eosinophilia is a short-lived illness in which cough and a slight fever are associated with transient pneumonic shadowing (4.104) and blood eosinophilia. It appears to be an allergic response, and the provoking allergen may be the result of worm infestation or drug therapy, though often no allergen can be identified. The condition is usually self-limiting.

Allergic aspergillosis (*see* p. 63) occurs in asthmatics and may produce chronic symptoms with the risk of permanent lung damage (1.166); as may tropical pulmonary eosinophilia, which is probably usually caused by a reaction to *Wuchereria bancrofti* infection (*see* p. 72), and the 'hypereosinophilic' syndrome, in which the provoking cause in unknown.

4.104

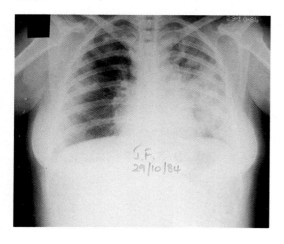

4.105

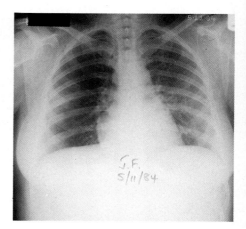

4.104, 4.105 Pulmonary infiltration with eosinophilia (also known as Löffler's syndrome) (4.104). In this patient the infiltration was mainly in the left lung, and it persisted for 2–3 weeks. The patient had a mild fever and a cough, but no other symptoms. **4.105** shows the appearance of the chest 4 weeks after **4.104**. Spontaneous clearing of the lung shadowing within one month is usual, and the condition produces few, if any, symptoms.

Goodpasture's syndrome

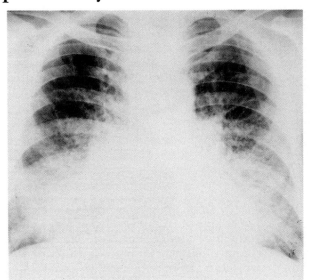

4.106

This is a disease of unknown aetiology which often presents after an upper respiratory infection. The patient usually has small repeated haemoptyses with progressive dyspnoea and cough, followed by massive intrapulmonary bleeding, which may present acutely with dyspnoea and massive haemoptysis (4.106). These appearances may precede the development of acute glomerulonephritis, which often progresses to renal failure (*see* p.286). The disease is mediated by anti-glomerular basement membrane antibodies. Treatment is generally unsatisfactory in the established case (*see* p. 286).

4.106 Goodpasture's syndrome. Massive intrapulmonary bleeding has led to opacities ('white-out') of both mid and lower zones on chest X-ray. The mortality rate is high as a result of pulmonary and renal involvement.

Pulmonary oedema: cardiogenic and non-cardiogenic

In patients with heart disease, a rise in the hydrostatic pressure within the pulmonary capillaries produces pulmonary oedema. This is most commonly seen acutely, following a myocardial infarction, pulmonary embolus, arrhythmia or hypertension, or may happen chronically in patients with valve disease or a rise in pulmonary or systemic pressure (5.14, 5.23).

Acute pulmonary oedema may also be the result of a range of non-cardiac conditions, the end result of which is to increase the permeability of the pulmonary capillaries (**Table 4.5**). Most of these patients are admitted with an acute medical or surgical condition which is later followed, in hours or days, by progressive hypoxia, and dyspnoea associated with scattered rhonchi and crepitations over the lung fields (the 'adult respiratory distress syndrome'). X-rays show diffuse patchy 'infiltrates' (4.107). These findings often progress rapidly to cardiorespiratory failure and death, and assisted ventilation may be urgently required.

4.107

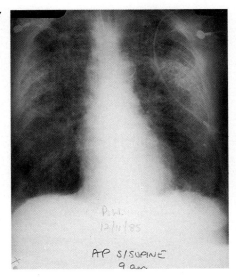

4.107 Adult respiratory distress syndrome. The chest X-ray appearances are similar to those seen in cardiogenic pulmonary oedema, but the condition results from an increase in pulmonary capillary permeability rather than from heart failure. This patient had inhaled smoke in a domestic fire.

Table 4.5 Causes of the adult respiratory distress syndrome.

Inhaled smoke
Overwhelming infections
Aspiration of gastric contents
Drowning
Uraemia
Pancreatitis
Massive blood transfusion
Disseminated intravascular coagulation (DIC)
Poisoning with paraquat
Post-cardiopulmonary bypass
Acute radiation pneumonia

Pulmonary fibrosis

Many different lung diseases may result in pulmonary fibrosis, which may be localised or generalised. For example:

- Localised unilateral fibrosis may result from a destructive pneumonia.
- Localised bilateral fibrosis may occur in tuberculosis, histoplasmosis and other chronic infections.

- Generalised fibrosis may occur as the end-stage of a range of parenchymal lung disorders, including industrial lung diseases, connective tissue diseases and sarcoidosis; and in cryptogenic fibrosing alveolitis and extrinsic allergic alveolitis.

Cryptogenic fibrosing alveolitis

CFA (idiopathic pulmonary fibrosis) is the most common of the interstitial lung diseases. Alveolitis leads to the destruction of alveoli and the laying down of scar tissue (fibrosis), which further disrupts the function of the lung. There is wide variation in the tempo of the illness. Patients may die from respiratory failure within a few months of presentation, or the disease may be identified by chance and show little progression over many years. Most commonly, the disease progresses to respiratory failure over a few years. The principal symptoms are dyspnoea and cough, generally unproductive. Gross clubbing of the fingers is characteristic (4.108) and crackles are heard, particularly at the lung bases. Chest X-ray shows predominantly lower zone shadowing (4.109) and comparison of x-rays over time often shows a loss of lung volume (if taken correctly in full inspiration, the chest X-ray is a good indicator of total lung capacity). Pulmonary function tests show a restrictive defect, often with a greater reduction in transfer factor than would be expected for the loss of lung volume. Blood tests may show positive autoantibodies and there is an association with other autoimmune diseases (4.102). The response to treatment with immunosuppressive agents is better if active inflammation is more marked than fibrosis in the lung histology. Younger and otherwise fit patients with severe disease should be considered for heart–lung transplantation.

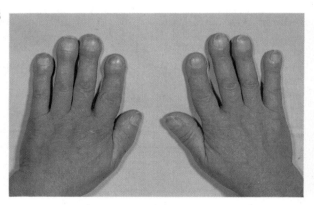

4.108 Gross clubbing of the fingers is characteristic of cryptogenic fibrosing alveolitis (*see also* **2.89, 2.90**). Note also the tar staining of the fingers in this patient who continued to smoke despite his precarious respiratory state.

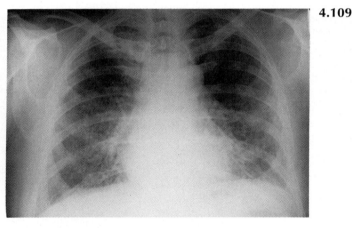

4.109 Cryptogenic fibrosing alveolitis typically causes predominantly basal pulmonary shadowing. Note that the appearance is very similar to that found in rheumatoid fibrosis (**4.102**).

Extrinsic allergic alveolitis

Extrinsic allergic alveolitis (EAA, allergic bronchioalveolitis, hypersensitivity pneumonitis) develops as a result of a hypersensitivity reaction in the lungs, provoked by a wide range of organic dusts. Many of these are encountered at work, and a large number of occupational lung diseases fall within this classification; while other causes relate to hobbies, especially the keeping of birds. Some common causes are listed in **Table 4.6**.

Repeated exposure of a susceptible individual to the offending antigen leads to the production of circulating precipitating antibodies and immune complexes and ultimately to macrophage activation and epithelioid cell granuloma formation.

The factors which predispose to allergic alveolitis are poorly understood. There is some evidence of genetic susceptibility, but no link with atopy, or with elevated IgE or eosinophil levels.

Symptoms may develop within six hours of heavy exposure to the antigen, and the most common presentation is with breathlessness, dry cough and influenza-like symptoms (malaise, fever and muscle pains). Chest X-ray in the acute phase shows a fine nodular shadowing (**4.110**), but repeated exposure may lead to chronic respiratory impairment caused by pulmonary fibrosis (**4.111**), which radiologically tends to be more marked in the upper zones, as with sarcoidosis, than in the lower zones, as with cryptogenic fibrosing alveolitis.

Table 4.6 Some common causes of extrinsic allergic alveolitis.

Disease	Provoking activity	Antigens
Farmer's lung	Forking mouldy vegetable matter, especially mouldy hay	Thermophilic actinomycetes *Micropolyspora faeni*
Bird fancier's lung	Handling pigeons or cleaning pigeon lofts and budgerigar cages	Proteins from feathers and excreta
Maltworker's lung	Turning germinating barley	*Aspergillus clavatus*
Humidifier fever	Working in offices or factories with contaminated air-conditioning or humidifying systems	Possibly bacterial or protozoal (esp. *Naegleria gruberi*)

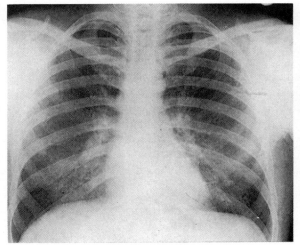

4.110

4.110 Acute extrinsic allergic alveolitis—in this case pigeon fancier's lung. This man presented with acute symptoms after cleaning out his pigeon loft. The X-ray shows diffuse, hazy opacification in both lung fields which partially obscures the normal vascular markings.

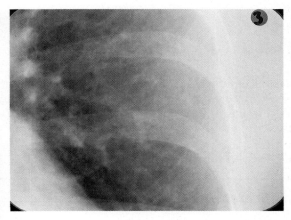

4.111

4.111 Chronic extrinsic allergic alveolitis—budgerigar fancier's lung. Budgerigar fanciers may develop similar X-ray changes to pigeon fanciers (**4.110**) or to those with farmer's lung. Because they often keep their birds indoors, their exposure to antigen is more constant and they usually present with insidious chronic lung disease. This X-ray shows diffuse fibrosis and some bullae towards the hilum. The changes led to a permanent severe ventilatory restrictive and diffusion defect.

Iatrogenic lung disease

The most common iatrogenic lung lesion results from radiotherapy, usually given for diseases such as cancer of the breast, bronchus, thymus or lymph nodes. The determining factors in lung damage are total radiation dose, duration of time over which the dose is given and the number of treatments. Acute radiation pneumonitis occurs a few days to some weeks after exposure and presents with a cough, fever and progessive dyspnoea. Corticosteroids may ameliorate these acute symptoms. Fibrosis may develop over many months (**4.112**) and there is evidence of a progressive restrictive defect in the pulmonary function tests with a decrease in transfer of carbon monoxide.

A large number of drugs, alone or in combination, may produce a range of respiratory problems which include:

- Asthma.
- Infiltration/fibrosis.
- Eosinophilia.
- SLE-like syndromes.
- Respiratory depression.
- Opportunistic infection.

4.112

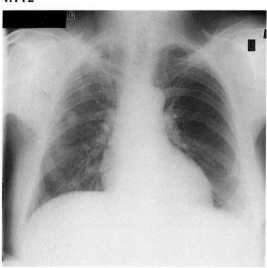

4.112 Radiation fibrosis. This patient had undergone a right mastectomy (note missing breast shadow) for breast cancer, followed by a course of radiotherapy. There are fibrotic changes in the lung, with upper lobe shrinkage, especially on the right, and the trachea is pulled to the right. She also had some ununited rib fractures on the right, resulting from secondary deposits.

Occupational lung disease

Lung diseases associated with industrial exposure are a common problem. They can be avoided if appropriate occupational regulations are enforced, especially efficient ventilation and individual protection by ventilators or masks. A range of common disorders related to dust inhalation are listed in **Table 4.7**. Asthma (p. 176) and extrinsic allergic alveolitis (p. 197) are other common problems.

Table 4.7 Lung diseases caused by dust inhalation.

Disease	Dust	Notes
Coal workers' pneumoconiosis	Coal	Simple/complicated
Silicosis	Crystalline silica	Simple/complicated
Asbestosis	Serpentine (Chrysolite) Amphibole (Crocidolite, amosite, anthophyllite)	
Pneumoconiosis	Talc, slate, kaolin	Rarely produces nodular fibrosis and pleural plaques
Stannosis	Tin oxide	Rare
Baritosis	Barium sulphate	Rare
Berylliosis	Beryllium	May produce acute bronchiolitis, pneumonia and pulmonary oedema

Coal workers' pneumoconiosis

Pneumoconiosis is lung disease resulting from exposure to coal dust. Coal workers' pneumoconiosis (CWP) was commonplace until dust exposure was reduced. Initially, it was believed that the disease was caused by the inhalation of silica (silicosis), but it is now clear that the disease can be caused by silica-free coal dust, although the mineral make-up of the dust influences the incidence and progression. CWP and silicosis are defined radiologically as **simple** where there is fine micronodulation, usually in the upper lobes (**4.30, 4.113**), or as **complicated** where the nodules coalesce to masses greater than 1 cm in diameter causing lung damage and significant functional impairment (**4.114**). These diseases attract industrial compensation in many countries, and a spectrum of functional and radiological lung changes is recognised for this purpose. Tests of lung function show a reduction in lung volume, with some obstruction and restrictive defects. Patients who are developing complicated CWP complain of progressive dyspnoea on exertion and eventually at rest. Cough with black sputum is a common feature (melanoptysis). No treatment prevents the progression of the disease. The picture is often clouded by the effects of chronic cigarette smoking and in some cases by coincidental infection with tuberculosis. Many of these patients also have chronic bronchitis and emphysema.

Caplan's syndrome is the association of rheumatoid arthritis with CWP. The nodules may grow rapidly and may cavitate (**4.115**). These appearances are usually associated with the presence of subcutaneous nodules, active joint disease and high titres of rheumatoid factor.

4.113

4.114

4.115

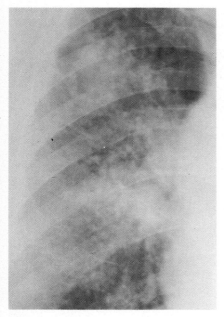

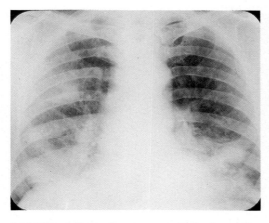

4.114 Complicated pneumoconiosis. Large fibrotic masses, which are irregular in shape, are present, mainly in both lower zones the upper and right middle lobes. Similar appearances may occur in complicated silicosis.

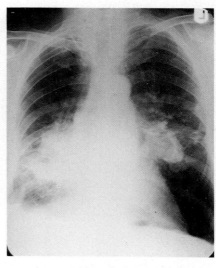

4.115 Progressive massive fibrosis (PMF) in Caplan's syndrome. There is progression in the formation of fibrotic tissue to form large masses, as seen in both midzones. Central necrosis has led to a fluid-filled cavity in the right lung, and the necrotic material may be coughed up.

4.113 Simple pneumoconiosis. A close-up view shows the fine, reticular pattern associated with the repeated inhalation of coal dust. The appearance is very similar to that of other forms of miliary mottling. It may not be associated with symptoms.

Silicosis

This is a disease of miners, tunnellers and stonemasons, which results from inhalation of crystalline silica. The result is progressive pulmonary fibrosis that ranges in appearance from micronodular fibrosis to progressive massive fibrosis, as in coal workers' pneumoconiosis. The time taken for development of the changes depends on the amount of inhaled silica. With **simple silicosis** there are usually no clinical features and the condition is diagnosed on routine X-ray. **Complicated silicosis** is associated with progressive dyspnoea, weight loss, cough and recurrent chest infections. The X-ray appearance is of progressive fibrosis (**4.114**), there may be a pleural reaction and the hilar lymph nodes may be enlarged. Pulmonary function tests become abnormal as the disease progresses and the defects are a mixture of restriction and obstruction. The disease may be compounded by cigarette smoking and infection with tuberculosis, fungi or bacteria. There is no specific treatment for the fibrous reaction. Prevention of exposure to silica dust is the key to prevention.

Asbestosis

Asbestos can exist in a variety of chemical forms which are associated with different disease patterns in the lung. Inhalation of the fibres as a result of industrial or occupational exposure was relatively common in certain industries, especially shipbuilding, insulation and demolition. The risks are greatest with the chemical forms crocidolite (blue asbestos) and chrysolite (white asbestos). The long-term effects include pulmonary fibrosis, pleural effusion, pleural thickening and eventual calcified pleural plaques, mesothelioma and bronchial carcinoma. These effects are compensatable in many countries. The diagnosis depends on a history of exposure to the fibres, usually at work. There may be evidence of a restrictive lung defect which progresses over a period of years. X-rays are important and may show a spectrum of abnormalities (4.116 –4.119). Examination of the sputum may show asbestos bodies (4.14). A history of cigarette smoking is important, as tobacco smoke and asbestos exposure seem to have a synergistic action in promoting subsequent onset of bronchial carcinoma. Mesothelioma is a highly malignant tumour of the pleurae which requires a pleural biopsy for diagnosis. Treatment of asbestos-related disease is ineffective and this underlines the importance of preventing exposure.

4.116

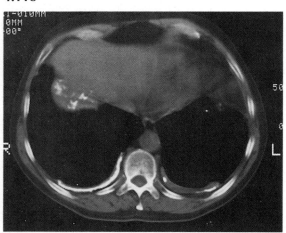

4.117

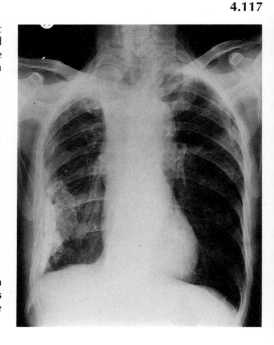

4.116 Asbestosis. The fairly early fibrotic changes in the lungs are best seen around the heart and in the lower zones. The patient's occupational exposure was as a shipyard worker.

4.117 Extensive pleural calcification following long-term industrial asbestos exposure. There are many plaques in the parietal pleura on the right.

4.118

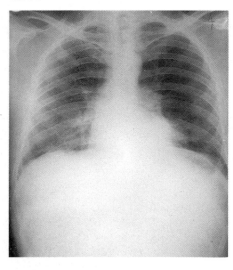

4.119

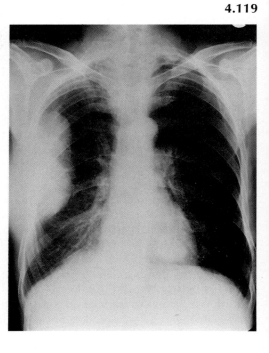

4.118 Pleural calcification shown by CT scan in the patient seen in **4.117**. The pleural calcification is particularly obvious in this cut posteriorly on the right; and anteriorly, the calcification in the right diaphragmatic pleura is clearly seen.

4.119 Mesothelioma of the right pleura. The patient had a long history of asbestos exposure and has now developed a large pleural mass which can be seen by soft tissue shadowing to have extended through the chest wall (see **4.46**).

4.120 Carcinoma of the bronchus in asbestosis. Reticulo-nodular shadowing is present throughout both lungs, especially basally. A mass is seen behind the heart in the left lower lobe. Percutaneous needle biopsy showed a squamous cell carcinoma. The patient was a retired shipbuilder.

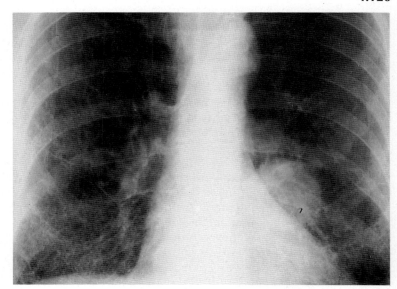

Tumours of the lung

Benign tumours

Benign tumours of the lung account for about 2% of all tumours of lung and present either as solitary nodules on the chest X-ray or, if endobronchial, with cough, haemoptysis or pneumonia. The most common type is a hamartoma, which is usually found as a solitary nodule in a young asymptomatic adult (**4.34, 4.121**). Other benign tumours are rarely seen. Endobronchial carcinoid tumours may give rise to atelectasis, recurrent infections and sometimes bronchiectasis. The carcinoid syndrome may occasionally be seen, and carcinoid tumours may ultimately metastasise.

The treatment of all these tumours is surgical removal whenever possible.

4.121 A pulmonary hamartoma, presenting as a solitary nodule. Biopsy or surgical removal is usually essential, but the benign nature of hamartomas can occasionally be inferred from the characteristic 'popcorn' calcification of their cartilaginous element, which occurs in up to 40% of cases, and is well seen here. A lateral view of the same patient can be seen in **4.34**.

Bronchial carcinoma

Bronchial carcinoma (lung cancer) is the most common type of malignant disease in developed countries. It causes about 35,000 deaths annually in England and Wales, almost 80% of which are men. In the last few years the steady rise in male mortality from bronchial carcinoma seems to have peaked and begun its decline, but female mortality continues to increase. The development of lung cancer has been associated with exposure to a number of substances, but the over-riding aetiological agent is tobacco. Cigarette smoking is associated with about 85% of bronchial carcinoma, but since only a minority of smokers develop bronchial carcinoma other factors must be important. There is some evidence that genetic and dietary factors may play a role.

Presentation

Intrathoracic manifestations

The clinical presentation of bronchial carcinoma can vary enormously:

- In about 5% of patients, a symptomless abnormality is found on a 'routine' chest X-ray (**4.23**), whereas other patients present with extensive disease and die rapidly (**4.122**).
- Cough is the most common presenting symptom. Since the majority of cases are in smokers, a change in the character of the cough is more important than the cough itself.
- Haemoptysis occurs as an initial symptom in up to 50% of patients, and in a smoker over the age of 40 is an indication for bronchoscopy (**4.43**), even in the absence of a radiological abnormality.
- Dyspnoea occurs commonly and may be caused by large airway obstruction with tumour, the development of pneumonia or collapse distal to the tumour (**4.122, 4.123**), the development of a large pleural effusion or, more rarely, involvement of the lung lymphatics (lymphangitis carcinomatosa) (**4.124**) or pericardium.
- Chest discomfort is a common symptom. It is often of an ill-defined aching nature, but may be localised to the chest wall where there is direct invasion of the chest wall, metastasis to the ribs or pleurisy associated with infection.
- Pain in the shoulder, radiating down the upper inner arm, can be the first sign of a Pancoast tumour situated in the apex of the lung, causing symptoms by invasion of the ribs, vertebrae, sympathetic trunk, brachial plexus and artery (**4.125–4.128**).
- Wheeze is described by 10% of patients, and is often stridor caused by narrowing of a major airway.
- A hoarse voice may be caused by paralysis of the left recurrent laryngeal nerve as it loops round the arch of the aorta. In contradistinction to the hoarse voice of chronic laryngitis associated with smoking, the patient with a paralysed vocal cord is unable to produce an explosive cough, producing instead a 'bovine' cough (**4.129**).
- Superior vena caval obstruction is most commonly caused by small cell carcinoma, and presents with swelling of the head and neck, engorgement of the neck veins without visible pulsation and the development of collateral venous circulation over the chest wall (**4.130, 4.131**).
- Another feature of mediastinal glandular involvement is compression of the oesophagus causing dysphagia.

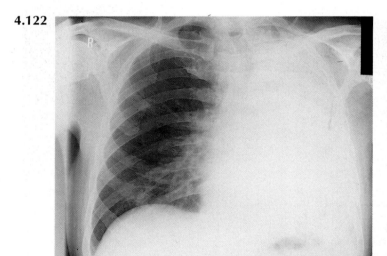

4.122 Carcinoma of the bronchus presenting with complete collapse of the left lung as a result of total occlusion of the left main bronchus. Note the marked deviation of the trachea and mediastinum to the left, and the compensatory hyperinflation of the right lung. The patient presented with rapid-onset dyspnoea.

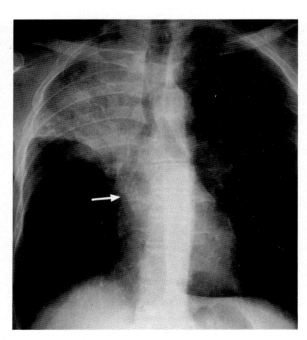

4.123 Bronchial carcinoma with right upper pneumonic consolidation. The carcinoma can be seen as a mass at the right hilum (arrowed), and the consolidation follows obstruction of the right upper lobe bronchus.

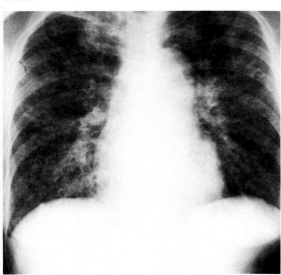

4.124 Lymphangitis carcinomatosa. Micronodular shadows are seen throughout the lungs, and there is a streaky appearance, which results from tumour infiltration of lymphatic vessels.

4.125 Right apical carcinoma of the bronchus (Pancoast tumour). In this location, the tumour may cause other symptoms (*see* **4.126–4.128**).

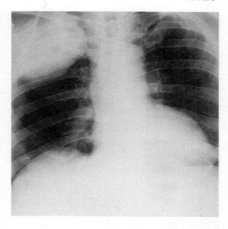

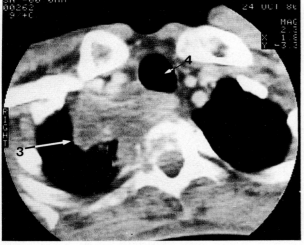

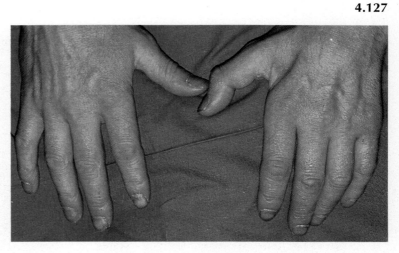

4.127 Wasting of the small muscles of the left hand (most noticeably the first dorsal interosseus) as a consequence of a left apical tumour.

4.126 Right apical bronchial carcinoma. The CT scan shows the extent of the tumour (3) between the trachea (4) and the spine, and it also shows that the tumour is invading the vertebral body.

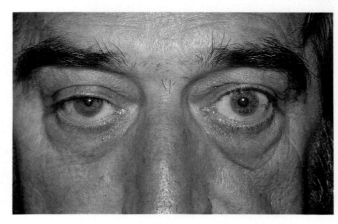

4.128 Horner's syndrome resulting from a right Pancoast tumour. The patient had a right ptosis and a constricted right pupil, caused by tumour infiltration of the inferior cervical sympathetic ganglia.

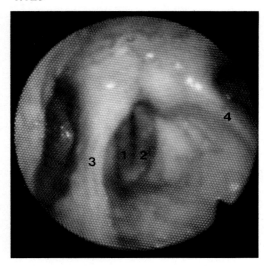

4.129 Left vocal cord paralysis during phonation in a patient with recurrent laryngeal nerve involvement by a bronchial carcinoma. This endoscopic view shows that during phonation the normal right vocal cord (1) adducts to the midline, while the left vocal cord (2) appears bowed and lies at a lower level than the right vocal cord. Adduction to the midline is partial, resulting in incomplete glottic closure, so the patient has a breathy voice and a bovine cough. The right aryepiglottic fold (3) is tense and appears in the normal position during phonation, whereas the left aryepiglottic fold (4) has lost its tone and cannot conform to the normal position.

4.130

4.131

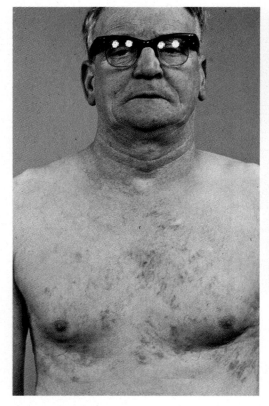

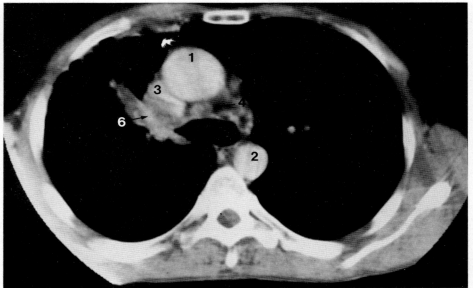

4.131 Superior vena caval obstruction caused by bronchial carcinoma. The superior vena cava (3) is severely compressed by the tumour (6), which has also invaded and enlarged a pre-tracheal lymp node (4). The ascending aorta is marked 1 and the descending aorta is marked 2. The mediastinal involvement demonstrated by this CT scan shows that the tumour is inoperable.

4.130 Superior vena caval obstruction in bronchial carcinoma. Note the swelling of the head and neck, engorgement of the neck veins and the development of a collateral circulation in the veins of the chest wall.

Extrathoracic manifestations

About one-third of patients present with symptoms resulting from metastases; 20% of patients have bone pain at presentation (*see* p.159). The lung is the most common origin of cerebral metastases (4.132); liver (*see* p.407), adrenal and para-aortic lymph node involvement is also common.

A number of non-metastatic syndromes are associated with bronchial carcinoma. Inappropriate secretion of ADH and ectopic ACTH secretion are seen with small cell lung cancer, whereas hypercalcaemia and more rarely gynaecomastia (4.133) and hyperthyroidism are associated with squamous cell cancer. Neuromyopathies (11.104, 11.105), dermato-myositis, encephalopathy and myelopathy have all been associated with bronchial carcinoma. Finger clubbing (2.90, 2.91, 4.3, 4.108) is common, except in small cell cancer, and may progress to hypertrophic pulmonary osteoarthropathy, where there is pain in the wrists and ankles associated with periosteal new bone formation in the long bones (4.134). Anaemia and weight loss are common accompaniments of bronchial carcinoma. Thrombophlebitis, venous thrombosis and skin lesions such as acanthosis nigricans occur much less commonly.

4.132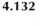

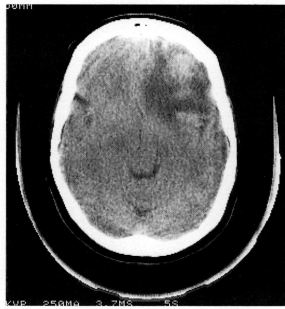

4.132 Large secondary deposit in the frontal lobe of the brain demonstrated by an unenhanced CT scan. The patient was a 45-year-old woman smoker, and the primary was a small cell carcinoma of the lung.

4.133

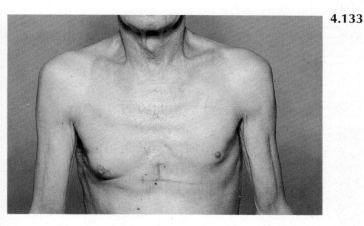

4.133 Unilateral gynaecomastia developed in this male patient with squamous cell carcinoma of the bronchus. Note the positioning line for radiotherapy. The patient shows signs of weight loss and possible early generalised hyper-pigmentation.

4.134

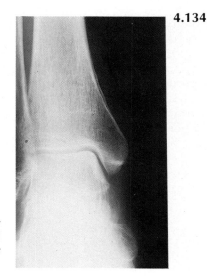

4.134 Hypertrophic pulmonary osteoarthropathy (HPOA) at the ankle in a patient with bronchial carcinoma. New bone formation is shown by the double margin seen at the medial border of the tibia.

Diagnosis and treatment

Most tumours are visible on chest X-ray, and a firm diagnosis is made by microscopic examination of sputum (4.16) or of specimens obtained at bronchoscopy, or by the biopsy of metastatic lesions. Occasionally, closed or open lung biopsy is required. Although there are many types of lung tumour, the most simple, clinically useful classification is to distinguish between small cell lung cancer, non-small cell lung cancer and benign tumours.

- Small cell carcinoma has almost always metastasised by the time of diagnosis, and it is rare for surgical resection to be performed if this diagnosis is known. The tumour is sensitive to chemotherapy and radiotherapy, both of which can lead to a significant prolongation of useful life but rarely a cure.
- In non-small cell lung cancer, the patients with the best outcome are those who undergo a successful resection. Two criteria must be satisfied before a patient undergoes surgery: firstly, they must be fit enough to survive the operation and have sufficiently good lung function to have good-quality survival after lung removal; secondly, the surgery must be likely to remove all of the tumour and therefore it is usual to perform scanning before operation to identify metastases. Radiotherapy is valuable for the treatment of bronchial bleeding, superior vena caval obstruction, and painful bony metastases.

Many patients with cancer fear a painful death, but simple analgesics, morphine, radiotherapy and techniques such as transcutaneous nerve stimulation will control pain in almost all patients. The prognosis of bronchial carcinoma is poor. About 5% of patients will survive 5 years, and the majority of these are patients who undergo successful surgery.

Secondary tumours

Metastases in the lung are common. They may present as one or more discrete nodules (4.24), as a finer pattern of multiple metastases (4.26) or as lymphangitis carcinomatosa (4.124). The most common primary sites are the kidney, breast, prostate, gut, cervix and ovary. Discrete metastases are often asymptomatic, but their presence is generally a bad prognostic sign. Surgical removal of secondaries is only very rarely possible.

Diseases of the pleura

Pleural effusions

Pleural effusions are a common clinical problem and can be divided into transudates and exudates (*see* p. 173).

- Transudation of fluid occurs with increased capillary pressure and reduced plasma oncotic pressure, and therefore is most common in cardiac failure and hypoalbuminaemic states.
- An exudative pleural effusion is caused by an inflammatory process, such as carcinoma, pneumonia (4.29), tuberculosis (4.81), rheumatoid arthritis (3.32), asbestosis or pulmonary infarction. Pleural fluid cytology, Gram stain, culture, glucose, amylase, LDH, and pH and pleural biopsy can all contribute to the identification of aetiology.
- A bloody effusion is most commonly seen with tumour involvement of the pleura (4.119), but can also occur in pulmonary infarction, tuberculosis, trauma, coagulation disorders or ruptured aneurysm.
- Damage to the thoracic duct, usually by trauma or mediastinal malignancy leads to drainage of chyle into the pleural cavity, a chylothorax.

Large pleural effusions may require aspiration to improve the patient's respiratory state, but in general, it is most important to treat the underlying condition.

Pneumothorax

In pneumothorax air leaks into the pleural cavity, usually from the lung but occasionally from penetration of the chest wall (e.g. during surgery, penetrative trauma, etc.). The most common medical problem is a 'spontaneous' pneumothorax. This results from rupture of a congenital 'bleb' in the lung, which is usually apical and may be multiple. These are relatively common in young, tall, thin, healthy athletic males and pneumothoraces may come on at rest or after some major respiratory effort. Spontaneous pneumothorax also occurs in Marfan's syndrome (*see* p. 318), in divers, asthmatics, in chronic bronchitics with emphysema, following lung abscess, in bronchial carcinoma and following adhesions resulting from pleurisy.

Clinical presentation is usually dramatic, with the sudden onset of unilateral pain of a pleuritic type and sometimes progressive dyspnoea. It is probable that most small pneumothoraces remain undiagnosed and resolve rapidly. Larger ones can be readily diagnosed by clinical examination, and chest X-rays usually confirm the diagnosis (**4.30, 4.135**). Rarely, rupture of a bleb may leave a valve-like abnormality on the pleural surface, so that air continues to fill the pleural space which expands and pushes over the mediastinum (tension pneumothorax). Urgent decompression is necessary and this may be done with an intrapleural catheter attached to an underwater seal drain (**4.136, 4.137**). Most patients rapidly seal the ruptured bleb and spontaneous resolution occurs. Rarely a pleurodesis or pleurectomy is required to prevent recurrence.

4.135

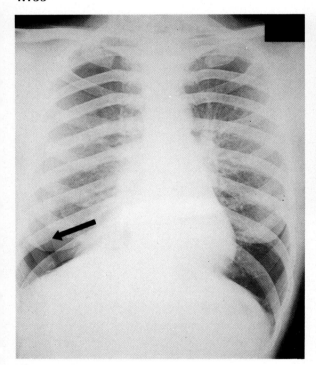

4.135 Right-sided pneumothorax in an adult woman with asthma. The edge of the collapsed lung is not so obvious as in **4.30** and **4.100**, and it is important to consider pneumothorax whenever examining the chest X-ray of a patient with an acute respiratory problem. The edge of the collapsed lung is marked with an arrow.

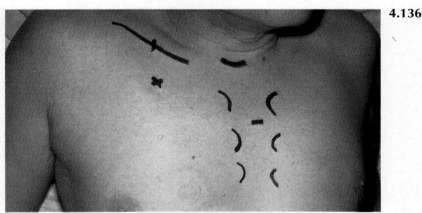

4.136

4.136 The surface marking for the drainage of a pneumothorax is usually the second intercostal space in the midclavicular line (marked with an X).

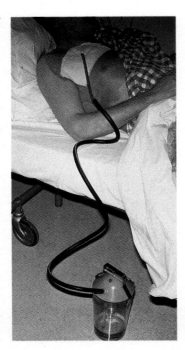

4.137 Drainage of a pneumothorax. The drainage tube can be attached to a one-way valve or, as here, to an underwater seal drain. If a tension pneumothorax is present, or if a large air leak from the lung persists, suction may be applied to the underwater seal.

5. Cardiovascular Disorders

History

Many patients with heart disease are symptom-free until a relatively late stage in the illness when a catastrophic event may occur. This is particularly the case when the progression of atheroma is concerned. Early lesions may be present from the early teens, but patients usually present with myocardial infarction, stroke or peripheral arterial disease in middle or old age. Valve diseases, congenital lesions, hyperlipidaemia and hypertension may also be asymptomatic for many years.

Most of the symptoms of heart disease result from myocardial ischaemia, abnormalities of rhythm or impaired pumping action. Many patients have non-specific symptoms such as tiredness, easy fatiguability and anorexia, but the two main symptoms are chest pain and breathlessness.

There are two main causes of **cardiac pain**: myocardial ischaemia and pericarditis. Ischaemic pain is usually of sudden onset, located centrally and stabbing or constricting; it may radiate to the left arm, occasionally to the right, into the neck and to the back. It may be brought on by exercise, emotion, fright or sexual intercourse. Angina pectoris usually lasts less than 30 minutes and may be relieved by rest or administration of trinitrin. The pain of myocardial infarction usually lasts for more than 30 minutes, often as long as several hours.

Failure of the heart to pump efficiently may lead to the accumulation of blood in the lungs and **dyspnoea** (breathlessness). Heart failure should be defined in the four categories of the New York Heart Association (**Table 5.1**). **Orthopnoea** is the feeling of being out of breath when lying flat, which improves on sitting up. **Paroxysmal nocturnal dyspnoea** occurs when the patient lies flat in bed at night; as a result of redistribution of oedema from the periphery to the lungs there is sudden dyspnoea which makes the patient sit up or lean out of the window to get 'fresh air'.

Palpitations are an awareness of the heart beating. They can be normal in excitement, anxiety or after exercise, but may also result from rhythm disturbances.

Syncope results from failure to maintain an adequate circulation to the brain. The attacks may come on suddenly without any warning and result in sudden collapse.

Always note any **family history** of congenital heart disease or other genetic disorders with cardiac implications. Premature death in near relatives from myocardial infarction or stroke, or hyperlipidaemia or hypertension in family members are important findings.

Table 5.1 Functional grading of heart disease (New York Heart Association).

Grade I	No limitation of activities, i.e. free of symptoms.
Grade II	No limitation under resting conditions, but symptoms appear on severe activity.
Grade III	Limitation of activities on mild exertion.
Grade IV	Limitation of activities at rest, restricting the person to bed or a chair.

Examination

The most acute presentation of heart disease is cardiac arrest. The patient collapses, respiration ceases and no pulse can be felt (**5.1**). Death results unless resuscitation is carried out successfully (*see* p. 225).

Examination should start with the general appearance. There may be obvious breathlessness, even at rest, as a result of heart failure; this may make the patient sit up in bed, propped up on pillows. The skin of the face may have the bluish discoloration of cyanosis. Severe central cyanosis, best seen in the tongue and lips, is often a feature of congenital heart

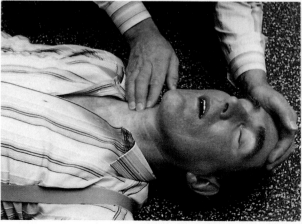

5.1

5.1 Cardiac arrest. The diagnosis is established clinically by feeling for the carotid (or femoral) pulse. The head should be slightly extended if possible, and the neck should be palpated for evidence of a carotid pulse on one side of the thyroid cartilage for 10 seconds. An absent carotid or femoral pulse indicates probable cardiac arrest, but peripheral pulselessness or the absence of heart sounds are unreliable signs.

disease (4.5). A facial flush may be present in mitral valve stenosis (5.2). Arcus cornealis in a young patient (7.112), xanthelasmas (7.113) or skin and tendon xanthomata (7.114–7.117) point to hyperlipidaemia. Jaundice may reflect hepatic disturbance from heart failure.

Finger clubbing may be caused by infective endocarditis or, more commonly, cyanotic congenital heart disease (5.3). Infective endocarditis may cause splinter haemorrhages in the nails (3.28) and tender nodules in the tips of fingers and toes (5.102).

Distended internal and external jugular veins (5.4) and abnormalities of the jugular venous wave-form occur in right heart failure, with abnormalities of the tricuspid valve, and in arrhythmias where the right atrium contracts against a closed tricuspid valve.

Patients with the disproportionately long arms and fingers of Marfan's syndrome (7.48–7.51), are susceptible to the development of aortic aneurysm and aortic regurgitation.

The abdomen may be distended in chronic heart failure, because of the presence of ascites, and there may be pitting oedema of the legs (5.5) and the skin over the sacrum. Unilateral leg swelling is usually caused by deep venous thrombosis (5.6). Arterial embolism into the legs causes gangrene, which may also result from diffuse atherothrombotic arterial disease.

Examination of the radial artery pulse gives information about heart rate and rhythm, and the character of the pulse may suggest abnormalities of the aortic valve or pericardium, or cardiomyopathies.

The position of the apex beat can indicate cardiac enlargement, and auscultation of the heart allows the detection of abnormal heart sounds and murmurs caused by valve disease and congenital malformations (5.7–5.9).

Crepitations in the lung fields which persist after coughing usually indicate cardiac failure. In hypertensive patients, the fundi may show evidence of retinal arterial damage (*see* p. 251).

5.2

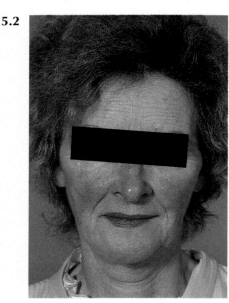

5.2 Malar flush in mitral stenosis. Redness of the cheeks used to be described as a specific sign of mitral stenosis, but a similar appearance can be seen in normal people. It is important to distinguish malar flush from the butterfly rash of systemic lupus erythematosus (**3.72, 3.73**) and from acne rosacea (**2.70**).

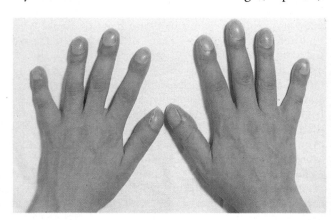

5.3 Severe finger clubbing in a patient with cyanotic congenital heart disease. The drumstick appearance of the fingertip is similar to that seen in clubbing from other causes (**2.90, 2.91**), but the nailbeds are obviously cyanotic.

5.4

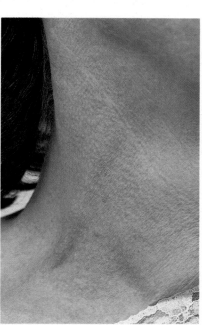

5.4 Elevated external jugular venous pressure. The pressure in the internal and external jugular veins is elevated in right heart failure. Abnormalities in wave-form may provide evidence of tricuspid valve disease or cardiac arrhythmia, although these abnormalities are more reliably noted in the internal than the external jugular vein, which may be affected by position.

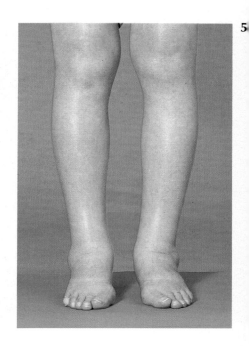

5.5 Bilateral leg oedema in a patient with cardiac failure. Note the 'pitting' effect of the patient's shoes on both feet.

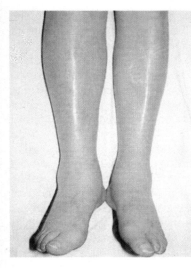

5.6 Unilateral oedema in the right leg, which developed 6 days after abdominal surgery, and was caused by deep vein thrombosis (DVT). Congestive heart failure is another common cause of DVT.

5.7 Common systolic murmurs. 1 = first heart sound; 2 = second heart sound (A = aortic component; P = pulmonary component).

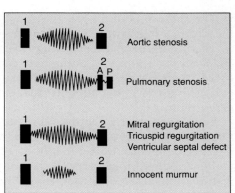

5.7

Aortic stenosis

Pulmonary stenosis

Mitral regurgitation
Tricuspid regurgitation
Ventricular septal defect

Innocent murmur

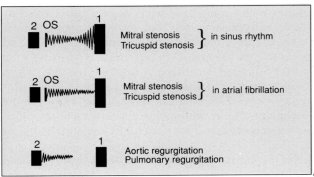

Mitral stenosis } in sinus rhythm
Tricuspid stenosis

Mitral stenosis } in atrial fibrillation
Tricuspid stenosis

Aortic regurgitation
Pulmonary regurgitation

5.8 Common diastolic murmurs. 1 = first heart sound; 2 = second heart sound; OS = opening snap.

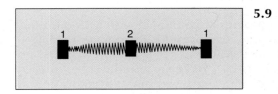

5.9

5.9 A continuous murmur. The most common cause is patent ductus arteriosus. 1 = first heart sound; 2 = second heart sound.

Investigations

The main investigatory techniques in cardiovascular disorders are electrocardiography, chest radiography, echocardiography, colour-flow Doppler, nuclear cardiology, cardiac catheterisation, angiography and magnetic resonance imaging.

The heart generates electrical activity which can be recorded on an **electrocardiogram** (ECG or EKG):

- The resting ECG is useful in the diagnosis of myocardial infarction, cardiac hypertrophy or abnormalities in rhythm. Characteristic ECG abnormalities usually develop soon after coronary artery occlusion occurs, and some abnormalities usually persist after the patient's recovery (*see* p. 227). The resting ECG can also detect ventricular hypertrophy and abnormalities of conduction, such as bundle branch block.
- The resting ECG is often normal in patients with angina pectoris, but a recording during exercise, on a bicycle or treadmill, usually reveals characteristic changes indicating myocardial ischaemia (**5.10, 5.11**).
- Ambulatory electrocardiography is useful when heart rhythm disturbances occur only intermittently. The recording is made on a portable tape recorder (**5.12**), usually over 24 hours, and it can be analysed in a computer. Correlation is made between symptomatic episodes, e.g. palpitations, and the ECG record.

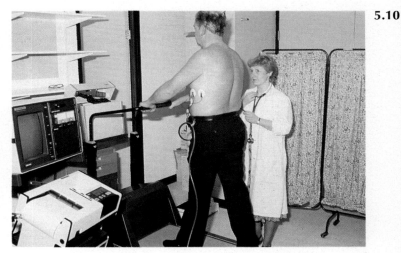

5.10

5.10 The exercise treadmill test may reveal signs of ischaemia on the ECG when the resting trace is normal (**5.11**).

211

The **chest X-ray** is important in diagnosing and assessing the severity of many cardiac abnormalities (5.13). It is superior to the stethoscope in revealing heart failure and shows characteristic features of pulmonary congestion and oedema (5.14). It indicates whether the heart and great vessels are enlarged and whether there is calcification or fluid in the pericardium.

Echocardiography, Doppler flow studies and **colour-flow Doppler** involve the analysis of reflected high-frequency sound directed at the heart from a transducer on the chest wall. They permit real-time visualisation of the heart valves, to determine if they are stenosed or incompetent, and examination of the walls of the left ventricle, providing an index of the function of the left ventricle during systole.

- The original technique, M-mode echocardiography, is one-dimensional, but it allows the assessment of intracardiac dimensions and the simultaneous monitoring and visualisation of the ECG (5.15).
- Doppler flow studies can be combined with M-mode or two dimensional echocardiography to provide further dynamic information (5.16).
- Two-dimensional (2D) imaging produces clearer anatomical images (5.17), and allows simple diagnosis of a range of cardiac abnormalities including valvular heart disease, congenital abnormalities, cardiac tumours and pericardial effusions.
- Colour-flow Doppler echocardiography allows further evaluation of blood flow within the heart. It has further improved the diagnosis of valvular stenosis and incompetence (5.18) and the study of the function of the left ventricle during diastole.

Nuclear cardiology is a useful method of assessing the function of cardiac muscle. Technetium 99m may be bound to albumin or red cells from the patient's blood and thallium-201 may be injected intravenously. Radioactivity can be assessed from within the cavities of the heart (technetium erythrocyte or albumin technique), permitting evaluation of cardiac function (5.19), or from the walls of the heart (thallium technique), allowing assessment of ischaemia and infarction (5.20).

Cardiac catheterisation and **angiography** are invasive techniques. Catheters are advanced to the right and left heart under X-ray screening. Pressures are measured at the tips of the catheters, permitting evaluation of valvular stenosis; and oxygen saturations can be assessed to diagnose septal defects. During angiography, radio-opaque contrast medium is injected through the catheters into the heart or vessels. Left ventriculography outlines the inside of the left ventricle and assesses systolic function and mitral regurgitation. Many of these catheter techniques have been largely superseded by (non-invasive) echocardiography, but coronary angiography is still the only accurate method of assessing the severity and extent of coronary disease—an essential preliminary to coronary artery surgery. A catheter is inserted into the mouth of a coronary artery and the vessel is injected with radio-opaque contrast (5.21). Digital subtraction angiography permits the use of smaller amounts of contrast medium which can be given intravenously. This is useful in imaging peripheral arteries.

Magnetic resonance imaging is still being evaluated, but has major potential as a non-invasive tool which can be synchronised with the ECG to allow diastolic and systolic images to be produced (5.22).

5.11

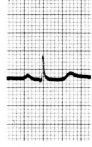

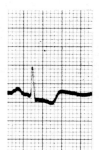

5.11 A positive exercise test as shown in lead II. The trace taken before exercise is normal, but the second trace, recorded 2 minutes after the end of exercise, shows ST segment depression with T-wave inversion. Analysis of the full trace may show further evidence of ischaemia (**5.50**).

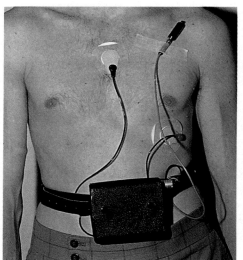

5.12

5.12 Ambulatory electrocardiography ('Holter monitoring'). The patient undertakes a range of normal activities over a 24-hour period while wearing this lightweight ECG monitoring equipment. He can mark symptomatic episodes on the recording tape by pushing a button on the recorder, and the entire 24-hour recording can then be analysed for ischaemia or arrhythmias in a computer.

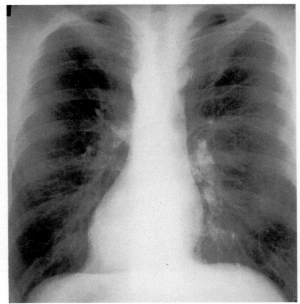

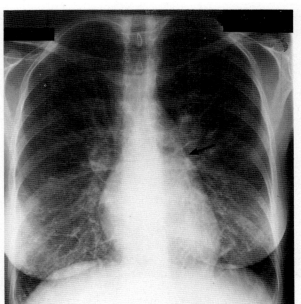

5.13 Situs inversus revealed by chest X-ray. The apex of the heart lies in the right side of the the thorax (dextrocardia). The left dome of the diaphragm is higher than the right, because the liver is on the left and the spleen and the stomach are on the right. Dextrocardia and situs inversus are usually harmless abnormalities associated with a normal life-expectancy. However, situs inversus may be associated with ciliary abnormalities in Kartagener's syndrome, a hereditary disorder in which the patient also has sinusitis, bronchiectasis and, if male, infertility resulting from immotile spermatozoa.

5.14 Heart failure in a patient with mitral stenosis. The left atrial appendage is enlarged (arrowed), the upper zone blood vessels are distended, and there are linear densities in the periphery of the lower zones (interstitial or Kerley's B lines). The lung-field changes are typical of moderate pulmonary oedema.

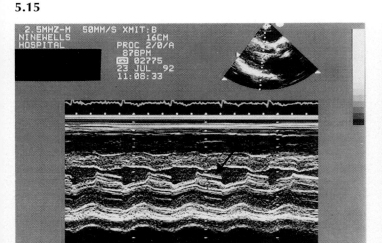

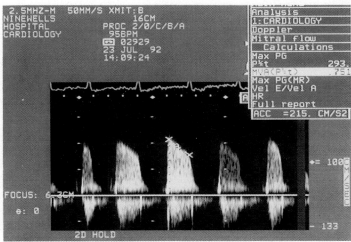

5.15 M-mode echocardiogram in mitral stenosis. Ultrasound waves are transmitted into the body in a 1-dimensional ('ice-pick') form. They are reflected back each time they reach an interface between tissues of different acoustic impedance. This allows an assessment of the relative movement of different parts of the heart. This tracing shows impaired movement of the mitral valve leaflets, which is revealed as flattening of the normal mitral valve trace (arrow).

5.16 Doppler flow study in mitral stenosis. In Doppler studies, ultrasound is reflected back from the red cells in the blood. This allows further assessment of haemodynamics. In this patient (the same patient as in **5.15**) the flow through the mitral valve is diminished, and—when analysed against the cardiac cycle—the velocity of flow during early diastole relates to the degree of stenosis. In this patient the velocity (A) has been used to calculate the valve area, which is 0.75cm^2, compared with a possible normal value of 3.5cm^2.

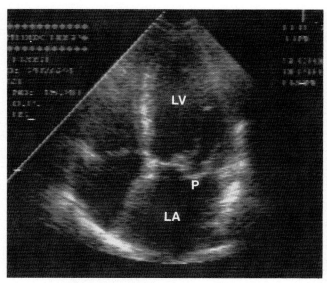

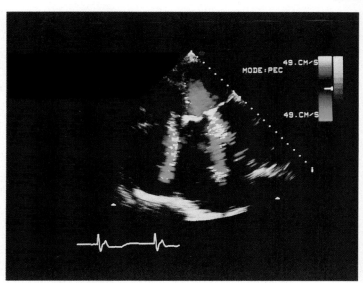

5.17 2D cardiac ultrasound allows imaging which can be monitored in real time. This apical four-chamber view is from a patient with mitral valve prolapse. The central portion of the mitral valve is seen to prolapse backwards into the left atrium in this systolic frame. LV = left ventricle; LA = left atrium; P = prolapsed valve.

5.18 Colour-flow mapping results from the parallel processing of both 2D and Doppler flow data, which are combined in real time to provide a dynamic image of anatomical, functional and haemodynamic status. This systolic apical four-chamber view corresponds to that seen in **5.17**. This patient has both mitral and tricuspid regurgitation. The left ventricle is the blue area at the top of the image, and the regurgitant flow through the mitral valve is seen on the right. Tricuspid regurgitation is seen as a narrower band of flow on the left.

5.19

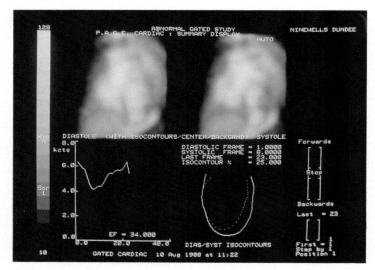

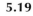

5.19 Technetium blood pool study in a patient with poor left ventricular function after myocardial infarction. Typical systolic and diastolic frames are shown top left and top right, and the contours of the left ventricle are displayed graphically at bottom right. The area of the blood pool at each of 16 frames of the cardiac cycle is plotted bottom left and allows the calculation of the LV ejection fraction, which is very low at 34%. The LV wall movement is best seen kinetically. It was poor at the interventricular septum and there was early aneurysmal dilatation at the apex.

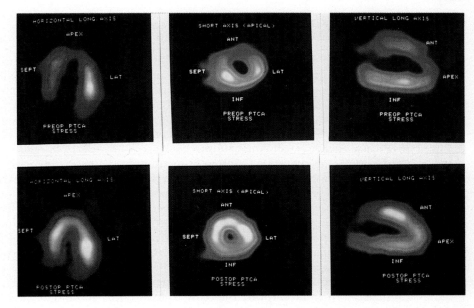

5.20 Exercise nuclear tomograms following the injection of radioactive thallium in a patient before (top) and after (bottom) percutaneous transluminal coronary angioplasty (PTCA) of a 90% stenosis of the left anterior descending coronary artery. Before the procedure, the distal anterior wall and apex were poorly perfused during exercise. After PTCA, the images are all normal.

5.21

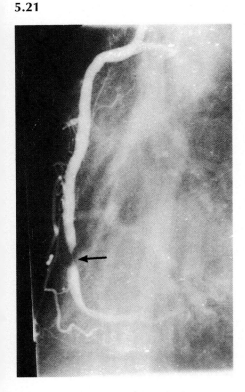

5.21 Coronary arteriogram showing a severe stricture of the right coronary artery (arrowed). This isolated lesion may be amenable to treatment by percutaneous transluminal coronary angioplasty (PTCA).

5.22

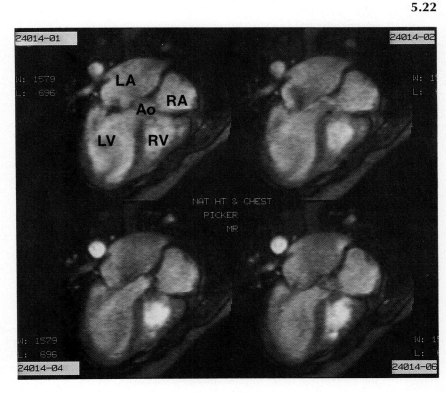

5.22 Magnetic resonance cine gradient echo scan (horizontal long axis plane) in dilated cardiomyopathy showing a grossly hypertrophied left ventricle (LV) which contracts poorly. These four frames show extremely poor systolic left ventricular thickening and motion, and a small jet of mitral regurgitation can be seen in the top right image by virtue of loss of signal (black) from the turbulent jet. LV = left ventricle; LA = left atrium; RV = right ventricle; RA = right atrium; Ao = aortic root.

Circulatory failure

Circulatory failure occurs when an adequate blood flow to the tissues cannot be maintained. This may be caused by inadequate cardiac output (heart failure) or by a markedly reduced intravascular volume, e.g. after major haemorrhage, acute dehydration or in septicaemic shock.

Heart failure may develop because the heart muscle itself is diseased or because excessive demands are placed on it. The main myocardial disease is ischaemia resulting from atheromatous narrowing of the coronary arteries. Others include cardiomyopathies and hypertension. Excessive demands on the heart may occur with regurgitant or stenotic valves, atrial fibrillation, outflow tract obstructions and with obstruction caused by cardiac tamponade or constrictive pericarditis. High-output states such as anaemia, thyrotoxicosis, beriberi and Paget's disease have a similar effect.

When cardiac output is inadequate, compensatory mechanisms develop in an attempt by the body to maintain blood flow. These mechanisms are responsible for many of the signs of heart failure and may have other deleterious effects. Increased sympathetic tone causes tachycardia, and increased aldosterone levels stimulate salt and water retention. The signs of heart failure depend to a great extent on its chronicity. It is conventional to describe heart failure as mainly right- or left-sided, but usually features of both are present.

In **left ventricular failure**, the dominant symptom is dyspnoea, which may be present at rest or after exercise, or may be associated with paroxysmal nocturnal dyspnoea. There may be episodes of acute pulmonary oedema during which the patient coughs up copious volumes of frothy white sputum that may be tinged with blood, and Cheyne–Stokes respiration may also be observed. The clinical signs in the heart vary with the cause of the failure, but most patients have a marked tachycardia and occasionally pulsus alternans and a third heart sound during diastole (gallop rhythm). The basal areas of both lungs may reveal fine moist crepitations.

In **right heart failure** there is engorgement of the venous tree. This leads to distension of the jugular veins (5.4); distension of the liver, which is enlarged and tender; and retention of fluid, producing dependent oedema of the legs (4.65, 5.5), ascites, hydrothorax and sometimes pericardial effusion. The patient may be deeply cyanosed (4.5)

The degree of failure can be confirmed by chest X-ray (5.14, 5.23), and echocardiography demonstrates reduced motion of the walls of the failing heart during systole. Doppler echocardiography can demonstrate impaired filling of the ventricles in diastole.

The drug treatment of heart failure is largely concerned with improving or abolishing the unwanted effects of pulmonary congestion and fluid retention. In heart failure, an attempt is also made to increase cardiac output.

Diuretics, nitrates and angiotensin-converting enzyme (ACE) inhibitors reduce cardiac work, while a variety of inotropes can increase cardiac output.

5.23

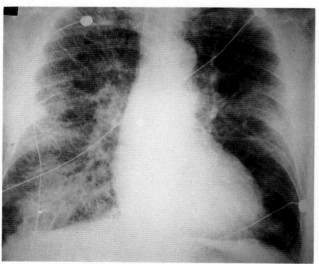

5.23 Heart failure following myocardial infarction. The changes are more severe than in **5.14**: there is distension of the upper zone vessels, interstitial (Kerley B) lines are present at both bases; and there are some areas of apparent consolidation, indicating alveolar pulmonary oedema.

Arrhythmias

Abnormal heart rhythms may be classified according to the mechanism of origin of the rhythm disturbance, by the site of origin or by their effect on heart rate. Because the mechanisms are often not clear and the precise site is often unknown, this section will classify those rhythms into **tachycardias** (heart rate greater than 100 bpm) and **bradycardias** (heart rate less than 60 bpm). The rhythm is usually investigated by a standard 12-lead ECG with a rhythm strip (usually a prolonged section of lead II).

Typical examples of ECG traces in the tachycardias are seen in 5.24–5.37, and typical bradycardia traces are seen in 5.38–5.40.

Heart block, a failure of conduction, may occur at the AV node (5.41–5.45). When complete, it may need to be treated by cardiac pacing (5.46–5.48). Intraventricular block may be the result of conduction failure in the right or left branches of the His bundle, or in the hemi-branches of the left branch. Left bundle branch block (5.49) and right bundle branch block give typical ECG appearances, but these may often be modified by myocardial infarction or other underlying causes. Bifascicular block (where any two of the three main intraventricular conduction pathways are wholly or partially blocked) may also occur. The treatment of bundle branch block is usually that of the underlying disease and its haemodynamic complications.

5.24

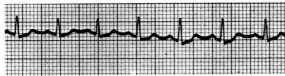

5.24 Sinus tachycardia - a regular tachycardia in which the beats originate in the SA node. This may represent a physiological response to exercise, emotion, fear or anxiety; or it may accompany fever, blood loss, thyrotoxicosis, a falling blood pressure or heart failure. Each beat is preceded by a normal P wave, the upper limit of rate is about 180/minute and, in contrast to paroxysmal tachycardia, the rate tends to fluctuate. Carotid sinus compression usually slows the rate.

5.25

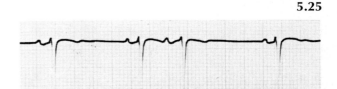

5.25 Atrial ectopic beat. The ectopic is arrowed. Its QRS complex is identical to those of normal beats, but the P wave differs slightly in shape and deforms the T wave of the preceding beat. The next sinus beat follows after an interval which is close to the inter-beat interval of the basic sinus rhythm. Like other ectopics, atrial ectopics are caused by an electrical discharge from an irritable focus, but atrial ectopics are usually of little clinical significance.

5.26

5.27

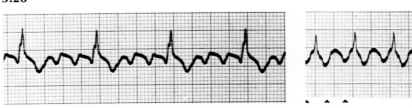

5.26, 5.27 Atrial flutter is always associated with organic heart disease and is characterised by a rapid regular atrial rate between 220 to 360 beats/minute. There is a fixed or variable degree of A-V block, which results in one, two or three atrial impulses being blocked for each one transmitted. On the ECG the flutter (F) waves produce a 'saw tooth' pattern, though some may be buried in the QRS complex. **5.26** shows atrial flutter with 4:1 A-V block. **5.27** shows atrial flutter with 2:1 A-V block. The usual associations are with ischaemic heart disease, rheumatic valvular disease and cor pulmonale. Chronic atrial flutter is usually treated with digoxin.

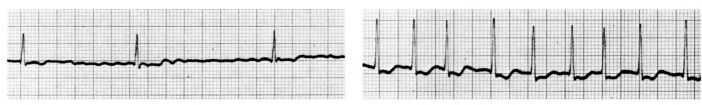

5.28, 5.29 Atrial fibrillation. There is chaotic atrial activity at a frequency of 400–600/minute. There is little or no mechanical activity of the atria and few of the beats are conducted by the A-V node, so the ventricular response is totally irregular and may be slow (**5.28**) or as rapid as 150 beats/minute (**5.29**). The pulse is 'irregularly irregular' on palpation and the ECG has absent P waves, which are replaced by rapid irregular waves (f waves). Note the irregularity of the QRS response. This is one of the most common arrhythmias and is found in rheumatic heart disease, ischaemia, hypertension and thyrotoxicosis. It is also found in about 15% of elderly people who are otherwise symptom-free. Atrial fibrillation of acute onset can often be reversed by DC shock or drug therapy, but in chronic AF, drug therapy may be used to modify the ventricular response.

5.30   **5.31**

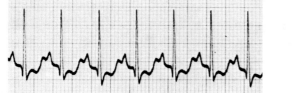 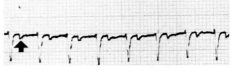

5.30, 5.31 Junctional tachycardias are brought about by re-entry of the cardiac impulse often via an accessory pathway between atria and ventricles. These rhythms are usually paroxysmal, and they may be precipitated by coffee or alcohol. The patient may be aware of palpitations, and the tachycardia may lead to dyspnoea and polyuria. There is usually no major structural heart disease. In atrio-ventricular re-entry tachycardia (**5.30**) there is a large circuit comprising the A-V node, the His bundle, the ventricle, an abnormal connection and the atrium. The rhythm is absolutely regular, but the rate may vary from 140 to 280 beats/minutes—in **5.30** it is roughly 150/minute. In **5.30**, the P waves can be clearly seen preceding the QRS complexes. The appearance is that of a regular atrial tachycardia. In **5.31**, inverted P waves can be seen buried in the QRST complex (arrowed), so there has been retrograde atrial activation from a focus in the A-V node. These tachycardias may be terminated by vagotonic manoeuvres such as carotid sinus massage, by drug therapy or, occasionally, by DC shock.

5.32

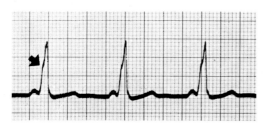

5.32 Wolff–Parkinson–White (WPW) syndrome. In this congenital condition, there is an abnormal myocardial connection between atrium and ventricle (the bundle of Kent). The activating impulse from the atria can pass down this pathway, as well as across the A-V node, so the ventricles are activated without the usualy delay introduced by the A-V node, and the PR interval is short. There is a characteristic wide QRS complex that begins as a slurred part, the 'delta wave' (arrowed). WPW may be associated with re-entrant tachycardia or atrial fibrillation. With severe or frequent paroxysmal attacks, patients require treatment, which may involve surgery or electrical ablation of the aberrant pathway.

5.33 Ventricular ectopic beats are beats resulting from an abnormal irritable focus in the ventricle. Occasional ectopics are usually of little clinical significance, but in acute abnormalities such as myocardial infarction they may be the prelude to the 'coupled' ectopic beats seen here (where each sinus beat is followed by an ectopic) and to ventricular tachycardia or fibrillation. Coupled beats like this can cause serious disturbance of cardiac performance, since the ectopic beat may contribute little or nothing to cardiac output.

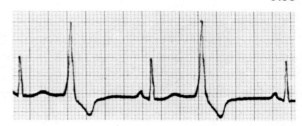

5.34

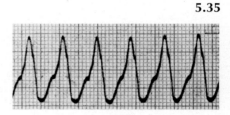

5.35

5.34, 5.35 Ventricular tachycardia. This serious arrhythmia may have a range of appearances and two examples are shown here. The QRS complexes are broad and they merge into one another, and the heart rate is commonly in the range 150–200/minute. VT may be caused by the repetitive discharge of an irritable focus in the ventricles; it may be sustained or end rapidly in ventricular fibrillation. VT occurs in ischaemia, rheumatic heart disease, cardiomyopathy and digoxin toxicity, and requires urgent treatment.

5.36

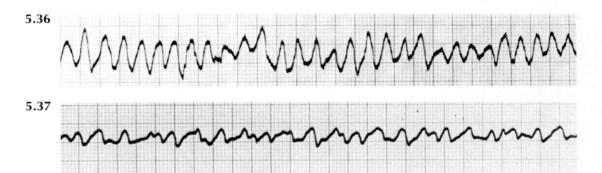

5.37

5.36, 5.37 Ventricular fibrillation. This is a terminal rhythm in which co-ordinated activity of the ventricles ceases. Despite continuing electrical activity, the heart does not pump. The patient rapidly becomes unconscious and pulseless, and emergency treatment for cardiac arrest is essential. The ECG shows irregular, ill-defined waves which vary in size. In **5.36** the fibrillation waves are of good amplitude and there are periods suggestive of ventricular flutter. Defibrillation by DC shock is more likely to be successful with this appearance than with that seen in **5.37**, where there are very variable low-voltage waves.

5.38

5.38 Sinus bradycardia. The complexes are normal, but the heart rate is below 60/minute (here about 45/minute). This may be a normal finding in healthy athletes, but after myocardial infarction it may be more sinister, producing a reduction in coronary blood flow, hypotension and decreased cardiac output. In these circumstances it can be treated with atropine.

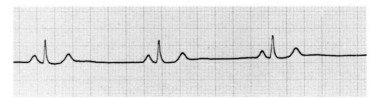

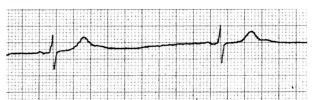

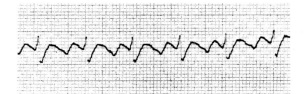

5.39, 5.40 Sinus node disease (the 'sick sinus syndrome'). This syndrome is caused by ischaemia, infarction or degenerative disease of the sinus node, and is characterised by long intervals between consecutive P waves. These intervals may allow tachycardias to emerge, often resulting in alternating periods of bradycardia and tachycardia (the tachy-brady syndrome). In this patient, extreme sinus bradycardia (**5.39**) was followed by atrial flutter with 2:1 block (**5.40**).

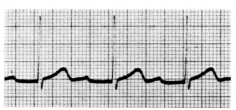

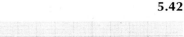
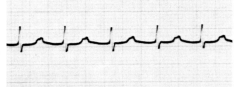

5.41, 5.42 First degree A-V block. The PR interval exceeds 0.22 seconds, so there is a delay in A-V conduction, but all impulses pass on and result in a QRS complex and ventricular contraction. In **5.41** the PR interval is easily measured, but in **5.42** the P wave is hidden in the T wave of the preceding beat and could easily be missed.

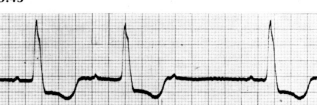

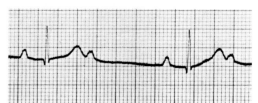

5.43, 5.44 Second degree A-V block occurs in two forms. In the first, there is progressive lengthening of the PR interval until finally one P wave is not conducted (the Wenckebach phenomenon, **5.43**). In the second form, there is intermittent blockage of P-wave conduction to the ventricles without any preceding lengthening of the PR interval, as in **5.44** which shows regular 2:1 conduction. This type is particularly likely to be followed by complete heart block.

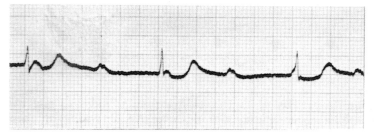

5.45 Third degree A-V block, in which the atria and ventricles beat completely independently of one another and there is no transmission of atrial activity to the ventricles. The ventricular rhythm is usually regular at 40–50/minute, and the P waves are not always easy to see (they are arrowed here). The most common cause of complete heart block is acute myocardial infarction, but it may occur in a range of other congenital and acquired conditions. Definitive treatment usually requires temporary or permanent cardiac pacing.

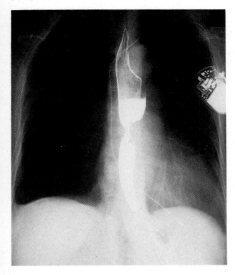

5.46 Chest X-ray showing an implanted pacing system. The pacing generator is in the left pectoral region, and the endocardial pacing wire is positioned in the right ventricle, in contact with the endocardium. This patient also has a carcinomatous stricture of the oesophagus, and the film was taken during a barium meal examination (*see* p.361).

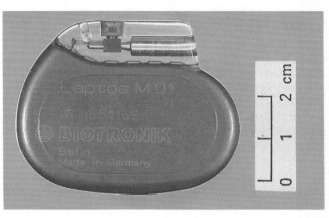

5.47 A modern permanent cardiac pacemaker unit. These pacemakers are small and easily and inconspicuously implantable beneath the skin. They may, however, be large enough to set off security alarms and are a hazard in the presence of microwaves or magnetic resonance imaging equipment. They should be removed before cremation.

5.48

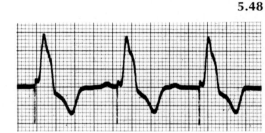

5.48 Endocardial pacing produces a pacing artefact on the ECG as here, where the patient is being paced with a unipolar electrode at the apex of the right ventricle.

5.49

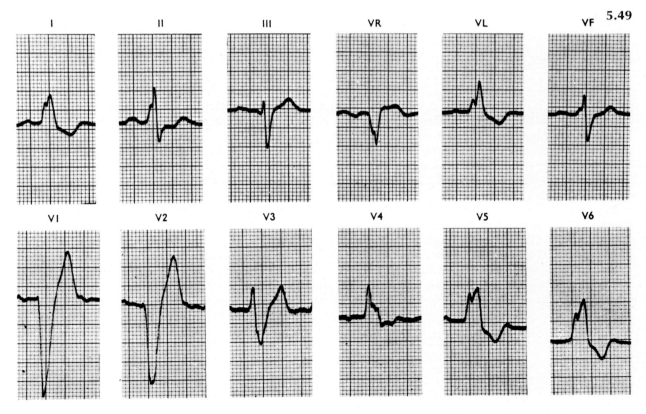

5.49 Left bundle branch block. The QRS complex is widened and notched over the left ventricle as a result of abnormal activation via the right bundle. Repolarisation is also abnormal, so the T waves are sharply inverted in these leads. The small Q wave normally seen in V6 is missing, because the septum is no longer activated from the left side.

Coronary artery disease

Coronary artery disease (coronary heart disease, CHD) is the main cause of death in Western society and is usually a result of a combination of genetic and lifestyle factors (**Table 5.2**). Cigarette smoking has a major causative effect.

Coronary artery disease is characterised by the deposition of plaques of atheroma, a fatty deposit, in the subendothelium of the coronary arteries. Atheroma has a patchy distribution, usually in the proximal parts of the vessels, and the atheromatous plaques narrow the lumen of the arteries, limiting blood flow through them. Further narrowing can result from spasm of the vessel wall near the site of the plaques and from the formation of platelet-fibrin thrombus on the surface. Symptoms are usually experienced when the cross-sectional area of the artery is reduced by about 75%. Atheromatous plaques may fissure and heal spontaneously or a thrombus may form on the surface of the fissure. Thrombosis usually underlies the development of unstable angina or myocardial infarction.

Coronary artery disease produces three main syndromes:

- Angina pectoris
- Unstable angina
- Myocardial infarction.

Cardiac failure may accompany any of these syndromes, and sudden death may result from arrhythmia without the onset of other symptoms.

Table 5.2 Risk factors for coronary heart disease (CHD).

Fixed risks
- Male sex
- Family history of CHD
- Increasing age

Modifiable risks
- Cigarette smoking
- High blood cholesterol (LDL) level
- Hypertension
- Obesity
- 'Western' diet
- Diabetes mellitus
- Physical inactivity
- Use of oral contraceptive pill
- High plasma fibrinogen level

Other factors still await identification

Angina pectoris

Angina is a painful constricting sensation felt in the middle of the chest, which radiates to the arms, the throat, back and epigastrium. It is usually provoked by activity which increases heart rate and blood pressure, thereby increasing myocardial oxygen demand, e.g. exercise, emotion, stress, fear or sexual intercourse. The pain or tightness of 'stable' angina typically starts while walking and is relieved in a few minutes by rest or sublingual trinitrin.

Patients with stable angina frequently have a normal electrocardiogram at rest, but changes may occur during angina attacks (**5.50**) and an exercise ECG usually shows characteristic changes (**5.10, 5.11**).

Drug therapy for angina may include nitrates, beta-blockers and calcium antagonists. If optimum drug therapy does not permit a patient to lead a near-normal life, then coronary angiography should be performed to identify the site of atheromatous narrowing or occlusion of the coronary arteries (**5.21**), as a prelude to possible coronary angioplasty or bypass surgery.

Coronary angioplasty involves dilating a stenosed coronary artery with a balloon-tipped cardiac catheter (usually inserted via the femoral artery) (**5.51–5.54**). The technique often relieves angina (**5.20**), but 30% of patients experience recurrent pain within six months and need repeated angioplasty or coronary artery surgery.

In coronary artery surgery, the patient's own saphenous vein or internal mammary artery is used to bypass the blocked segment (**5.55–5.57**). The operation carries a mortality rate of 1–2%. After surgery, almost all patients are free of angina for several years and their life expectancy may also be improved.

5.50 Angina pectoris associated with ECG changes. During anginal pain, there are usually ST segment changes on the ECG. This ECG was taken during an episode of exercise-induced angina, and it shows ST segment depression (4mm) in leads V4-6 and standard leads II and III.

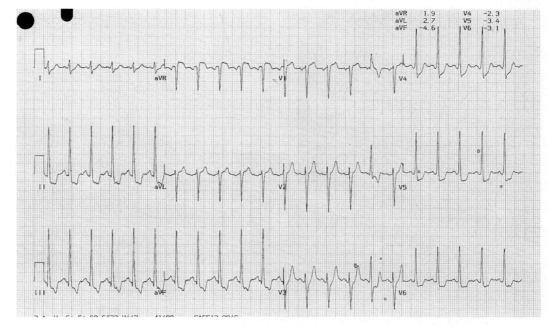

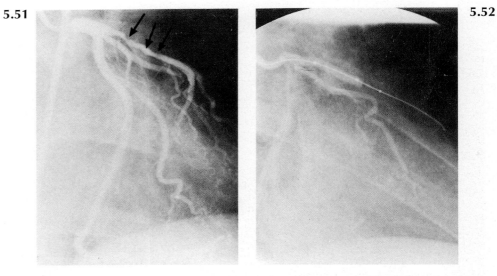

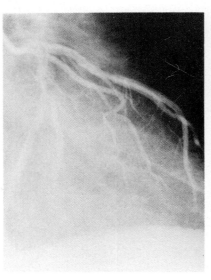

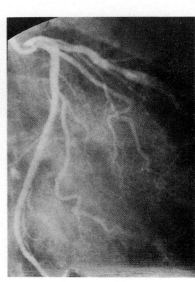

5.51–5.54 Percutaneous transluminal coronary angioplasty of a left anterior descending coronary stricture: **5.51** is the pre-angioplasty coronary arteriogram—a long stricture is arrowed; **5.52** shows the balloon of the angioplasty catheter inflated in situ across the stricture; **5.53** shows the coronary arteriogram taken immediately after the angioplasty catheter had been removed. The stricture has been successfully dilated; **5.54** shows the appearance 1 month after angioplasty. There is a slight residual narrowing, which is a normal finding at this stage and does not indicate re-stenosis. The patient's angina was dramatically improved by the manoeuvre.

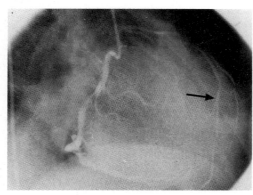

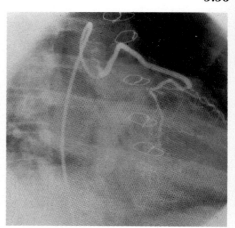

5.55, 5.56 Coronary angiogram before and after saphenous vein grafting in a patient with angina. **5.55** shows the appearance pre-surgery. There is a significant stenosis in the right coronary artery, but this fills by the normal route. By contrast, the left anterior descending artery (arrowed) fills only by collaterals. The origin of the artery is completely obstructed. **5.56** shows the post-surgical appearance. The saphenous vein graft is arrowed, and it fills the left anterior descending artery. The patient's angina was relieved.

5.57

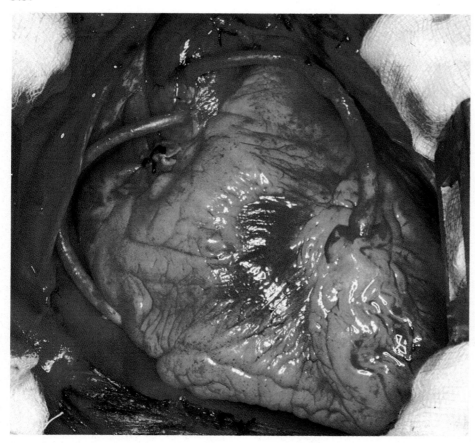

5.57 Coronary artery surgery. Bypass grafts to the right and left anterior descending coronary arteries are in position, and the anastomoses are checked for leaks immediately before closing the chest.

Unstable angina

In unstable angina, anginal pain occurs at rest or with less provocation than previously, but there is no evidence of myocardial infarction. ST-segment changes may be seen on the ECG during episodes of pain or at rest.

Unstable angina is a serious development requiring bed rest and intensive drug therapy. If pain persists, immediate coronary angiography is performed, followed by angioplasty or coronary artery surgery.

Myocardial infarction

Myocardial infarction (MI) usually results from the complete occlusion of one or more coronary arteries by atheroma and thrombus. It presents with severe central chest pain, having the same site and character as the pain of angina pectoris but usually lasting for more than 30 minutes. Pallor, anxiety, sweating and vomiting are usually present. Occasionally, myocardial infarction occurs without any pain.

Acute ischaemia often provokes changes of rhythm. Ventricular fibrillation (5.36, 5.37) is the most important, as it rapidly leads to death from circulatory arrest. Immediate cardiopulmonary resuscitation is required (5.58–5.63). More rarely, cardiac arrest is due to asystole.

Acute myocardial infarction produces a distinctive ECG pattern. The appearances depend upon the site and the time from the onset of the infarct. Within a few minutes, the T waves become tall, pointed and upright and ST segment elevation follows rapidly. Within a few hours the T waves invert. With full-thickness infarcts, the R-wave voltage diminishes and pathological Q waves develop (5.64). The ST segment usually returns to normal within a few days. The T wave usually becomes upright within a few weeks, but the pathological Q waves persist as a marker of previous infarction.

The diagnosis of recent infarction can be confirmed by detecting enzymes released from the damaged heart muscle into the blood, e.g. creatine kinase (CK) and its isoenzymes (especially CK-MB), aspartate aminotransferase (AST) and lactate dehydrogenase (LDH) (5.65).

Myocardial infarction should usually be managed in hospital, but treatment can begin before admission. Pain relief by morphine or diamorphine is usually necessary. Aspirin should be given immediately, and when the diagnosis has been confirmed by an ECG, a thrombolytic agent should usually be administered. This dissolves the thrombus responsible for the occlusion in the coronary artery, improves blood flow to the myocardium, limits left ventricular dysfunction and improves the prognosis. Aspirin and heparin may prevent the diseased vessel reoccluding after successful thrombolysis. Further treatment may be needed for arrhythmias.

5.58–5.63 Treatment of cardiac arrest.

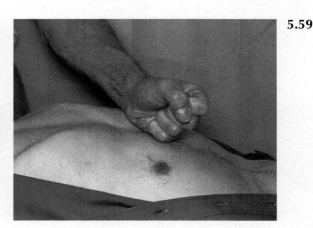

5.58 The cardiac arrest patient should be placed flat on a hard surface. His head and neck should be extended by holding the angles of the jaw well forward to maintain an airway, and the airway should be cleared using suction.

5.59 The sternum should be thumped hard once, using a closed fist. This may sometimes restart the heart.

225

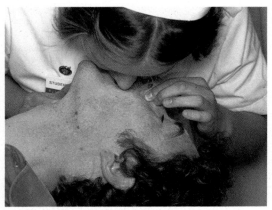

5.60 Artificial respiration should be started using the mouth-to-mouth technique. The nose is occluded with the thumb and index finger, and the movement of the chest provides an index of the efficacy of ventilation.

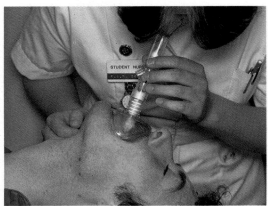

5.61 To avoid mouth-to-mouth contact and to ensure a clear airway, artificial respiration may be established using a Brooke airway. As soon as possible, ventilation should be carried out with 100% oxygen using a bag and mask. The next stage in respiration is to intubate the trachea with a cuffed endotracheal tube.

5.62

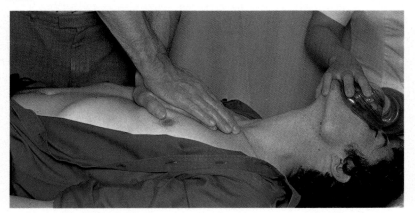

5.62 Cardiac massage. The heel of one hand is placed on the lower third of the sternum and the other hand is rested on top of the first with the arms straight. Sixty to ninety strokes per minute are administered using a sharp jerky movement, aiming to move the sternum 3–5 cm at each stroke. After each stroke it is important to lift the hands quickly to allow the chest to expand and the heart to fill. An assistant should set up an intravenous line and administer sodium bicarbonate, and the patient's ECG should be monitored as soon as possible.

5.63

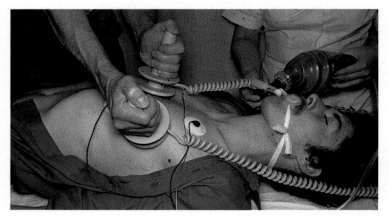

5.63 External DC defibrillation should be performed if the heart has not restarted and/or the ECG shows ventricular fibrillation. The electrodes must be well separated to avoid a short circuit, and all personnel should stand clear of the patient to avoid receiving an electric shock.

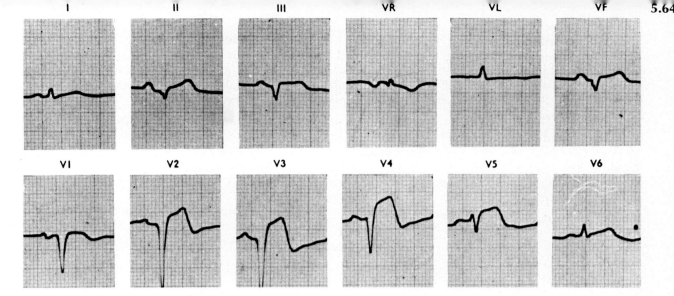

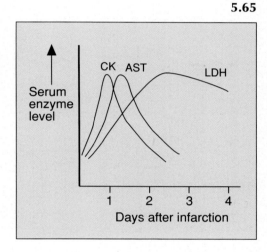

5.64 Acute anterior myocardial infarction extending inferiorly—three hours after onset. The changes of acute full thickness infarction, the ST segment has normally returned to the isoelectric line within 3–6 weeks; persistence of ST elevation beyond this time is a pointer to possible aneurysm. This ECG was taken 10 weeks after infarction in a patient who had signs of heart failure. The QRS complexes in all precordial leads show that the patient had an extensive full-thickness infarct.

5.65 The pattern of serum enzymes after acute myocardial infarction. CK = creatine kinase and its MB fraction (CK-MB); AST = aspartate aminotransferase; LDH = lactate dehydrogenase.

Other complications of acute myocardial infarction

Cardiac failure and shock (*see also* p.216)

Mild left ventricular failure is a common sequel to acute infarction and the only apparent features are bilateral basal crepitations that respond rapidly to diuretic therapy. More severe heart failure carries a poor prognosis and cardiogenic shock has a mortality of over 90% despite therapy.

Cardiac rupture

This is an uncommon feature after infarction and usually occurs about 7–10 days later as the muscle necroses. It may vary from papillary-muscle rupture, producing acute mitral regurgitation, to rupture of the left ventricular wall producing acute cardiac tamponade (and rapid death).

Left ventricular thrombosis

Anterior myocardial infarction is associated with an incidence of about 30% of mural thrombus formation. This may be detected by ultrasound (**5.66**) or ventriculography. Surprisingly, only about 5% of these thrombi throw off clinically significant emboli to the brain, kidneys, mesentery or limbs. Heparin may prevent this complication.

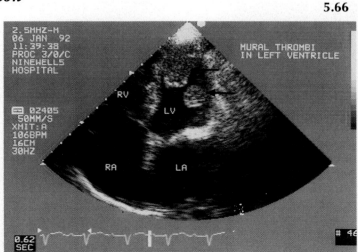

5.66 Left ventricular thrombus after myocardial infarction. The apical four chamber view shows at least two large thrombi on the apical and anterior walls of the left ventricle (arrowed). Left ventricular thrombosis is common after myocardial infarction, and its incidence, and the risk of embolism, can be dramatically reduced by heparin therapy.

Deep vein thrombosis

Immobility associated with tissue breakdown and cardiac failure produces an incidence of venous thrombosis of 5–10% (*see* p.261), and a small number of these thrombi embolise to the lung (*see* p. 262). These complications may be prevented by low-dose heparin therapy.

Shoulder–hand syndrome

The cause of this disability is unknown, but stiffness of the shoulder and upper arm joints may follow an infarct. Physiotherapy and non-steroidal anti-inflammatory drugs are useful in treatment.

Dressler's syndrome

This is an autoimmune response to acute myocardial infarction in which autoantibodies are formed and produce a febrile illness with pericarditis and effusion about 10–14 days after the acute episode.

Left ventricular aneurysm

Death of myocardial fibres and replacement by fibrous tissue may result in a severely weakened left ventricular wall that becomes aneurysmal. This produces persistent ST-T changes on the ECG (**5.67**) and a typical appearance on chest X-ray (**5.68**).

Isotope scans (**5.69**), ultrasound or ventriculography show part of the left ventricle to be non-contractile. Some of these aneurysms can be surgically resected.

5.67

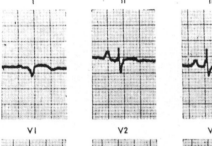
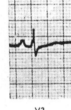
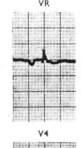
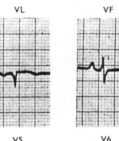
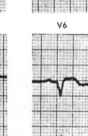

5.67 Left ventricular aneurysm produces a persistence of the pattern of acute myocardial infarction in the ECG. In uncomplicated myocardial infarction, the ST segment has normally returned to the isoelectric line within 3–6 weeks; persistence of ST elevation beyond this time is a pointer to possible aneurysm. This ECG was taken 10 weeks after infarction in a patient who had signs of heart failure. The QRS complexes in all precordial leads shows that the patient had an extensive full-thickness infarct.

5.68

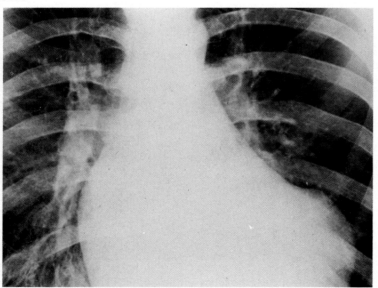

5.68 Ventricular aneurysm, revealed on chest X-ray 3 weeks after acute myocardial infarction. Note the bulge in the left cardiac border. On screening, this would be found to move paradoxically—outwards during systole.

5.69 Left ventricular aneurysm revealed in a nuclear 'MUGA' scan.
The 'amplitude' analysis shows that only a small part of the left ventricle has good amplitude of movement; the large segment which does not move is shown not to be in phase in the phase analysis. The ejection fraction of the left ventricle is only 14% (very low), but the ejection fraction of the contracting segment of the left ventricle is 32%. This raises the possibility that surgical removal of the LV aneurysm may improve overall left ventricular function.

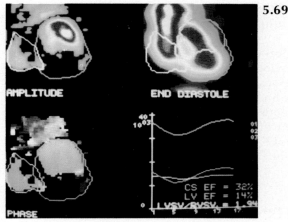

Rehabilitation and secondary prevention of coronary heart disease

After about a week in hospital, most patients with myocardial infarction are fit to return home, but they should be offered a rehabilitation programme of graduated exercise and lifestyle advice. Regular aspirin and beta-blocker therapy may lessen the chances of subsequent infarction. It is usually possible to identify individuals with a poor prognosis after myocardial infarction by exercise ECG, nuclear exercise tests and coronary angiography. Where appropriate, coronary artery surgery may improve their prognosis.

All patients with symptomatic coronary disease must be given appropriate lifestyle advice, as reduction of blood cholesterol by diet alteration or drugs, stopping smoking and an exercise programme can improve prognosis, even when coronary artery disease has already developed; indeed there is evidence that these measures may lead to reduction in size (regression) of occluding atheromatous plaques.

Rheumatic fever

This is an acute inflammatory disease of connective tissue which is a sequel to infection with Group A streptococci (*see* p.38) and may involve the heart, skin, central nervous system and joints. It is now a rare disease in the developed world but is still endemic elsewhere; and even in the West there is still a large residue of patients with rheumatic valve disease which has resulted from childhood infection.

The cardinal skin signs are erythema marginatum (**5.70**) and subcutaneous nodules, which are firm, painless and discrete, about 0.5–1 cm in diameter, and are found mainly over bony prominences and tendons. They resolve after a few weeks.

The arthritis varies from arthralgia to a flitting polyarthritis, mainly affecting are the larger joints such as the knees, ankles, wrists and elbows. These joints may become acutely swollen, hot and tender, and the synovial fluid is full of polymorphs.

Carditis is the most important aspect of this disease as it has major long-term implications. Endocarditis, myocarditis and pericarditis are all often present. The diagnosis of carditis requires the finding of:

- new cardiac murmurs
- cardiomegaly
- pericarditis
- congestive cardiac failure.

The murmurs may include an apical systolic murmur (caused by mitral regurgitation), a transient apical mid-diastolic (Carey–Coombs) murmur (caused by turbulent flow across the inflamed mitral valve), and a basal diastolic murmur (caused by aortic regurgitation). Other cardiac signs may

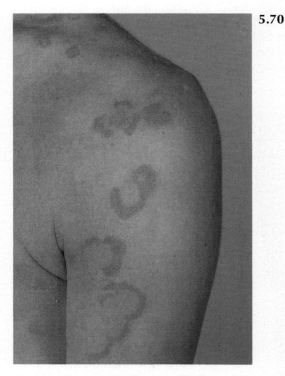

5.70 Erythema marginatum is a characteristic skin rash which may follow any streptococcal infection, especially tonsillitis. It is one of the common signs of acute rheumatic fever, and its presence should raise the possibility of cardiac involvement.

include tachycardia, pericardial friction rub, muffled heart sounds resulting from pericardial effusion and evidence of heart failure.

Neurological involvement (Sydenham's chorea) is uncommon and develops after a latent period of several weeks. The patient develops rapid purposeless involuntary movements mostly in the limbs and face (*see* p. 504).

Investigations should include throat-swab culture and the measurement of antibody response to *Streptococcus* (anti-streptolysin 'O' titre). There is usually a leucocytosis and elevation of the ESR and C-reactive protein levels. X-ray of the chest may show a pericardial effusion and rarely pneumonia or lobar collapse. ECG often shows first degree heartblock (5.41, 5.42).

Treatment should be directed towards the elimination of any residual streptococcal infection with penicillin. Aspirin is an effective anti-inflammatory and anti-pyretic agent for the other features. Prevention of recurrence may be necessary with long-term oral penicillin.

The long-term damage resulting from rheumatic fever may require further lifelong treatment.

Acquired valve diseases

The most common forms of heart valve disease affect the mitral and aortic valves, causing left heart failure and pulmonary congestion. The valves may fail to open fully (stenosis) or to close (regurgitation or incompetence). Both stenosis and regurgitation can co-exist. The effects of both types of lesion are haemodynamic with major implications for cardiac function.

The presence of heart valve disease is suspected from a heart murmur. An electrocardiogram and chest X-ray may provide additional clues, but the main diagnostic technique for valve disease is echocardiography. Doppler echocardiography is particularly useful in establishing the severity of valvular stenosis or regurgitation. Where valve surgery is planned, the diagnosis in adults is usually confirmed by cardiac catheterisation and angiography, which also permits evaluation of the coronary arteries.

Mitral stenosis

The most common cause of mitral stenosis is rheumatic fever; and mitral stenosis occurs in about half of all patients with chronic rheumatic heart disease. The mitral valve usually narrows slowly and the pulmonary vasculature adapts to the rising pressure of blood within the pulmonary capillaries, pulmonary veins and the left atrium.

The walls of the pulmonary vessels thicken, reducing blood flow and cardiac output but protecting the patient from pulmonary oedema. Patients notice only a gradual decline in exercise tolerance, although they may be aware of a brisk deterioration if their heart rhythm changes from sinus rhythm to atrial fibrillation. Episodes of acute pulmonary oedema occur as the cross-sectional area of the valve diminishes and the patient may have episodes of acute dyspnoea and orthopnoea and paroxysmal nocturnal dyspnoea. As the pulmonary blood pressure rises there are episodes of haemoptysis. Systemic embolism is common from thrombi in the large left atrium, especially in the presence of atrial fibrillation. The common sites for embolism are cerebral (*see* p.454), mesenteric, renal and limb arteries (**5.71**).

Two-thirds of the patients are female. They may have a malar flush (**5.2**) or central cyanosis; there may be signs of weight loss or peripheral oedema. Jugular venous pulsation becomes obvious only when right heart failure appears. The key cardiac findings are a tapping apex beat, and a rumbling mid-diastolic murmur at the apex (**5.8**). There may be pre-systolic accentuation and the murmur may be preceded by an opening snap. Exercise and positioning the patient in the left lateral position will accentuate the murmur. As pulmonary hypertension develops, the pulmonary second sound becomes accentuated and a right ventricular heave becomes apparent. Bilateral basal pulmonary crepitations may herald the onset of left heart failure.

Radiography of the chest shows a generally small heart with an accentuation of its left upper border from the enlarged left atrium and often signs of pulmonary oedema (**5.14**). The ECG shows a bifid P wave (P mitrale) (**5.72**) and there may be features of right ventricular hypertrophy and atrial fibrillation (**5.28, 5.29**). The diagnosis should be confirmed by echocardiography

5.71

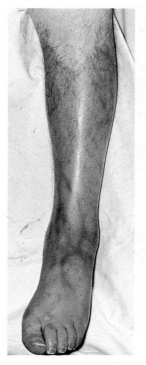

5.71 Arterial embolism causing acute ischaemia of the leg in a patient with mitral stenosis. The patient was in atrial fibrillation, and the source of the embolus was the left atrium (see **5.74**). Initial pallor of the leg and foot is replaced by reactive hyperaemia as the collateral circulation opens up.

which will show the immobility of the mitral valve cusps (**5.15, 5.16, 5.73**), and may show atrial thrombus (**5.74**), and cardiac catheterisation is usual if surgery is contemplated.

Treatment includes diuretics for heart failure and digoxin

for atrial fibrillation. Warfarin reduces the chances of thrombosis in the left atrium and of embolism. In severe cases, the fused cusps may be separated surgically (valvotomy) or the valve can be replaced (**1.9**).

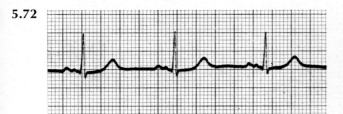

5.72

5.72 P mitrale. The P wave is bifid and has a duration of 0.12 seconds or more. The appearance results from delayed activation of the enlarged left atrium: the first peak represents right atrial, and the second left atrial activation.

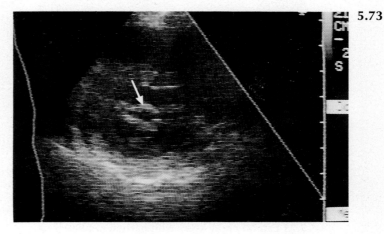

5.73

5.73 Echocardiogram (short-axis view) showing tight mitral stenosis. The tight orifice of the mitral valve is arrowed.

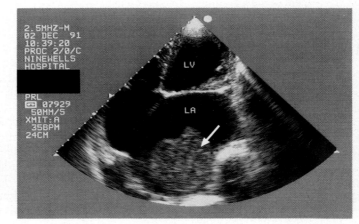

5.74

5.74 Echocardiogram (parasternal short-axis view) in a patient with rheumatic mitral stenosis, showing a very large thrombus attached to the walls of the left atrium (arrow). The patient presented with a stroke (see p. 454) and was found to have atrial fibrillation and a diastolic murmur. Anticoagulation is required to prevent further emboli.

Mitral regurgitation

There are many causes of mitral regurgitation. Rheumatic fever is rarely responsible unless there is associated mitral stenosis. The valve cusps may be damaged by myxomatous degeneration, SLE, or endocarditis, the chordae may rupture, and the papillary muscles may malfunction as a result of coronary artery disease. The result of mitral regurgitation is dilatation of the left atrium. Eventually this leads to atrial hypertrophy and pulmonary hypertension and oedema. The same picture may develop acutely with rupture of the chordae tendineae. Infective endocarditis may also occur.

Symptoms may appear only after some time has elapsed—usually dyspnoea on exertion (later at rest) and palpitations. With the onset of pulmonary hypertension, there may be symptoms from right heart failure.

Signs are dominated by left ventricular dilatation, with the heaving apex beat displaced to the left, a systolic thrill at the apex and a high-pitched pansystolic murmur at the apex, transmitted to the left axilla (**5.7**). Later in the disease, there

may be a right ventricular heave associated with accentuation of the pulmonary second sound. The diagnosis is confirmed by:

- Chest X-ray shows enlargement of left ventricle and atrium (**5.75**), and sometimes calcification of the mitral valve.
- ECG shows left ventricular hypertrophy (**5.121**), and often atrial fibrillation (**5.28, 5.29**).
- Echocardiography shows the position of the valve leaflets at closure (**5.76**), and colour-flow Doppler shows the regurgitant jet (**5.18**).
- Cardiac catheterisation can define the pressure differences between chambers, and ventriculography will confirm the presence of regurgitation.

Medical treatment includes prevention of endocarditis, control of heart failure, and anticoagulation to prevent thromboembolism. A severely damaged valve will need surgical replacement.

231

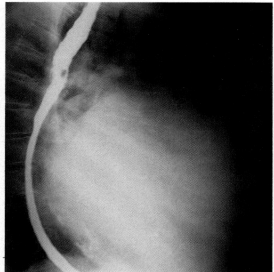

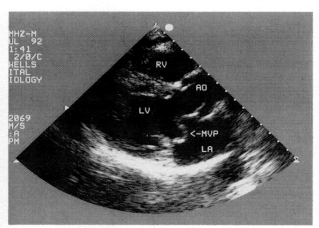

5.76 Mitral regurgitation associated with a floppy, prolapsing mitral valve seen on 2D echocardiography (parasternal long-axis view) in systole. Note the open cusps of the aortic valve. The posterior leaflet of the mitral valve is prolapsing backwards into the left atrium in systole (MVP). This abnormality is fairly common in young women for no obvious caused. It may also be a feature of Marfan's syndrome (p. 318) and other connective tissue disorders. LA = left atrium; LV = left ventricle; Ao = aorta; RV = right ventricle.

5.75 Lateral chest X-ray with barium swallow in a patient with mitral regurgitation. This technique has been superseded by echocardiography, but it provides graphic evidence of the extent of enlargement of the left atrium, which is bulging backwards and distorting the oesophagus.

Aortic stenosis

Acquired aortic valve stenosis often results from progressive degeneration and calcification of a congenitally bicuspid valve. Rheumatic fever and arteriosclerotic degeneration are rarer causes. Aortic stenosis leads to left ventricular hypertrophy and relative left ventricular ischaemia, so patients may present with angina, infarction, left ventricular failure or arrhythmias. Ventricular fibrillation is a common cause of sudden death. Calcification around the valve may extend into the conducting tissue causing heart block and syncope.

The dominant clinical features of aortic stenosis are a low-volume, slow-rising pulse; a forceful apex beat; a systolic thrill at the base of the heart; and a mid-systolic murmur at the aortic area, which radiates to the neck (5.7).

The diagnosis is supported by features of left ventricular hypertrophy on the chest X-ray and ECG (5.121). Echocardiography confirms the diagnosis by showing thickened and calcified valve cusps (5.77). Doppler echocardiography and/or cardiac catheterisation (5.78) establish the severity of the stenosis.

The valve is usually replaced with a prosthetic valve. Alternatively, the narrowed valve may be stretched by balloon valvuloplasty, although the long-term benefits of this procedure are unclear.

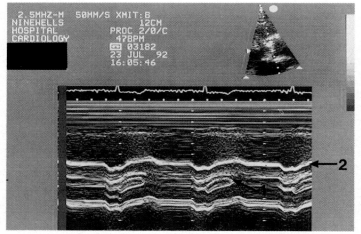

5.77 Aortic stenosis with calcification. This M-mode parasternal long axis view shows the characteristic box shape of valve opening during systole (1). Calcification of the valve and annulus is suggested by the density of whiteness of the tracing (2).

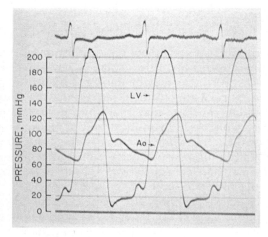

5.78 Pressure gradient across the aortic valve in aortic stenosis, as measured at cardiac catheterisation. Note the low aortic (Ao) pressure compared with the left ventricular pressure (LV) and the delayed peak in aortic pressure—both characteristic of severe aortic stenosis.

Aortic regurgitation

Aortic regurgitation occurs if the aortic valve ring dilates, as a result of dissecting aneurysm, ankylosing spondylitis or syphilis for example, or if the valve cusps degenerate, e.g. after rheumatic fever or endocarditis. Aortic regurgitation leads to hypertrophy of the left ventricle and ultimately left ventricular failure. Clinical symptoms often occur late and the patient may present with significant heart failure or angina. There may have been a preceding history of palpitations, syncope or headaches because of the high systolic blood pressure, especially during exercise.

Many of the physical signs are a reflection of the size of the leak, e.g. collapsing pulse, capillary pulsation, visible carotid pulsation, head bobbing and the Duroziez's murmur heard over the femoral artery. On examination, there is left ventricular hypertrophy, and an early diastolic murmur down the left side of the sternum which is best heard by sitting the patient upright, leaning forward in full expiration. A diastolic thrill is rarely felt down the left sternal edge.

X-ray of chest (5.79), ECG (5.121) and echocardiogram show left ventricular enlargement. Aortography (5.80) or colour-flow Doppler (5.81) shows the regurgitant jet.

Medical treatment is directed at managing the angina, correcting the failure and preventing endocarditis. Definitive treatment consists of replacing the valve with a prosthetic one.

5.79 Left ventricular hypertrophy and dilatation in a patient with severe aortic regurgitation. Left ventricular hypertrophy alters the shape of the heart, making the left heart border more convex than normal, but hypertrophy alone does not increase the size of the heart. The cardiac enlargement seen here is indicative of ventricular dilatation.

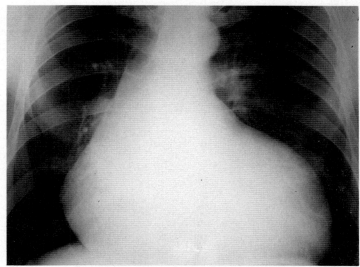

5.79

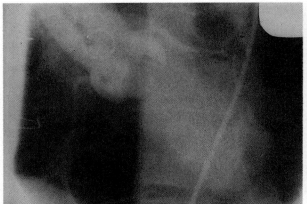

5.80

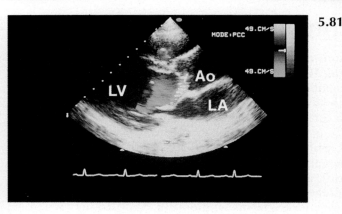

5.81

5.80 Aortogram in severe aortic regurgitation. Contrast medium has only been injected into the aorta, but even in this systolic view it is clear that it has regurgitated into the left ventricle. The aortic valve is arrowed. The 'ring' over the aortic root is due to an ECG skin electrode.

5.81 Colour-flow Doppler mapping in a patient with mild aortic regurgitation (parasternal long axis view). The aortic regurgitant jet (in blue) is directed posteriorly at an acute angle from the aortic valve, and it impinges directly on the anterior mitral valve leaflet. Colour-flow Doppler has revolutionised the non-invasive investigation of these patients. LV = left ventricle; LA = left atrium; Ao = aorta.

Tricuspid and pulmonary valve disease

These valves are rarely stenosed by rheumatic fever and they may be slightly incompetent in quite healthy individuals. Severe pulmonary regurgitation is usually secondary to left heart failure or lung disease, through the effects of a raised pulmonary arterial pressure, which causes dilatation of the pulmonary artery and stretching of the pulmonary valve annulus. The resultant murmur of pulmonary regurgitation has the same early diastolic characteristics as the murmur of aortic regurgitation (5.8), but the characteristic findings in the arterial pulse are absent.

Tricuspid regurgitation usually follows dilatation of the right ventricle. Once it develops, signs of right heart failure become prominent, e.g. distended jugular veins, enlarged liver, ascites and oedema. A pansystolic murmur may be audible at the lower left sternal border (5.7). Chest X-ray may show right atrial enlargement (5.82). Echocardiography is the most effective method of diagnosing pulmonary and tricuspid valve disease (5.18).

Obstruction to right ventricular outflow may occur above, below or at the level of the pulmonary valve. The clinical problems which result from pulmonary stenosis depend on the severity of the obstruction rather than on the acutal site. Patients are usually asymptomatic and symptoms appear only if there is progression of the stenosis. These include fatigue, symptoms of right ventricular failure and syncope. The clinical signs are those of right ventricular hypertrophy (a right ventricular heave) and a loud systolic murmur in the second left intercostal space, with a preceding click if valvular stenosis is responsible. Chest X-ray may show right ventricular enlargement or post-stenotic dilatation. Pulmonary stenosis can be diagnosed by echocardiography and its severity assessed by Doppler. Pulmonary valvuloplasty corrects valvular stenosis.

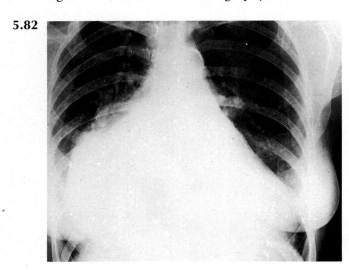

5.82

5.82 Chest X-ray in a patient with tricuspid regurgitation. The enlargement of the right heart shadow is caused by a grossly enlarged right atrium. Note also the calcified aortic arch (and the incidental bilateral hilar calcification, resulting from old tuberculosis). This woman's tricuspid regurgitation resulted from ischaemic heart disease.

Congenital heart disease

Serious congenital heart disease is found in 1 per 1,000 live births. Congenital bicuspid aortic valve is much more common but usually only becomes a problem when it calcifies. With advances in surgical and medical care, many patients with congenital heart disease now live into adult life.

Congenital lesions may result from a variety of maternal and fetal factors including maternal alcohol or drug abuse, maternal rubella (diminishing in importance in the developed world), and occasionally single gene mutations. A range of syndromes which include cardiac abnormalities are described elsewhere, e.g. Down's syndrome (p. 352), Turner's syndrome (p. 317), Ehlers–Danlos syndrome (p. 151), Friedreich's ataxia (p. 509) and Noonan's syndrome (p. 317). Congenital cardiac lesions may also be associated with other, less well defined anomalies (5.83).

Patients with congenital heart disease may present at birth (5.84), with cyanosis or associated symptoms in childhood (5.85, 5.86, 7.145), or sometimes in adult life. They commonly have finger clubbing (5.3).

Congenital cardiac anomalies may be divided into two main types:

- Communications between cardiac chambers or blood vessels.
- Lesions which obstruct blood flow.

Combinations of both types of anomaly may occur, as in Fallot's tetralogy and other complex congenital conditions.

Communications between the left and right sides of the heart cause blood to flow from the high-pressure left side to the low-pressure right side. This happens when an atrial septal defect or ventricular septal defect is present, or where there is a patent ductus arteriosus causing blood to flow from the aorta to pulmonary artery. Pulmonary blood flow increases and, in extreme cases, the pulmonary capillaries and arterioles may respond by thickening their walls and narrowing their lumens. This increases the work of the right ventricle, which must raise its systolic pressure to maintain normal cardiac output (pulmonary hypertension). The elevated pressure may then reverse the shunt, causing blood to flow from right to left through the abnormal communication, so that unoxygenated blood bypasses the lungs (Eisenmenger syndrome).

5.83

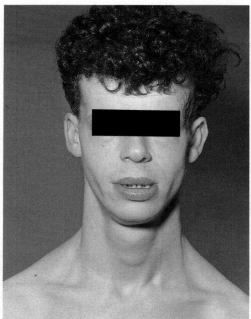

5.84

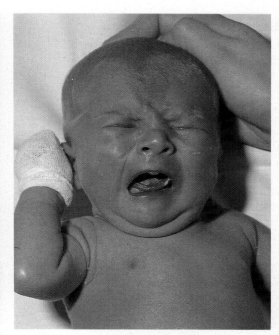

5.83 Congenital heart disease may be associated with many other congenital anomalies. This young man with congenital aortic stenosis also had a webbed neck, a small face, with a hypoplastic mandible, low set ears and a range of other musculoskeletal abnormalities (not part of any named syndrome). Note also the presence of dental caries—a risk factor for infective endocarditis and brain abscess. Antibiotic prophylaxis should be given before dental treatment commences.

5.84 Congenital heart disease commonly presents with cyanosis at or soon after birth (a 'blue baby'). Urgent assessment and consideration for cardiac surgery is necessary, and feeding is often particularly difficult in these neonates. This baby had transposition of the great arteries (p. 240).

5.85

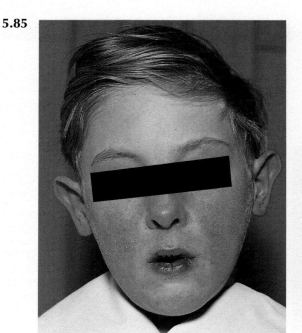

5.86

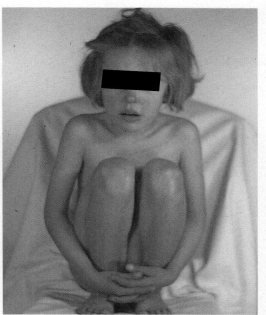

5.85 Severe central cyanosis in a boy with Fallot's tetralogy, photographed just before surgical correction. Fallot's tetralogy is the commonest cause of cyanotic congenital heart disease in patients over the age of 1 year.

5.86 Squatting is a common feature in children with cyanotic congenital heart disease, especially Fallot's tetralogy. The child usually squats after exercise, apparently to relieve breathlessness. The mechanism by which squatting achieves symptomatic relief is not clear, but it may involve an increase in systemic vascular resistance which decreases the right-to-left shunt, a pooling of desaturated blood in the legs or an increase in systemic venous return and pulmonary blood flow.

Atrial septal defect

Atrial septal defects (ASDs) most commonly occur in the middle of the inter-atrial septum (a secundum defect), although they may occur in the upper part (sinus venosus defect) or lower part (primum defect) where associated abnormalities of the mitral and tricuspid valves make the condition more serious. The history and findings depend on the age at presentation and the severity of the defect or defects. Children with secundum defects seldom experience symptoms, but in adult life, heart failure and cardiac arrhythmias, usually atrial fibrillation, develop, so the defects should often be closed. If presentation is late, the main features are those of right heart failure. There is usually a marked right ventricular impulse and wide fixed splitting of P2, with a systolic pulmonary ejection murmur resulting from increased flow across the normal pulmonary valve. These findings change as pulmonary vascular resistance increases and a right to left shunt appears. The X-ray of the chest may show evidence of right ventricular hypertrophy and dilatation, with a prominent pulmonary artery with pulmonary plethora (5.87). The ECG shows a characteristic right bundle branch block pattern. Echocardiography confirms right ventricular hypertrophy and dilatation of the pulmonary artery and may define the anatomical site and dimensions of the defect (5.88). These findings may be confirmed by cardiac catheterisation or by MRI (5.89). Treatment is surgical.

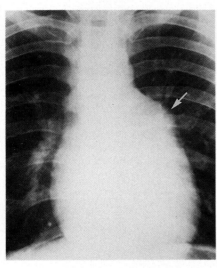

5.87 Atrial septal defect with a large left-to-right shunt. The pulmonary arteries are prominent, especially on the left (arrow).

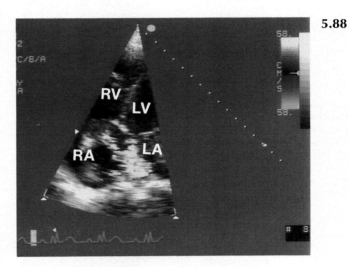

5.88 Atrial septal defect. This colour flow doppler apical four chamber view shows blood flow from the left to the right atrium through a moderate sized atrial septal defect. LA = left atrium; RA = right atrium; LV = left ventricle; RV = right ventricle.

5.89 Atrial septal defect. This MRI (transverse spin echo) image shows an ostium secundum atrial septal defect (arrow). The right ventricle and right atrium are dilated, there is a small part of the atrial septum present at the atrioventricular valve plane but the rest of the septum is absent. RA = right atrium; RV = right ventricle; LA = left atrium; LV = left ventricle.

Ventricular septal defect

Ventricular septal defects (VSDs) are common and the most frequent type is a single opening in the membranous portion of the septum. The symptoms and signs are dependent on the size of the defect, the state of the pulmonary vasculature and the presence of other abnormalities. Most defects are small, cause no symptoms and close spontaneously during childhood. Initially, the greater pressure in the left ventricle is associated with a left-to-right shunt that is present throughout systole and is heard as a loud systolic murmur to the left side of the sternum (maladie de Roger). With moderate-sized shunts, fatigue and dyspnoea on exertion may occur; and with larger shunts, there may be recurrent pulmonary infections, growth retardation and cardiac failure at an early age. Large defects cause right and left heart failure and, if they are not closed surgically, the Eisenmenger syndrome ensues, with cyanosis, finger clubbing and polycythaemia. Once this has developed survival is poor and heart and lung transplantation is the only possibility.

Clinical signs in these large defects include the signs of right ventricular hypertrophy and pulmonary hypertension. There is cardiomegaly with a forceful apex beat and a prominent systolic thrill at the left sternal edge. The pulmonary second sound is accentuated and there is a characteristic pansystolic murmur best heard at the third and fourth interspaces to the left of the sternum with radiation across the anterior chest wall (5.7). With a small VSD, the chest X-ray and ECG are both normal. With larger defects, the chest X-ray may show an enlarged left atrium, left and right ventricular hypertrophy, a large pulmonary artery and increased pulmonary vascular markings (5.90). The ECG shows evidence of biventricular hypertrophy. The diagnosis can be confirmed by echocardiography (5.91), colour-flow Doppler (5.92) or MRI and cardiac catheterisation may be required if the defect is complicated by other pathology. There is a risk of bacterial endocarditis in all VSD patients, especially in those with smaller defects. Surgery is required in all patients with a moderate or large left-to-right shunt.

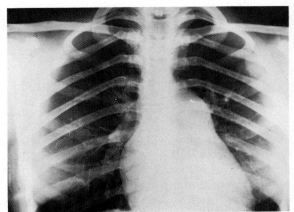

5.90 Large ventricular septal defect. The chest X-ray shows cardiomegaly with prominent pulmonary arteries and some pulmonary plethora. With a smaller VSD, the chest X-ray may be completely normal or may show simply a slight increase in pulmonary vascular markings.

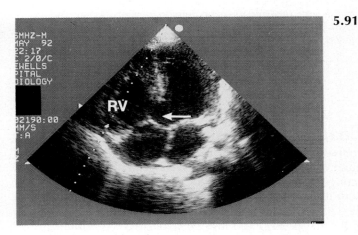

5.91 Ventricular septal defect. This apical four chamber echocardiogram view clearly shows the anatomical defect in the interventricular septum (arrowed). There is also enlargement of the right ventricle (RV) due to the left-to-right shunt. This patient had Down's syndrome.

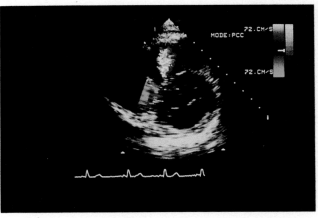

5.92 Ventricular septal defect. This colour-flow Doppler echocardiogram (parasternal short-axis image) shows a high-velocity jet of blood flowing through a small septal defect from the left ventricle (below) to the right ventricle (above). This small defect could not be visualised using conventional 2D echo.

Patent ductus arteriosus

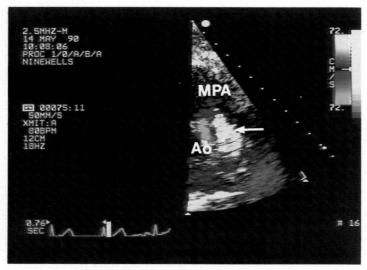

5.93 Patent ductus arteriosus. This colour flow doppler (short axis view) shows a characteristic ductal jet (arrowed), which represents flow from the aorta (Ao) into the main pulmonary artery (MPA). The patient was a 43 year old woman from a developing country, who presented in Dundee with shortness of breath and signs of heart failure.

Normal closure of the ductus arteriosus (joining the aorta to the bifurcation of the pulmonary artery) occurs immediately after birth, probably as a result of changes in production of vascular prostaglandins. Patency of the ductus (PDA) may be an isolated lesion or it may be combined with other lesions so that the ductus remains the only route for maintenance of the pulmonary or systemic blood flow. The amount of flow in the ductus is a reflection of its size and of the pulmonary and systemic pressures. The clinical signs depend on the extent of the pathology and its duration. With a large PDA there may be rapid onset of heart failure. Examination often shows a typical thrill at the left sternal edge, and on auscultation, there is a characteristic 'machinery' murmur at the upper left sternal border over the first intercostal space (5.9). In a large ductus, there is an enhanced differential in pulse pressure, felt as a bounding pulse. The X-ray of the chest may show left ventricular and left atrial enlargement, a prominent aorta and pulmonary artery and pulmonary plethora (appearances similar to 5.90). The ECG and echocardiogram show evidence of left ventricular and atrial hypertrophy and the duct may be seen on echo (5.93). Catheterisation of the aorta may be necessary to demonstrate the defect. Heart failure indicates an urgent need for surgical correction.

Coarctation of the aorta

Coarctation of the aorta is a relatively uncommon lesion, found in 5–10% of patients with congenital heart disease. It is a congenital narrowing of the aorta which can occur at any point in its length but is usually found just after the origin of the left subclavian artery. It is often found in Turner's syndrome (p. 317) and may be associated with other cardiac and vascular abnormalities. Most children are asymptomatic and the patient is often found to have hypertension in the upper half of the body on routine physical examination. Severe cases may present with intermittent claudication, cold lower limbs or headache and epistaxis from hypertension. The dominant clinical feature is absence, diminution or delay of the pulse at the femoral artery compared to the radial artery. There is also a marked difference between the blood pressure in the upper and lower limbs. In the adult, pulsating collateral vessels may be found in the interscapular area, the axillae and the intercostal spaces. Auscultation of the heart reveals a mid-systolic murmur over the anterior chest and back.

X-ray of the chest may show left ventricular hypertrophy with a dilated ascending aorta. The stenotic area may occasionally be visible. Rib notching caused by dilated collateral vessels is common (5.94). The ECG shows left ventricular hypertrophy (5.121). Aortography is necessary to define accurately the position and length of the coarctation, though MRI can produce elegant results (5.95). Echocardiography and cardiac catheterisation may be needed to exclude other lesions, especially bicuspid aortic valve, congenital aortic stenosis and patent ductus arteriosus.

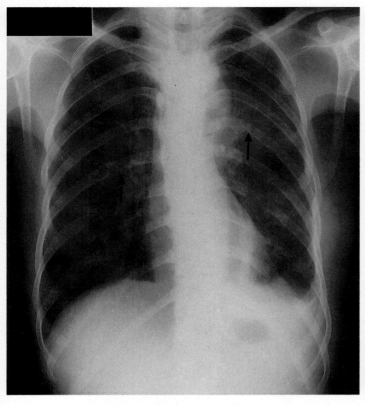

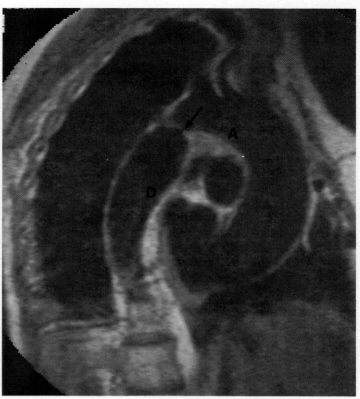

5.94 Coarctation of the aorta. The heart is not enlarged, but there is obvious bilateral rib notching as a result of dilated intercostal arteries (arrows).

5.95 Coarctation of the aorta. This oblique MRI view through the arch of the aorta shows the coarctation as a thin shelf across the whole of the aorta (arrow). There was a small lumen, allowing blood to flow past the obstruction, which was out of plane in this view. A = ascending aorta; D = descending aorta.

Aortic and pulmonary stenosis

Aortic stenosis accounts for 2–4% of congenital heart disease. Congenital narrowing of the aortic valve is present from birth, and calcification of the valve may occur later in life (5.77). The signs, investigatory findings and treatment are similar to those in acquired disease (*see* p. 232). Pulmonary stenosis may also be an isolated congenital lesion (*see* p. 234) or part of a complex congenital lesion.

Fallot's tetralogy

Fallot's tetralogy forms about 10% of all cases of congenital heart disease and is the most common cardiac cause of cyanosis in infants over 1 year of age. The four characteristics of this syndrome are:

- Ventricular septal defect.
- Over-riding of the aorta over the defect.
- Pulmonary outflow tract obstruction.
- Right ventricular hypertrophy resulting from the stenosis.

Affected children are cyanosed from birth (5.84, 7.145) and have dyspnoea on exertion (5.86) (and later at rest), retarded growth, finger clubbing (5.3) and secondary polycythaemia. The cardiac signs are those of right ventricular hypertrophy and dilatation, and a systolic thrill may be felt along the left sternal edge. There is a loud ejection systolic murmur often maximal in the second left interspace as a result of disturbed flow across the stenotic pulmonary outflow tract.

The chest X-ray shows a normal-sized heart which is boot-shaped (coeur-en-sabot) because of prominence of the right ventricle and the small pulmonary arteries (5.96). The ECG shows right ventricular and later right atrial hypertrophy. Echocardiography may show the defect and angiocardiography is necessary to define the extent of the abnormalities (5.97).

Affected children invariably died before the advent of complete surgical repair of both the septal defect and stenosis. Before surgery, patients are cyanosed (5.85, 5.86) and require repeated venesections for polycythaemia. They are susceptible to endocarditis and cerebral abscesses. Total correction of the lesions is required and this may be done in two stages. The first-stage operation is designed to increase pulmonary blood flow and this may involve aortopulmonary or subclavian-pulmonary anastomosis. The second-stage operation—to correct the remaining defects—can then be carried out more safely in adolescence.

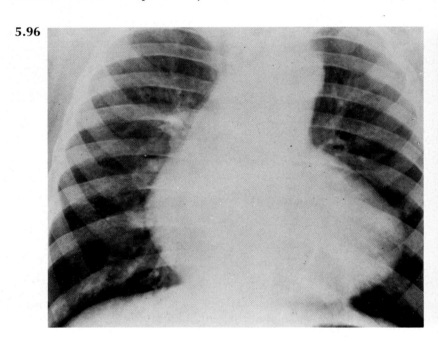

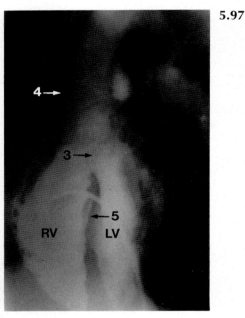

5.96 Fallot's tetralogy. The classic boot-shaped heart (coeur-en-sabot). The appearance is brought about by gross right ventricular hypertrophy, associated with small pulmonary arteries. The absence of the normal pulmonary arterial markings produces a 'bay' or indentation in the left cardiac border. The lung fields retain some vascular markings, because of their supply by systemic rather than pulmonary arteries.

5.97 Fallot's tetralogy. A right ventriculo-gram (left anterior oblique view) shows right ventricular hypertrophy, a sub-aortic ventricular septal defect (3) and the aorta (4) overriding the ventricular septum (5). LV = left ventricle; RV = right ventricle.

Complete transposition of the great arteries

This is a relatively common congenital anomaly (5.84) but few patients survive to adult life. The aorta arises from the right ventricle, and the pulmonary artery arises from the left ventricle so that the systemic and pulmonary circulations are quite distinct. Death is inevitable without a communication between the two circulations to oxygenate systemic blood.

Fortunately, many patients have an associated ventricular septal defect, and in others an atrial septal defect can be created immediately after birth, by pulling a balloon-tipped cardiac catheter across the inter-atrial septum. Further surgery is necessary later if life is to be maintained.

Pulmonary hypertension

Pulmonary hypertension is a common consequence of a variety of lung and heart conditions (**Table 5.3**). The long-term result is right ventricular and atrial hypertrophy and dilatation. Such patients may present with ischaemic-type chest pain, features of right heart failure, syncope and occasionally hoarseness caused by pressure on the left recurrent laryngeal nerve from the enlarging pulmonary artery. Sudden cardiac death is relatively common and may occur during diagnostic instrumentation. On examination, the clinical picture is that of right heart failure with a prominent right ventricular heave, jugular venous congestion with a prominent A wave, peripheral oedema, and hepatic congestion. The pulmonary second sound is accentuated and may be felt. Incompetence of the pulmonary valve may be a late feature.

The chest X-ray usually shows cardiac enlargement with right ventricular and right atrial enlargement and dilatation of the pulmonary arteries (4.66). The lung fields may be oligaemic. The ECG shows features of right-axis deviation, right ventricular hypertrophy and strain (5.98) and occasionally right bundle branch block. Echocardiography and colour-flow Doppler may show the cause of hypertension, e.g. atrial or ventricular septal defects or mitral stenosis. Cardiac catheterisation is of value to determine the site of the lesion and measure pressures and degree of oxygenation. Treatment is directed at the underlying cause. Diuretics, oxygen, vasodilators and anticoagulants have a place in management, as does heart-lung transplantation as a last resort.

Table 5.3 Diseases associated with pulmonary hypertension.

Chronic obstructive lung diseases
Chronic parenchymal lung disease
Recurrent pulmonary embolism
Chronic left ventricular failure
Mitral valve disease
Congenital heart diseases (VSD, ASD, PDA and pulmonary
  artery stenosis)
Idiopathic (primary) pulmonary hypertension
Connective tissue diseases (SLE, systemic sclerosis, etc.)
Peripheral arterio-venous shunts
Left atrial myxoma
High-altitude living
Pulmonary veno-occlusive disease

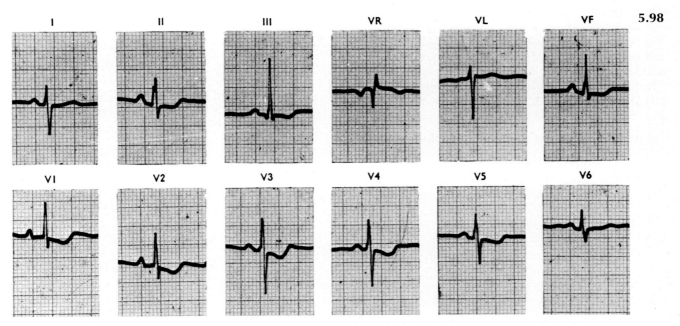

5.98

5.98 Right ventricular hypertrophy in a patient with pulmonary hypertension. Note the tall R wave (7mm +) in V1 which is taller than the S wave, a combined voltage of R in V1 and S in V6 of 10mm or more, and the ST depression and T-wave inversion from V1 to V5 - a manifestation of right ventricular strain. Right ventricular hypertrophy may also be manifested as dominant S waves across all the chest leads. P pulmonale (tall, peaked P waves at least 2.5mm in height) is another common finding, though absent on this trace.

Infective endocarditis

In infective endocarditis, a bacteraemia is complicated by the development of 'vegetations' on the endocardium of the heart (endocarditis). Vegetations usually form on aortic and mitral valves which are already damaged following rheumatic fever, but they may be associated with congenital abnormalities such as ventricular and atrial septal defects and coarctation of the aorta (where they may cause aortitis). The organisms involved are usually commensals of the mouth and pharynx (*Streptococcus viridans*) or the bowel (*Streptococcus faecalis*). Rarely, virulent organisms such as *Streptococcus pyogenes* or *Staphylococcus aureus* may infect a previously normal heart valve, especially in intravenous drug abusers and in patients with in-dwelling cannulae and pacing lines. Prosthetic heart valves are more susceptible to endocarditis than normal valves and they may become infected with unusual organisms, such as *Staphylococcus epidermidis*, Gram-negative organisms and fungi such as *Candida albicans, Histoplasma* and *Aspergillus*. Although episodes of bacteraemia may apparently occur spontaneously, especially in patients with dental caries (**5.83, 5.99**), dental procedures, endotracheal intubation and bronchoscopy, genitourinary and colonic endoscopy and surgery are especially likely to provoke bacteraemia. Patients with diseased valves or congenital cardiac abnormalities should therefore be given prophylactic antibiotics before these procedures.

Infective vegetations produce clinical features in four ways:

- They induce febrile symptoms, such as sweating and weight loss.
- They may erode heart valves and rupture chordae tendineae, causing valvular incompetence and heart failure. The infection may extend beyond the valve into the conducting tissue of the heart, causing heart block.
- They can embolise causing stroke, limb ischaemia, renal and splenic infarcts and occasionally myocardial and pulmonary infarction.
- Their presence can stimulate the formation of immune complexes in the blood. These complexes can produce focal glomerulonephritis and vasculitis in the eye and skin.

Untreated endocarditis is usually fatal. Numerous signs are traditionally associated with the disorder, but many are seldom seen in modern medicine. Most patients feel generally unwell, with a low-grade fever. If this is associated with the development over a few weeks of a murmur caused by an incompetent heart valve, the diagnosis is very likely. In addition, there may be weight loss, anaemia, haematuria, an enlarged spleen, petechiae and vasculitic lesions under the nails (splinter haemorrhages, **3.28**), in the sclerae (**5.100**), conjunctivae, retinae (Roth spots) (**5.101**) and in the finger and toe pulps (Osler's nodes) (**5.102**). Finger clubbing is now extremely rare, as patients are usually treated before it develops.

When the diagnosis is suspected, an echocardiogram should be performed. Small vegetations are often not identifiable, but large vegetations can be visualised (**5.103, 5.104**) and the extent of the valvular incompetence clarified. Vegetations are particularly difficult to identify on prosthetic heart valves and colour-flow or trans-oesophageal echocardiography may be valuable in these patients. Blood tests often show a normochromic, normocytic anaemia, there may be a polymorph leucocytosis and the ESR and C-reactive proteins are elevated. Circulating immune complexes are found and there is a rise in immunoglobulin levels and a fall in total complement.

Multiple blood cultures are required and sampling should coincide with peaks of fever. This permits identification of the infecting organism, so that appropriate combinations of antibiotics can be given in high dosage intravenously for several weeks. Less aggressive therapy is usually ineffective. If cultures are negative, other causes of endocarditis should be sought by appropriate serological tests, e.g. for fungi, Q fever or psittacosis.

Antibiotics may not eradicate the infection and emergency surgery may be required. The infected valve is removed and replaced with a prosthetic one. Other indications for emergency valve replacement are the development of severe valvular incompetence causing heart failure or a dangerous embolic episode, e.g. cerebral embolism. The mortality rate associated with emergency valve replacement during endocarditis is higher than for elective surgery involving a sterile valve.

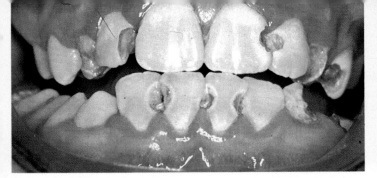

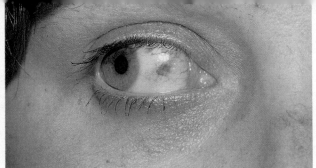

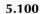

5.99 Severe dental caries predisposes patients to episodes of bacteraemia, and thus to infective endocarditis in the presence of a congenital or acquired cardiac abnormality. Full treatment of caries or appropriate dental extraction should be carried out with antibiotic prophylaxis in all such patients.

5.100 Scleral and conjunctival haemorrhages are a recognised but rare feature in established infective endocarditis. They are probably the result of infected microemboli from cardiac vegetations, but may also be associated with thrombocytopenia.

5.101

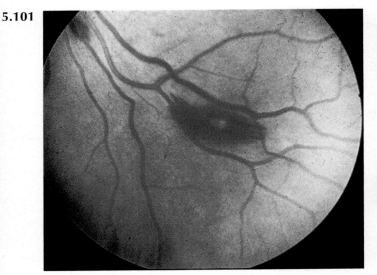

5.102

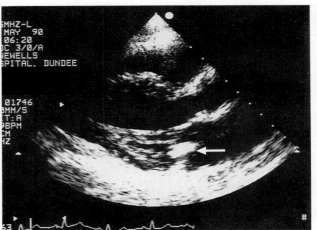

5.102 Small dermal infarcts in infective endocarditis. When palpable, these are known as Osler's nodes. These infarcts are usually tender. They may be caused by septic emboli from the cardiac vegetations, but similar appearances may result from vasculitis associated with circulating immune complexes.

5.101 A Roth spot in the retina in infective endocarditis. These oval haemorrhagic lesions with white centres are thought to result from septic emboli, but similar appearances may sometimes occur in patients with anaemia or leukaemia.

5.103

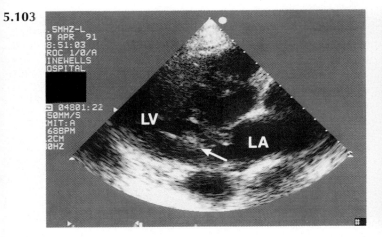

5.104

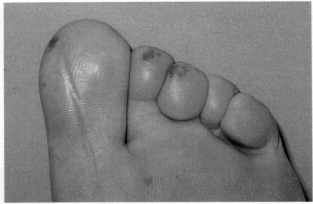

5.103 Echocardiogram in infective endocarditis. This parasternal long axis view shows a large vegetation on the anterior leaflet of the mitral valve (arrowed). The patient had recently been unwell with diverticulitis and a local intra-abdominal abscess. *Streptococcus faecalis* was grown on blood culture. LA = left atrium; LV = left ventricle.

5.104 Calcified mitral valve vegetation in infective endocarditis. This long axis parasternal view across the mitral valve shows a large calcified vegetation attached to the posterior leaflet (arrowed). This young man had had several previous episodes of infective endocarditis.

Myocarditis

'Myocarditis' is a general term for any inflammatory process involving the heart. It is usually infective but can be caused by chemicals, physical agents or drugs (**Table 5.4**).

The history depends on the cause. The most common type of myocarditis in the developed world follows a viral infection, typically an upper respiratory tract infection. The onset is usually insidious with features of right and left heart failure, fever and general malaise. There is tachycardia with a low-volume pulse, hypotension, faint heart sounds, a third heart sound and features of pericarditis. The chest X-ray shows cardiomegaly (**5.105**), sometimes with a pericardial effusion; the ECG may show arrhythmias, diffuse ST-segment and T-wave changes and heart block. Cardiac enzymes are elevated if the acute inflammatory process is ongoing. Serology may show a rising titre of viral antibodies. Treatment involves bed rest and control of failure and arrhythmias. Steroids can be of value.

Myocarditis usually remits but it may progress and behave like a chronic cardiomyopathy.

Table 5.4 Causes of myocarditis.

Infections	Viruses	Coxsackie
		Influenza
		Adenoviruses
		Echovirus
		Rubella
	Bacteria	*Corynebacterium diphtheriae*
		Chlamydia
		Rickettsia
		Coxiella burnetii
	Protozoa	*Trypanosoma cruzi*
		Toxoplasma gondii
Physical	Radiation	From therapy for breast or lung cancer, lymphoma or thymoma
Chemical	Lead	
	Alcohol	
Drugs	Emetine	In treatment of amoebiasis
	Chloroquine	In malaria prophylaxis

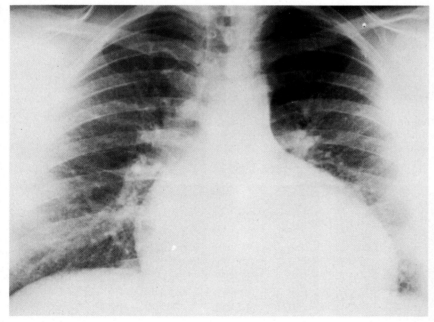

5.105

5.105 Acute myocarditis causing marked enlargement of all cardiac chambers and pulmonary venous congestion. The ECG showed generalised T-wave inversion. Serology showed the cause to be a coxsackievirus infection, and the patient made a complete recovery within a few weeks. An identical chest X-ray appearance may be seen in dilated cardiomyopathy.

Cardiomyopathies

The most common causes of diseased heart muscle are coronary disease, hypertension and heart valve disease. However, the myocardium may also be damaged in other conditions, e.g. prolonged alcohol abuse, hypothyroidism, acromegaly, phaeochromocytoma, inherited neuromuscular disorders, connective tissue and storage diseases and by some drug therapy (e.g. adriamycin).

Idiopathic cardiomyopathies are primary heart muscle disorders of indeterminate cause. They can be divided into three pathophysiological types which produce distinctive clinical syndromes:

- Dilated cardiomyopathy.
- Hypertrophic cardiomyopathy.
- Restrictive cardiomyopathy.

Dilated cardiomyopathy

In dilated cardiomyopathy, the heart muscle weakens and the chambers progressively dilate. The aetiology of idiopathic dilated cardiomyopathy is unknown, but previous coxsackievirus infection may be causally related. Patients become breathless and develop signs of right and left heart failure, with pulmonary congestion, cardiomegaly and, sometimes, arrhythmias and emboli. Ventricular dilatation may lead to functional mitral or tricuspid regurgitation.

Chest X-ray (5.105), echocardiography and MRI (5.22) confirm dilated cardiac chambers and inefficient LV wall motion in systole. The ECG may show ST segment changes and arrhythmias, but has no diagnostic value.

Patients with idiopathic dilated cardiomyopathy may fail to respond to diuretics and vasodilator drugs and the heart failure may progress to death within a few years. Cardiac transplantation is feasible in some younger patients.

Hypertrophic cardiomyopathy

In hypertrophic cardiomyopathy, a localised segment of the heart muscle becomes thickened; the interventricular septum is usually involved and the abnormal muscle restricts filling of the left ventricle during diastole. If it also obstructs the flow of blood from the ventricle to the aorta during systole, the condition is termed 'hypertrophic obstructive cardiomyopathy' (HOCM). The abnormal muscle is a focus for dangerous arrhythmias, especially ventricular tachycardia which may convert to ventricular fibrillation. Hypertrophic cardiomyopathy is potentially fatal, and patients should avoid strenuous exercise which may provoke arrhythmias. Patients with hypertrophic cardiomyopathy may be asymptomatic. However, some have angina, as their hypertrophied muscle requires more oxygen, even in the absence of coronary disease. Some also have a low cardiac output causing dizziness and syncope. These patients may also develop an ejection systolic murmur, best heard over the left sternal border, caused by the obstruction. As the obstruction develops, it also distorts the mitral valve and a regurgitant murmur may be heard.

The diagnosis is best made by echocardiography (5.106, 5.107). The ECG classically shows a combination of left ventricular hypertrophy and pathological Q waves resulting from hypertrophy of the inter-ventricular septum. Treatment is directed at preventing serious arrhythmias and relieving angina. Where there is severe obstruction to left ventricular outflow, surgical removal of the hypertrophied muscle below the aortic valve may be beneficial.

The condition is inherited in about half the reported cases, and family members should be studied by echocardiography to determine if they have an asymptomatic form of the condition. Long-term follow-up of these family members is required for early diagnosis and treatment of complications.

5.106

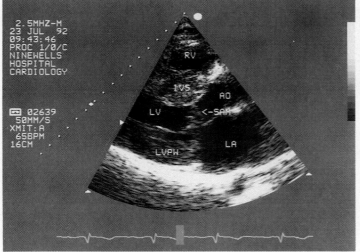

5.107

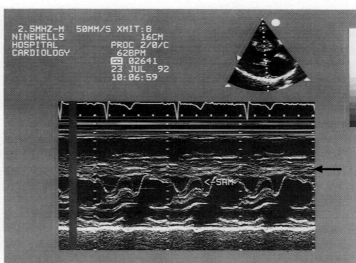

5.106 and 5.107 Hypertrophic obstructive cardiomyopathy. The 2D long axis parasternal view (**5.106**) shows the chambers of the heart (LA = left atrium; RV = right ventricle; LV = left ventricle). The left ventricle posterior wall (LVPW) is thickened, and the most striking abnormality is the hypertrophy of the interventricular septum (IVS). Another characteristic feature is a Venturi effect: as blood leaves the left ventricle it sucks the anterior leaflet of the mitral valve forward—systolic anterior motion (SAM). This phenomenon is more clearly shown (SAM) in the parasternal long axis M-mode echocardiogram (**5.107**). The massive thickening of the septum is also obvious in the M-mode (arrowed).

Restrictive cardiomyopathy

Restrictive cardiomyopathy is very rare in developed countries. It is associated with a range of conditions including amyloidosis, sarcoidosis and leukaemic infiltration. Endomyocardial fibrosis is the most common cause in the tropics.

The myocardium is infiltrated by abnormal tissue, which renders the chambers stiff and non-compliant. This is particularly evident in diastole and can be confirmed by Doppler echocardiography. Patients develop congestive cardiac failure, with ascites and ankle swelling. The physical signs are similar to those of constrictive pericarditis (p. 249) with raised jugular venous pressure and cardiac enlargement. The X-ray (5.105) and ECG show cardiac enlargement. The echocardiogram shows the thickening of the myocardium with impaired ventricular filling.

Cardiac tumours

Primary cardiac tumours are rare, but secondary deposits are often found incidentally at post mortem, infiltrating the pericardium and, less commonly, the myocardium. Pericardial deposits may produce a pericardial effusion which can constrict the heart and cause death from tamponade.

The most common primary tumour of the heart is an atrial myxoma. It usually grows in the cavity of the left atrium and is attached by a stalk to the left atrial wall just behind the mitral valve. If it obstructs blood flow from the left atrium to the left ventricle, syncope can occur. Portions of the tumour may also become detached and embolise. This association of peripheral emboli with a heart murmur may lead to the mistaken diagnosis of infective endocarditis, but a myxoma is easily demonstrable by echocardiography (5.108) or MRI (5.109). Myxomas can be removed surgically with good long-term results.

Tumours in the myocardium are usually secondaries and the bronchus and breast are the most common primary sites. These malignant deposits may have haemodynamic effects, and they often interfere with the conducting system, causing heart block, or may be a focus for ventricular or supraventricular tachyarrhythmias. Curative treatment is usually impossible.

5.108

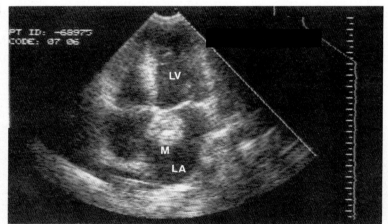

5.108 Left atrial myxoma. This apical four-chamber echocardiogram shows a circular mass (M) arising in a typical position from the interatrial septum just above the mitral valve. LA = left atrium; LV = left ventricle).

5.109

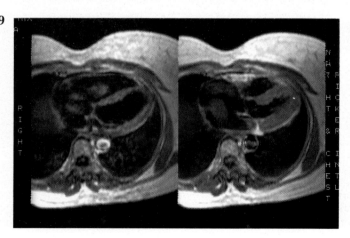

5.109 Right atrial myxoma, demonstrated by MRI. Diastolic (left) and systolic (right) transverse images show that the mass has three lobes. It prolapses through the tricuspid valve in diastole and is fully within the right atrium in systole.

Pericardial disease

Pericardial disease may present in one of three ways: pericarditis, pericardial effusion or constrictive pericarditis.

Pericarditis

Causes of pericarditis include:

- Acute and chronic infections.
- Myocardial infarction.
- Metabolic.
- Connective tissue disorders.
- Acute rheumatic fever.
- Malignancy.
- Radiation.
- Idiopathic.

The usual clinical presentation is with acute, sharp, central chest pain which may radiate to the neck and shoulders and may be brought on by movement. There is usually associated fever and occasionally myalgia. The most common causes are Coxsackie B virus infection (*see* p. 21) and acute myocardial infarction (p. 225). A friction rub may be heard. Investigations show leucocytosis and elevation of the ESR, and in the absence of myocardial infarction the ECG shows a typical pattern of ST elevation without QRS changes (**5.110**). The T wave becomes inverted in most leads after several days. There may also be an increase in levels of cardiac enzymes and echocardiography may show an increase in pericardial fluid. The chest X-ray usually shows a normal cardiac outline which may enlarge as the amount of pericardial fluid increases. There may also be associated inflammatory lung changes. Analgesia and anti-inflammatory drug treatment are often helpful.

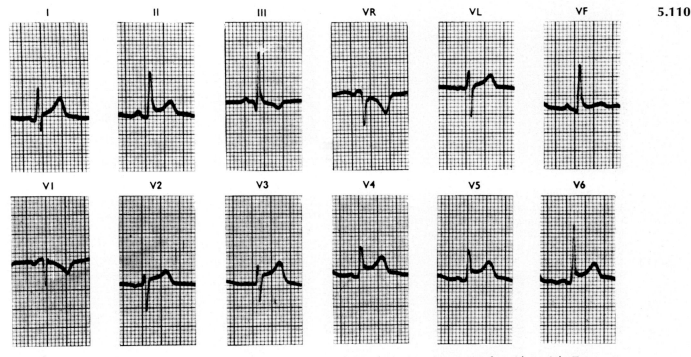

5.110

5.110 Acute pericarditis. In the first few days, the ECG shows ST elevation, concave upwards, with upright T waves in most leads. Classically it is more obvious in lead II than in I or III. There are no pathological Q waves, and the widespread distribution of ST-T changes, without reciprocal depression, distinguishes acute pericarditis from early myocardial infarction. In the later stages of pericarditis, the T waves become inverted in most leads. The ECG changes in pericarditis are caused by the superficial myocarditis which accompanies it.

Pericardial effusion

A pericardial effusion is an accumulation of excess fluid within the pericardium, often as a result of acute or chronic pericarditis. The implications for cardiac function depend on the rate at which the fluid accumulates. The first effect is to reduce the venous return to the heart—this is reflected in elevation of the jugular venous pressure, hepatic congestion and peripheral oedema. As the amount of pericardial fluid increases, cardiac filling is progressively diminished and cardiac output reduced; so a vicious circle is established (cardiac tamponade) that leads to declining cardiac function and death. The diagnosis can be made clinically because of the features of heart failure (JVP elevation, peripheral oedema,

hepatomegaly) and diminished output (thready 'paradoxical' pulse, central cyanosis, low BP). There may be an increased area of cardiac dullness and the heart sounds may be muffled. Pericardial rub is usually absent.

X-ray of the chest shows an enlarged cardiac shadow (5.111) and may give clues to the underlying cause (5.112). The ECG shows low-voltage complexes, often with T-wave inversion (5.113). Echocardiography shows the size of the effusion (5.114). If there is impairment of cardiac function, urgent aspiration is required (5.115). Examination of the aspirate may give a clue to aetiology and the need for further treatment.

5.111

5.112

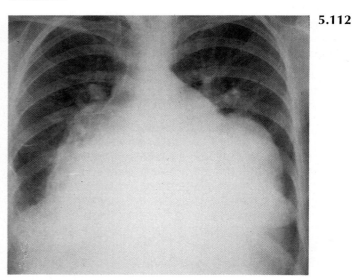

5.111 Pericardial effusion. The heart shadow appears generally enlarged, but the appearance is not diagnostic. A similar appearance can be seen in cardiac failure, in myocarditis or in dilated cardiomyopathy.

5.112 Malignant pericardial effusion. The heart shadow is generally enlarged, but the odd, irregular outline of the enlargement suggests the presence of secondary tumour deposits in the pericardium. This patient had a primary ovarian carcinoma.

5.113

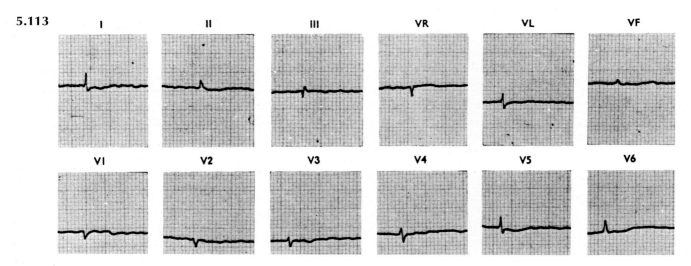

5.113 Pericardial effusion. Large quantities of pericardial fluid produce an ECG of generally low voltage, with generalised T-wave flattening or inversion—partly the result of the insulating effect of the fluid, and partly because of superficial myocarditis. Note that this patient has also developed atrial fibrillation.

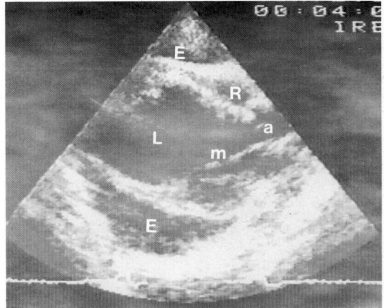

5.114 Pericardial effusion. This echocardiogram (parasternal long-axis view) shows effusion (E) surrounding the heart. The left ventricle (L) is dilated, but the right ventricle (R) is compressed—the patient had developed pericardial tamponade. (m = mitral valve; a = aortic valve).

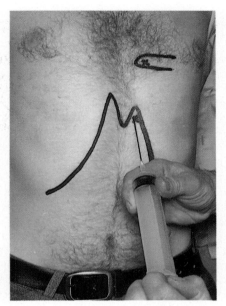

5.115 Aspiration of pericardial fluid in cardiac tamponade. A wide-bore needle is inserted in the epigastrium between the left border of the xiphoid process and the lower left ribcage and advanced in the direction of the medial third of the right clavicle. (Ignore the mark over the left chest.) If the needle is connected to the V lead of an ECG monitor, ST elevation will usually be seen if the needle touches the epicardium. This can be useful in distinguishing a bloody pericardial effusion from accidental puncture of the heart.

Constrictive pericarditis

Fibrosis and calcification of the pericardium may follow an episode of acute pericarditis or may develop insidiously over a period of time. The end result is impaired cardiac filling and ventricular function. The dominant features are distension of the neck veins, peripheral oedema, ascites and hepatic congestion. There may be a striking increase in jugular venous distension on inspiration (Kussmaul's sign). Pulsus paradoxus is present. Chest X-ray shows a small heart shadow and there may be pericardial calcification (**5.116**). The ECG shows non-specific changes, often with low-voltage complexes, and atrial fibrillation is frequently found in the late stages of the disease. Echocardiography shows a thickened pericardium with small ventricular and atrial chambers. Treatment is by pericardiectomy.

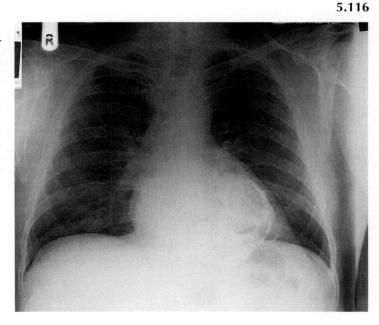

5.116 Pericardial calcification is clearly seen around the left and inferior borders of the heart. This patient has a normal sized heart, but the calcification may progress further, leading to constrictive pericarditis.

Hypertension

Hypertension is high blood pressure in the systemic arterial circulation, which can damage the walls of arteries, arterioles and the left ventricle of the heart with serious consequences, chiefly affecting the brain, heart, kidneys and eyes.

Large and medium-sized arteries respond to high blood pressure by thickening of the media and disruption of the elastic tissue within their walls. The vessels may become tortuous and dilated and may rupture because of the high pressure in the lumen. If this occurs in the brain, cerebral haemorrhage usually leaves the patient dead or paralysed from a 'stroke'. Hypertension also promotes the formation of atheroma in medium-sized and large arteries, so a stroke may also be caused by occlusion of a cerebral artery by thrombus formed on an atheromatous plaque, or by embolisation of atheromatous material from plaques in the extra-cranial segments of the carotid arteries or aorta (*see* p. 494). Atheroma formation in the coronary arteries renders hypertensive patients susceptible to angina pectoris, myocardial infarction and sudden death.

In smaller arteries and arterioles, hypertension causes prominent thickening of the intima, in addition to medial hypertrophy. In cases of 'accelerated' or 'malignant' hypertension, where the blood pressure is very high or has risen quickly, these intimal changes can occlude the vessels, producing distal tissue ischaemia. This particularly affects the kidneys, causing renal failure (see p. 294). The walls of the small arteries in the brain may be damaged so that their permeability is increased and cerebral oedema results, causing 'hypertensive encephalopathy' characterised by headache, confusion, fits and coma. There may also be visual disturbances due to retinal arterial damage, which may be seen on examination of the fundi.

The left ventricle responds to high blood pressure by hypertrophy. Initially, this increases its force of contraction and maintains a normal cardiac output, but eventually the hypertrophied muscle outgrows its oxygen supply and angina and cardiac failure result.

An identifiable cause of high blood pressure is only apparent in 1–2% of hypertensive individuals. They are said to have 'secondary' hypertension. In the remainder, no single cause of high blood pressure has been found. These individuals are said to have 'primary' or 'essential' hypertension. Constitutional factors are important, as shown by the relevance of a family history of hypertension and by racial variations in prevalence. Lifestyle patterns also influence blood pressure, and obesity, alcohol intake, insufficient physical activity and possibly excessive salt consumption all contribute to hypertension. Smoking does not cause hypertension, but it accelerates atherogenesis.

Many patients with hypertension are asymptomatic, and the elevated blood pressure is picked up by chance on routine screening or following a stroke, infarct or other vascular catastrophe. Those with more severe disease may not present until they have features of renal failure, heart failure or angina. Only when there is a rise in intracranial pressure is headache a feature. Blurred vision may result from retinopathy.

Examination of the patient with uncomplicated hypertension usually reveals few abnormal findings, but it is important to look for signs of 'end-organ' damage (renal failure, cerebrovascular disease, cardiac failure) and to 'stage' any changes in the fundi (5.117–5.120).

It is also important to look for signs of possible causes of 'secondary' hypertension (**Table 5.5**).

Table 5.5 Causes of secondary hypertension.

Renal disease

Bilateral	Chronic glomerulonephritis
	Chronic pyelonephritis (reflux nephropathy)
	Polycystic kidneys
	Analgesic nephropathy
Unilateral	Chronic pyelonephritis (reflux nephropathy)
	Renal artery stenosis

Endocrine disorders
Conn's syndrome
Cushing's syndrome
Phaeochromocytoma
Acromegaly
Hyperparathyroidism

Cardiovascular disorders
Coarctation of the aorta

Pregnancy
Pre-eclampsia and eclampsia

Drugs
Oral contraceptives
Corticosteroids
Carbenoxolone
Monoamine oxidase inhibitors (interaction with tyramine)

Investigations should usually include an ECG for signs of LVH (5.121) and ischaemia, and a chest X-ray for cardiac size (5.122) and (rarely) signs of coarctation of the aorta (5.88). Echocardiography can also provide an accurate assessement of the severity of ventricular hypertrophy.

Proteinuria is an indicator of possible renal disease. Plasma electrolytes, urea and creatinine will show changes where there is renal failure and these and other specific investigations may be required in patients with renal disease (p. 294) and to exclude other causes of secondary hypertension.

Treatment must be decided on an individual basis. This depends on several baseline blood pressure recordings, age, sex and whether complications of hypertension are already present. Patients with diastolic pressure in excess of 105 mmHg are usually treated and those with diastolic pressure between 90 and 105 mmHg may be treated. Many antihypertensive drugs are available, and they act in different ways, so drugs may be used in combination. Reduction of blood pressure reduces the risks of stroke, heart failure and renal failure but a significant beneficial effect in reducing mortality from coronary events has not yet been clearly demonstrated.

In those relatively rare patients where hypertension is 'secondary' to an identifiable cause, there is the possibility of treatment of the cause, or of curative surgery.

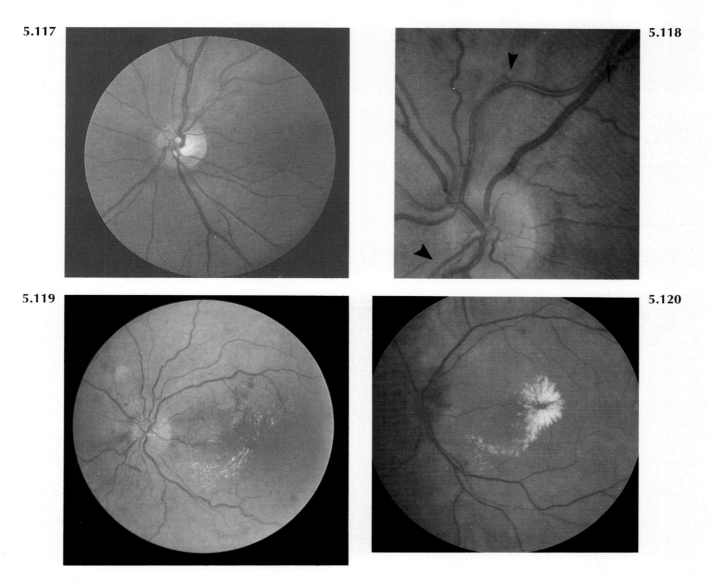

5.117–5.120 Hypertensive retinopathy is traditionally divided into four grades. **Grade 1 (5.117)** shows very early and minor changes in a young patient: increased tortuosity of a retinal vessel and increased reflectiveness (silver wiring) of a retinal artery are seen at 1 o'clock in this view. Otherwise, the fundus is completely normal. **Grade 2 (5.118)** again shows increased tortuosity and silver wiring (coarse arrows). In addition there is 'nipping' of the venules at arteriovenous crossings (fine arrow). **Grade 3 (5.119)** shows the same changes as grade 2 plus flame-shaped retinal haemorrhages and soft 'cotton-wool' exudates. In **Grade 4 (5.120)** there is swelling of the optic disc (papilloedema), retinal oedema is present, and hard exudates may collect around the fovea, producing a typical 'macular star'.

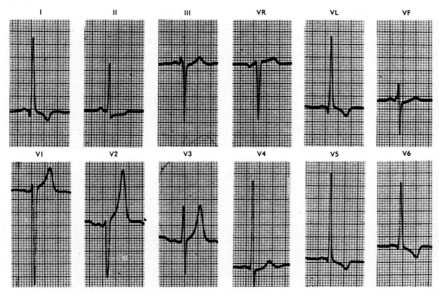

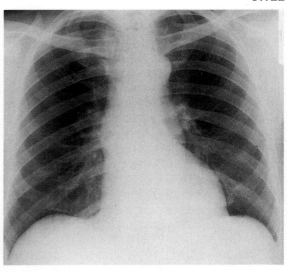

5.121 Left ventricular hypertrophy in hypertension. This ECG shows severe hypertrophy. Left ventricular hypertrophy (LVH) is present when the R wave in V5 or V6 or the S wave in V1 or V2 exceeds 25mm in an adult of normal build. This ECG also shows the characteristics of LV 'strain', with T-wave inversion over the left ventricle (V5–6) and, as the heart is relatively horizontally placed, in I and VL.

5.122 Hypertension. The chest X-ray is usually normal in mild to moderate hypertension, but cardiac enlargement associated with left ventricular hypertrophy (as here) may occur in the later stages. There is no evidence of cardiac failure in this patient.

Peripheral vascular disease (PVD)

Peripheral arterial obstruction in the legs is a common problem in the ageing population of the Western world. Atheroma is the most common cause and patients often have other arterial manifestations, including coronary artery disease, stroke, transient ischaemic attacks and intestinal ischaemia. Atheroma usually has a patchy distribution in the aorta and the femoral and popliteal vessels. It is found particularly at the aortic bifurcation and around the origins of smaller vessels. The lesions tend to enlarge slowly and gradually reduce blood flow.

Symptoms usually occur when the obstruction is 50–75%. The most common symptom is a cramp-like pain in the calf and thigh muscles on exercise, which disappears on resting for a few minutes ('intermittent claudication'). There is often a history of progressive shortening of the distance walked without pain as the disease progresses. The level of the arterial block dictates the muscle group in which pain is felt, e.g. an obstructive lesion in the profunda femoris artery will present with buttock, hip and thigh claudication (and impotence).

Patients may also complain of weakness of muscle groups and numbness or paraesthesiae. Ulceration and gangrene may appear with constant pain at rest. Diabetics usually have extensive atheroma and their presentation is more complex as they often also have peripheral neuropathy and small vessel disease, and have lost deep pain sensation and sympathetic tone.

Clinical examination in PVD shows:

- Atrophy of the skin, loss of hair, trophic nail changes (**5.123**).
- A cold limb, which may be pallid or cyanosed (**5.124, 5.125**).
- Slow capillary return when finger pressure is released.
- Loss or diminution of pulses in the affected leg (**5.123**).
- A bruit over the affected segment of vessel.
- Ulceration or gangrene, particularly of the toes (**5.126**).
- Loss of sensation.

Special investigations include measurement of arm/leg systolic blood pressure (lower in the leg), blood pressure measurement at the ankle after exercise (it falls to very low levels) and arteriography (**5.127**) to localise the site and extent of the block and the presence of collaterals. The site of block may also be found non-invasively with colour-flow Doppler. Thermography may have a place in determining skin blood flow in patients in whom amputation is being considered (**5.128**).

Treatment includes lifestyle advice about stopping smoking, weight reduction, cholesterol and blood pressure control, and graded exercises. Sympathectomy may have a place in selected patients. Skilled foot care is important, especially in the diabetic. Drug therapy is generally unsatisfactory. The circulation may be improved by angioplasty or vessel grafting, but gangrene requires amputation (**5.129**).

5.123

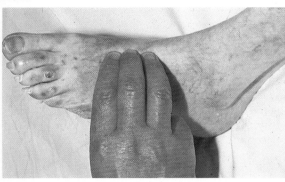

5.124

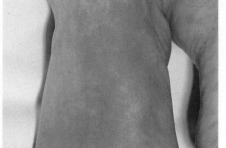

5.123 Peripheral vascular disease. Typical changes in the skin include atrophy, pallor, loss of hair and, in some patients, trophic nail changes. This patient also has early ulceration on the dorsum of three toes. It is important to examine the peripheral pulses. In this patient the dorsalis pedis pulse was impalpable.

5.124 Ischaemic pallor of the patient's right foot. Note the colour difference between the two feet, which has been accentuated by elevation of the legs.

5.125

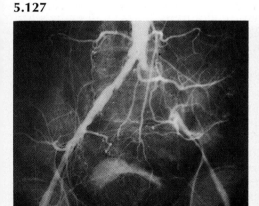

5.126

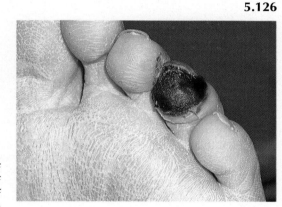

5.125 'Critical' ischaemia of the foot. The patient had a sudden onset of discomfort, with coldness and loss of sensation in the toes and the dorsum of the foot, He had previously suffered from intermittent claudication and has evidence of chronic ischaemia, including absence of hair and thinness of the skin. Arteriography is necessary to define the nature of the lesion.

5.126 Typical dry gangrene of a toe in a patient with diffuse atheroma. The patient had a history of intermittent claudication. The treatment is amputation.

5.127

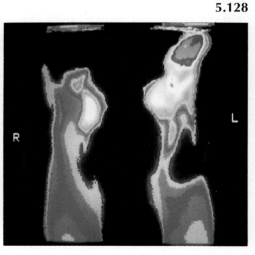

5.128

5.129

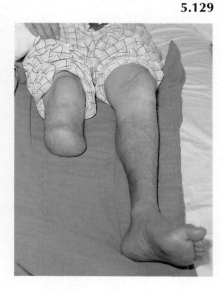

5.127 Multiple atheromatous deposits and complete occlusion of the left external iliac artery with collateral formation, in a patient with severe left-sided intermittent claudication and ischaemic skin changes.

5.128 Thermography may be useful in assessing the skin circulation is ischaemic limbs. This patient has severe ischaemia of the right foot.

5.129 Amputation is still often necessary in patients with severe peripheral vascular disease. This patient developed massive gangrene of the leg and foot.

Thrombo-angiitis obliterans (Buerger's disease)

This is a disease of young male smokers who develop ulceration and gangrene of their digits, caused by spasm of the digital arteries associated with an intense inflammatory response, which may also involve veins and nerves (5.130). There is no evidence of excessive atheroma. The major symptoms are referable to ischaemia of the fingers and toes, but many patients also have intermittent claudication, usually affecting the calf and often the 'instep' of the foot, and also occasionally claudication of the hand. Ultimately, there may be severe rest pain and gangrene (5.131). Examination may show cold digits, digital ulcers, a migratory phlebitis of hands and feet and absent foot and hand pulses. Patients should stop all use of tobacco and may be helped by vasodilator drugs. Sympathectomy may be of value, but amputation of digits may become necessary.

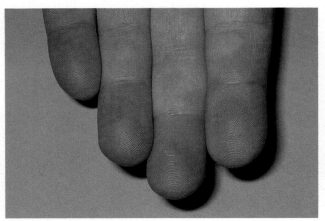

5.130

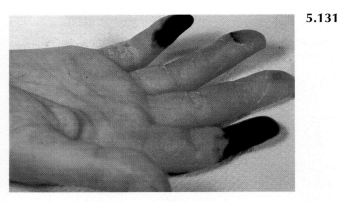

5.131

5.131 Digital gangrene in Buerger's disease. This young male smoker required treatment by amputation.

5.130 Digital ischaemia in Buerger's disease. The fingertips are cyanotic, though no irreversible changes have yet occurred. This man continued to smoke, against all advice, and subsequently developed gangrene.

Acute ischaemia

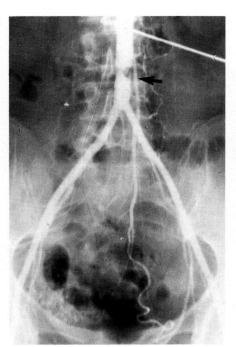

5.132

Thrombosis on an atheromatous plaque or embolism may produce acute ischaemia very rapidly. The sources of emboli include the left atrium when the mitral or aortic valves are damaged by rheumatic endocarditis (5.74), especially when the rhythm changes from sinus to atrial fibrillation; mural thrombus in the left ventricle following myocardial infarction (5.66); prosthetic valves (1.9); vegetations in infective endocarditis (5.103, 5.104); and atheromatous plaques or aneurysms in the aorta (5.144). The features are acute onset of pain, pallor of the limb and lack of pulses and capillary return, followed by reactive hyperaemia (5.71) or cyanosis and gangrene (5.124–5.126). The level of the block may be defined by colour-flow Doppler or angiography (5.132). Distal emboli or thrombosis may be treated with a thrombolytic agent. More proximal lesions may be amenable to angioplasty or thrombectomy. Prevention of recurrence requires treatment with aspirin and anticoagulants.

5.132 An aortic thrombus (arrowed) caused ischaemia and embolism to the leg in this patient. The thrombus had developed on the site of a pre-existing atheromatous plaque, but it was successfully removed by surgery.

Raynaud's syndrome

Raynaud's syndrome mainly affects young women and is characterised by recurrent vasospastic episodes in which one or more fingers becomes white and numb, followed after a few minutes by a blue/purple cyanosis and then by redness caused by reactive arterial dilatation (3.29, 5.133). The toes are rarely affected. The attacks are usually bilateral and symmetrical and may have a familial incidence. These attacks (primary Raynaud's syndrome) are often precipitated by exposure to cold or by emotion. Most patients have no evidence of any other disease process and are only inconvenienced by the attack. Rarely the signs progress to finger tip ulceration and gangrene (5.134).

Secondary Raynaud's syndrome implies that the features are a result of an underlying disease (Table 5.6). This is the most likely diagnosis if the condition starts later in life, is seen in a man, is unilateral, or has an abrupt onset with rapid onset of digital ulceration and gangrene.

It is important to enquire about cigarette smoking and the use of beta-blocking drugs, oral contraceptives or ergot derivatives, and about the handling of vibrating tools such as drills, chain saws or electric hammers (vibration white finger) (5.135). The position of the arm before the onset of symptoms may suggest a thoracic outlet syndrome (see p. 260).

In the primary form, the prognosis is very good and treatment is directed at prevention of attacks by keeping the hands (and feet) warm. Electrically heated gloves are usually effective. The patient should stop smoking and stop taking any relevant drugs that predispose to the condition.

In secondary Raynaud's, an attempt must be made to identify and treat the underlying condition. Cervical sympathectomy is rarely of value. Treatment with a calcium-channel blocker and transdermal prostacyclin is often effective.

5.133

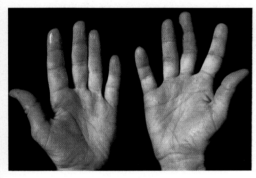

5.133 Raynaud's phenomenon in a patient with scleroderma (see p.144). In this patient the bases of the fingers are pale and the tips are congested and cyanotic (compare this with the common appearance seen in **3.29**).

5.134

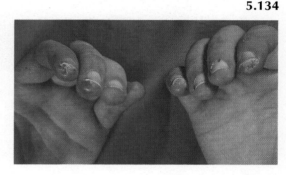

5.134 Primary Raynaud's syndrome occasionally progresses to fingertip ulceration or even gangrene. This 36-year-old woman had small, painful recurrent necrotic ulcers of the fingertips, wasting of the pulps and irregular nail growth.

Table 5.6. Diseases associated with secondary Raynaud's syndrome.

- Connective tissue disorders especially SLE and scleroderma
- Drug-associated — especially nicotine, oral contraceptives, beta- blockers and ergot derivatives
- Vibration tool associated ('vibration white finger')
- Thoracic outlet syndrome
- Neurogenic
- Malignancy
- Hyperviscosity syndromes
- Polycythaemia

5.135

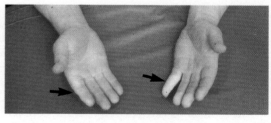

5.135 Vibration white finger. This patient developed painful vasospasm (arrowed) as a result of continual use of a power saw. His symptoms appeared within a year of starting this work.

Cold injury

Cooling of tissues produces vasoconstriction, increase in plasma and whole blood viscosity, and impairment of oxygen transport. Below freezing point, these changes are compounded by the formation of ice crystals which produce irreversible cell death.

'Immersion' or 'trench' foot is a result of wet, cold exposure of the feet over a prolonged period. There are recognisable phases: initially, an ischaemic phase when the feet are cold, white and pulseless; followed by a hyperaemic response, when they become painful, red and oedematous. They may eventually recover, but superficial areas of skin gangrene may require grafting. In frostbite, the blood supply is permanently damaged and tissue necrosis occurs in the exposed extremities. The area is usually numb and bloodless. Rewarming is associated with local pain (5.136) and the development of a demarcation zone between viable and non-viable tissues. Gangrene may result (5.137). Chemical or surgical sympathectomy may be of value.

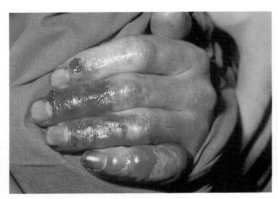

5.136

5.136 Frostbite of the hand in a mountaineer. On rewarming, the hand became painful, red and oedematous, with signs of probable gangrene in the fifth finger.

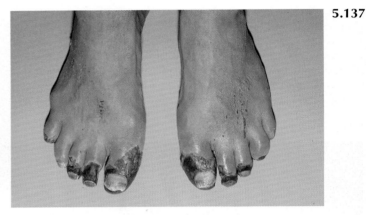

5.137

5.137 Gangrene following frostbite. The patient had been sleeping rough in the winter in London. He developed symmetrical changes in both feet, requiring the amputation of some toes.

Hypothermia

A fall in the body's core temperature may result from a variety of illnesses such as myxoedema, Addison's disease, hyperglycaemia, stroke, myocardial infarction and the ingestion of drugs or alcohol. It is especially likely to occur in the elderly. Hypothermia may also occur accidentally in those injured or immersed in snow or icy water or exposed to cold, wet and windy conditions. Often multiple factors play a role, e.g. the alcoholic lying comatose outside in the winter, or the isolated elderly stroke patient falling in an unheated house. The rate of loss of heat depends on factors such as nutritional status, clothing, recent alcohol or drug ingestion and the ambient temperature.

The clinical features depend on the core temperature. Mild hypothermia (core temperature 35–37°C) usually only causes discomfort: the patient feels cold and shivers, but remains mentally alert and is often able to take appropriate action to reverse the decline in temperature. Below this level there is progressive impairment of higher cerebral function with loss of co-ordination, judgement and eventually loss of consciousness. Below a temperature of 32°C there is an exponential rise in mortality.

Patients usually appear cold and pale, with bradycardia, hypotension, slow respiration and an appearance of rigor mortis. Laboratory investigations show acidosis, haemo-concentration and renal impairment. There is peripheral hypoxia as the low temperature drives the oxygen dissociation curve to the left—there is decreased unloading of oxygen in the periphery. Central nervous reflexes (e.g. pupillary responses) become progressively impaired. Ventricular arrhythmias (tachycardia or fibrillation) are the common cause of death, but a variety of changes may be found on the ECG, e.g. bradycardia, slow atrial fibrillation and a characteristic J wave (5.138).

Treatment of minor degrees of hypothermia can be achieved by gradual rewarming in a heated room or bed, use of a 'space blanket' (5.139) and general supportive measures. Most patients with temperatures over 32°C respond to these simple measures. In severe hypothermia the patient should also be well oxygenated and attention should be paid to correction of the fluid and metabolic disturbance. External warming with an electric blanket is contraindicated, but intravenous fluids and peritoneal dialysis fluid (if needed for renal failure) should be warmed. Antibiotics should be given, as these patient are likely to develop pneumonia.

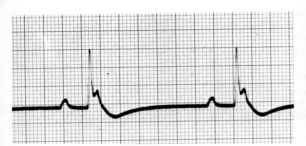

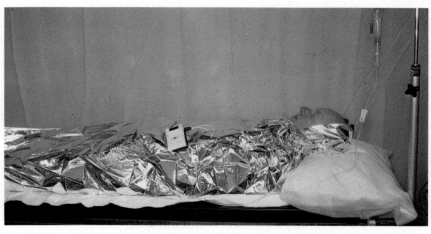

5.138 Hypothermia. The characteristic finding is the J wave, a positive wave occurring between the QRS and ST segment. It appears in all leads and broadens and increases its size as the body temperature drops.

5.139 Treatment of hypothermia. A 'space' blanket is useful for slow rewarming. A constant-reading digital electronic rectal thermometer is in place. An intravenous infusion and a central venous pressure line are established, so that any hypotension caused by vasodilatation as warming occurs can be safely corrected.

Aortic diseases

Aneurysms

An aneurysm is an abnormal widening of an artery which involves all four coats. In the aorta they may occur in the thoracic and abdominal segments.

Abdominal aneurysms

Abdominal aneurysms are most common in men over 50 years whose vessels are arteriosclerotic. They may be found by chance on routine abdominal palpation or on x-ray. Occasionally, patients complain of pain in the epigastrium with radiation into the flanks. Rarely, they present with a dramatic onset of abdominal pain and severe hypotension (leading to death) caused by rupture. As an aneurysm enlarges, concentric layers of thrombus are laid down; in a large aneurysm this may be the source of disseminated intravascular coagulation (DIC) with consumption of clotting factors and platelets. Multiple emboli may also originate from this thrombus and occlude the vessels of the toes and feet. Occasionally, the enlarging aneurysm may erode into the vena cava or bowel to form a fistula.

The diagnosis may be made on plain X-ray (**5.140**), ultrasound (**5.141**) or angiography (**5.142**), which enables the precise dimensions to be defined, and surgery to be planned if necessary. Elective surgery carries a mortality of 5–10% and emergency surgery has a mortality of over 50%.

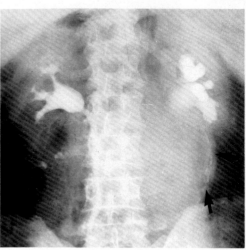

5.140 Abdominal aortic aneurysm. Aortic dilatation and calcification (arrowed) was an incidental finding during an IVU examination (the IVU also shows dilatation of the left renal pelvis).

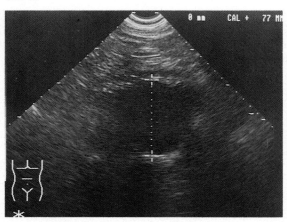

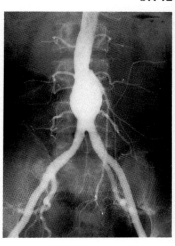

5.141 Abdominal aortic aneurysm revealed by ultrasound. The aorta is grossly and irregularly dilated. Note the presence of echogenic material in the lumen, representing layers of thrombus. The diameter of lumen was 6.2 cm (a diameter over 4 cm is an indication for operative intervention). Examination at a higher level showed that the aneurysm started below the renal arteries, so immediate aortic bifurcation grafting was indicated.

5.142 Small abdominal aortic aneurysm revealed on aortography. The diagnosis was suspected by the presence of an abdominal bruit.

Thoracic aneurysms

Thoracic aneurysms are historically associated with the long-term complications of syphilitic aortitis (1.235) and may involve the ascending or descending thoracic aorta or the arch. Aneurysms of the ascending aorta may involve the ostia of the coronary arteries and the aortic valve, so that diastolic filling of the coronary arteries is defective and the patient has angina pectoris. Massive enlargement may lead to a pulsatile painful mass in the anterior chest wall as the ribs and sternum are eroded. Aneurysmal dilatation of the arch may compress the left main bronchus to produce respiratory difficulty from atelectasis, a 'brassy' cough, a tracheal tug and paralysis of the left recurrent laryngeal nerve, and occasionally a left-sided Horner's syndrome. Compression of the oesophagus may cause dysphagia, and rupture may occur into the oesophagus, bronchus or externally. The diagnosis of syphilis should be confirmed serologically and treated with an appropriate antibiotic regime. These aneurysms are now extremely rare in the developed world, but non-syphilitic aneurysms of the descending thoracic aorta may be found at routine X-ray examination (5.143, 5.144) and are often symptomless.

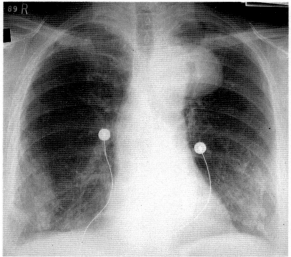

5.143 An aortic aneurysm at the level of the aortic knuckle. This PA film alone does not allow a firm diagnosis, and the differential diagnosis could include a mass in the mediastinum or lung. The appearance of the film is complicated by the presence of extensive bilateral lower-zone pleural calcification, which resulted from previous tuberculous pleurisy.

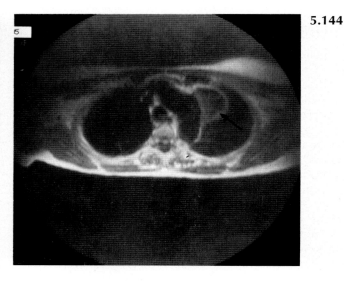

5.144 Transverse MRI scan of the patient in **5.143**. The mass on the chest X-ray can be seen to be an aortic aneurysm containing a thrombus (arrowed).

Other aneurysms

Aneurysms may develop in many other situations in the arterial tree.

- Berry aneurysms in the circle of Willis result from genetic weakness at the bifurcation of vessels and probably represent developmental defects in the media and elastic fibres. The aneurysmal sac gradually enlarges, and rupture may occur with extravasation of blood into the subarachnoid space (*see* p. 498).
- Mycotic aneurysms may form in any part of the arterial tree, but they are found most commonly in the cerebral circulation. They are associated with damage to the arterial wall caused by sepsis, which may be embolic in nature. They are rare in developed countries.
- Polyarteritis nodosa may be associated with the formation of multiple microaneurysms (*see* p. 148, 193, 287).
- Kawasaki syndrome is probably an infectious disease caused by an unknown agent, which causes arteritis and aneurysms of the coronary arteries.

Dissecting aneurysm of aorta

Dissection of the aorta often begins with an intimal tear which allows blood to dissect into the media, forming a 'false channel' which may re-enter the lumen at a point further down. About half the cases involve the ascending aorta, one-third the arch and the rest are found in the descending aorta. The initial tear may occur spontaneously in patients with defects in the aortic wall (as seen in Marfan's syndrome, Ehlers–Danlos syndrome and cystic medial necrosis), in patients with coarctation of the aorta and in patients with hypertension: or it may be iatrogenic, following angiography or coronary artery surgery.

The clinical presentation is usually a sudden onset of severe pain in the chest, abdomen or back. Ascending aortic dissection may involve the coronary ostia and the aortic valve which may become acutely incompetent and the patient may present with acute left ventricular failure or with acute myocardial infarction. Dissection of the arch may involve the arteries to the brain and upper limbs with hemiplegia or an ischaemic arm. Rupture may occur into the pericardium, mediastinum, left pleural cavity or abdomen.

The diagnosis can often be made clinically by the finding of absent or diminished pulses with differences in blood pressure, and it is confirmed by X-ray (**5.145**), angiography, ultrasound, CT scan (**5.146**) or MRI. ECG and normal serum enzyme levels exclude acute infarction. The high mortality varies with the site and length of dissection. Surgery is the only treatment and involves replacement or repair of the damaged wall if possible.

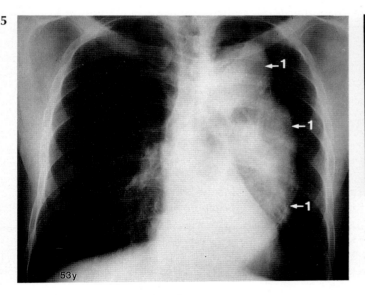

5.145 Dissecting aneurysm of the aorta. The edge of the grossly dilated descending aorta is marked (1) in this 53-year-old hypertensive man who presented with vague chest pains. Further investigation could include angiography, ultrasound, MRI or CT scan (see **5.138**).

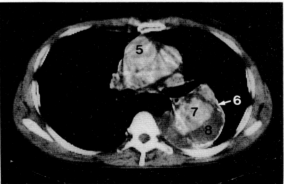

5.146 Dissecting aneurysm of the aorta revealed by a contrast enhanced CT scan (same patient as **5.145**). The scan shows a normal ascending aorta (5), a dilated descending aorta (6), the opacified true lumen (7) and a clot-filled false lumen (8).

259

Aortic arch syndrome

This is a general term given to diseases of the aortic arch that interfere with blood flow in the major vessels of the arch, the innominate artery, the left common carotid artery and the left subclavian artery. A range of pathologies may produce this effect (**Table 5.7**). The usual presentations result from cerebral ischaemia and impairment of upper arm circulation.

Table 5.7 Causes of aortic arch syndrome.

Arteriosclerosis
Dissecting aneurysm
Takayasu's arteriopathy
Syphilis (aortitis and aneurysm)
Mycotic aneurysm
Relapsing polychondritis
Giant cell aortitis
Ankylosing spondylitis
Kawasaki syndrome

Thoracic outlet syndromes

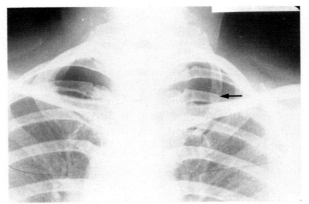

5.147

5.147 Cervical rib (arrowed). Most patients with cervical ribs are asymptomatic, but some may develop Raynaud's phenomenon or other thoracic outlet syndromes.

The neurovascular bundle that supplies the upper limb lies in the angle between the scalenus anterior muscle and the first rib. An extra rib ('cervical rib'), or a fibrous band equivalent to it, may compress the lower trunk of the brachial plexus (C8, T1) and the subclavian artery when the shoulder is abducted. Patients are often aware of the association between symptoms of paresthesiae, numbness and blanching of the fingers and arm position and their immediate disappearance when the arm is returned to the side. Eventually aneurysmal dilatation of the artery occurs, which may be associated with peripheral ischaemic episodes and emboli.

The diagnosis is made clinically by abducting the arm to 90° and rotating it externally. This leads to disappearance of the radial pulse and the appearance of symptoms (Adson's test). X-ray of the thoracic inlet may show unilateral or bilateral cervical ribs or a rudimentary cervical rib, which is often associated with a fibrous band (**5.147**). Treatment is surgical removal of the rib(s).

Venous thrombosis and pulmonary embolism

One of the most common causes of preventable death in developed countries is pulmonary embolism following deep vein thrombosis. Autopsies carried out in hospitalised patients show that up to 25% of all deaths are associated with pulmonary embolism, and it is estimated that in over half of these deaths venous thrombosis and pulmonary embolism were the main cause of death. One per cent of all hospitalised patients may die from pulmonary embolism. Most emboli originate in the deep veins of the legs; only a small number originate from the pelvis and the inferior vena cava. The types of patients who are at risk of deep vein thrombosis are shown in **Table 5.8** and these risks are important when considering patients for prophylaxis, which has now been shown to prevent deep vein thrombosis and pulmonary embolism without significant side-effects in most patients. Prophylaxis also prevents the development of the post-phlebitic limb, which is estimated to affect about 5% of the population.

Table 5.8 Risk factors for thromboembolic complications following surgery or during medical care.

Over 40 years old	Oestrogen therapy
Obesity	Renal transplant recipients
Malignancy	Paralysis
Infection	Types of surgery:
Previous thromboembolism	Knee surgery
Family history of thrombo–embolism	Hip fracture surgery
	Elective hip surgery
Heart failure	Retropubic prostatectomy
Varicose veins	General abdominal surgery
Trauma	Gynaecological surgery
Re-operation	Neurosurgery

Deep vein thrombosis (DVT)

DVT is common, but its clinical history and signs are very unreliable. Up to half the patient group may have no leg symptoms or signs before presenting with a pulmonary embolism. A high index of suspicion is essential, especially in the 'at risk' patients listed in **Table 5.8**. Symptoms that may be relevant include pain in the calf, cramps and tenderness on touching or attempting to bear weight. The patient may be aware of changes in skin colour, from normal to a dusky blue or a waxy white, and this is usually associated with swelling. Signs may include a 'boggy' swelling of the leg, increased warmth, tenderness on palpation over the course of the deep veins, venous dilatation, cyanosis or pallor of the limb (**5.6**) and superficial phlebitis. Varicose veins (**5.148**) are a common association. Superficial thrombophlebitis that migrates is often a sign of internal malignancy (**9.60**).

Massive occluding thrombosis in the femoral veins may lead to 'phlegmasia cerulea dolens' and venous gangrene. This is heralded by acute pain in the leg, woody hard oedema and deep cyanosis from the toes to the groin (**5.149**). Multiple petechial haemorrhages develop, followed by exquisitely painful areas of gangrene of skin and subcutaneous tissue on the dorsum of the foot and skin.

The diagnosis of DVT is made by venography (**5.150**) or, for DVT above the knee, by ultrasound scanning. The differential diagnosis includes muscle strain, muscle haematoma, ruptured Baker's cyst, cellulitis, lymphatic obstruction and other causes of oedema.

Treatment of deep vein thrombosis is with heparin followed by warfarin for at least 3–6 months. Analgesics, support stockings, and occasionally surgery or fibrinolytic therapy may also be of value. Prevention of DVT should be considered in all hospitalised patients at medium to high risk and this involves the use of support stockings and low doses of heparin or related compounds.

Deep vein thrombosis is very uncommon in the upper limbs. When it does occur, there may be a history of recent physical activity or of rest or coma in which the arms may have been held in an unusual position or compressed. Underlying malignant disease is another important cause. The presenting features are similar to those in the lower limb, but there are rarely any significant sequelae. Treatment is with a short course of anticoagulants.

5.148

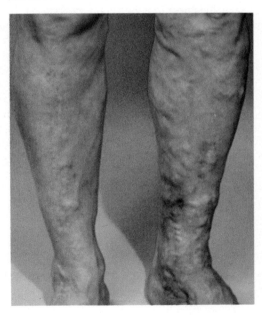

5.149

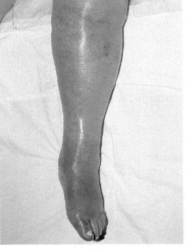

5.150

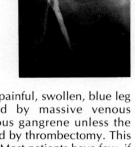

5.148 Varicose veins are a risk factor for deep vein thrombosis and may also result from it.

5.149 Phlegmasia cerulea dolens. The painful, swollen, blue leg results from vascular stasis caused by massive venous thrombosis, and it may lead to venous gangrene unless the resulting high tissue pressure is relieved by thrombectomy. This is a relatively rare presentation of DVT. Most patients have few, if any, signs, and the appearance seen in **5.6** is much more typical.

5.150 DVT in the iliac vein. Venography is still the 'gold standard' in the diagnosis of DVT. All DVTs are potentially dangerous, but this example seems particularly likely to embolise as it is not obviously attached to the wall of the vein.

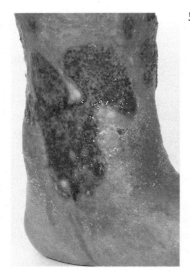

5.151

5.151 'Varicose' ulceration of the leg is probably usually a long-term complication of DVT. These ulcers can be extensive and indolent.

Thrombosis in the leg veins is usually centred around venous valve cusps. Resolution of the thrombus often leaves the valve leaflets damaged and incompetent; retrograde flow occurs, and this increased venous pressure distends the distal veins and makes the blood follow different pathways, especially after prolonged standing and following exercise. The long-term result is varicose veins which are under increased pressure (5.148). Recurrent minor haemorrhages lead to deposition of iron in the skin, which becomes brown-stained and firm from the deposition of fibrous tissue. Local anoxia and oedema lead to ulceration, often around the medial malleolus, which tends to be resistant to healing (5.151). Treatment should be directed at reduction of the hydrostatic pressure by the use of support hose and healing of the ulcer by elevation of the limb and, if necessary, by plastic surgery.

Pulmonary embolism

Acute pulmonary embolism is the impaction of one or more emboli in the pulmonary circulation. It is usually the sequel of venous thrombosis in the legs, is a major cause of morbidity and causes significant avoidable mortality. The clinical presentation is often dramatic, with the sudden death of a patient who was expected to recover uneventfully from major surgery. Sometimes there are preceding symptoms, such as chest discomfort, wheeze, cough or syncopal attacks. These result from small emboli ('herald' emboli), but the symptoms are often ignored. Often there are no specific symptoms or signs, and it is the suspicious mind of the vigilant clinician that will trigger the appropriate investigations.

Symptoms that may be present in established embolism include dyspnoea, pleuritic chest pain, cough, apprehension, haemoptysis, sweating and syncope. Signs are not specific, but may include increased respiratory rate (>20/min) ,pulmonary crackles, an accentuated pulmonary second sound, a rapid pulse rate (>100 beats per minute), fever, phlebitis, sweating,

pleural friction rub and cyanosis. A range of abnormalities is usually present in the ECG, reflecting the sudden increase in right ventricular strain (e.g. arrhythmias, axis deviation and right bundle branch block, acute cor pulmonale (S1, Q3, T3), the development of P pulmonale and T-wave abnormalities (5.152)). The plain X-ray of the chest may be totally normal or, in a minority of cases, may show an infiltrate or consolidation, a high hemidiaphragm, pleural effusion, atelectasis or focal oligaemia (5.153).

The diagnosis depends on a ventilation/perfusion X-scan of the lungs (V/Q) using radioactive xenon gas for the ventilation part and technetium-labelled macroaggregates of human serum albumin for the perfusion part (4.39, 4.40, 5.154). The 'gold standard' test is pulmonary angiography (5.155), but this is invasive and carries a small morbidity and mortality. Treatment is with anticoagulant doses of heparin followed by warfarin for at least 3–6 months. Fibrinolytic agents may be used in the acute stage and emergency surgery to remove a massive embolus is occasionally life-saving.

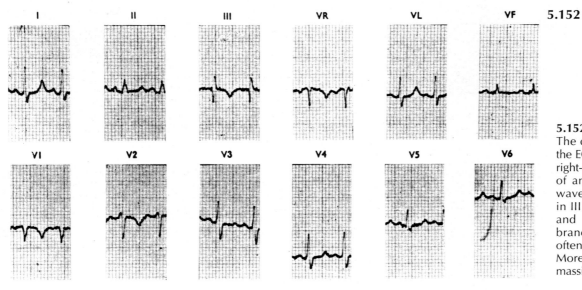

5.152

5.152 Acute pulmonary embolism. The classical changes are seen in the ECG. They include tachycardia, right-axis deviation, the appearance of an S wave in lead I and a Q wave in lead III, T-wave inversion in III and over the right ventricle, and incomplete right bundle branch block. The changes are often slight and easily overlooked. More major changes may occur in massive pulmonary embolism.

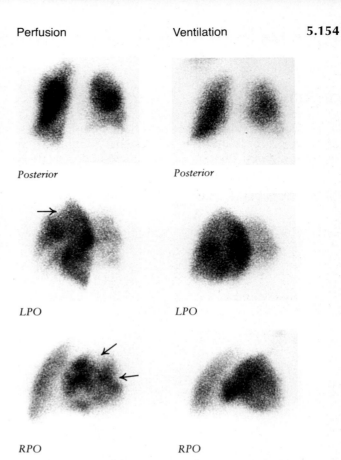

Posterior   *Posterior*

LPO   *LPO*

RPO   *RPO*

5.153 Pulmonary embolism. The chest X-ray is rarely diagnostic. In this patient it showed a raised right hemidiaphragm, some right basal shadowing and blunting of the fight costophrenic angle. The diagnosis is unclear, but the combination of a history of right-sided chest pain and slight haemoptysis with these findings was an indication to proceed to lung scanning (**5.154**).

5.154 Pulmonary embolism. Ventilation/perfusion scintigram in the patient seen in (**5.153**). Note that there were multiple perfusion defects (arrowed) with normal ventilation in the same areas. This combination gives a high probability of a diagnosis of pulmonary embolism. LPO = left posterior oblique view; RPO = right posterior oblique view.

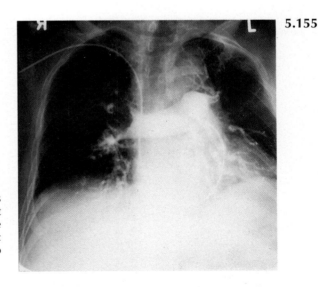

5.155 Acute massive pulmonary embolism. This pulmonary angiogram shows some filling of the left upper and lower segmental vessels only. The remaining vessels show near total of embolic occlusion. This patient responded dramatically to streptokinase infusion.

Disorders of peripheral lymphatics

Lymphangitis

This is an acute inflammation of peripheral lymphatic vessels in which a focus of infection, usually on the skin and usually caused by streptococci, drains to the regional lymphnodes and causes an acute inflammatory reaction, with redness, swelling, oedema and pain in the lymphatic vessels and nodes (*see* p. 39).

Lymphoedema

5.156

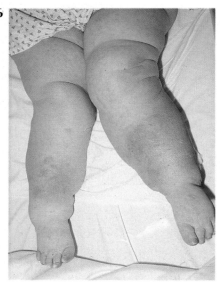

5.156 Bilateral lymphoedema of unknown cause. Lymphoedema mainly involves the subcutaneous tissues, where many of the lymphatic channels run; and in chronic lymphoedema it is often more severe above the ankle than below it.

Oedema that results from blockage of the lymphatic drainage of a limb is termed lymphoedema. It may be secondary or primary. Secondary causes are more common and include infiltration with neoplasm, parasitic infiltration (**1.196**, **1.197**), and surgical operations or radiotherapy that remove or damage lymphatics. Primary disorders result from a hereditary abnormality in the formation of the lymphatics. The most common of these is Milroy's disease but lymphoedema may also be found in ovarian dysgenesis and in Noonan's syndrome.

The onset of the condition varies according to the cause. Oedema is usually easily pitted, but as the disease becomes more chronic, the limb becomes hard and woody and the skin thickened and wrinkled (**5.156**). The diagnosis is made on lymphangiography.

This is a difficult condition to treat adequately, but elevation of the limb or compression bandages may help. Surgery has little to offer.

6. Renal Disease

History and Examination

A full medical history is important in any patient with suspected renal disease. Remember that the kidney has endocrine as well as excretory functions.

Specific questions should be asked about current features and symptoms, including:

- Urine volume—high in diabetes mellitus, diabetes insipidus or with loss of renal concentration; low in advanced renal failure or urinary tract obstruction.
- Frequency of micturition and/or presence of nocturia—high frequency associated with high urine volume or urinary infection.
- Urine appearance and colour—may be affected by a range of disorders or ingested substances (**Table 6.1**). Painless haematuria may be a sign of urological malignancy and requires urgent investigation.
- Pain—in loins, back, abdomen, suprapubic area? Constant or intermittent? Related to micturition? Pain may result from infection, stones, tumour or inherited renal or urinary tract disorders.
- Non-specific symptoms associated with renal failure, including tiredness, nausea, weight loss, pallor, easy bruising and symptoms associated with heart failure (*see* p. 216).

On general examination, there may be few, if any, abnormal findings in patients with urinary infections, renal calculi or other uncomplicated renal disorders. Even some patients with acute renal failure may appear physically normal.

In acute nephritis, the patient (often a child) develops acute facial puffiness (**6.1**) and hypertension in association with haematuria, proteinuria and oliguria; while in the nephrotic syndrome, there is usually severe oedema and ascites (**6.2**).

Chronic renal failure is usually associated with a wide range of signs (**6.3–6.6**).

Where renal disease is part of a multisystem disorder (diabetes mellitus, systemic lupus erythematosus, etc.), there may be other signs of the primary disease.

Table 6.1: Macroscopic appearance of the urine.

Appearance	Cause
Milky	Acid urine: urate crystals Alkaline urine: insoluble phosphates Infection—pus Spermatozoa Chyluria
Smoky pink	Haematuria (>0.54 ml blood /l urine)
Foamy	Proteinuria
Blue/green	Pseudomonas urinary tract infection Bilirubin Methylene blue
Pink/red	Aniline dyes in sweets Porphyrins (on standing) Blood, haemoglobin, myoglobin Drugs, e.g. phenindione, phenolphthalein Anthocyaninuria (beetroot—'beeturia')
Orange	Drugs: anthraquinones (laxatives) rifampicin Urobilinogenuria
Yellow	Mepacrine Conjugated bilirubin Phenacetin Riboflavin
Brown/black	Melanin (on standing) Myoglobin (on standing) Alkaptonuria
Green/black	Phenol Lysol

Brown	Drugs: phenazopyridine, furazolidone,
	  L-dopa, niridazole
	Haemoglobin and myoglobin
	  (on standing)
	Bilirubin

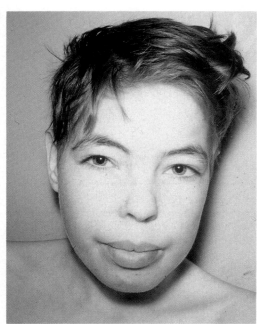

6.1 Acute nephritis. The generalised facial puffiness and the erythematous periorbital oedema are typical, and this boy also had ankle oedema and hypertension.

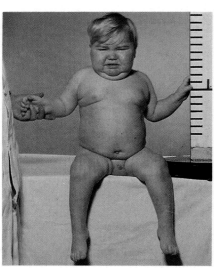

6.2 Nephrotic syndrome in a young boy. Note the severe generalised facial and body oedema. The facial oedema gives him a cushingoid appearance, but this picture was taken before he started on steroid therapy. He also had ascites.

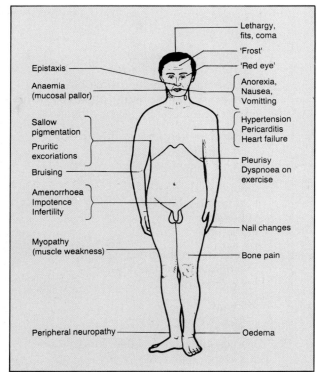

6.3 Chronic renal failure: common symptoms and signs.

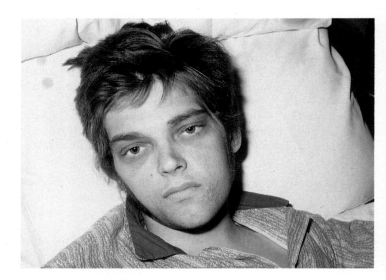

6.4 Uraemic facies. Note the pale, sallow, yellow-brown appearance of the skin and the anaemic pallor of the sclerae.

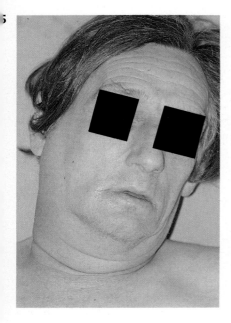

6.5 Parotitis is a common complication of chronic renal failure. This patient also shows the characteristic pale, sallow skin, and anaemic pallor of the lips.

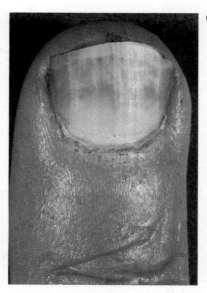

6.6 The nail in chronic renal failure. Various nail changes may be observed including those seen here: discoloration of the distal nail, pallor of the proximal nail and lunula and pigmentation of the skin at the base of the nail.

Investigations

Investigations in renal disease have three main purposes:

- To establish a diagnosis.
- To assess the complications of impaired renal function.
- To monitor the progress of the disease and/or its response to therapy. The ideal sequence of investigations depends upon the clinical picture, but a widely applicable approach is summarised in **Table 6.2**.

Table 6.2 The investigation of patients with suspected renal disease.

Initial investigations	
Urine stick test:	blood
	protein
	glucose
	pH
Urine microscopy:	cells
	casts
Mid-stream urine for culture	
Plasma:	urea
	creatinine
	electrolytes:: sodium, potassium, chloride, bicarbonate, calcium, phosphate
Haematology:	full blood count

Investigations used selectively	
24-hour urine collection:	creatinine clearance
	protein excretion
Ultrasound	
Plain X-ray of renal tract:	kidney
	ureter
	bladder (KUB)
Intravenous urogram (IVU)	

Specialised investigations
Further radiology
Isotope scans
Specialised renal tubule function tests
Biopsy
Endoscopy
Tests for multisystem diseases

Investigations on urine and blood

- **Urine stick testing (6.7, 6.8).** As a minimum, sticks should test for pH, glucose, blood and protein, and usually also for ketones, bilirubin, urobilinogen and nitrites. The nitrite test is a simple screening test for the presence of infection, as most urinary pathogens convert dietary nitrates to nitrites.
- **Urine microscopy** may identify red cells (6.9), white cells, casts (6.10) or parasites.
- **Urine culture.** In women, samples must be collected with care to avoid contamination—usually in mid-stream after washing the external genitalia. Urine may be cultured on a plate or on a dip-slide impregnated with culture medium (6.11). If there is a suspicion of urinary tract tuberculosis, three early-morning samples may be required for concentration and culture.
- **Plasma biochemistry** provides an initial assessment of renal function. As most laboratories now use automated systems, the urea, creatinine, sodium, potassium, chloride and bicarbonate levels are usually accompanied by calcium, phosphate and alkaline phosphatase results and the albumin level, which allows correction of the calcium value. Complement (C3, C4) values may be helpful. Cholesterol elevation is found in nephrotic syndrome.
- **Haematology profile**—a fall in haemoglobin is invariable, as renal function and the production of endogenous erythropoietin decline. A normochromic normocytic anaemia is often complicated by acute episodes of haemolysis (microangiopathic haemolytic anaemia, MAHA) or by iron deficiency. Elevation of the white-cell count is a good indicator of renal tract infection, and a decline reflects the response to antibiotic therapy. Thrombocytopenia is found in the consumption coagulopathies associated with haemolytic uraemic syndrome.
- **Urine biochemistry** is used selectively to measure 24-hour excretion of creatinine, and thus calculate the creatinine clearance. The 'selectivity' of proteinuria can also be assessed. Electrophoresis may show the presence of kappa or lambda light chains and suggest a diagnosis of multiple myeloma (*see* p. 465).
- **Passage of a stone** or 'gravel' may reflect a metabolic abnormality and all such materials passed should be analysed (p. 301).

6.7

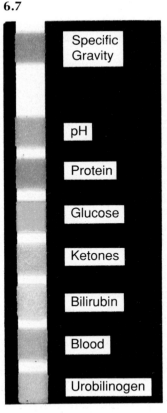

6.7 A typical urine test stick, which provides instant measurement of a range of possible abnormalities in the urine.

6.8

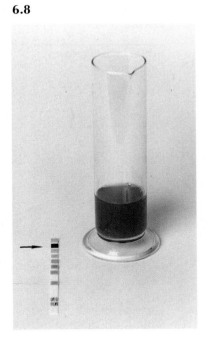

6.8 A positive result for blood (arrowed) occurred when this reddish-brown urine was tested with a standard stick.

6.9

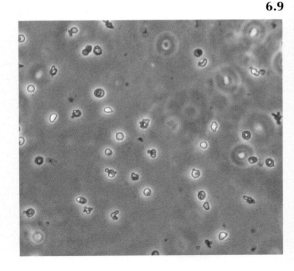

6.9 Phase contrast microscopy of urine sediment, showing a wide range of dysmorphic red cells. In fresh urine, dysmorphic red cells imply glomerular bleeding. In lower urinary tract bleeding, the red cells appear similar to one another (isomorphic). Patients with isomorphic red cells in the urine require further detailed urological investigation, whereas patients with dysmorphic red cells require further investigation for possible renal disease.

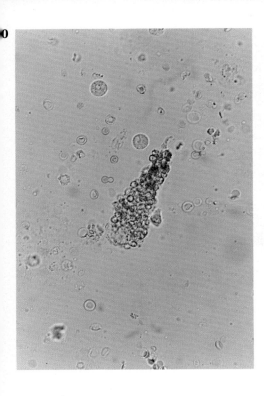

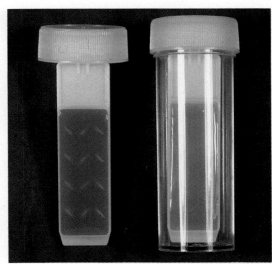

6.10 A red-cell cast, seen on direct microscopy of urine from a patient with the acute nephritic syndrome. The presence and nature of casts in the urine provide clues to the nature of the underlying renal disease: for example, red-cell casts imply bleeding at the glomerular level, while white-cell casts are seen most commonly in acute bacterial pyelonephritis.

6.11 A dip slide coated with culture medium (CLED—green; MacConkey—brown) may be used to start urine culture away from the laboratory, in general practice or in the clinic.

Imaging

- **Ultrasound** is the preferred initial investigation, as it is a cheap, non-invasive and repeatable technique which determines kidney size, shape and position and the presence or absence of obstruction or space-occupying lesions. It is an ideal tool for screening relatives of patients with polycystic kidneys (**6.12**). Enlargement of the prostate may be further investigated by an ultrasound probe inserted into the rectum. This allows repeated examination of patients with prostatic carcinoma to assess the extent of possible local invasion (**6.13**).
- **Plain X-ray of kidney, ureter and bladder** (KUB) is a preliminary to specialised imaging. It is of value in detecting calcification in the kidney or stone in the renal tract (**6.14**) and may reveal other abnormalities.
- **Intravenous urogram or pyelogram** (IVU, IVP) requires the injection of a radio-opaque contrast medium. Serial pictures reveal a nephrogram phase that shows lesions in the parenchyma and a pyelogram phase that outlines the renal calyces, ureters and bladder (**6.15, 6.16**). In patients with diminished renal function, films taken many hours later may still show contrast, but tomography may be necessary to visualise the kidneys (**6.17**).
- **Renal arteriography** allows precise anatomical demonstration of the branches of the renal arteries. This is of value in detecting stenosis (**6.78**), aneurysms (**6.62**) or a tumour circulation (**6.18**).
- **Digital subtraction images** enable high-quality images to be obtained following intravenous injection of contrast

medium, or a small arterial bolus, by computerised subtraction analysis. This technique has replaced arteriography in many patients as it is cheaper, less invasive and readily repeatable (**6.19**).
- **Renal vein venography** allows the anatomy of the renal vein to be seen and samples of blood to be collected for assays (e.g. of renin in the investigation of suspected renovascular hypertension).
- **Retrograde pyelography** is carried out in conjunction with cystoscopy. A ureteric catheter is threaded into the lower end of the ureter and contrast injected. Retrograde pyelography can usually define the site and cause of obstruction (**6.20**).
- **CT scanning** is valuable in defining retroperitoneal lesions and urinary tract obstruction. It is especially valuable in locating and staging tumours and will also show abnormalities such as polycystic kidneys (**6.21**).
- **Micturating cystogram** is used to demonstrate reflux of urine from the bladder to the ureter(s) during emptying of the bladder. The bladder is catheterised and filled with contrast, and films are then taken during and after micturition (**6.22**).
- **Radionuclide scans** are of value in both static and dynamic imaging. The usual isotope is 99m-technetium attached to dimercaptosuccinic acid (99mTc-DMSA) (static, **6.23**), or to diethylene triamine-penta-acetic acid (99mTc-DTPA) (dynamic, **6.24**). These tests are repeatable, simple and relatively non-invasive.

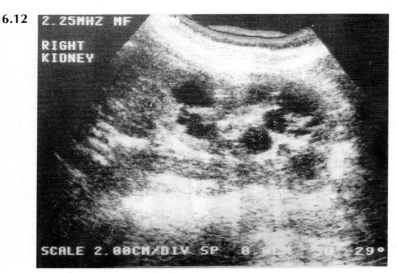

6.12 Ultrasound is the preferred initial investigation for kidney size, shape and position. This patient's large kidneys showed the typical appearance of polycystic kidneys. The multiple parenchymal cysts are clearly shown.

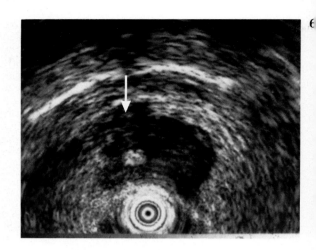

6.13 A rectal ultrasound probe can be used to define and stage carcinoma of the prostate. In this case, the right lobe of the capsule of the prostate is distorted, and anteriorly a capsular breach is evident (arrow), suggesting extra-capsular spread of the tumour.

6.14

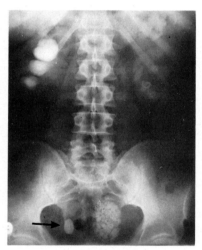

6.14 Plain X-ray of the kidney, ureter and bladder (KUB) is a useful initial investigation in many patients. Here it has revealed a rather unusual combination of calculi in both kidneys (more prominent on the right), in the lower right ureter (arrowed) and in a bladder diverticulum.

6.15

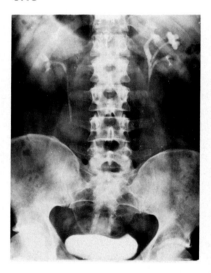

6.15 Intravenous urogram showing a normal right kidney and ureter, but marked calyceal clubbing in the left kidney. Note the gross dilatation of the calyces, especially in the middle and upper poles of the kidney. These changes were the result of unilateral reflux of urine and chronic infection.

6.16

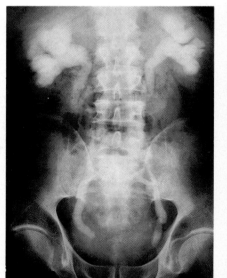

6.16 IVU showing bilateral hydronephrosis and hydroureter with a large bladder. The changes are typical of an elderly patient with chronic urinary retention as a result of prostatic enlargement. Unless the bladder outflow obstruction is surgically relieved, the patient will develop progressive chronic renal failure.

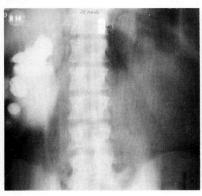 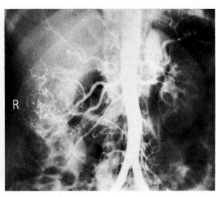 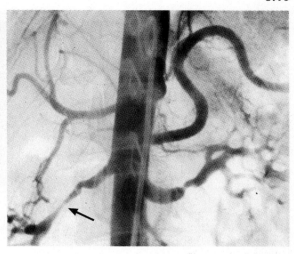

6.17 Tomography was necessary to reveal the left kidney in this patient's IVU. The grossly hydronephrotic right kidney was visible on a normal film, but the nephrogram, which reveals a large left kidney, can be seen only on tomography.

6.18 Renal arteriography. This 'flood' film, in which dye is allowed to enter both kidneys simultaneously from the aorta, demonstrates a normal arterial circulation in the left kidney and an abnormal tumour circulation in the right kidney. Selective arteriography can also be performed by catheterising individual renal arteries, and digital subtraction imaging (**6.19**) allows further detailed assessment.

6.19 Renal arteriogram (digital subtraction technique) showing bilateral renal artery stenosis. The appearances are typical of stenosis caused by fibromuscular hyperplasia rather than atheroma, and the stenosis is more marked on the right (arrow). The stenoses were successfully treated by balloon angioplasty.

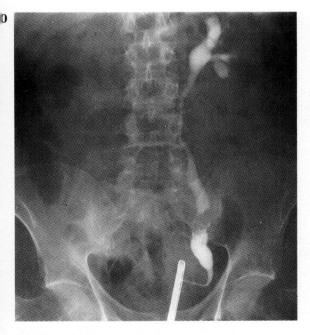

6.20 Retrograde pyelogram revealing a large filling defect in the left ureter caused by a transitional cell carcinoma. The technique is particularly useful in defining the nature and site of ureteric obstruction.

6.21 CT scan revealing bilateral congenital polycystic kidneys, larger on the patient's left (to the right of the picture). The liver also contains multiple cysts. The pancreas can be clearly seen in this view, but does not seem to contain cysts in this patient.

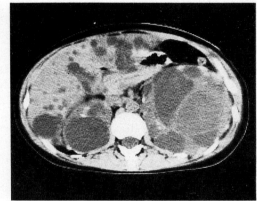

6.22 Micturating cystogram, showing bilateral ureteric reflux. Reflux is categorised in three grades: Grade I, in which contrast medium enters the ureter only; Grade II, in which the pelvicalyceal system is filled with dye; Grade III, where dilatation of the calyces and ureter also occurs. In this patient, there is some ureteric dilatation and early calyceal clubbing, so there is Grade III reflux.

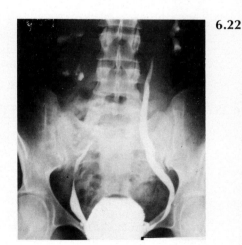

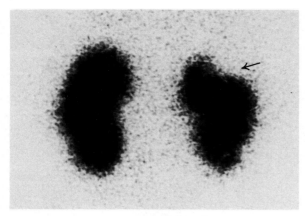

6.23

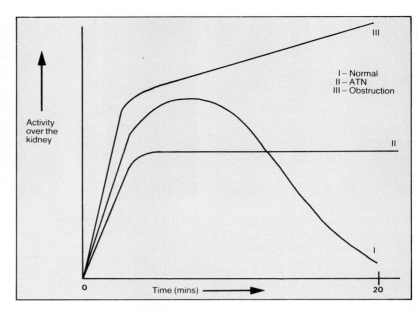

6.23 A 99mTc-DMSA scintigram, showing a defect in the upper pole of the right kidney (arrowed). The patient was a young girl with a urinary tract infection. The most common cause of this appearance is reflux nephropathy with pyelonephritis scarring, and this was confirmed by micturating cystogram in this patient.

I – Normal
II – ATN
III – Obstruction

Activity over the kidney

Time (mins)

0   20

6.24 99mTc-DTPA renogram. Activity over the kidney is measured after initial injection of the isotope and plotted against time. Typical results in normals, acute tubular necrosis (ATN) and obstruction are shown here.

Other investigations

Renal biopsy can be performed percutaneously in patients who can co-operate and hold their breath, have normal coagulation, have two kidneys, have a reasonably controlled blood pressure and have a haemoglobin >8g/dl (**6.25**). Open biopsy is advisable if these criteria are not met.

Renal biopsy is valuable in patients with nephrotic syndrome, nephritic syndrome and unexplained renal failure. Light microscopy with special stains will often lead to a diagnosis but may be complemented by immunofluorescence and electron microscopy.

Electron microscopy of glomeruli from patients with glomerulonephritis determines the location of electron-dense deposits in relation to the glomerular basement membrane (subepithelial, intramembranous, subendothelial) or mesangium. Immunofluorescence microscopy, using cryostat sections treated with fluorescein-labelled antiserum, determines the pattern of deposition (granular, linear, mesangial) of different classes of immunoglobulin and complement within glomeruli.

Cystoscopy allows for direct vision and biopsy of bladder wall pathology (**6.26**) and the insertion of ureteral catheters for retrograde pyelography or the direct removal of ureteric stones.

Tests for systemic disease may be needed, including a search for infection elsewhere (throat swab, ASO-titre, hepatitis B markers, syphilis serology, etc.), an auto-antibody screen, including antinuclear factor, rheumatoid factor, anti-ds-DNA antibody, cryoglobulins, anti-neutrophil cytoplasmic antibody (ANCA) and anti-glomerular basement membrane antibody, and investigations into diabetes mellitus or other underlying disorders.

6.25

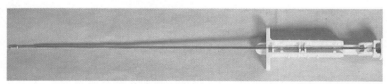

6.25 A Trucut biopsy needle, of the type commonly used for percutaneous renal biopsy (and for other biopsies including liver and prostate). Renal biopsy is an important technique in the assessment of many patients with renal, especially glomerular, disease.

6.26 Cystoscopy revealing a transitional cell carcinoma of the bladder. The patient presented with painless haematuria.

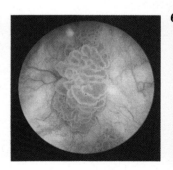

Clinical presentations of renal disease

Acute renal failure

Acute renal failure is defined as a recent rapid and profound decline in renal function, whereas **rapidly progressive renal failure** refers to renal failure developing over weeks rather than days. These disorders, therefore, can be diagnosed only by serial observations of serum creatinine levels and urine flow rates.

Patients commonly present because of oliguria, but more than 25% of patients with acute renal failure are non-oliguric (urine volumes remain greater than 400 ml per day). There are no characteristic clinical signs.

The causes of acute renal failure are usually considered in three groups (pre-renal, renal or post-renal), depending on whether the main component of the initiating event is renal hypoperfusion, intrinsic renal disease or urinary outflow obstruction (**Table 6.3**). Pre-renal failure may be prevented from evolving to established acute renal failure by correction of hypovolaemia or impaired cardiac output. Pre-renal failure is likely to be present if urinary concentrating ability (urine to plasma osmolality >1.7) or urinary sodium retention (urinary sodium concentration >20 mmol/l) are demonstrated.

Established acute renal failure which is caused by nephrotoxins (myoglobinuria, haemoglobinuria, aminoglycosides, organic solvents, contrast material), ischaemia (hypovolaemia or cardiac failure), septicaemia, surgery or obstetric complications is potentially reversible and acute tubular necrosis is usually shown if the kidneys are examined morphologically.

In these forms of reversible acute renal failure, a diuretic phase usually begins spontaneously during the second or third week after the onset of renal failure and the functional and histological abnormalities may completely resolve. Acute renal failure caused by glomerular lesions is less likely to recover without specific treatment and renal biopsy should be performed promptly in suspected cases. Post-renal failure is potentially reversible, so obstruction should be excluded in all cases of acute renal failure.

The causes of acute renal failure can usually be identified from a full history, examination, urinalysis, urine microscopy and renal ultrasound.

The management of established acute renal failure requires careful attention to fluid and dietary intake; dialysis to correct and thereafter prevent hyperkalaemia (**6.27**), fluid overload, acidosis or uncontrolled uraemia; and treatment of the underlying cause if possible (**6.28**). Immunosuppressive therapy is often needed in patients with rapidly progressive or acute renal failure caused by biopsy-proven glomerular, interstitial, vasculitic or multisystem disease.

Table 6.3 Common causes of acute renal failure.

Pre-renal failure	Intrinsic renal failure	Post-renal failure
Hypovolaemia	Rhabdomyolysis	Obstructive uropathy
Low cardiac output	Haemolysis	
Sepsis	Drugs/nephrotoxins	
Trauma	Glomerulonephritis	
	Interstitial nephritis	
	Multisystem diseases	
	Malignant hypertension	
	Arterial occlusion	

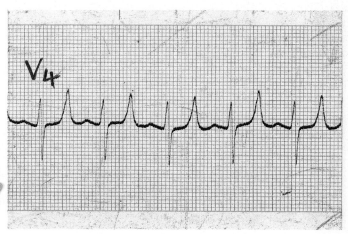

6.27

6.27 Severe hyperkalaemia is a common complication of acute renal failure and can be diagnosed on ECG, which shows peaked and symmetrical T waves. Hyperkalaemia is an indication for urgent dialysis; other indications include pulmonary oedema, severe acidosis and pericarditis.

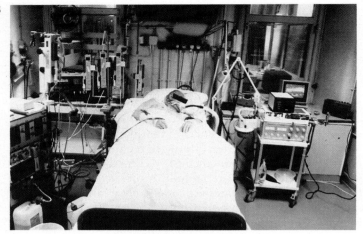

6.28 Patients with acute renal failure are often severely ill. They may require both ventilation and haemodialysis. The percentage survival of patients with acute renal failure has not improved significantly over the past decade, but this may be explained, at least in part, by an increasing proportion of patients with multi-organ failure surviving to a stage at which they develop renal failure.

Chronic renal failure

Chronic renal failure (CRF) is defined as a progressive decline in renal function for at least three months. Loss of functioning nephrons in chronic renal disease often results in an exponential rise in serum creatinine as end-stage renal failure is approached. Consequently, the decline in renal function is frequently linear when the reciprocal of serum creatinine is plotted against time (**6.29**). Progressive impairment of the excretory, homeostatic, metabolic and humoral functions of the kidneys produces a range of non-specific symptoms and signs (**6.3, 6.29**), so chronic renal failure may be diagnosed only after biochemical investigation. The syndrome of advanced uraemia includes anaemia, osteodystrophy (p. 156), metabolic acidosis, pruritus, nausea and vomiting, pericarditis (p. 247) and fluid overload. When renal disease progresses insidiously, patients may not present until they develop end-stage renal failure (**6.4, 6.5, 6.30**). Long-standing pre-existing renal disease may be suspected in such patients by the presence of anaemia or evidence of hyperparathyroidism (p. 154) and confirmed radiologically by the presence of bilateral shrunken kidneys (**6.31**). Chronic renal failure may result from a range of primary diseases (**Table 6.4**).

Progression of chronic renal failure can be arrested when there is treatable urinary tract obstruction, urinary tract infection, hypertension, or dehydration. In the absence of these reversible factors or effective therapy for the primary renal disease, conservative management of chronic renal failure requires restriction of dietary protein and potassium intake, maintenance of correct fluid and sodium balance, and the use of phosphate-binding agents and active metabolites of vitamin D to control hyperparathyroidism. Anaemia in chronic renal failure results mainly from inappropriately low production of erythropoietin by the diseased kidneys but other factors, such as iron or folate deficiency, chronic blood loss, aluminium toxicity or hyperparathyroidism, may also often contribute. Renal anaemia can now be corrected by the regular administration of human recombinant erythropoietin and treatment of any co-existing causal factors.

Table 6.4 Primary renal disease in 2143 patients accepted for renal replacement therapy in the UK.

Renal disease	% of patients
Chronic glomerulonephritis	19
Unknown	19
Diabetes mellitus	13
Pyelonephritis/interstitial nephritis	13
Renal vascular disease	12
Cystic diseases	9
Multisystem disease	7
Amyloidosis	1.5
Hypoplastic kidneys	1
Other hereditary diseases	1
Miscellaneous	3.5

1987 figures, adapted from Combined Report on Regular Dialysis and Transplantation in Europe, XIX, 1988

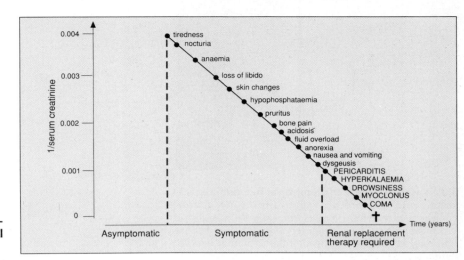

Graph labels (top to bottom along the declining line):
tiredness
nocturia
anaemia
loss of libido
skin changes
hypophosphataemia
pruritus
bone pain
acidosis
fluid overload
anorexia
nausea and vomiting
dysgeusis
PERICARDITIS
HYPERKALAEMIA
DROWSINESS
MYOCLONUS
COMA

Y-axis: 1/serum creatinine (0, 0.001, 0.002, 0.003, 0.004)
X-axis: Time (years)
Bottom axis categories: Asymptomatic | Symptomatic | Renal replacement therapy required

6.29 The typical progressive onset of the non-specific symptoms and signs of chronic renal failure.

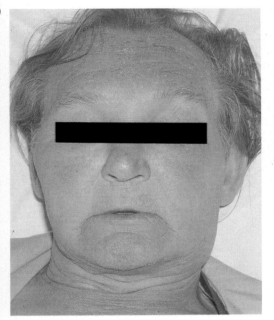

6.30 Uraemic facies. Another patient (see **6.4**) demonstrating sallow brown pigmentation, pallor and facial puffiness associated with long-standing renal failure.

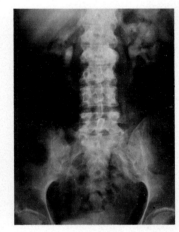

6.31 IVU demonstrating two small contracted kidneys. The cortical scarring and calyceal dilatation and deformity are features of reflux nephropathy (chronic pyelonephritis), but shrunken kidneys without these appearances may also occur in end-stage glomerular or interstitial disease.

Renal replacement therapy

Most patients with chronic renal failure require renal replacement therapy when renal function declines to approximately 5% of the normal expected for age, usually with a creatinine clearance of 5–10 ml/min.

The treatment options for patients with end-stage renal failure are hospital or home haemodialysis, continuous ambulatory peritoneal dialysis or renal transplantation:

- **Haemodialysis.** Most patients on regular haemodialysis have an arterio-venous fistula created for vascular access (**6.32**) and require approximately 12 hours dialysis per week, usually divided into three treatment periods. This may be carried out in hospital (**6.33**) or in the patient's home. Even with this regimen, patients still need to follow dietary and fluid restriction.
- **Continuous ambulatory peritoneal dialysis (CAPD).** Patients on a standard CAPD regime perform exchanges of 2-litre volumes of dialysis solution through a permanent in-dwelling peritoneal catheter (**6.34, 6.35**) usually four times every day using an aseptic technique. CAPD is less restricting than haemodialysis and may be carried out at home. Patients do not usually need to restrict their dietary or fluid intake.
- **Renal transplantation.** Haemodialysis and CAPD are both associated with significant physical and psychological demands on the patient and his or her family. Near-normal renal function and much improved quality of life can result from successful renal transplantation (**6.36, 6.37**) and the inclusion of cyclosporin in immunosuppression protocols has increased the percentage of functioning grafts one year after transplantation to over 80%.

Most patients with CRF are keen to undergo transplantation, but the feasibility of this approach is limited in most countries by the supply of kidneys for transplantation.

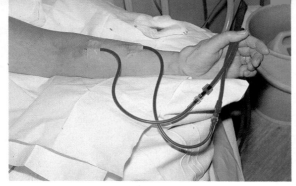

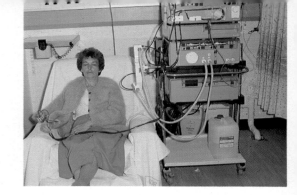

6.32 Vascular access for long-term haemodialysis is usually provided through a surgically created arterio-venous fistula. Blood leaves the patient through the distal needle to pass through the dialyser before returning to the patient through the proximal needle. Patients usually become adept at inserting their own needles.

6.33 Typical patient with chronic renal failure undergoing haemodialysis in a hospital setting. In some countries, including the UK, many patients carry out this treatment on a long-term basis in a specially converted room at home.

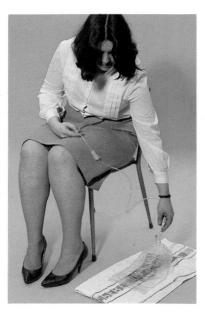

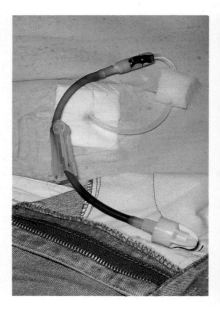

6.34 Continuous ambulatory peritoneal dialysis (CAPD) is a simpler and less restricting technique than haemodialysis, and is compatible with a virtually normal lifestyle. Bags need only be connected to the peritoneal catheter four times per day during exchanges of fluid.

6.35 The Tenckhoff peritoneal dialysis catheter remains implanted in the CAPD patient, but it can be simply strapped to the abdominal wall when not in use for fluid exchanges.

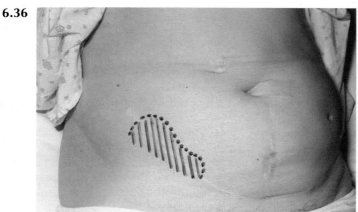

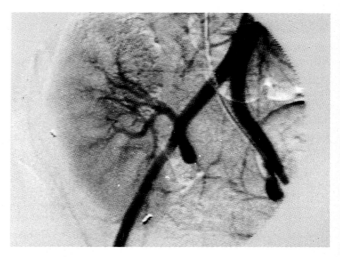

6.36 Renal transplant—typical surface markings. The kidney is usually implanted extraperitoneally in either the right or left iliac fossa, and it can be easily palpated. Percutaneous biopsy is also simple when necessary.

6.37 Normal renal transplant in situ. This digital substraction angiogram shows the normal site for a renal transplant. The renal artery has been anastomosed to the right external iliac artery.

Acute nephritic syndrome

In the acute nephritic syndrome (acute nephritis) there is an abrupt onset of haematuria and proteinuria accompanied by evidence of salt and water retention and reduced renal function. The clinical features are periorbital puffiness (**6.1**), ankle oedema, brown or cola-coloured urine (**6.8**) and hypertension. Sometimes the patient or his or her parents may also notice a reduction in urine volume. All patients have haematuria and proteinuria on urinalysis, but the degree of renal impairment is variable. Glomerular bleeding in patients with nephritis can be confirmed by demonstrating red-cell casts in the urinary sediment (**6.10**).

Acute nephritis may result from:

- **Infection:** post-streptococcal glomerulonephritis, infective endocarditis or shunt nephritis.
- **Multisystem disease:** systemic lupus erythematosus, Henoch–Schönlein disease, vasculitis or Goodpasture's syndrome.
- **Primary glomerulonephritis:** mesangiocapillary glomerulonephritis, IgA nephropathy or crescentic glomerulonephritis.

Evidence of infection or extrarenal involvement should therefore be sought in all patients with acute nephritis. It is important to establish the underlying cause of the nephritic syndrome as soon as possible, since renal outcome can be improved when specific therapy is started promptly.

Nephrotic syndrome

The nephrotic syndrome is characterised by the combination of heavy proteinuria, hypoalbuminaemia and oedema (**1.186, 6.2, 6.38, 6.39**) and is a common mode of presentation in a variety of glomerular diseases. Prolonged proteinuria leads to hypoalbuminaemia, decreased plasma oncotic pressure, hypovolaemia, subsequent retention of sodium and water by the kidney caused by activation of the renin-angiotensin-aldosterone axis and accumulation of fluid in the extravascular space. Hypercholesterolaemia is frequently present and may be a consequence of increased hepatic synthesis of cholesterol as well as albumin. Serious complications of the nephrotic syndrome include bacterial infections, particularly cellulitis and peritonitis, and arterial and venous thrombotic episodes.

The major causes of the nephrotic syndrome are listed in **Table 6.5**. No systemic cause is evident in 80% of cases and renal biopsy in such patients shows a variety of primary glomerular diseases (minimal change glomerulonephritis, focal and segmental glomerulosclerosis, membranous glomerulonephritis, mesangiocapillary glomerulonephritis and mesangial proliferative glomerulonephritis). Almost 20% of cases of nephrotic syndrome are caused by renal involvement from systemic disease (e.g. diabetes mellitus, amyloidosis, systemic lupus erythematosus) and the remainder are caused by drugs, neoplasia or rare heredofamilial disorders.

The non-specific treatment of the nephrotic syndrome involves fluid and dietary sodium restriction, high protein intake and judicious use of diuretics. A mild degree of ankle oedema late in the day while on treatment is desirable, in order to avoid complications from hypovolaemia. Infusions of albumin should be reserved for patients with gross hypovolaemia or refractory oedema. Renal outcome is dependent on the underlying cause of the nephrotic syndrome. Corticosteroid treatment is of value in patients with minimal change glomerular lesions (*see* p. 280), and may have a role in some other forms of glomerulonephritis; but high-dose steroid therapy may produce cushingoid features (**6.40**) and its use should be carefully controlled.

Table 6.5 Causes of nephrotic syndrome.

Glomerulonephritis
Diabetes mellitus
Amyloidosis
Multisystem disease
Drugs: gold, penicillamine, heroin, captopril
Neoplasia
Infection
Heredofamilial disorders

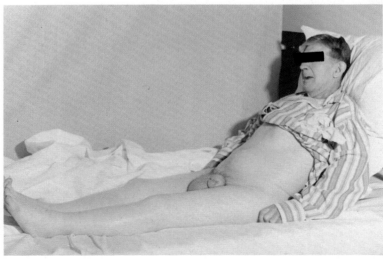

6.38

6.38 Nephrotic syndrome—a typical adult patient. He is breathless as a result of pulmonary oedema and has oedema of the ankles, calves, scrotum and penis. He has abdominal swelling as a result of oedema of the abdominal wall, and ascites.

6.39

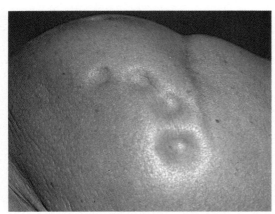

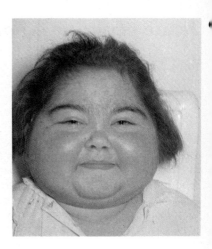

6.39 Nephrotic syndrome—gross pitting oedema of the abdominal wall, secondary to severe hypoalbuminaemia.

6.40 Gross cushingoid features (*see also* p. 310) in a 7-year-old girl with the nephrotic syndrome who was treated with corticosteroids. Although steroid treatment is of value in children with minimal change glomerular lesions, such gross features of steroid excess should be avoided if possible by careful planning of dosage and timing of therapy.

Asymptomatic proteinuria

6.41

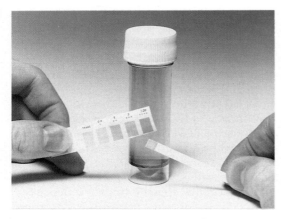

6.41 Asymptomatic proteinuria may be found on 'routine' urine testing. Although it may be benign, further investigation is indicated to exclude progressive renal disease.

Screening investigations in apparently healthy patients may show persistent asymptomatic proteinuria (**6.41**) and/or microscopic haematuria, which may be the only evidence of underlying renal disease. The presence of urinary abnormalities in patients with hypertension strongly suggests that they are suffering from renal disease. Asymptomatic proteinuria always requires further investigation to exclude treatable causes of progressive renal disease.

Glomerular Diseases

Glomerular diseases may be classified on a three-tier basis:

- Clinical syndromes.
- Histological appearances.
- Aetiology.

Glomerular disease may lead to a variety of clinical syndromes including asymptomatic proteinuria, haematuria, acute nephritis, nephrotic syndrome and slowly or rapidly progressive renal failure.

There is a degree of correlation between the histological appearance of the glomeruli (**Table 6.6**) and the clinical presentation (**Table 6.7**). The histological appearance often provides a valuable guide to prognosis and likely response to therapy.

In primary glomerular disease, the aetiology is usually unclear; but 'aetiological' classification is useful in secondary glomerulopathies.

Investigations in glomerular disease should usually include the 'initial' investigations listed in **Table 6.2**, together with renal ultrasound or an IVU, serum complement levels, auto-antibodies and appropriate tests for multisystem disorders. In adults, these will usually be followed by renal biopsy, with assessment of light-microscopic (**6.42**) and, often, electron microscopic (**6.43**) and immunofluorescence microscopic appearances.

In children, biopsy may often be postponed until after a trial of steroid therapy.

Table 6.6 Terminology used in the histological description of glomerular lesions.

Diffuse:	all of the glomeruli are uniformly involved
Focal:	some of the glomeruli are involved
Segmental:	only part of the glomerular tufts are involved
Crescentic:	at least 70% of the glomerular tufts are compressed by crescents (proliferation of macrophages and epithelial cells of Bowman's capsule)

Light microscopy of renal tissue also assesses pathological involvement in the interstitium, tubules and blood vessels.

Table 6.7 Correlation between histology and clinical picture in primary glomerulopathy.

Histological type	Clinical features
Minimal change glomerulonephritis	Nephrotic syndrome
Focal and segmental glomerulosclerosis	Nephrotic syndrome, progressive renal failure
Membranous glomerulonephritis	Nephrotic syndrome
Mesangiocapillary glomerulonephritis	Haematuria, proteinuria, acute nephritis, progressive renal failure
Mesangial proliferative glomerulonephritis	Haematuria, proteinuria
Diffuse endocapillary proliferative glomerulonephritis	Acute nephritis, progressive renal failure

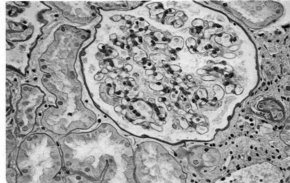

6.42 A normal glomerulus and normal proximal tubules (top right) (*PAS x352*).

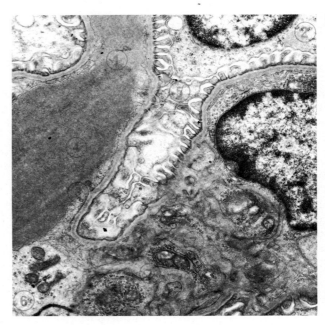

6.43 The ultrastructure of the normal glomerulus as seen on electron microscopy: 1 = capillary lumen; 2 = epithelial cell; 3 = basement membrane; 4 = red blood cell; 5 = epithelial foot processes; 6 = endothelial cell; 7 = mesangial matrix; 8 = mesangial cell.

Primary glomerulopathies

Minimal change glomerulonephritis

The nephrotic syndrome (p. 277) is the clinical presentation in almost all cases of minimal change glomerulonephritis, but rarely asymptomatic proteinuria may be the only abnormality. Hypertension and haematuria are both rare. The disease is the underlying cause in more than 80% of children and almost 20% of adults with the nephrotic syndrome. Auto-antibody and complement studies are normal and proteinuria is usually highly selective (high urinary transferrin to IgG ratio). On renal biopsy, the glomeruli are normal (**6.44**) except for the presence of epithelial foot process fusion on electron microscopy (**6.45**), which is found in all causes of proteinuria of glomerular origin.

Since remission of proteinuria can be induced in virtually all cases by a course of prednisolone, this is usually prescribed to all childhood nephrotics without first performing a renal biopsy. Renal biopsy is reserved for children with steroid-resistant or frequently relapsing nephrotic syndrome. In adults minimal change glomerulonephritis is a less frequent cause of nephrotic syndrome and a biopsy is indicated in all cases. When relapses are frequent or unacceptable steroid side-effects develop, an eight-week course of cyclophosphamide (2 mg/kg) may produce prolonged remission. On rare occasions, the disease is associated with lymphoma, and remission is usually induced on successful treatment of the underlying disease. Renal prognosis in this condition is very good, even though a few patients may develop acute renal failure as a result of overuse of diuretics.

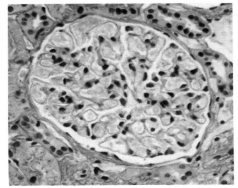

6.44 Minimal change glomerulonephritis showing a normal glomerulus on light microscopy of a renal biopsy (*MSB x224*).

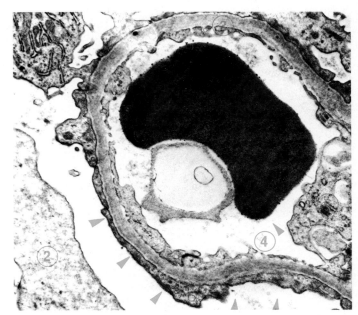

6.45 Minimal change glomerulonephritis. Electron micrograph showing fusion of the epithelial foot processes (arrowed) and absence of electron-dense deposits (magnification *x10,750*): 2 = epithelial cytoplasm; 3 = basement membrane; 4 = red blood cell in capillary lumen; 6 = endothelial cell.

Focal and segmental glomerulosclerosis

Patients with this disease most commonly present with nephrotic syndrome, and focal and segmental glomerulo-sclerosis is the underlying cause in almost 10% of child nephrotics. Auto-antibodies and complement studies are normal. Renal biopsy shows segmental areas of sclerosis, initially only in the juxtamedullary glomeruli without evidence of cellular proliferation or necrosis (**6.46**). Immunofluorescence microscopy often shows deposition of IgM and C3 in affected glomeruli. Since glomerular involvement is at first focal, early cases may be indistinguishable from minimal change glomerulonephritis, even on renal biopsy. This disease may be suspected if the nephrotic syndrome in childhood is resistant to steroid therapy or runs a relapsing and remitting course. Cyclophosphamide or cyclosporin may induce partial or complete remission of proteinuria, but in more than 50% of patients renal function declines progressively and 20–40% of patients reach end-stage renal failure after 10 years. The long-term renal prognosis may be further compromised by recurrence of the disease in around one-third of patients after renal transplantation.

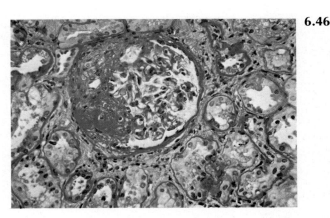

6.46 Focal and segmental glomerulosclerosis. The segmental sclerosis is clearly seen on light microscopy of a renal biopsy (*PAS x330*).

6.47

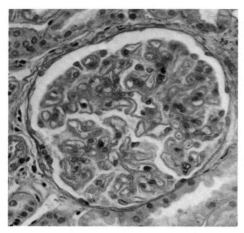

6.47 Membranous glomerulonephritis. The renal biopsy shows uniform thickening of the capillary basement membranes. Compare with **6.42** and **6.44** (*MSB x224*).

This disease is the most common cause of adult-onset nephrotic syndrome, but is rare in childhood. Microscopic haematuria is common and hypertension is present in around one-third of patients at presentation. The diagnosis is confirmed by the presence of diffuse uniform thickening of the glomerular capillary wall in all glomeruli (**6.47**) associated with subepithelial electron-dense deposits on electron microscopy (**6.48**) and diffuse granular capillary loop IgG on immunofluorescence microscopy (**6.49**). Most cases are idiopathic, but it is important to exclude associated infection (syphilis, hepatitis B), neoplasia, SLE or drug therapy (gold, penicillamine, captopril). Renal outcome in the secondary type depends on the underlying cause. If untreated, 20% of the idiopathic group remit spontaneously and 50% reach end-stage renal failure after 10 years. Corticosteroids are of no benefit. Recent clinical studies in nephrotic patients have shown reduction in proteinuria and improvement in renal function after treatment with combined courses of prednisolone and chlorambucil.

6.48

6.49

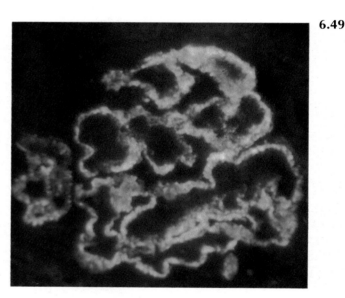

6.49 Membranous glomerulonephritis. Immuno-fluorescence microscopy showing diffuse granular deposition of IgG in the capillary loops (*x300*).

6.48 Membranous glomerulonephritis. Electron micrograph showing markedly thickened basement membrane with electron-dense deposits (arrowed) representing deposits of antigen-antibody complexes located subepithelially, i.e. beneath the fused epithelial cell foot processes (5). 3 = basement membrane; 5 = epithelial cell foot processes; 6 = endothelial cell; 13 = mesangium. (Magnification *x10,750.*)

Mesangiocapillary glomerulonephritis

The mode of presentation of this disease is variable: 20% of patients have the acute nephritic syndrome, while all of the remaining patients have proteinuria; 50% have hypertension, 50% have renal failure and 30% have haematuria. The disease mainly affects school-age children and young adults and is more common in females. Serum C3 levels are reduced transiently in Type 1 and are persistently low in Type 2. These are differentiated from each other on renal biopsy. The histological feature common to both types of disease is a combination of mesangial cell proliferation and thickening of the glomerular capillary wall on light microscopy (**6.50**). In the subendothelial type (Type 1) there is interposition of mesangial matrix between the endothelial cells and glomerular basement membrane; subendothelial deposits on electron microscopy (**6.51**); and granular deposition of IgG and C3 on immunofluorescence microscopy. In the dense-deposit type (Type 2) there are linear dense intramembranous deposits on electron microscopy (**6.52**); and only deposition of C3 on immunofluorescence microscopy. There is no specific therapy for this form of glomerulonephritis and the renal prognosis is relatively poor with more than 50% of patients reaching end-stage renal failure after 10 years. Type 2 mesangiocapillary glomerulonephritis may recur in patients following renal transplantation.

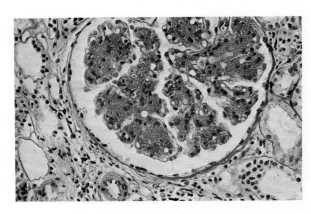

6.50

6.50 Mesangiocapillary glomerulonephritis. Light microscopy showing an increase in mesangial cells and matrix and patchy thickening of the basement membrane. This glomerulus also shows marked lobulation of the glomerular tufts (*PAS x330*).

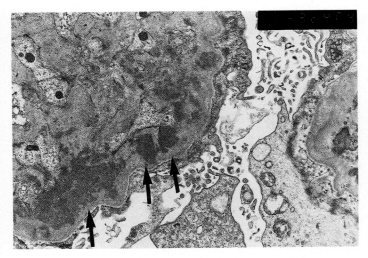

6.51 Mesangiocapillary glomerulonephritis. Electron micrograph showing subendothelial electron-dense deposits (arrowed) in a patient with Type 1 mesangiocapillary glomerulonephritis. (Magnification *x13,200.*)

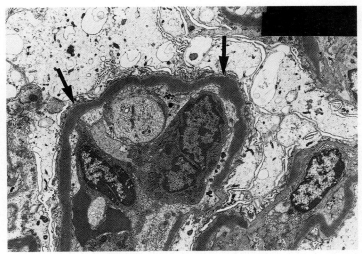

6.52

6.52 Mesangiocapillary glomerulonephritis. Electron micrograph from a patient with Type 2 mesangiocapillary glomerulonephritis (dense-deposit disease) showing linear dense intramembranous deposits (arrows). (Magnification *x5,200.*)

6.53

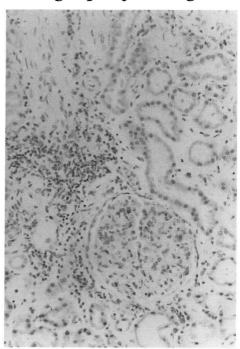

6.53 Mesangial proliferative glomerulonephritis. Light microscopy of a glomerulus from a patient with microscopic haematuria and asymptomatic proteinuria showing an increase in mesangial cells and matrix (*H & E*).

Recurrent macroscopic haematuria, often within two days of an upper respiratory tract infection, was the most common mode of presentation of this disorder, but as a result of routine urinalysis many patients are now detected with microscopic haematuria and/or asymptomatic proteinuria. Peak incidence is in young adults, and men are more commonly affected. Renal failure at presentation is uncommon. Auto-antibodies and complement studies are usually normal, unless the disorder is a manifestation of systemic lupus erythematosus. Serum IgA levels may be elevated in Henoch–Schönlein disease. Renal biopsy shows increased mesangial cells and mesangial matrix (**6.53**). These light microscopic appearances are associated with the presence of mesangial deposits on electron microscopy (**6.54**) and commonly with mesangial deposition of IgA on immunofluorescence microscopy (**6.55**), so-called IgA nephropathy (Berger's disease). Less frequently, immunofluorescence microscopy shows mesangial deposition of either IgG or IgM. The electron and immunofluorescence microscopy appearances of IgA nephropathy are indistinguishable from those of Henoch–Schönlein nephritis. The latter is usually associated with purpura (**2.116**), abdominal pain or arthropathy, is more common in children, and is more likely to present with the nephritic syndrome and to have glomeruli containing crescents on biopsy.

There is no specific treatment for either IgA nephropathy or Henoch–Schönlein nephritis, but the overall prognosis is good. Only 5–10% of patients with IgA nephropathy reach end-stage renal failure after 10 years, and progressive renal failure is more likely in patients with hypertension or nephrotic syndrome at presentation.

6.54

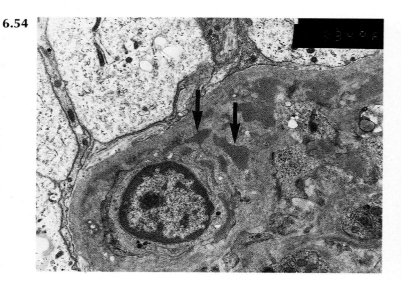

6.54 Mesangial proliferative glomerulonephritis. Electron micrograph showing electron-dense deposits distributed within the mesangium (arrows). (Magnification *x13,200.*)

6.55

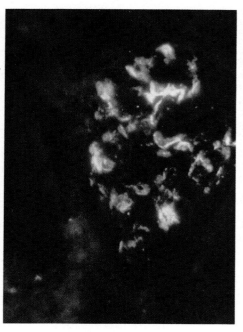

6.55 Mesangial proliferative glomerulonephritis. Immunofluorescence microscopy from the same patient as in **6.54** showing mesangial deposition of IgA, indicating that this patient has IgA nephropathy (Berger's disease).

Diffuse endocapillary proliferative glomerulonephritis

Patients with this form of glomerulonephritis usually present with acute nephritis, although not all features may be evident. The condition is more frequent in children and young adults. In some patients, the onset of renal disease is associated with an extrarenal infection 10–14 days earlier, but most cases are idiopathic.

Classically, this disease is preceded by a nephritogenic group A streptococcal infection, usually of the throat or skin. However, the frequency of isolating streptococcus from the presumed site of infection, or demonstrating a rise in antibody titre to streptococcal antigens (anti-streptolysin O titre), is relatively low. Auto-antibodies are negative and serum C3 levels are usually transiently decreased. Renal biopsy is characterised by hypercellularity in all of the glomeruli (**6.56**),

not infrequently associated with crescent formation (**6.57**). Electron microscopy in the acute stage shows large subepithelial electron-dense deposits (**6.58**) and immunofluorescence microscopy shows granular staining of IgG and C3 within the glomeruli. The prognosis in post-streptococcal glomerulonephritis is generally good, and the only specific treatment recommended is a seven-day course of penicillin. Complete recovery is common, and less than 5% of patients reach end-stage renal failure at 10 years. The latter is more likely in adult patients with persistent hypertension or nephrotic syndrome, and in patients with rapid progressive renal failure. The long-term outcome for the larger idiopathic group is less well defined, but is again generally good if there is early regression of features of renal disease.

6.56

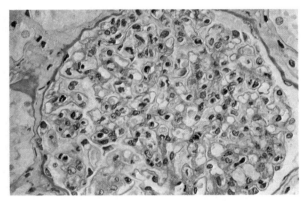

6.56 Diffuse endocapillary proliferative glomerulonephritis. The glomerulus shows increased cellularity, caused by endothelial and mesangial cell proliferation and polymorph infiltration. (*PAS x330.*)

6.57

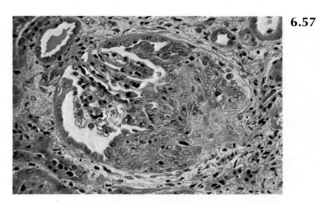

6.57 Diffuse endocapillary proliferative glomerulonephritis with crescents. Glomerulus shows a large cellular crescent compressing the glomerular tuft (*H & E x330*). Crescentic glomerulonephritis may be found in all types of acute nephritis with rapidly progressive renal failure.

6.58

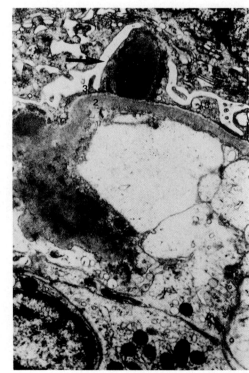

6.58 Diffuse endocapillary proliferative glomerulonephritis. The electron micrograph shows a large subepithelial electron-dense deposit (arrowed): 1 = endothelial cell; 2 = basement membrane; 3 = epithelial cell.

Secondary glomerulopathies

Anti-glomerular basement membrane disease

Anti-glomerular basement membrane disease (anti-GBM disease) usually presents with rapidly progressive renal failure, haematuria and proteinuria. The haematuria may be macroscopic and, if associated with haemoptysis, is termed Goodpasture's syndrome (p. 195). The disease has a peak incidence in young adults, and is more common in males. There is often an association with recent infection or exposure to hydrocarbons at the onset, or prior to relapses of the disease. The disease is mediated by an anti-glomerular basement membrane antibody present in the serum, and the antibody titre is used for diagnostic purposes and to assess the adequacy of treatment. Other auto-antibodies and complement levels are usually normal. The diagnostic feature on renal biopsy is linear deposition of IgG and occasionally C3 along the capillary loops of the glomeruli (6.59). Light microscopy usually shows a focal necrotising glomerulitis with crescent formation (6.60).

The prognosis is dependent on the degree of renal failure at the time of diagnosis and on whether pulmonary haemorrhage is present. Two major features of the natural history of the disease determine treatment strategies. Pulmonary haemorrhage is almost invariably fatal if untreated, and recovery of renal function is rare if the patient is already dialysis-dependent when immunosuppressive therapy is begun. Consequently, immunosuppression with pulsed intravenous methylprednisolone, oral prednisolone, cyclophosphamide and plasma exchange is reserved for patients with Goodpasture's syndrome or patients not yet receiving dialysis. The risks of intensive immunosuppression in patients already requiring dialysis and without pulmonary haemorrhage outweigh the small chance of improvement in renal function.

6.59

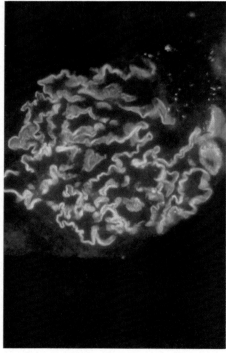

6.60

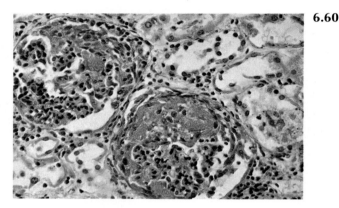

6.60 Anti-glomerular basement membrane disease. Light microscopy shows focal necrotising glomerulitis with a small crescent. (*H&E x308.*)

6.59 Anti-glomerular basement membrane disease in a patient with renal failure, proteinuria and haematuria. Immuno-fluorescence microscopy of the renal biopsy shows IgG distributed in a linear pattern along the capillary loops. The serum was positive for anti-glomerular basement membrane antibody.

Renal vasculitides

The renal vasculitides should be suspected in patients with symptoms and signs of multisystem disease in addition to renal disease. The clinical features depend to some extent on the type of vasculitis. Weight loss, anaemia, malaise, fever, high ESR and raised C-reactive protein are found in most cases. Peak incidence is in the middle-aged or elderly and patients are more often male. The more common forms of renal vasculitis can be conveniently classified according to the size of the vessels involved, the presence or absence of granulomata, and whether there is evidence of either gastrointestinal or respiratory tract disease (**Table 6.8**). Churg–Strauss syndrome (allergic granulomatosis, p. 193) is relatively rare, and renal disease is usually associated with asthma and eosinophilia. Evidence of vasculitis may also be found histologically in patients with severe renal disease caused by systemic lupus erythematosus or Henoch–Schönlein disease.

Table 6.8 Classification of renal vasculitides.

| | Vessel size involved | | |
	Medium	Small	
Granulomata absent	Polyarteritis nodosa Kawasaki disease	Microscopic polyarteritis Henoch–Schönlein disease SLE	Gastrointestinal involvement common
Granulomata present	Churg–Strauss syndrome	Wegener's granulomatosis	Respiratory involvement common

Polyarteritis nodosa

In polyarteritis nodosa (classical polyarteritis), there is segmental necrosis and fibrinoid change within the walls of medium-sized arteries, often associated with intraluminal thrombosis (**6.61**). Ischaemia distal to occluded vessels may produce infarcts in virtually any organ. The clinical features depend on the extent and location of the lesions (*see* p. 148). Mesenteric, splenic, myocardial, cerebral or renal infarction are common modes of acute presentation. Renal infarcts, often multiple, may lead to the development of loin pain, macroscopic haematuria and hypertension. The diagnosis is best confirmed by selective renal arteriography which may show both aneurysms of the intra-renal vessels and renal infarcts (**6.62**). The prognosis without treatment is poor, and less than half of untreated patients survive more than one year. Treatment with high doses of prednisolone and cyclophosphamide produces rapid symptomatic improvement and appears to improve patient survival.

6.61

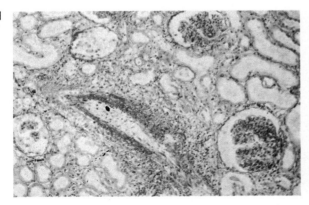

6.61 Polyarteritis nodosa. There is fibrinoid necrosis (stained red) of an interlobular artery. The glomeruli are usually normal outside the areas of renal infarction.

6.62 Polyarteritis nodosa. A selective left renal arteriogram shows aneurysms of the intra-renal vessels (small arrows) and subcapsular renal infarcts (large arrows).

6.62

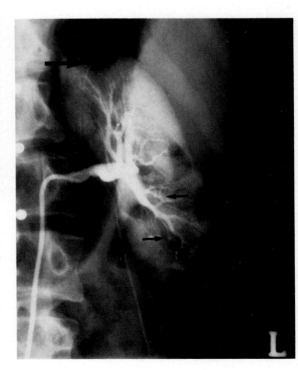

Microscopic polyarteritis

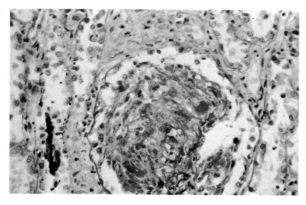

6.63 Microscopic polyarteritis. There is focal fibrinoid necrosis (red) and proliferative change in a glomerulus (*MSB x330*).

Microscopic polyarteritis (hypersensitivity angiitis) involves mainly the arterioles and capillaries. Many organs may be involved, but the kidneys, skin and lungs are most often affected. Patients with renal disease commonly present with rapidly progressive renal failure associated with microscopic haematuria and proteinuria. Serological investigations may show positive titres for rheumatoid factor and antinuclear factor in up to one-third of patients. Serum from patients with microscopic polyarteritis may also be positive for anti-neutrophil cytoplasmic antibody (ANCA), showing a perinuclear staining pattern. Renal biopsy shows diffuse proliferation and focal fibrinoid necrosis in the glomeruli (**6.63**), often associated with crescent formation. Electron and immunofluorescence microscopy usually show absence of deposits. Arteriolitis or capillaritis is seen in only a minority of renal biopsies, but may be demonstrated on biopsy of skin lesions. Prognosis is poor without treatment and is worst in patients who are already oliguric at presentation, or who have more than 70% crescent formation in the glomeruli on renal biopsy. Treatment with pulsed intravenous methylprednisolone, oral prednisolone and cyclophosphamide has significantly improved both patient and renal survival. Some centres also perform short-term daily plasma exchange in patients who are already dialysis-dependent when therapy is started.

Wegener's granulomatosis

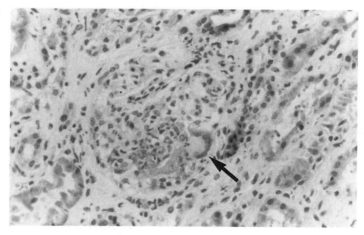

6.64 Wegener's granulomatosis. Renal biopsy showing focal necrosis in the glomerulus, associated with a small granuloma including a Langhan's type giant cell (arrowed) (*H&E x330*).

The presence of nasal symptoms, haemoptysis, pleurisy or deafness combined with renal disease is highly suggestive of Wegener's granulomatosis (*see* p. 149, 193). In many cases renal involvement is detected only during the course of investigation of either the respiratory tract or ear and nasal symptoms. Renal disease in this disorder commonly presents as rapidly progressive renal failure associated with haematuria and proteinuria. Serum is usually positive for anti-neutrophil cytoplasmic antibody (ANCA) and the diagnosis can be confirmed by nasal mucosa or renal biopsy. Renal biopsy may show similar histological appearances to microscopic polyarteritis, with features of necrotising glomerulitis, crescent formation and arteritis. Granulomata are present only in the minority of renal biopsy specimens (**6.64**), but may be found on biopsy of the nasal mucosa. Indirect immunofluorescence microscopy for ANCA shows a cytoplasmic pattern in Wegener's granulomatosis. This test may prove helpful in differentiating Wegener's from microscopic polyarteritis. Patient and renal survival in this condition have improved considerably since introduction of treatment with pulsed methylprednisolone, cyclophosphamide and prednisolone. Long-term immunosuppression with cyclophosphamide or azathioprine is required, since clinical relapse is common on withdrawing cytotoxic agents.

Renal systemic lupus erythematosus

Renal involvement is evident in up to 75% of patients with other features of SLE (*see* p. 142), and some patients may present with renal disease before the onset of extrarenal symptoms of SLE. The severity of renal disease varies greatly; some patients may have only asymptomatic proteinuria or microscopic haematuria, while others may develop nephrotic syndrome or rapidly progressive renal failure. The diagnosis is confirmed serologically by the presence of serum antibodies to double-stranded DNA and a reduced concentration of C3 in the serum.

Several histological types of renal disease are evident on renal biopsy. Mesangial proliferative and membranous glomerulonephritis in SLE patients have clinical and histological features akin to idiopathic types of these disorders (p. 282, 284).

SLE patients with nephrotic syndrome or renal failure often have a diffuse proliferative glomerulonephritis (6.65) with subepithelial, intramembranous and subendothelial deposits on electron microscopy (6.66) and peripheral deposition of IgG and complement components on immunofluorescence microscopy. Patients with this form of glomerulonephritis who have more severe renal impairment may also show evidence of crescent formation (6.67), vasculitis and interstitial fibrosis on renal biopsy.

Treatment depends on the severity of renal disease and the histological findings on renal biopsy. Patients with mesangial proliferative glomerulonephritis usually have mild renal disease, and treatment is required only for extrarenal involvement. Patients with membranous glomerulonephritis often improve with prednisolone alone, and the prognosis for renal function is good. Evolution to end-stage renal failure is relatively common in diffuse proliferative glomerulonephritis, and treatment with azathioprine or cyclophosphamide in addition to prednisolone is usually necessary. Female patients with SLE should be warned that renal function may worsen with use of the oral contraceptive pill or post-partum.

6.65

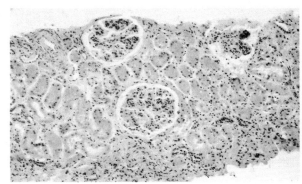

6.65 Systemic lupus erythematosus. This renal biopsy shows proliferative changes within three glomeruli (*H&E x 143*).

6.66

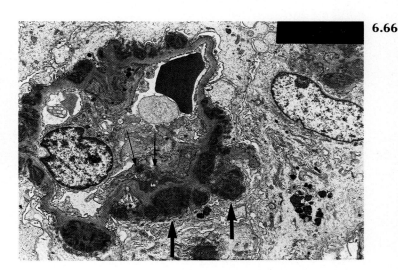

6.66 Systemic lupus erythematosus with the nephrotic syndrome. This electron micrograph shows both subendothelial deposits (small arrows) and subepithelial deposits (large arrows). The subepithelial deposits show classical 'fingerprinting'. (Magnification *x 5,200.*)

6.67

6.67 Systemic lupus erythematosus. This renal biopsy shows proliferative change and crescent formation in both glomeruli (*HV x110*).

Renal amyloidosis

The most common mode of presentation of amyloidosis in the kidney is the nephrotic syndrome associated with renal failure. Even in advanced renal failure, the kidneys may remain relatively large because of the deposition of amyloid. Clinically-evident renal disease is more frequent in primary than secondary amyloidosis. Congestive cardiomyopathy, hepatosplenomegaly, peripheral neuropathy and malabsorption may result from systemic deposition of amyloid.

At the ultrastructural level, amyloid consists of protein fibrils and a glycoprotein known as amyloid P component. Two forms of fibril protein are found: amyloid light-chain (AL) proteins are found in myeloma-associated and primary amyloidosis; and amyloid A (AA) fibril proteins are found in amyloidosis secondary to chronic infections, rheumatoid arthritis or familial Mediterranean fever. Rectal or renal biopsy confirms the diagnosis. Renal biopsy sections stained with Congo Red show pink-red deposition within the glomeruli and blood vessel walls (**6.68**), which under polarised light exhibits apple-green birefringence (**6.69**). Electron microscopy of the amyloid deposits shows a characteristic arrangement of fibrils, and immunofluorescence microscopy for immunoglobulin and complement is negative. Monoclonal antibodies can be used to differentiate amyloid light-chain and amyloid A proteins.

There is no specific treatment for amyloidosis, although renal function may stabilise following chemotherapy in patients with myeloma-associated amyloidosis, or colchicine in patients with familial Mediterranean fever. The prognosis for renal function in most cases is poor, and more than 50% of patients with biopsy-proven amyloidosis reach end-stage renal failure within one year.

6.68

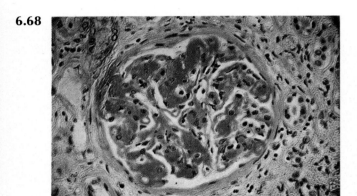

6.68 Renal amyloidosis. The glomerulus shows amyloid deposition, stained by Congo Red, in the glomerular capillaries (*x330*).

6.69

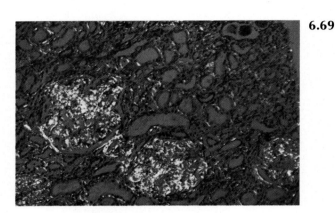

6.69 Renal amyloidosis. This Congo Red stained renal biopsy has been examined by polarised light to show the apple-green birefringence caused by amyloid deposition within the glomeruli and around the tubules (*x198*).

Diabetic nephropathy

Renal disease is evident in around 40% of patients 20 years after developing insulin-dependent diabetes mellitus (IDDM, *see* p. 327) and, until recently, was a major cause of death in diabetic patients. The aetiology of diabetic nephropathy is multifactorial; both metabolic and genetic factors appear to be important, since more than 40% of patients with IDDM do not develop microvasculopathy in spite of the presence of long-term hyperglycaemia. Renal involvement in IDDM usually evolves through a number of stages:

- **Stage I.** At diagnosis, the glomerular filtration rate is increased, because of poor metabolic control.
- **Stage II.** With improved glycaemic control, renal function remains within the normal range, and urinary albumin excretion (UAE) is normal.
- **Stage III.** Within the first 10 years after onset of diabetes, a proportion of patients develop microalbuminuria, defined as a persistent elevation in the urinary albumin excretion rate to <20 μg/min but without evidence of proteinuria on urinalysis.
- **Stage IV.** Most patients with microalbuminuria progress to overt nephropathy, which is characterised by the onset of clinical proteinuria and hypertension and is usually associated with retinopathy. The nephrotic syndrome commonly develops at this stage.
- **Stage V.** Renal impairment from Stage IV almost invariably progresses to end-stage renal failure.

The evolution of renal disease in non-insulin dependent diabetes mellitus (NIDDM) is less well defined, because of difficulty in ascertaining the exact onset of diabetes in this group.

Patients with suggestive clinical features and associated retinopathy are usually assumed to have diabetic nephropathy without performing a renal biopsy. Renal biopsy is performed only if renal disease unrelated to diabetes is suspected. The most common feature on renal biopsy is diffuse glomerulosclerosis (**6.70**) which may be associated with the classical lesions of diabetic nephropathy (**6.71**, **6.72**). Electron microscopy in diabetic nephropathy shows thickening of the glomerular membrane in all patients. It is important to exclude other urological diseases associated with diabetes, such as renal papillary necrosis (**6.73**), urinary tract infection, perinephric abscess/pyonephrosis and neurogenic bladder.

Progression of renal failure in patients with overt proteinuria can be retarded by achieving good control of hypertension, but the benefits of good glycaemic control and low-protein diets in this group remain to be confirmed. The efficacy of maintenance of normal blood pressure levels and optimal glycaemic control are currently undergoing assessment in patients with microalbuminuria. Early aggressive control of blood pressure, using angiotensin-converting enzyme inhibitors, has shown a reduction in microalbuminuria in patients with incipient nephropathy, and a decrease in proteinuria and improvement in renal function in patients with clinical nephropathy in preliminary trials. These therapeutic strategies, introduced at an early stage of diabetic nephropathy, may help prevent progression of renal failure in future.

Once chronic renal failure develops, patients almost inevitably require renal replacement therapy, unless reversible factors such as urinary tract infection or obstruction are present. Continuous ambulatory peritoneal dialysis has been preferred to haemodialysis for most diabetic patients, since it provides steady-state control of biochemistry and fluid balance, stable blood pressure, and avoids the need for either vascular access or heparin. Quality of life and patient survival are better with renal transplantation than with either mode of dialysis.

6.70

6.70 Diffuse glomerulosclerosis is the most common glomerular lesion in diabetic nephropathy. There is generalised thickening of the capillary walls throughout the glomerular lobules (*MSB x250*).

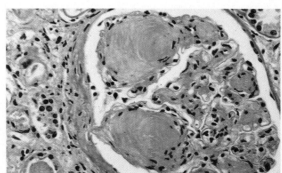

6.71

6.71 Kimmelstiel–Wilson nodules are the classic lesions of diabetic nephropathy. Their presence is virtually diagnostic of diabetes mellitus. Note the nodular intercapillary glomerulosclerosis (*MS x250*).

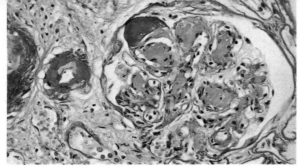

6.72 Glomerulus in diabetes showing a fibrin cap lesion (red) associated with Kimmelstiel–Wilson nodules (blue). The afferent arteriole has been infiltrated with hyaline (*MS x 330*).

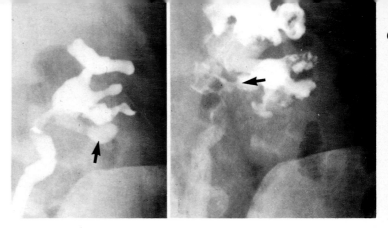

6.73 Renal papillary necrosis may be a feature of diabetic renal disease. The retrograde pyelogram on the left shows marked calyceal clubbing and distortion. One month later (right) there has been sloughing of calyceal tissue into the renal pelvis.

Tubulointerstitial diseases

This generic term refers to all diseases of the interstitium and tubules with little or no evidence of concomitant glomerular disease.

Acute interstitial nephritis

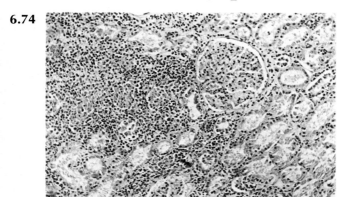

Acute interstitial nephritis frequently presents as acute renal failure and may be idiopathic, associated with infection or drug-induced (antibiotics, non-steroidal anti-inflammatory drugs, diuretics). Acute renal failure is frequently accompanied by the presence of fever, rash, eosinophilia, non-nephrotic range proteinuria and microhaematuria. On renal biopsy, there is interstitial infiltration with lymphocytes, plasma cells, polymorphs and eosinophils; interstitial oedema; and variable degrees of damage to the renal tubules (**6.74**). Renal function usually recovers on withdrawal of the putative drug or treatment of the associated infection. Treatment with prednisolone induces recovery of renal function in the idiopathic cases.

6.74 Acute interstitial nephritis. This renal biopsy shows interstitial oedema and infiltration with lymphocytes, plasma cells and polymorphs, without evidence of concomitant glomerular disease (*H&E x80*).

Chronic interstitial nephritis

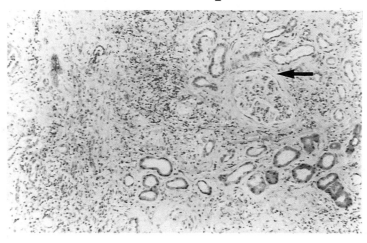

Chronic interstitial nephritis usually presents with chronic renal failure associated with non-nephrotic range proteinuria and evidence of tubular dysfunction. Polyuria, renal salt wasting, hypokalaemia and renal tubular acidosis are common, but there may be a surprising lack of symptoms even in the presence of severely impaired renal function. Renal biopsy in long-standing cases shows interstitial fibrosis, tubular atrophy and a variable degree of interstitial infiltration (**6.75**). A search for an underlying cause may reveal analgesic abuse, chronic pyelonephritis, radiation nephritis, Sjögren's syndrome, gout, sickle cell disease or heavy metal exposure, but many cases are idiopathic. Control of fluid and electrolyte balance may require sodium, potassium or bicarbonate supplementation.

6.75 Chronic interstitial nephritis. The renal biopsy shows a diffuse lymphocytic infiltrate and fibrosis in the interstitium with focal tubular atrophy and periglomerular scarring (arrow) (*H&E × 80*).

Analgesic nephropathy

Analgesic nephropathy results from the long-term ingestion of large quantities of analgesic drugs, such as phenacetin combined with aspirin. Analgesic abuse is a common cause of chronic renal failure in Australia and Switzerland, and is more common in women than men. Tubulointerstitial damage occurs along with papillary necrosis. Patients may present with chronic renal failure, sterile pyuria, haematuria, renal colic resulting from ureteric obstruction by a fragment of necrotic tissue, or hypertension. Anaemia is often more severe than expected for the degree of chronic renal impairment. On IVU, the kidneys are usually bilaterally shrunken with deformed calyces and the appearance of a 'ring sign' on the pyelogram, representing a sloughed papilla within a dilated calyx, is typical of this disorder (6.76). The main therapeutic endeavour is in convincing the patient to stop ingesting analgesics, since continued intake invariably leads to end-stage renal failure.

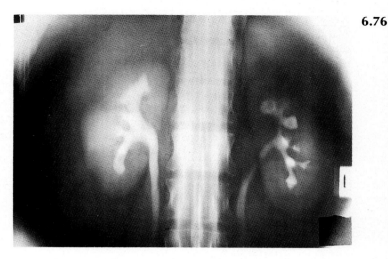

6.76 Analgesic nephropathy. This IVU shows bilaterally shrunken kidneys with typical calyceal distortions—the classic 'ring sign' plus the appearance of 'horns' and 'egg in cup'.

Myeloma kidney

Myeloma kidney is the most common cause of renal failure in patients with multiple myeloma (*see* p. 465), and is more frequent in patients with Bence–Jones proteinuria. Renal failure in such patients is almost invariably associated with anaemia, and the diagnosis can usually be established by serum and urine electrophoresis, bone marrow examination and skeletal survey. Histologically, myeloma kidney is characterised by eosinophilic intraluminal casts, atrophic renal tubules and multinucleated giant cells within the tubule walls or interstitium (6.77). Renal failure in myeloma may also be caused by AL amyloidosis, light-chain nephropathy, hypercalcaemia, hyperuricaemia, or it may follow dehydration or intravenous urography. Management of renal impairment in myeloma includes maintaining hydration, bicarbonate supplementation to improve solubility of light chains in the urine, and allopurinol to prevent hyperuricaemia following chemotherapy.

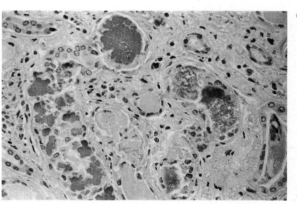

6.77 Myeloma kidney. There are prominent casts in the renal tubules, and a giant cell reaction is seen (bottom right) (*MSB x330*).

Renal tubular disorders

Most patients with renal disease have some abnormality in renal tubular function, but other manifestations of renal disease usually dominate the clinical picture. In some patients, however, renal tubular dysfunction occurs in isolation and results in clinical disorder.

There are many rare inherited and acquired disorders of renal tubular function. Their classification and management is a specialised field. The main categories of renal tubular disorders are summarised in **Table 6.9**.

Table 6.9 Renal tubular disorders: a simplified classification.

Renal glycosuria
Aminoaciduria
    Single, e.g. cystinuria
    Multiple
Phosphate transport defects
Multiple tubular defects (Fanconi syndrome)
    Inherited
    Acquired
Renal tubular acidosis
    Type I (distal)
    Type II (proximal)
    Type IV (distal with hyperkalaemia and hyperchloraemia)
Salt-losing nephropathy
Nephrogenic diabetes insipidus

Hypertension and the kidney

Renal hypertension

Renal disease is the most common cause of secondary hypertension and should be excluded in all young hypertensive patients (*see also* p. 250). Causes of renal-mediated hypertension can be classified into vascular diseases and parenchymal diseases (**Table 6.10**).

The clinical features associated with hypertension depend on the underlying disease. Renal artery stenosis may be caused by atheroma or fibromuscular hyperplasia. Atheromatous renal artery stenosis should be suspected in patients with severe hypertension presenting in middle-age or later without other evidence of renal disease. Often these patients are heavy smokers and there is evidence of widespread atherosclerosis. Fibromuscular hyperplasia is more common in women, appears most often in the third or fourth decades, and is frequently bilateral. A bruit may be heard over the flank, and biochemical investigation often reveals evidence of secondary hyperaldosteronism. Screening for unilateral renal artery stenosis is best performed by a DTPA isotope renogram, before and after captopril. The renogram shows delayed perfusion, delayed uptake, and a reduced rate of excretion of isotope from the affected kidney, which is further accentuated following captopril. Identification of renal artery stenosis can then be accomplished by arteriography (**6.19, 6.78**). Hypertension caused by fibromuscular disease is cured in more than 90% of patients after renovascular surgery. In patients with atherosclerotic disease, the failure rate following either surgery or angioplasty is much higher and corrective procedures are often restricted to patients who have severe renal failure or poorly controlled hypertension on medical therapy.

Renal disease may ultimately develop in about half of patients with systemic sclerosis (*see* p. 144), often with the sudden onset of severe hypertension and progression to end-stage renal failure within months. Renal biopsy shows gross intimal thickening and reduction in the lumen of the interlobular arteries. Control of hypertension may be difficult and, if renal failure develops, recovery of renal function is unlikely.

The other causes of renal hypertension are described elsewhere in this chapter.

Table 6.10 Causes of renal hypertension.

Vascular diseases
Atheromatous renal artery stenosis
Fibromuscular renal artery hyperplasia
Renal infarction
Renal vasculitis
Systemic sclerosis

Parenchymal diseases
Glomerulonephritis
Chronic pyelonephritis
Polycystic kidney disease
Multisystem disease
Hydronephrosis

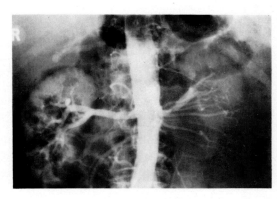

6.78

6.78 Renal artery stenosis. There is an atheromatous stricture of the left renal artery with slight post-stenotic dilatation and a reduction in left renal size.

Hypertensive nephropathy

In hypertensive nephropathy, renal failure results from inadequately treated hypertension in the absence of primary renal disease. Long-standing moderate hypertension in itself can lead to hyaline thickening of the intra-renal arterial walls, patchy ischaemic atrophy and glomerulosclerosis. Patients with benign hypertensive nephrosclerosis usually present with chronic renal failure and mild proteinuria, without haematuria or other evidence of glomerulonephritis. Renal impairment often stabilises if adequate, long-term control of hypertension is achieved.

Accelerated nephrosclerosis is a dramatic complication of malignant hypertension, which commonly caused progressive or acute renal failure before effective antihypertensive drugs were available. The two essential clinical features are the presence of severe hypertension and grade IV retinopathy (**5.120**). Cardiac failure, hypertensive encephalopathy, renal failure, secondary hyperaldosteronism and microangiopathic haemolytic anaemia may accompany the onset of malignant hypertension. The malignant phase may complicate essential and all forms of secondary hypertension. Renal biopsy may be required to determine whether there is underlying renal disease or whether renal failure is a direct consequence of severe hypertension. The histological features of malignant hypertension are fibrinoid necrosis of the afferent arterioles, and endarteritis of the interlobular and arcuate arteries which result in ischaemic atrophy or infarction distal to the abnormal vessels (**6.79**).

High blood pressure should be lowered gradually, to lessen the risk of a sudden drop in blood pressure either precipitating cerebral infarction or worsening renal function. In many patients, renal function may recover or at least stabilise after blood pressure is controlled and the prognosis depends on whether or not there are cardiac or cerebral complications.

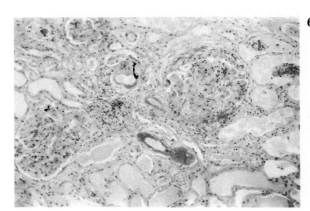

6.79

6.79 Malignant hypertension. The renal biopsy shows fibrinoid necrosis in the arterial and glomerular capillaries (red) and haemorrhage into the renal tubules (yellow) (*MSB x132*).

Familial disorders

There are many inherited disorders of renal structure and function. Some gross structural disorders, such as unilateral or bilateral duplex kidneys and ureters or a single horseshoe kidney, may predispose patients to ureteric reflux or obstruction and to recurrent urinary tract infections, with a long-term risk of renal failure. Others, such as polycystic kidneys, may lead more directly to renal failure, by reducing the volume of functional renal tissue.

Inherited disorders may also cause both glomerular disease and tubular disorders.

Two inherited conditions are particularly important causes of chronic renal failure: adult polycystic kidney disease and Alport's syndrome

Adult polycystic kidney disease

6.80

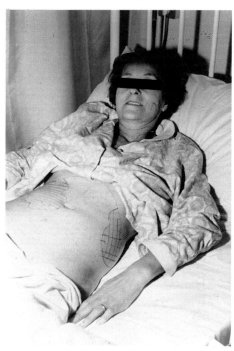

6.80 Adult polycystic kidney disease. The kidneys are huge and easily palpable as the skin markings show. Cysts are often also present in the liver and pancreas.

Adult-type polycystic kidney disease may be detected during the investigation of hypertension, loin pain or haematuria in young adults. Patients without these symptoms may not present until they develop chronic renal failure when middle-aged or older. The condition is inherited as an autosomal dominant with high penetrance, and many patients are now diagnosed during screening of the proband's family. The kidneys are almost invariably symmetrically enlarged because of the presence of multiple cysts. They may often be palpable clinically (**6.80**) and the diagnosis is best confirmed by ultrasound (**6.12**), or by CT scan (**6.21, 9.42**), both of which may also demonstrate cysts in the liver and pancreas. Intravenous urogram may show characteristic stretching and distortion of the calyces but is a less sensitive test than ultrasound. Haemorrhage or infection in a cyst, haematuria leading to clot colic, urinary tract infection and renal calculi are not uncommon. Hypertension develops in more than 75% of patients, and renal function usually declines slowly until end-stage renal failure is reached from middle-age onwards. Patients with end-stage renal failure caused by adult polycystic kidney disease, tend to be less anaemic than patients with renal failure resulting from other disorders. Genetic counselling is an important aspect of patient management, especially in families undergoing screening. Detection of carriers has now become possible with the availability of a gene probe. The enlargement of the kidneys does not usually lead to problems in performing peritoneal dialysis or renal transplantation.

Alport's syndrome

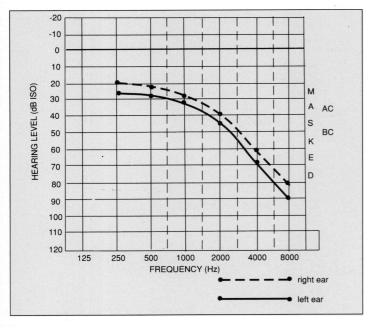

6.81 Alport's syndrome. Audiogram showing bilateral high-frequency nerve deafness. Lens abnormalities and deafness often co-exist with renal failure in patients with Alport's syndrome.

Alport's syndrome is characterised by hereditary glomerulo-nephritis, nerve deafness (**6.81**) and, in some cases eye abnormalities (spherophakia, cataracts). Inheritance is autosomal dominant, but males are more severely affected. It is uncommon for females to be symptomatic before the age of 40, while most males have reached terminal renal failure by the age of 30. Most male patients present with recurrent or persistent haematuria in childhood, non-nephrotic range proteinuria, hypertension and chronic renal failure. Renal biopsy shows a proliferative glomerulonephritis which on electron microscopy shows characteristic splitting and lamellation of the glomerular basement membrane. Renal failure is uncommon in women, but affected males usually require renal replacement therapy when adolescents or young adults.

Urinary tract infection

Urinary tract infection (UTI) is defined as the presence of micro-organisms within the urinary tract with or without symptoms or signs of inflammation.
Bacteriuria is considered significant if the numbers of bacteria in urine voided per urethram exceed 100,000 colony-forming units/ml in a properly collected specimen. Dip slide urine culture (**6.11**) should be performed if delay is anticipated in a mid-stream urine specimen reaching the laboratory. A suprapubic aspiration may be needed to obtain a urine sample in infants, and any growth of bacteria from a suprapubic specimen of urine signifies the presence of infection.

Table 6.11 Organisms which commonly cause UTI.

E. coli
Klebsiella sp.
Proteus sp.
Streptococcus faecalis
Pseudomonas aeruginosa
Coagulase-negative *Staphylococcus*
Staph. aureus
Corynebacterium sp.

The urinary tract may also be infected by *Mycobacterium tuberculosis* (p. 298) and by the trematode *Schistosoma haematobium* (p. 77).

The organisms which commonly cause UTI are listed in **Table 6.11**.

Urinary tract infection is important because of its frequency and its association with reflux nephropathy. In females, the incidence of urinary tract infection increases with age and approximately 5% of adult women will, at some time, develop infection. In males, there is a high incidence in the neonatal period, associated with developmental anomalies of the lower urinary tract, a low incidence in childhood and adult life, and an increase with advancing age. Investigation of the structure of the urinary tract is indicated in children and adult males found to have a symptomatic or asymptomatic urinary tract infection. Adult women with recurrent infection also merit investigation (**6.82**).

Urinary tract infection is usually adequately treated with a course of antibiotics but long-term prophylaxis may be required in patients with structural abnormalities or recurrent infections.

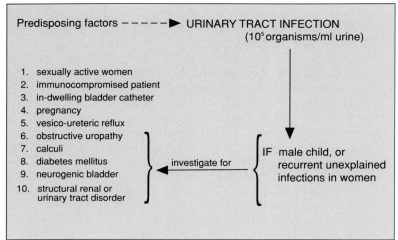

6.82 Predisposing factors in urinary tract infection.

Chronic pyelonephritis (reflux nephropathy)

Chronic interstitial nephritis which is thought to result from bacterial infection of the kidney has been termed chronic pyelonephritis. It may occur in patients with predisposing urological abnormalities (vesico-ureteric reflux, obstruction or neurogenic bladder) or in patients with apparently normal urinary tracts. The pathogenesis of pyelonephritic renal scarring in children is attributed to both parenchymal damage and impaired renal growth, which result from intra-renal reflux of infected urine. A history of recurrent urinary tract infection during childhood and evidence of vesico-ureteric reflux are therefore risk factors for the development of focal cortical scars.

During micturating cystography, reflux of contrast from the bladder may be limited to the ureter (Grade I), reach the kidney but not distend the calyces (Grade II) or reach the kidney and cause calyceal distension (Grade III) (**6.22, 6.83**). Vesico-ureteric reflux is present in 85% of patients with coarse scarred kidneys and 35% of children with symptomatic urinary tract infections.

Reimplantation of the ureters to correct reflux and long-term antibiotic prophylaxis to prevent infection have been the main interventions utilised to try and prevent development of chronic pyelonephritis in children, but studies have shown no proven benefit from operative treatment of reflux when compared to antibiotic prophylaxis alone. Surgery to correct reflux is therefore now reserved for patients who have urinary infection despite antibiotic prophylaxis. Further renal scarring is unlikely after 7 years of age, so children with vesico-ureteric reflux and urinary tract infections are often treated with prophylactic antibiotics until they reach this age and are encouraged to keep up a liberal fluid intake and to practise double voiding.

Chronic pyelonephritis may be unilateral or bilateral and the characteristic appearance on IVU is clubbing of the calyces with overlying cortical scars, most commonly in the upper poles but ultimately generalised (**6.15, 6.84**). Scarring of the renal outline may also be demonstrated by DMSA isotope scan, and unilateral scarring is not uncommon (**6.23**). Chronic pyelonephritis may be detected during the investigation of patients with non-specific ill-health, recurrent urinary tract infections, hypertension or chronic renal failure. End-stage renal failure may develop in patients with bilateral renal scarring (**6.31**), even when hypertension is treated and further UTI prevented.

Renal tuberculosis is uncommon, but should be considered in all patients with sterile pyuria. The most common symptoms are fever, dysuria, haematuria, weight loss and general malaise (*see* p. 46 for a general account of tuberculosis). At least three early-morning urine samples should be sent for culture of *Mycobacterium tuberculosis* and IVU may show calyceal changes (**6.85**), hydronephrosis, a contracted bladder or calcification at any point in the renal tract (**6.86**). Treatment with antituberculous drugs should continue for at least six months and surgery may be required in some cases to relieve obstruction or to remove a non-functioning kidney.

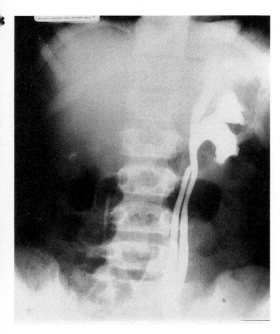

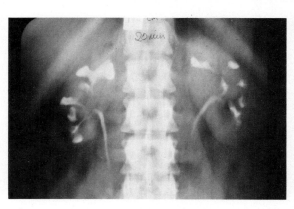

6.84 Bilateral chronic pyelonephritis. The IVU shows shrunken kidneys with gross calyceal clubbing and adjacent cortical scarring.

6.83 Unilateral Grade III vesicoureteric reflux with left bifid ureters, demonstrated by micturating cystogram.

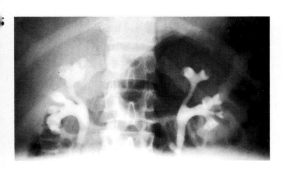

6.85 Renal tuberculosis affecting the right kidney. An initial minor lesion in the upper pole has become more invasive, and the disease has spread to affect more than one calyx, with irregularity and papillary cavitation.

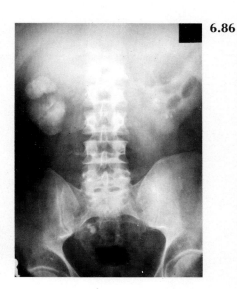

6.86 Renal tuberculosis may lead to progressive renal destruction and calcification, as here, where two-thirds of the right kidney has been destroyed and calcified.

Obstructive uropathy

Obstruction to the flow of urine results in increased urinary tract pressure and is a common cause of acute or chronic renal failure. Early relief of obstruction can allow renal function to recover completely, but chronic obstruction may produce cortical atrophy and permanent renal dysfunction. Obstructive uropathy should therefore be excluded promptly in all patients with acute or chronic renal failure of no established cause. Obstruction to urine flow may result from intrinsic or extrinsic mechanical blockade at any level of the urinary tract from the renal calyces to the external urethral meatus. Obstruction at or below the level of the bladder usually produces bilateral dilatation of the ureter (hydro-ureter) and renal pelvis and calyces (hydronephrosis), while obstruction may be unilateral if the site of blockage is above the level of the bladder. Mechanical causes of obstruction may be congenital (posterior urethral valves, ureterocele or pelvi-ureteric stricture), acquired intrinsic defects (calculi, tumour, blood clot, sloughed papilla, stricture) or extrinsic defects (retroperitoneal fibrosis, fibroids, retroperitoneal or pelvic tumour). Functional impairment of urinary flow, caused by neurogenic bladder, may also cause obstruction.

Acute obstruction may present with loin or suprapubic pain, renal colic, oliguria or anuria. Chronic obstruction, on the other hand, may progress insidiously, but on direct questioning patients often admit to having polyuria and nocturia as a result of impaired renal concentrating ability. Hesitancy, post-voiding dribbling, urinary frequency and overflow incontinence are common in patients with obstruction at or below the level of the bladder. The possibility of obstructive uropathy should always be considered in patients with unexplained urinary tract infection or calculi. Dilatation of the urinary tract may be demonstrated by ultrasound (**6.87, 6.88**) and functional obstruction confirmed by DTPA renography (**6.24**). Intravenous urography can be used to demonstrate obstruction anatomically and functionally, provided the patient does not have significant renal failure (**6.16, 6.17**), and retrograde pyelography may be needed in some cases (**6.89, 6.90**).

Treatment depends on the site of obstruction and the underlying cause. The renal prognosis following relief of obstruction depends largely upon the degree of irreversible renal damage that has already occurred. Pre-renal failure may develop because of a post-obstructive diuresis, which not uncommonly occurs after relief of bilateral urinary tract obstruction. Such patients may require intravenous fluids temporarily.

6.87

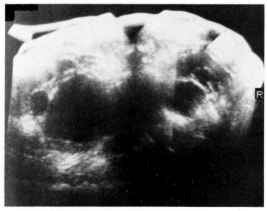

6.87, 6.88 Bilateral hydronephrosis demonstrated by ultrasound. The normal renal outlines are distorted by the dilated fluid-filled renal pelves.

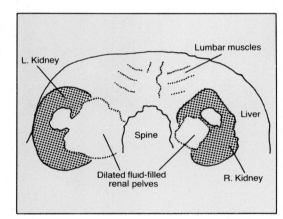

6.89

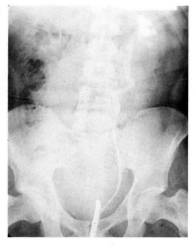

6.89, 6.90 Retroperitoneal fibrosis. This condition commonly affects both ureters, but it may be unilateral. In this patient, the left retrograde ureterogram (**6.88**) shows that retroperitoneal fibrosis has obstructed and distorted the left ureter and caused a left hydronephrosis; while the right retrograde ureterogram and pyelogram are normal (**6.90**).

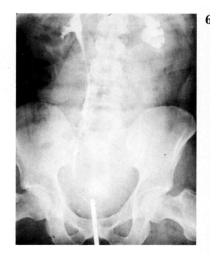

Renal calculi

Renal calculi are relatively common, affecting 1–5% of the population; they are most common in warm, dry countries and are composed of a mixture of chemicals, most commonly calcium oxalate alone or in combination with hydroxyapatite or calcium phosphate. Rarely, they may contain only uric acid or cystine. (Uric acid stones are radio-opaque.) About 20–40% of patients with calcium-containing stones have hypercalciuria and a small number have hypercalcaemia which should be investigated and treated (*see* p. 154). In the others, a search should be made for a cause of increased calcium absorption, e.g. vitamin D intoxication or renal tubular acidosis.

Clinical presentation is often dramatic, with the sudden onset of acute colicky pain resulting from impaction of the stone in the kidney, the ureter, bladder or urethra. There may also be haematuria and obstruction to urine flow. Passage of the stone produces instant relief, but if it obstructs either ureter or urethra it may cause progressive dull back pain. Infection is common (*see* p. 297) and may produce a pyonephrosis when combined with obstruction.

The diagnosis is usually suggested clinically and is confirmed by a plain X-ray of the abdomen (**6.14, 6.91, 6.92, 6.93**), an IVU (**6.94**), ultrasound or retrograde pyelography.

Urine should be cultured and examined microscopically for blood. Treatment of the pain is the over-riding necessity and an antispasmodic may be of value. Stones less than 5 mm will usually pass spontaneously. Surgical intervention or lithotripsy may be required for larger stones. Urinary tract infection requires an appropriate antibiotic.

Renal and urinary tract calcification may occur in renal tuberculosis (p. 298) and in medullary sponge kidney, a condition in which cystic change occurs in the collecting ducts in the renal papillae, with accompanying stone formation. This most commonly presents as haematuria or renal colic, or with UTI. Nephrocalcinosis, the deposition of calcium within the body of the kidneys, may also occur in conditions associated with hypercalcaemia, including sarcoidosis, hyperparathyroidism, myeloma, malignancy and Paget's disease, and in idiopathic hypercalciuria.

Bladder stones may grow to a massive size before presentation and need to be removed surgically. They may arise from stones formed in the kidneys which have migrated, from foreign bodies in the bladder (e.g. sutures) or from the same biochemical abnormalities as in renal stones.

6.91

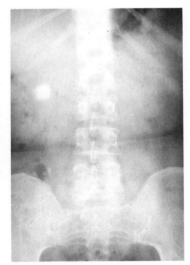

6.91 A single calculus in the renal pelvis is demonstrated on this plain (KUB) X-ray. The X-ray was performed to investigate an episode of renal colic.

6.92

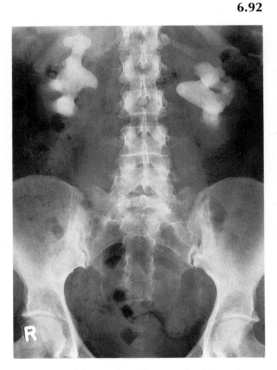

6.92 Large bilateral staghorn calculi are shown on this plain (KUB) X-ray. The patient presented with recurrent urinary infections.

6.93

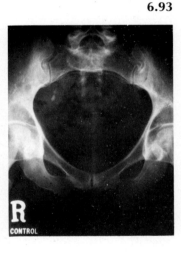

6.94

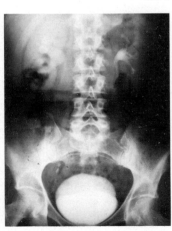

6.93, 6.94 Two small stones in the ureter are seen in **6.93**. Stones of this size may sometimes pass without symptoms or with only a transient effect, but in this patient they caused ureteric obstruction, as can be seen in the IVU (**6.94**).

Renal tumours

Neoplasms may develop at any point in the urinary tract, but they most commonly occur in the kidney or bladder and they should be excluded in all patients presenting with painless macroscopic or microscopic haematuria. Renal cell carcinoma (hypernephroma, adenocarcinoma of kidney) is the most common renal neoplasm and is of tubular epithelial origin. Patients may present with systemic symptoms (weight loss, malaise, fever) and/or urinary tract symptoms (haematuria, loin pain, abdominal mass). Renal cell carcinoma may be demonstrated by ultrasound, intravenous urography (6.95), abdominal CT scan (6.96) or renal arteriography (6.18). Metastases are common and, once the diagnosis is established, patients should be investigated to evaluate whether pulmonary (4.24), bony (3.124), hepatic (9.46) or cerebral (11.49) metastases are present. The prognosis depends largely upon the extent of tumour involvement at the time of diagnosis. The standard approach to treatment in patients without evidence of metastases is radical nephrectomy; in this group, the survival rate at 5 years approaches 65%. However, many patients have metastatic disease at the time of diagnosis and have a much poorer prognosis despite treatment with chemotherapy and radiotherapy.

Nephroblastoma (Wilms' tumour) is the second most common malignant tumour of the kidney and is the most common malignancy of the urinary tract in children, with a peak incidence between the ages of 2 and 4 years (6.97, 6.98). Aggressive treatment with nephrectomy, pre- or post-operative radiotherapy and post-operative chemotherapy have improved the prognosis and 5-year survival now exceeds 75%.

Neoplasms of the renal pelvis, ureter and bladder, derived from transitional urothelium, are relatively common and often occur or recur at multiple sites in the lower urinary tract. There is an increased incidence of bladder cancer in workers exposed to various aromatic amines employed in chemical, rubber or dye industries. Haematuria is the most common presentation and the site and extent of involvement is usually determined by a combination of cystoscopy (6.26) with biopsy, and intravenous urography (6.20). The prognosis is dependent upon the extent of local invasion and degree of anaplasia at the time of diagnosis. Treatments include cystoscopic removal, cystectomy and local radiotherapy. Patients with urothelial tumours of the renal pelvis or ureter usually require nephroureterectomy.

Diffuse infiltration of the kidneys by neoplastic cells in lymphomas or leukaemias may result in renal enlargement or renal failure. Retroperitoneal lymphoma may also cause renal failure as a result of bilateral ureteric obstruction.

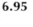

6.95

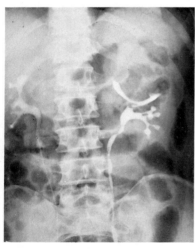

6.95 Renal cell carcinoma has caused calyceal distortion with stretching and separation of the calyces in the upper left kidney, as seen on this IVU.

6.96 Renal cell carcinoma as seen on CT scan. Compare the solid right renal tumour (arrowed) with the normal kidney seen on the left side.

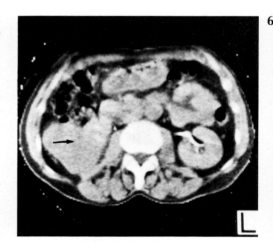

6.97

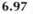

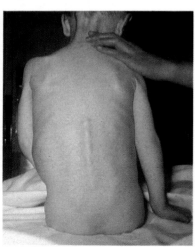

6.97 Nephroblastoma (Wilms' tumour). This 8-year-old boy had a mass in the left loin which moved on respiration and was ballotable. Its renal nature was confirmed on IVU (6.98) and a nephroblastoma was found at surgery.

6.98 Nephroblastoma (Wilms' tumour). This IVU shows a vast mass occupying the entire left loin.

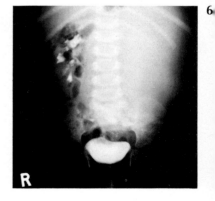

7 Endocrine, Metabolic and Nutritional Disorders

History, examination and investigation

The presentations of endocrine disease are diverse, and the findings in the history and on examination reflect this. Although multiple endocrine disorders may occur in the same patient, most have abnormalities of a single hormonal system, and the symptoms, signs and necessary investigations relate closely to those abnormalities.

A full history and examination is always advisable in any patient with suspected endocrine disorder. Common presentations that should raise the possibility of endocrine disease are listed in **Table 7.1**, and **Table 7.2** emphasises the common importance of aspects of the patient's previous medical and family history.

Necessary investigations depend upon the patient's clinical presentation and may include many different tests on blood

Table 7.1 Common presenting complaints in endocrine disease.

Body size and shape
 Short stature
 Tall stature
 Excessive weight or weight gain
 Loss of weight

'Metabolic' effects
 Tiredness
 Weakness
 Increased appetite
 Decreased appetite
 Polydipsia/thirst
 Polyuria/nocturia
 Tremor
 Palpitation
 Anxiety

Local effects
 Swelling in the neck
 Carpal tunnel syndrome
 Bone or muscle pain
 Protrusion of eyes
 Visual loss (acuity and/or fields)
 Headache

Reproduction/sex
 Loss or absence of libido
 Impotence
 Oligomenorrhoea/amenorrhoea
 Subfertility
 Galactorrhoea
 Gynaecomastia
 Delayed puberty
 Precocious puberty

Skin
 Hirsutes
 Hair thinning
 Pigmentation
 Dry skin
 Excess sweating

Table 7.2 Endocrine disease—past and family histories.

Previous medical history
 Previous pregnancies (ease of conception, postpartum haemorrhage)
 Relevant surgery (e.g. thyroidectomy, orchidopexy)
 Radiation (e.g. to neck, gonads, thyroid)
 Drug exposure (e.g. chemotherapy, sex hormones, oral contraceptives)
 In childhood, developmental milestones

Family history
Family history of:
 Autoimmune disease
 Endocrine disease
 Essential hypertension

Family details of:
 Height
 Weight
 Body habitus
 Hair growth
 Age of sexual development

and urine and imaging by radiological, nuclear or magnetic resonance techniques.

The diagnosis of endocrine diseases has been advanced by techniques which can measure low concentrations of hormones in body fluid by sensitive radiochemical means. As most hormones are produced in characteristic patterns, it is important to take appropriate samples at the relevant times, e.g. some hormones have a circadian rhythm with higher levels in the morning. Some hormones, especially the gonadotrophins, are produced intermittently. The pattern of release may vary with sex and with advancing age, with stress, diet and concurrent medication. Twenty-four-hour urine collections are of value for some hormones in measuring total output of the gland and overcoming the problems of rhythmic variations in level.

In addition to these static tests, it is often important to determine the response of a gland to stimulation and suppression.

- **Stimulation tests** assess the ability of the gland to increase its hormonal output. The response is diminished if the cells are structurally or functionally damaged.
- **Suppression tests** use the administration of purified hormone to test the negative feedback loop. Hormone production is normally suppressed in these tests, but persists where there is autonomy or a functional endocrine tumour.

Although isolated endocrine abnormalities are common, many are potentially related to abnormalities of the hypothalmic–pituitary axis, so initial investigations may lead on to a need for further tests.

Disorders of the pituitary and hypothalamus

The pituitary gland consists of an anterior and a posterior lobe. It lies at the base of the brain, in the sella turcica, within the sphenoid bone, and has a close anatomical and physiological relationship to the hypothalamus. Its anatomical relationship to the optic chiasma is important, as pituitary tumours often affect the visual fields. The hypothalamus has a major role in integrating and co-ordinating pituitary function, body temperature, water, mineral and calorie balance, and sexual and reproductive behaviour. This is achieved through the hypothalamo–hypophyseal portal system. The hypothalamus controls the secretion of the anterior pituitary hormones by secreting a number of regulatory factors (releasing or inhibitory hormones) (**Table 7.3**).

The posterior pituitary also functionally includes various hypothalamic areas. Oxytocin is released here. Antidiuretic hormone (ADH) is secreted by the supra-optic and para-ventricular nuclei, it passes down the neurohypophyseal tract to be linked with neurophysin and is stored in the posterior lobe, from where it is secreted into the general circulation.

Pituitary lesions may declare themselves by:

- Local space-occupying effects.
- Hypopituitarism.
- Hypersecretion of a pituitary hormone.
- An incidental radiological finding.

Both neuroradiological and endocrinological investigations are important in diagnosis and management.

Space-occupying effects. Large tumours commonly grow upwards, compressing the optic chiasma which is only 1 cm above the pituitary fossa (*see also* p. 491). The most common visual defects are a bitemporal upper quadrantic defect or a hemianopia as shown in 7.1. The patient may not notice the deterioration in eyesight until the central fields are affected. Expansion of the pituitary fossa is seen on a lateral skull radiograph in 90% of patients. Other important features are thinning and undercutting of the anterior and posterior clinoid processes and asymmetry of the fossa floor (7.2, 7.3). The extent of a pituitary tumour can be demonstrated by CT scan (7.4) or by magnetic resonance imaging (MRI) (7.5).

Less common effects of growth outside the pituitary fossa include:

- Diplopia (cranial nerve palsies with extra-ocular muscle dysfunction, 7.6, 11.14).
- Papilloedema (7.7) from raised intracranial pressure is very rare, as is optic atrophy from long-standing suprasellar extension with compression of the optic pathways (7.8).
- Personality changes, focal hemispheric neurological signs and epilepsy.
- Pituitary apoplexy (acute enlargement of a tumour caused by haemorrhagic infarction), resulting in depressed consciousness, sudden loss of vision, other focal signs and often meningism).

Table 7.3

Hypothalamic hormones	Pituitary hormones
Thyrotrophin releasing hormone (TRH)	Thyrotrophin (TSH) Prolactin
Gonadotrophin releasing hormone (GnRH)	Luteinising hormone (LH) Follicle stimulating hormone (FSH)
Somatostatin (GHRIH) Growth hormone releasing hormone (GHRH)	Growth hormone (GH)
Corticotrophin releasing hormone (CRH)	Corticotrophin (ACTH)
Dopamine	Prolactin

7.1

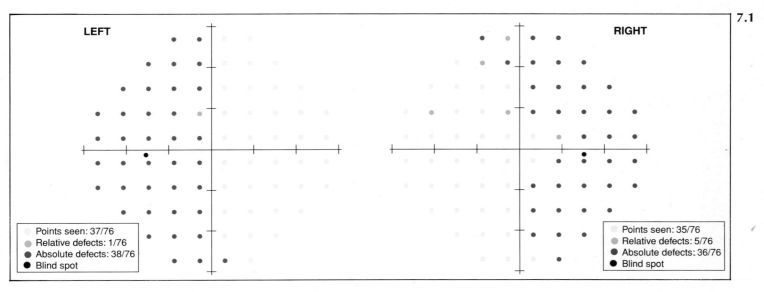

7.1 Typical visual field defects in advanced acromegaly, demonstrated using the Humphrey computer-based printout. The patient has bitemporal hemianopia as a result of compression of the optic chiasma by the enlarging pituitary tumour. In the earlier stages of tumour enlargement, asymmetric bitemporal upper quadrantic defects are typical.

7.2

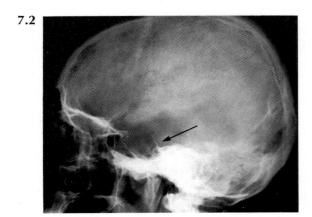

7.2 Enlargement of the pituitary fossa and virtual destruction of the posterior clinoid process (arrowed) resulting from progress of a chromophobe adenoma. The patient had a 6-year history of headache and a bitemporal visual field defect, but no clinical features of pituitary dysfunction.

7.3

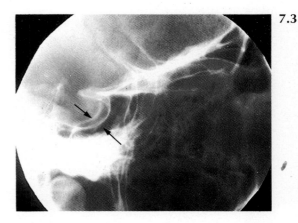

7.3 Pituitary fossa enlargement with a double floor (arrowed) on lateral X-ray. This patient had an acidophil tumour, with symptoms and signs of acromegaly.

305

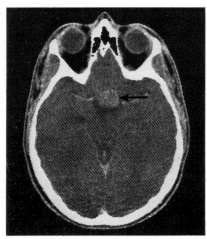

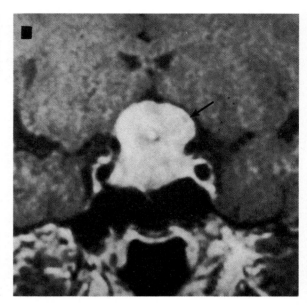

7.4 CT scan demonstrating a pituitary tumour with suprasellar extension (arrowed). This transverse cut shows the size and position of the tumour at a level at which pituitary tissue would not normally be seen.

7.5 MRI demonstration of a pituitary tumour. This view was obtained after contrast enhancement, and shows a large tumour with suprasellar extension (arrowed).

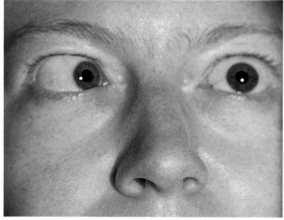

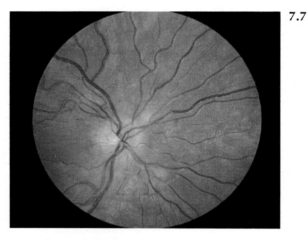

7.6 Sixth nerve palsy with lack of abduction of the right eye in a patient with a pituitary tumour. Invasion of the cavernous sinus by a pituitary tumour usually affects the sixth nerve first, because it is more medial than the third and fourth cranial nerves.

7.7 Early papilloedema in a patient with a pituitary tumour. There is hyperaemia of the optic disc, with blurring of the inferonasal margin. Papilloedema is a rare complication of pituitary tumours.

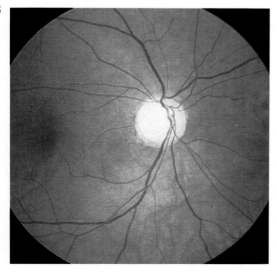

7.8 Optic atrophy in a patient with acromegaly. The flat, pale optic disc has a well-defined margin and the appearance of 'primary' optic atrophy. This type of optic atrophy results from compression of the optic pathways by the tumour, and is not a consequence of long-term papilloedema.

Hypopituitarism

Most lesions of the pituitary cause destruction of the anterior pituitary or the hypothalamus. The pattern of deficiencies depends on the nature of the lesion and its rate of progress. The clinical picture depends on the cause, the pattern of hormone loss and local effects of the pathology within the sella. Post-partum pituitary necrosis (Sheehan's syndrome, 7.9) was formerly the most common cause, but with improved obstetric practice this is now much less common. The main causes are peripituitary tumours, i.e. chromophobe adenomas in adults and craniopharyingiomas in children, and iatrogenic hypopituitarism following surgical or radiotherapeutic damage. Partial degrees of pituitary damage can occur, but symptoms are uncommon before at least 70% of the gland is destroyed.

The development of hypopituitarism often results in a progressive loss of function, starting with growth hormone (GH): this is important in children but probably not in adults. Gonadotrophin failure (initially luteinising hormone, LH, then follicle stimulating hormone, FSH) also occurs early and impotence in the male and amenorrhoea in the female are common symptoms. The clinical features in adults include fine wrinkling of the skin around the mouth with loss of facial and body hair (7.9), and atrophy of the genitalia in both sexes (7.10).

In childhood, gonadotrophin failure leads to delayed puberty and short stature (7.11). Isolated gonadotrophin deficiency associated with anosmia is seen in Kallman's syndrome (discussed later).

Next to be lost is ACTH. The features of this deficiency are asthenia, nausea, vomiting, postural hypotension, hypoglycaemia, collapse and coma, pallor of the skin and reduced sun-tanning ability. TSH is eventually lost, giving rise to features similar to those seen in primary hypothyrodism, although the skin is not dry and coarse. In childhood, TSH deficiency contributes to growth retardation. Finally, in large tumours, vasopressin production may be lost, leading to polyuria and polydipsia as patients are unable to concentrate their urine and they may pass 5–20 litres of dilute urine a day. Prolactin deficiency causes failure of lactation. A more common effect in hypopituitarism is hyperprolactinaemia, which occurs if a tumour prevents the prolactin inhibitor, dopamine, from reaching the pituitary by stalk compression.

Cranial diabetes insipidus (CDI) occurs uncommonly in pituitary disease and results from ADH (vasopressin) deficiency (or rarely, renal resistance to the hormone occurs in the nephrogenic form, NDI). It is most frequently associated with craniopharyngioma, which may cause destruction of the posterior pituitary. There may be other hypothalamic disturbances, such as sleep disorders, hyperphagia, disturbed thermoregulation and emotional lability. The main investigation is the water deprivation test. Treatment is with desmopressin by intranasal spray.

Pituitary hypofunction can be confirmed by 'basal' blood samples for cortisol, thyroxine and testosterone or oestradiol, followed by a pituitary stress test.

Treatment of panhypopituitarism is by hormone replacement. GH is replaced by daily injection until after puberty when growth has stopped. Cortisol is normally replaced by hydrocortisone, 20 mg in the morning and 10 mg in the evening to mimic the normal diurnal pattern. Thyroxine 100–200 µg a day and either testosterone or oestrogen, usually with progestogen, are prescribed to restore libido and prevent osteoporosis.

7.9

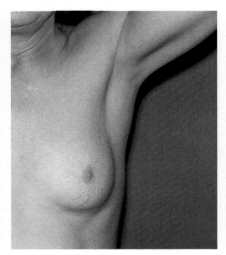

7.9 Lack of body hair in hypopituitarism. Twenty years earlier, this patient developed post-partum pituitary necrosis (Sheehan's syndrome). This resulted in many features of hypopituitarism, including a total absence of axillary and pubic hair.

7.10

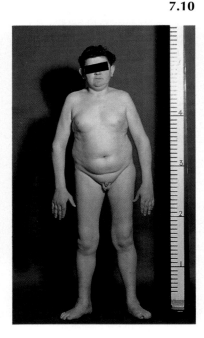

7.11

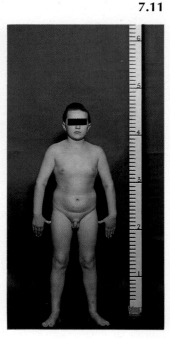

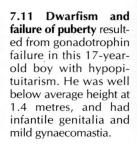

7.10 Hypopituitarism with gonadotrophin failure in a 39-year-old man. Note the extreme atrophy of the genitalia, the absence of body hair and the apparent gynaecomastia associated with obesity.

7.11 Dwarfism and failure of puberty resulted from gonadotrophin failure in this 17-year-old boy with hypopituitarism. He was well below average height at 1.4 metres, and had infantile genitalia and mild gynaecomastia.

Diseases associated with hypersecretion of pituitary hormones

Acromegaly and gigantism

The excessive secretion of GH is almost invariably caused by a pituitary tumour. If this occurs before fusion of the epiphyses, it leads to gigantism (**7.12**); after fusion, it produces the features of acromegaly.

Acromegaly is an uncommon condition with a prevalence of approximately 1.5 new cases/million/year. Some patients with multiple endocrine adenomatosis (MEA Type 1) may present this way. Some tumours are mixed and produce both prolactin or TSH and GH. The disease should be suspected on the finding of clinical features that include thickening of the soft tissues and skin, broadening of the nose, increased prominence of supraorbital and nuchal ridges, and prognathism, which leads to separation of the teeth (**7.13**–**7.15**).

Excessive sweating and acne (**7.13**) are common symptoms of acromegaly, and on examination large 'spade-like' hands are obvious (**7.16**, **7.17**). There is enlargement of the tongue (**7.18**) and all other viscera such as liver and spleen. Cardiomegaly and heart failure are major causes of death (**7.19**).

Diagnosis is based on demonstrating that GH is not suppressed during a 75 g oral glucose tolerance test.

Treatment is often difficult. Surgical removal of the tumour (trans-sphenoidal route) may reverse the disease, but complete removal without recurrence is rare and external radiotherapy to the pituitary fossa is indicated post-operatively. Radiotherapy alone leads to only a slow clinical improvement, causing GH to fall over 1–10 years. Surgery with or without radiotherapy often causes hypopituitarism; this should always be assessed and treated accordingly. Medical treatment is less effective in long-term management. Dopaminergic compounds lower GH in acromegaly, and 75% of acromegalic patients respond to bromocriptine in doses of 30–60 mg/day. Somatostatin lowers GH; although its action is too brief to be therapeutically useful, synthetic analogues have been developed that are long-acting and appear to offer a therapeutic option.

7.12

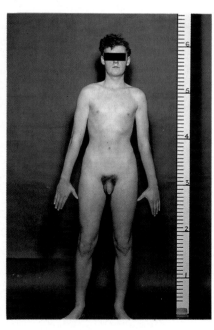

7.12 Mild gigantism resulting from the presence of increased growth hormone levels before epiphyseal fusion. The patient was 15 when this photograph was taken, and he reached a final height of 2.02 m.

7.13

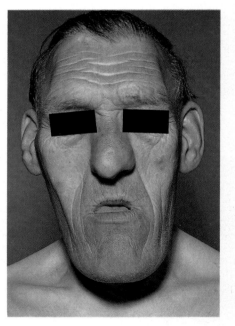

7.13 The characteristic facial features of acromegaly include thickening of the soft tissues and skin, enlargement of the nose and the supraorbital ridges, acne, thickening of the lips and prognathism.

7.14

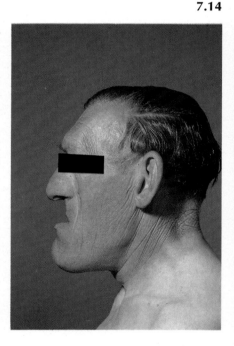

7.14 Acromegaly. Profile of the patient shown in **7.13**, showing prognathism, thickening of the soft tissues and skin, and increased prominence of the supraorbital ridge and nose.

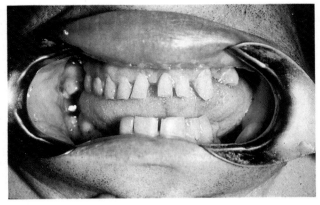

7.15 Malocclusion and separation of the teeth are commonly associated with the development of prognathism in acromegaly.

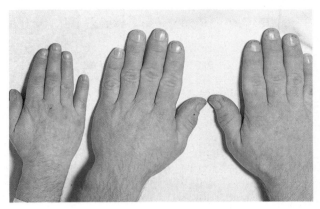

7.16 Spade-like hands are often an obvious abnormality in acromegaly. Compare the acromegalic hands on the right with the normal hand on the left. Overgrowth of the soft tissues may also cause compression of the median nerve at the wrist (carpal tunnel syndrome —see p. 515).

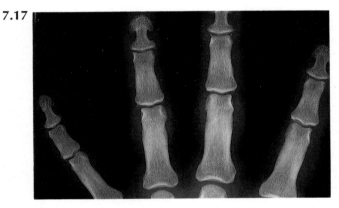

7.17 Acromegaly. This X-ray shows typical tufting of the terminal phalanges of the fingers, a common radiological associate of the clinical appearance seen in **7.16**.

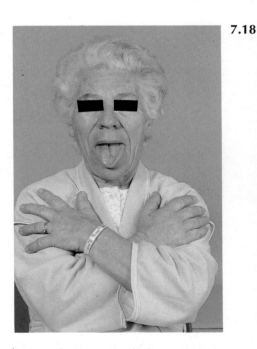

7.18 Enlargement of the tongue in acromegaly is obvious in this patient, who also shows other facial signs, and has classic changes in her hands.

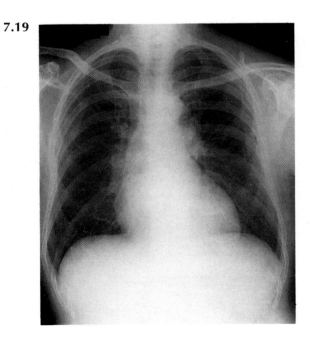

7.19 Acromegaly. The chest X-ray shows generalised cardiac enlargement (cardiothoracic ratio > 50%).

Hyperprolactinaemia

Sleep, stress, nipple stimulation, coitus, pregnancy and suckling are all associated with physiological elevation of circulating prolactin levels. Hyperprolactinaemia is associated with hypogonadism, either from pathological, physiological or iatrogenic causes. Therefore, the woman who breast feeds is often infertile and amenorrhoeic, and patients on drugs that raise prolactin may have infrequent periods (in women) or impotence (in men). Pituitary tumours secreting prolactin are four times more common than GH-producing tumours, and very much more common than those producing ACTH. Some non-functioning tumours may produce moderate elevations in prolactin by pituitary stalk compression. There are no specific signs of hyperprolactinaemia except hypogonadism, although galactorrhoea (inappropriate lactation 7.20) should always arouse suspicion. It should always be remembered however, that galactorrhoea may result from other causes, especially from malignant tumours producing prolactin or oestrogen, or from drug therapy with phenothiazines, antidepressants, haloperidol, methyldopa, metoclopramide or oral contraceptives.

Diagnosis of a prolactinoma is made from elevated prolactin levels above 4000 mU/l (upper limit of normal on most assays is 360 mU/l). Smaller tumours give lower levels. CT scan may show the presence of an adenoma (7.21), and it is important to note that these may undergo considerable expansion during pregnancy.

Treatment by a long-acting dopamine agonist such as bromocriptine will inhibit prolactin production and produce shrinkage of 80% of tumours, thus relieving pressure symptoms particularly on the optic chiasma. Fertility is regained and, although the drug is not teratogenic, once pregnancy has been established it is usually stopped; visual fields must be monitored regularly. Patients with macro-adenomas are best advised to have surgery or radiotherapy at least 3 months before attempts at conception, as these tumours may expand rapidly during pregnancy.

7.20

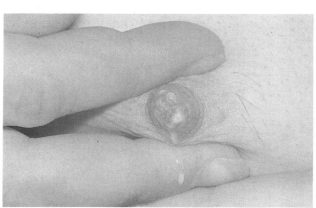

7.20 Galactorrhoea in a female patient with a prolactin-secreting pituitary tumour.

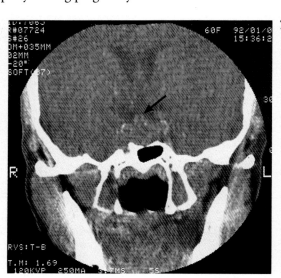

7.21 Pituitary tumour on a coronal CT scan (arrow). The tumour can be seen to extend above the level of the pituitary fossa. Visual field defects are likely to develop as the tumour expands. (**7.1**)

Over-production of ACTH ('Cushing's disease')

Cushing's syndrome refers to the clinical disorders resulting from an excess of circulating cortisol. The term Cushing's disease is used to describe patients in whom the syndrome results from excessive ACTH production by the pituitary; this is the most common cause of spontaneous Cushing's syndrome (60%). Other causes are ectopic ACTH production (15%), adrenal adenomata (15%) and carcinomata (10%). Cushing's disease is usually caused by a basophilic micro-adenoma (90%) and occurs more frequently in women, with a female:male sex ratio of approximately 10:1.

The clinical features of the syndrome that are of greatest discriminatory importance include thinning of the skin, easy bruising and bright purple striae (7.22–7.24), proximal muscle weakness and myopathy (7.25), facial plethora (6.40, 7.26), hirsutism (7.26, see also p. 110), acne and loss of scalp hair. Weight gain and obesity are the most common presenting features. The distribution of fat is central, involving the trunk and abdomen (7.27–7.29). This, together with the kyphosis that is often caused by osteoporosis (p. 152), results in a 'buffalo hump', with a 'moon face' and relatively thin limbs.

Pigmentation may occur, but this is more common in ectopic ACTH production (from a malignant bronchial tumour for example) or in Nelson's syndrome, where ACTH levels are very high (7.30). Nelson's syndrome may follow bilateral adrenalectomy for Cushing's disease if excesive ACTH production continues; expansion of the pituitary fossa may occur. Pigmentation is most marked in areas exposed to sunlight and friction, and in scars. Psychiatric symptoms, hypertension, glucose intolerance, diabetes and gonadal dysfunction (oligomenorrhoea and impotence) are all common.

Adrenal tumours may secrete cortisol and cause classical

Cushing's syndrome. However, the concomitant secretion of adrenal androgens may cause more virilisation, particularly in the case of carcinomas. Ectopic ACTH from highly malignant tumours causes gross elevations of cortisol: patients may present with fewer classic signs but with an illness of rapid onset with weight loss, profound proximal myopathy, pigmentation and a severe hypokalaemic alkalosis. Carcinoid tumours and other relatively benign sources of ectopic ACTH are clinically indistinguishable from other causes of Cushing's syndrome.

Diagnosis of Cushing's syndrome can be made by the detection of increased 24-hour urinary free-cortisol, by the loss of the normal circadian rhythm of cortisol at 24.00 hours or by use of a 48-hour low-dose dexamethasone suppression test. The differentiation between adrenal tumour, pituitary Cushing's disease and ectopic ACTH needs to be made with care.

If plasma ACTH is consistently undetectable, the condition is usually caused by an adrenal tumour. Diagnosis is established by ultrasound or CT scan of the adrenals (7.31) and carcinomas often show local invasion. Patients with adrenal tumours also show no suppression of serum cortisol with high-dose dexamethasone, and no response to the CRF test.

Plasma cortisol and ACTH are often grossly elevated in malignant tumours. Plasma potassium is almost always subnormal in patients with ectopic ACTH, so a hypokalaemic alkalosis is a pointer to this diagnosis. The high-dose dexamethasone suppression test is valuable in about 80% of cases. Patients with pituitary-dependent Cushing's show significant suppression of their cortisol, to less than 50% of the basal value at 48 hours, whereas those with adrenal tumours and ectopic ACTH do not suppress. Some ectopic tumours behave like a pituitary-dependent cause, but significant suppression is associated with a high probability (>50:1) that the condition is Cushing's disease. The CRF test provides further help in the differentiation.

Chest radiographs may reveal a branchial carcinoma (see p. 201), and CT scans of the pituitary in Cushing's disease may be helpful, as may scans of the lung fields, mediastinum, liver, pancreas and adrenals for detecting small carcinoids.

The treatment of choice for adrenal tumours is surgery, but metyrapone or o,p^1DDD may be necessary to achieve a clinical remission preoperatively. In Cushing's disease transsphenoidal surgery is the treatment of choice, achieving a biochemical cure in 75% of cases. Pituitary irradiation is now restricted to cases where surgery has been unsuccessful, and as it takes several years to be effective it needs to be combined with medical therapy. Ectopic ACTH production should be treated by eradicating the source if possible; bilateral adrenalectomy is an alternative.

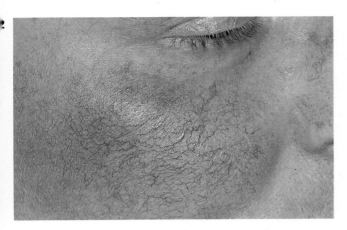

7.22 Cushing's syndrome is associated with typical thin skin and fragile blood vessels. Bruising commonly results from very minor trauma.

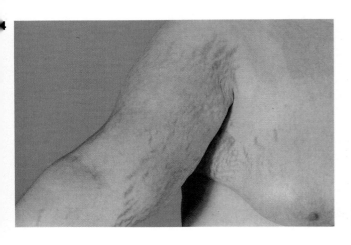

7.23

7.23 Thin, fragile skin in Cushing's syndrome and blood vessel fragility has resulted in extensive purpura.

7.24 Cushing's syndrome. This patient has typical purple striae on the breast and arm, associated with thinning of the skin.

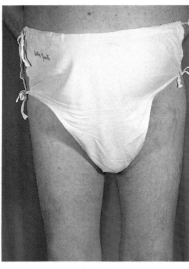

7.25 Proximal muscle wasting is common in Cushing's syndrome and leads to great difficulty in rising from the sitting position. Note the presence of striae on both thighs.

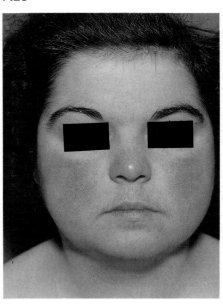

7.26 The typical facial features of Cushing's syndrome. The patient has a moon face with erythema and hirsutes. Identical appearances may result from corticosteroid therapy (*see* **6.40**).

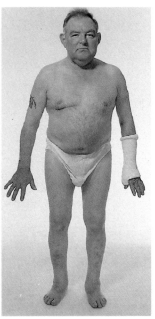

7.27, 7.28 Cushing's syndrome results in central rather than peripheral obesity. This patient's proximal myopathy resulted in a fall and fracture of his left wrist.

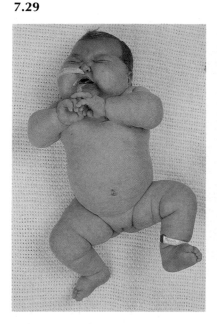

7.29 Gross Cushing's syndrome in infancy with classic central obesity and a moon face. and substantial growth retardation.

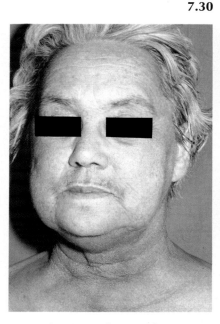

7.30 Nelson's syndrome. This woman underwent bilateral adrenalectomy for Cushing's disease, and subsequently became increasingly pigmented as a result of excessive ACTH secretion.

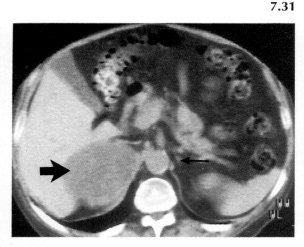

7.31 CT scan of a patient with an adrenal tumour causing Cushing's syndrome. The right-sided adrenal mass is extensive and is marked with a thick arrow. By contrast, the left adrenal gland (thin arrow) is atrophic.

Over-production of other pituitary hormones

Tumours which secrete TSH and produce hyperthyroidism are rare. Most tumours that secrete gonadotrophins are large, and they often do not produce a clinical syndrome (especially in menopausal women), although testicular enlargement in men has been described. Some tumours secrete the biologically inactive alpha subunit, which is common to FSH, LH and TSH. About 30% of all pituitary tumours are non-functioning.

Disorders of the adrenal glands

The adrenals are made up of cortex and medulla, which have separate embryological origins and different physiological functions.

Adrenal cortex

The cortex secretes glucocorticoids, mineralocorticoids and androgens.

Glucocorticoid-related disorders

- **Glucocorticoid excess** causes Cushing's syndrome (*see* p. 310).
- **Primary adrenocorticoid insufficiency** or Addison's disease is usually caused by an autoimmune process or, more rarely, by destruction of the cells by tuberculosis, other granulomatous disease, or infiltration by metastases.
- **Acute adrenal failure** follows withdrawal of suppressive doses of steroids or haemorrhage into the gland in the Waterhouse–Friderichsen syndrome or during anti-coagulant therapy.

The main clinical features of hypoadrenalism include tiredness, weight loss, gastrointestinal disturbances, hypoglycaemia and depression. The loss of negative feedback on the pituitary causes massive elevation in ACTH production with associated pigmentation. This is particularly seen in skin folds, areas of friction, light exposed areas, the buccal mucosa and often in scars (7.32–7.37). Aldosterone deficiency results in muscle cramps, dehydration and postural hypotension with the classic electrolyte disturbances of low serum levels of sodium and glucose and high potassium and urea. Androgen deficiency may lead to hair loss from the scalp and axillary and pubic regions in women. Associated vitiligo (*see* p. 106) may produce a striking contrast to the hyperpigmentation seen in other areas. The diagnosis is established by the short Synacthen test. Other investigations may reveal the underlying cause, e.g. adrenal auto-antibodies or adrenal calcification may be found (**7.38**).

Treatment in the acute crisis is intravenous hydrocortisone and 0.9% saline, with the addition of dextrose if hypoglycaemia is present. Long-term replacement is by oral hydrocortisone and fludrocortisone.

Synthesis of adrenal steroids is dependent on a number of enzymatically regulated stages. Congenital deficiences exist in six specific enzymes that can lead to congenital adrenal hyperplasias. The clinical features depend on where the block occurs, as biosynthesis is diverted down alternative metabolic pathways with effects predominantly on sexual development, mineralocorticoid or glucocorticoid balance.

7.32

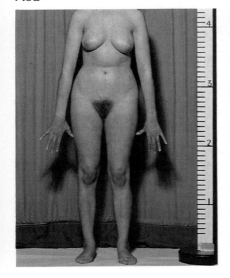

7.32 A patient with Addison's disease. Note the generalised increase in pigmentation, especially marked over the extensor surface of the knees.

7.33

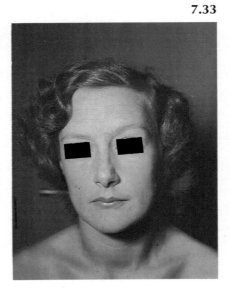

7.33 Facial appearance in Addison's disease. Note the generalised increase in pigmentation.

7.34

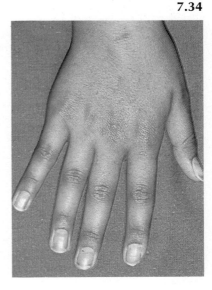

7.34 Addison's disease produces a generalised pigmentation of the hands, which—on the extensor surfaces—is often most marked over the knuckles.

7.35

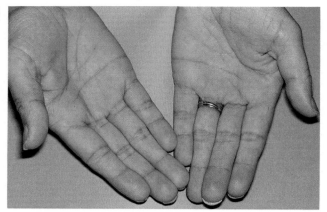

7.35 Addison's disease produces a similar increase in skin pigmentation in the skin creases of the palmar surface of the hands.

7.36 Buccal pigmentation in Addison's disease. There is a fairly general increase in mucous membrane pigmentation, and, in addition, there are some areas of much darker pigmentation. Both features are commonly seen in patients with Addison's disease.

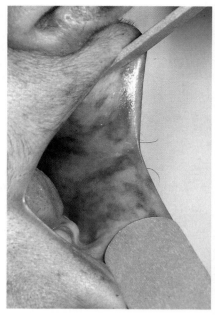

7.37

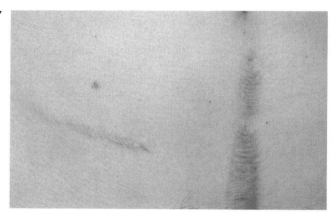

7.37 Pigmentation in scars is a common finding in patients with Addison's disease and with other causes of excessive ACTH production.

7.38

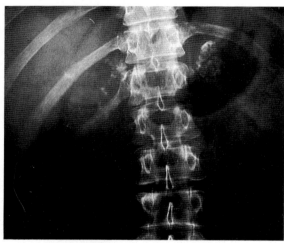

7.38 Adrenal calcification seen on plain abdominal X-ray in a patient with Addison's disease. The underlying pathology is almost certainly tuberculosis.

Mineralocorticoid-related disorders

Primary aldosteronism is caused by an adrenal adenoma (Conn's syndrome) in 70% of cases. In the remaining 30%, there is bilateral adrenal hyperplasia. Patients present with hypertension and hypokalaemia (<3.5 mmol/l) (**7.39**) and few if any symptoms. The characteristic biochemistry is a hypokalaemic alkalosis with a plasma sodium of 140–150 mmol/l, increased plasma aldosterone, suppressed plasma renin activity and an inappropriately high urinary potassium excretion. Differentiation between adenomas and hyperplasia is based on the effects of salt loading with fludrocortisone, adrenal CT scans, iodocholesterol radionuclide scanning and adrenal venous sampling. Treatment of adenomas should be surgical, 60% of patients are cured of hypertension post-operatively and a further 20% improved. In hyperplasia, the treatment of choice is spironolactone or amiloride.

7.39 Hypokalaemia in primary aldosteronism. The ECG provides a rapid means of diagnosis. Characteristic U waves are seen after the T waves, especially in the chest leads, as here in lead V3. In extreme hypokalaemia, the T wave may become flattened and the ST segment depressed, so that there is a risk of confusing the U wave with the T wave.

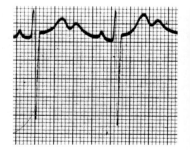

Adrenal medulla

Most phaeochromocytomas (80–90%) are found in the adrenal glands; 10% are malignant and 25% multiple. Their characteristic symptoms relate to catecholamine release. Symptoms include sustained or intermittent hypertension, tachycardia, palpitations and paroxysmal attacks of blanching and sweating. Diabetes and neuroectodermal diseases, such as neurofibromatosis are commonly associated. Diagnosis is based on clinical suspicion and the measurement of urinary metabolites such as vanillylmandelic acid and metanephrines. The tumour may be localised by selective venous sampling of catecholamines and/or by scanning techniques. Usually the tumours are large and can be localised by CT scan (7.40), ultrasound or radioisotope scanning with MIBG (metaiodobenzylguanidine) (7.41). Treatment should be surgical removal with pre-operative alpha and beta blockade.

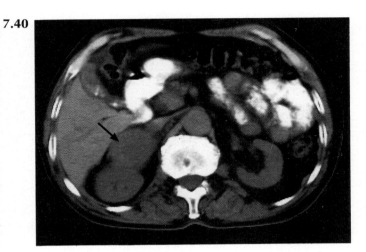

7.40

7.40 A large phaeochromocytoma demonstrated on CT scan (arrow). The close relationship of the adrenal phaeochromocytoma to the kidney is clear in this view.

7.41

7.41 A phaeochromocytoma was identified by its MIBG uptake in this patient. The renal uptake of Tc DMSA was also imaged, and the renal outline has been superimposed on this posterior view. Some liver uptake of MIBG can also be seen on the right.

Disorders of growth and sexual development

Growth assessment is an accurate and sensitive guide to child health. Growth velocity represents the dynamics of growth much better than a single measurement of stature. A healthy, adequately nourished and emotionally secure child grows normally. A slowly growing child has a disorder requiring diagnosis and, if possible, treatment.

Growth charts relating height to age are used to indicate the rate of growth in comparison to a reference population (7.42). From the fifth month of fetal life, repid growth begins to decelerate markedly over 3–4 years, there is a slight acceleration at 6–8 years, the mid-childhood growth spurt; and a pubertal growth spurt. There is a 4-year difference between when the earliest and latest 3% of normal children enter puberty. Abnormal height cannot be defined absolutely, but a child is usually considered abnormally short if height is below the 3rd centile, or too tall if above the 97th centile. Skeletal maturity is assessed by computing the maturation of bones in the wrist. This is useful in predicting final height and puberty timing. Final height is also contributed to by the child's parents, 95% of the children of given parents will have a height prognosis within ± 8.5 cm of the mid-parental centile.

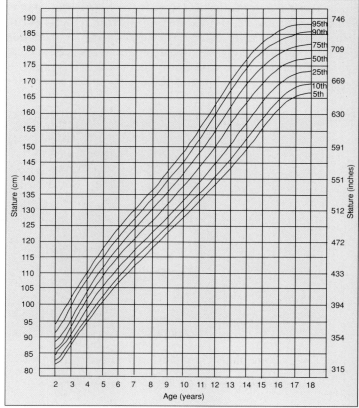

7.42 A typical growth chart, showing the normal age percentiles for boys aged from 2 to 18 years. The growth of an individual child should be plotted on such a chart. Response to therapy can be monitored in the same way.

Short stature

Short stature is a diagnostic challenge. A small child with normal growth velocity will be expected to achieve a normal final height, but may have growth delay, previous poor growth as a result of illness or short parents. Children with impaired growth velocity require careful examination for underlying disorders. Investigations include urinalysis, blood count, ESR, chromosome analysis, bone age and endocrine status — particularly GH, thyroxine and TSH, and sex steroids.

It is convenient to separate short children into those with normal proportions and those with abnormal proportions. Those with normal proportions form the largest group. There is a wide variety of causes of short stature:

- Any cause of intrauterine growth retardation and low birth weight leads to short stature.
- Numerous congenital syndromes lead to poor growth. The most common are the Silver–Russell syndrome (triangular facies, clinodactyly, facial and limb length asymmetry), the

Prader–Willi syndrome, Cornelia de Lange syndrome, progeria, Hallermann–Streiff syndrome, Seckel's syndrome, Ollier's disease, Aarskog's syndrome, Williams' syndrome and the mucopolysaccharidoses (p. 351).
- Nutritional and emotional deprivation leads to short growth as does systemic disease.
- Growth hormone deficiency may be congenital or acquired; it leads to short, plump children with immature facies and genitalia, and delicate extremities (7.43).
- Hypothyroidism should always be considered; the earlier the onset, the more severe the delay in growth, particularly in skeletal maturity.
- Cushing's syndrome delays growth, particularly when associated with precocious puberty.

The 'fat' short child is likely to have an endocrine cause for his short stature and obesity. The underlying endocrine condition should be treated and the growth response will be a

316

good sign of clinical response. In GH deficiency, treatment with recombinant growth hormone should continue throughout puberty.

Studies are underway to determine the benefits of accelerating the growth in 'short normal' children and in children with Turner's syndrome and Noonan's syndrome. Turner's syndrome (karyotype 45XO) and its many chromosomal variants (e.g. XO/XY mosaic in Noonan's) are always associated with impaired sexual development and short stature (7.44, 7.45). The combination of sex steroids and GH appears to increase the final height slightly.

Of the causes of short stature with abnormal proportions, achondroplasia, an autosomal dominant condition, is the most familiar with a frequency of 1 in 40,000 births (7.46, 7.47). There are many other forms of short limb and short trunk dwarfism.

7.43

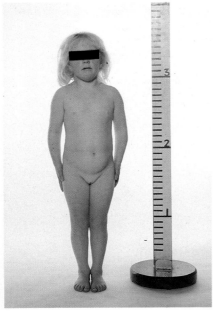

7.44

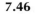

7.45

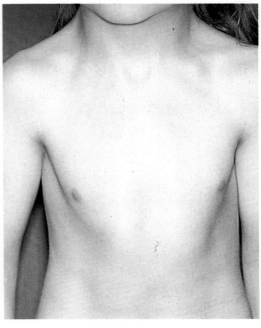

7.43 Pituitary dwarfism with growth hormone deficiency. This 10-year-old girl was 1.02 m tall, far below the 5th percentile for her age.

7.44, 7.45 Turner's syndrome is a genetic disorder with the chromosome configuration 45XO. This produces a phenotypic female with gonadal dysgenesis and primary amenorrhoea, retarded growth and short stature, webbed neck, absent breast development, an increased carrying angle at the elbow (cubitus valgus), congenital heart disease (especially coarctation of the aorta) and bilateral 'streak' gonads. These patients have a normal IQ. Noonan's syndrome has broadly similar appearances, but occurs in phenotypic males.

7.46

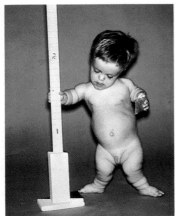

7.46, 7.47 Achondroplasia in infancy and adult life. Note the short stature, large head, prominent forehead and disproportion between the size of the body and limbs. Seventy to eighty per cent of cases of achondroplasia represent new mutations.

7.47

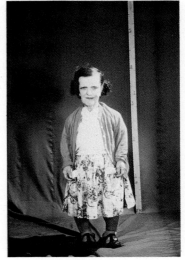

Tall stature

Tall stature is a much less common problem than short stature.

- Gigantism caused by GH excess precedes acromegaly and is investigated and treated as described on p. 308.
- Marfan's syndrome is a relatively common inherited cause of tall stature (7.48–7.51).
- Rarer causes include generalised lipodystrophy, Soto's syndrome and eunuchoidism.

7.48

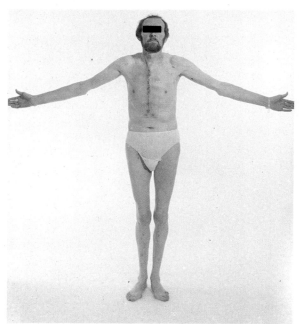

7.49

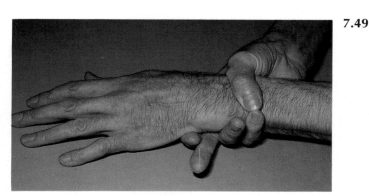

7.50

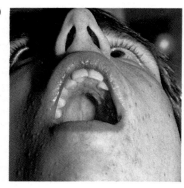

7.51

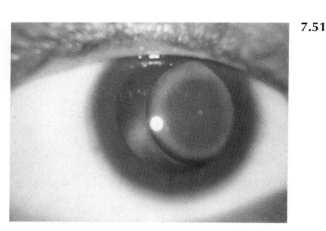

7.48–7.51 Marfan's syndrome is an autosomal dominant condition, in which there is tall stature, and reduced upper segment to lower segment ratio (**7.48**), long fingers (**7.49**) and toes, and often a high arched palate (**7.50**). It is commonly associated with laxity of the joints, dislocation of the lens in the eye (**7.51**), dissecting aneurysm of the aorta, aortic regurgitation and a floppy mitral valve. The patient in **7.48** has undergone surgery for aortic dissection. The length of the fingers can be demonstrated by the 'wrist sign' (**7.49**), in which the patient can encircle his wrist with the opposite thumb and fifth finger. The ability to do this is strongly suggestive of Marfan's syndrome.

Disorders of sexual development

At puberty, the growth of genitalia accelerates, secondary sexual characteristics develop and there is a general growth spurt. These changes are induced by pulsatile secretion of GnRH (gonadotrophin releasing hormone) which augments pituitary gonadotrophin output and promotes gonadal maturation and steroidogenesis.

Pubertal onset varies widely in different parts of the world, but in the UK the mean age of onset is 11.5 years for boys, and 10.5 years for girls with menarche occurring 2 years later. Delayed puberty in the UK for a boy is defined as a testicular volume below 4 ml by 14 years old, and for girls no breast development by 13.2 years of age. The most common cause is constitutional delayed puberty ('late developers').

The clinical features of hypogonadism depend on whether androgen secretion is impaired, and on the age of onset of the deficiency:

- **Fetal onset.** Differentiation of the external genitalia along male lines is androgen dependent within the first trimester of gestation. If testosterone fails to act pseudoherma-phroditism occurs, as is seen in testicular feminisation syndrome where XY males have an X-linked deficiency of androgen receptors (7.52). The testes, which may be found in the labia or inguinal canals, are hyperactive, producing high levels of testosterone and oestrogens. As negative feedback is ineffective, the LH levels are high. In congenital adrenal hyperplasia caused by 21-hydroxylase deficiency, the female child presents at birth with ambiguous genitalia, clitoral hypertrophy and partial or complete fusion of the labioscrotal folds (7.53) caused by the excess of androgenic cortisol precursors produced.

- **Prepubertal onset** of androgen deficiency leads to eunuchoidism as in Kallman's syndrome (hypogonadal hypogonodism, GnRH deficiency, anosmia, colour blindness, mid-line facial deformities) and Klinefelter's syndrome (7.54).

Diagnosis of hypogonadal states requires evaluation of visual fields and detection of anosmia, chromosome analysis, measurement of testosterone or oestradiol, LH and FSH.

7.52

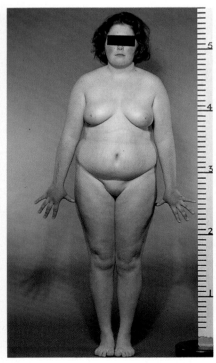

7.52 Testicular feminisation syndrome. The patient is genotypically male, but phenotypically female, because of an inherited X-linked deficiency of androgen receptors. Patients should usually be brought up as females, and the testes should be removed from their ectopic position as there is an increased risk of malignancy.

7.53

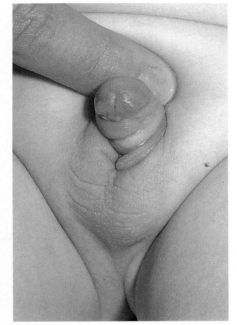

7.53 Congenital adrenal hyperplasia. A genotypically female patient presented at birth with ambiguous genitalia. The severity of the abnormalities varies considerably. In this case, there is clitoral hypertrophy and partial fusion of the labioscrotal folds.

7.54

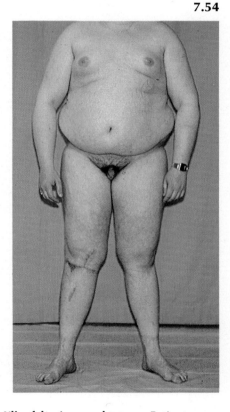

7.54 Klinefelter's syndrome. Patients are phenotypically male, but have two or more X chromosomes—most commonly 47XXY. They are eunuchoid with small, firm testes, gynaecomastia and a female distribution of body hair, and they may be unusually tall. They are infertile as a result of seminiferous tubule dysgenesis, which produces azoospermia.

Stimulation tests with GnRH or clomiphene and pituitary stress testing may be required. Treatment depends on cause; primary gonadal failure requires either cyclical oral oestrogen and progesterone preparations or intramuscular testosterone every month. This treatment will produce secondary sexual characteristics and prevent osteoporosis, but fertility can be produced only in secondary gonadal failure by the complex administration of human chorionic gonadotrophin (HCG), FSH or pulsatile GnRH in hypothalamic lesions.

Precocious puberty in males is generally defined as pubertal development before 10 years of age. Forty per cent of cases have no detectable organic disease, but there are rare associations with hypothyroidism, hepatoblastomas and cerebral tumours that affect the hypothalamus. In girls, the definition of precocious puberty is defined as sexual maturation before the age of 8 years; 80% of girls have no detectable organic disease.

Secondary amenorrhea and infertility are common post-pubertal presentations of gonadal failure. They may be caused by hypothalamic–pituitary axis disorders (p. 307–310), and hyperprolactinaemia is common. Weight loss is the underlying cause in 20% of cases, although when severe, as in anorexia nervosa, the gonadotrophin secretion reverts to a prepubertal pattern. Ovarian failure with a premature menopause often has an autoimmune basis and is associated with other auto-immune diseases such as Addison's disease (p. 313).

Polycystic ovary syndrome (PCO) commonly presents in the mid-twenties with menstrual irregularity, hyperandrogenisation (hirsutism, greasy skin and acne (**2.85, 2.86, 7.55**) and often obesity. The classic findings are a raised serum LH and slightly raised testosterone with normal FSH, prolactin and TSH. The ovaries contain multiple cysts. Other conditions, such as adrenal and ovarian tumours and late onset adrenal hyperplasia, present with virilisation (frontal baldness, deepening of the voice, breast atrophy, clitoral hypertrophy and masculine habitus), but in these conditions the testosterone concentration is in the normal male range. Management is of the primary cause, but in PCO hirsutism is treated with antiandrogens, such as cyproterone acetate, together with oestrogen. Effective treatment may take 12–18 months, during which time cosmetic treatments, shaving and electrolysis are required.

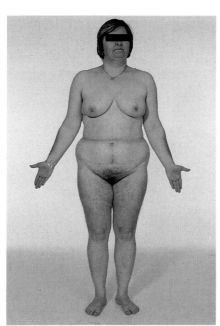

7.55

7.55 Virilisation with coarsening of the skin and hirsutism in a patient with the polycystic ovary syndrome.

Thyroid disorders

The thyroid secretes thyroxine (T4) and a small amount of tri-iodothyronine (T3). Approximately 85% of the biologically more-active circulating T3 is converted from T4 in the tissues (liver, muscle and kidney). The hormones are transported in the plasma almost entirely bound to thyroxine-binding globulin (TGB), pre-albumin and albumin. Production is stimulated by TSH in response to thyrotrophin-releasing hormone (TRH), and free T4 (FT4) has a negative feedback effect on TSH release. The thyroid para-follicular C-cells release calcitonin in response to an elevation in serum calcium. Enlargement of the thyroid gland from any cause is known as goitre.

Hyperthyroidism

Hyperthyroidism is caused by excess circulating T4 or T3. It is a common condition with a prevalence of about 20/1000 females; males are affected five times less frequently. Over 90% of cases are caused by either Graves' disease, toxic multinodular goitre or toxic solitary goitre. Graves' disease is the most common cause. The onset of the disease may be insidious. Atrial fibrillation is rare in young patients, but occurs in almost 50% of male patients over 60 years of age.

Graves' disease results from IgG antibodies against the TSH-receptor which bind and stimulate the gland via the adenylcyclase–cAMP system. These antibodies are termed thyroid-stimulating antibodies (TSAb). They may be responsible in part for thyroid enlargement in Graves' disease, but they do not appear to be responsible for the ophthalmopathy and pretibial myxoedema.

The cardinal signs of Graves' disease include a diffuse goitre, over which a vascular bruit can be heard (7.56), pretibial myxoedema (7.57), tachycardia with a bounding pulse, and a range of eye signs including exophthalmos (7.56, 7.58), lid retraction (7.59), lid lag on downward eye movement, periorbital puffiness (7.60), grittiness, increased lacrimation, chemosis (7.60), conjunctival oedema and

7.56

7.57

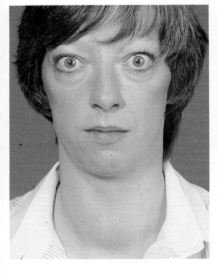

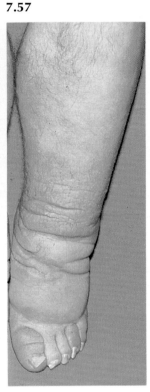

7.57 Pretibial myxoedema in Graves' disease. When this sign occurs, it may be combined with thyroid acropachy, in which there is oedema of the nail folds, producing a condition resembling clubbing.

7.58

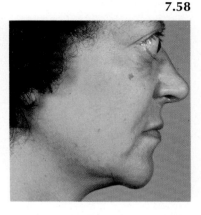

7.58 Exophthalmos (proptosis) in Graves' disease. This results from enlargement of the muscles, and fat within the orbit as a result of mucopolysaccharide infiltration.

7.56 Graves' disease. This usually affects women between the ages of 20 and 40 years. This patient presented classically with a diffuse goitre over which a vascular bruit could be heard, and with eye signs.

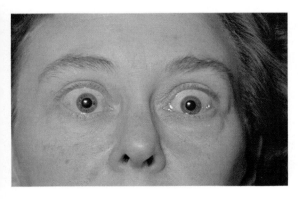

7.59 Lid retraction is a common eye sign in Graves' disease, which can be recognised when the sclera is visible between the lower margin of the upper lid and the cornea. Lid retraction is usually bilateral, but may be unilateral.

7.60

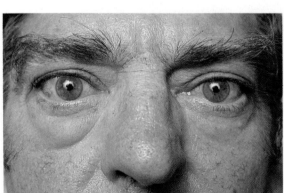

7.60 Periorbital swelling may be associated with other eye signs, giving an erythematous and oedematous appearance to the eyelids. Note that this patient also has chemosis, seen as reddening of the sclera.

ulceration (7.61), ophthalmoplegia (7.62), diplopia, papilloedema and loss of visual acuity.

Eye signs may be absent in thyrotoxicosis, especially in the elderly in whom 'masked' or 'apathetic thyrotoxicosis' is common. Atrial fibrillation, heart failure and weight loss may be the only signs in this group (7.63).

The diagnosis is made clinically, with confirmation by detecting biochemically raised T3 and T4, and undetectable TSH levels. Where a toxic multinodular goitre or a single toxic nodule (a toxic adenoma) in the thyroid is suspected clinically, a thyroid scan may provide useful information (7.64, 7.65).

Treatment options in thyrotoxicosis include:

- Antithyroid drugs — carbimazole or methimazole, followed by propylthiouracil.
- Beta-blocking drugs in the initial stages of management.
- Sub-total thyroidectomy.
- Radioactive iodine therapy.

The choice of therapy depends upon a number of factors, especially the age and previous history of the patient.

7.61

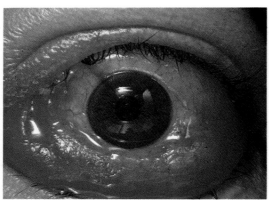

7.62

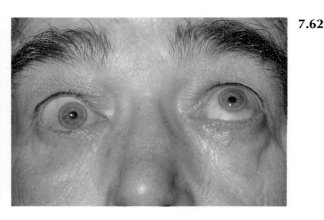

7.61 Severe conjunctival oedema associated with exophthalmos in a patient with Graves' disease. Tarsorrhaphy may be needed to aid lid closure and prevent damaging corneal exposure in patients with severe exophthalmos.

7.62 Ophthalmoplegia in Graves' disease. This is not caused by nerve palsy, but is the long-term result of swelling and infiltration of the extrinsic muscles of the eye. In this case, there is impaired upward and outward gaze in the patient's right eye. Ophthalmoplegia is usually accompanied by other eye signs. Note the presence of lid retraction. This patient also has markes corneal arcus.

7.63

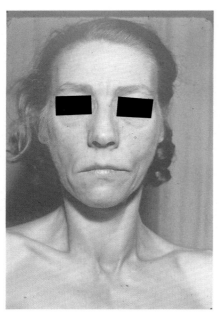

7.63 'Masked' hyperthyroidism. In the elderly, hyperthyroidism is commonly caused by a toxic multinodular goitre, but this does not necessarily result in significant thyroid enlargement. Because the patient does not have Graves' disease, the other signs associated with that condition are lacking. The clinical diagnosis is thus much less obvious, being suggested by a combination of tachycardia and/or atrial fibrillation, heart failure and weight loss in a patient over the age of 60 years.

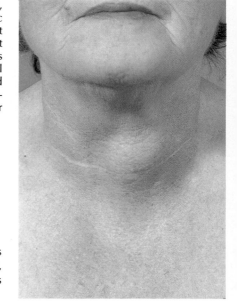

7.64 Toxic adenoma causing hyperthyroidism. This patient had a partial thytoidectomy 20 years previously, and a toxic nodule has now recurred. This was confirmed by isotope scanning.

7.65 Toxic adenoma in the right thyroid (a hot nodule), demonstrated using ^{99m}Tc scanning. The remainder of the gland does not take up significant amounts of isotope.

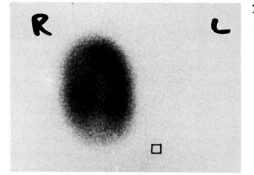

Hypothyroidism

Hypothyroidism (myxoedema) is the clinical syndrome which results from the reduced secretion of T3 and T4 from the thyroid.

Primary hypothyroidism is caused by an intrinsic disorder of the thyroid gland and is associated with a raised TSH. Spontaneous atrophic hypothyroidism and thyroid failure following surgery, radioactive iodine or Hashimoto's autoimmune thyroiditis account for over 90% of cases.

Secondary hypothyroidism is much less common and is caused by pituitary disease, where absence of TSH leads to atrophy of the gland.

Hypothyroidism affects all the systems of the body, but the wide range of clinical features means that the diagnosis will be missed if it is not positively considered. In children, the dominant features are a reduction in growth velocity and arrest of pubertal development. In adults, the presentation may vary from biochemical evidence with no clinical signs, to the insidious onset over many years of myxoedematous changes in the tissues with infiltration of mucopolysaccharides, hyaluronic acid and chondroitin sulphate (7.66, 7.67). Dermal infiltration gives rise to non-pitting oedema, most marked on the skin of the eyelids and hands. This is often associated with loss of scalp (7.68) and eyebrow hair. Dryness of the skin, and reduced body hair are other common features and systemic effects including pericardial and pleural effusions, ascites, cardiac dilatation, bradycardia and hypothermia may be life-threatening (*see* p. 256).

Diagnosis is based on clinical suspicion — prolonged relaxation time of peripheral reflexes and a low-voltage ECG may be helpful — biochemical estimation of T4 and TSH and an assessment of thyroid antibodies. Antibodies to thyroid microsomes and/or thyroglobulin are present in the serum of 90% of patients with Hashimoto's thyroiditis.

Hashimoto's disease is the most common form of goitrous hypothyroidism in the world. It usually presents in the sixth decade, and women are affected 15 times more frequently than men. The gland characteristically feels firm and rubbery and may range in size from being scarcely palpable to up to 10 times enlarged (7.69).

Spontaneous atrophic hypothyroidism is the most common form of non-goitrous hypothyroidism in the UK, with a prevalence of 10/1000 and an incidence that increases with age. Females are affected 6 times more commonly than males.

This is also an autoimmune condition—many patients have TSH-receptor blocking antibodies and some have a history of Graves' disease treated successfully with drugs 10–20 years previously. These patients may also have other autoimmune diseases such as pernicious anaemia, diabetes mellitus, Addison's disease or vitiligo.

Drugs may induce hypothyroidism. Lithium carbonate, which like iodide inhibits the release of thyroid hormones, may result in a TSH-induced goitre and prolonged administration of iodine, as in amiodarone given for the treatment of dysrhythmias, also occasionally induces goitrous hypothyroidism.

In certain parts of the world where there is iodine deficiency, such as the Andes, central Africa and the Himalayas, thyroid enlargement is common, affecting 10% of the population (**endemic goitre**, 7.70). Although most patients are euthyroid and have normal or only slightly raised TSH, the greater the iodine deficiency or the greater the demands (as in pregnancy), the greater the incidence of hypothyroidism.

Dyshormonogenesis is an unusual autosomal recessive defect in hormone synthesis. The most common form results from a deficiency in peroxidase enzyme (Pendred's syndrome: goitre, hypothyroidism, deaf mutism and mental retardation). Homozygotes present with congenital hypothyroidism, which needs to be distinguished from athyreosis or hypoplasia of the thyroid, the commonest causes of neonatal hypothyroidism.

Neonatal hypothyroidism (1 in 4,000 live births) is screened for by TSH measurement 5–7 days after delivery. If it is undetected, cretinism results. Prompt treatment with thyroxine has been shown to result in normal development, except in the rare cases of thyroid agenesis and impaired brain development caused by intrauterine hypothyroidism.

Treatment in all cases of hypothyroidism is with thyroxine. In patients with ischaemic heart disease, sudden introduction of T4 can cause myocardial infarction and therefore T4 is started in low doses (25 µg) and the dose increased very slowly every 4–6 weeks with intensified management of anti-anginal therapy. 'Myxoedema coma' is severe hypothyroidism in an elderly patient. Its presenting features may include hypothermia, cardiac failure, an altered conscious state often with convulsions, high CSF fluid pressure and protein content, hypotension, alveolar hypoventilation, intercurrent chest infection, and dilutional hyponatraemia. Mortality is around 50% and careful management is required.

7.66

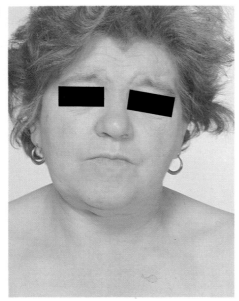

7.66 Hypothyroidism is not always clinically obvious. This patient shows some facial features, with a generalised pallor, puffiness andcoarsening of the features, and coarse , uncontrollable hair. She was grossly hypothyroid on biochemical testing.

7.67 Gross clinical hypothyroidism produces characteristic non-pitting oedematous changes in the skin of the face, giving rise to a characteristic clinical appearance. Note the dry, puffy facial appearance and the coarse hair. This patient was admitted with hypothermia. Her skin was cold and she showed mental apathy.

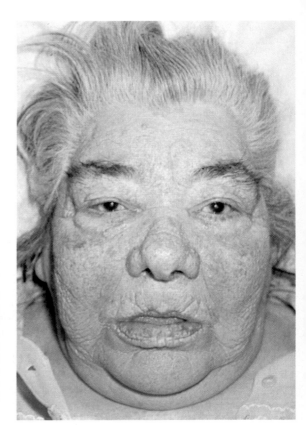

7.68

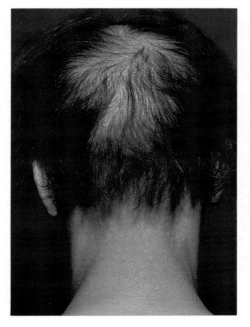

7.68 Hair loss is a common feature of hypothyroidism, as in this 48-year-old woman.

7.69

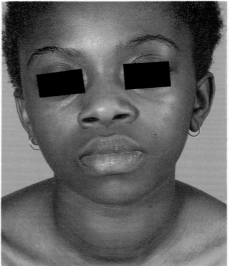

7.69 Hashimoto's disease is the most common cause of goitrous hypothyroidism in the world and is much more common in women than in men. This teenage patient has a marked goitre but few obvious signs of hypothyroidism. She is rather unusual, as the condition is much more common in older women.

7.70

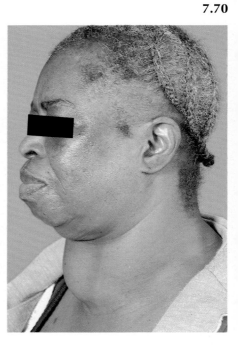

7.70 Endemic goitre. Large goitres like this are not unusual in areas of iodine deficiency, but they are not always associated with hypothyroidism. This African patient was euthyroid.

Thyroid nodules and thyroid cancer

A thyroid nodule is any discrete intrathyroidal lesion and nodules may be solitary or multiple. Palpable nodules can be found in 3–8% of European and American adults, and the incidence increases with age. In iodine deficient parts of the world, the prevalence is much greater. Clinically undiagnosed (occult) cases of thyroid cancer are found in up to 18% of routine autopsies. These are usually small (<1cm) papillary carcinomas without evidence of local invasion or metastases.

Thyroid nodules may be caused by involutional or degenerative changes, discrete inflammatory lesions or neoplasms. Colloid or adenomatous nodules are the most common type and consist of thyroglobulin-containing follicles. These are often multiple and may present as a multinodular goitre (7.71) or a simple non-toxic goitre. They are most common in women, and require no treatment unless they are cosmetically disfiguring or cause pressure effects such as tracheal compression.

Single thyroid nodules may be benign or malignant. The chance of a nodule being benign is at least 95%; and most thyroid cancers have a mortality rate similar to skin cancer and are not immediately life threatening. Malignancy may be suspected if there is a history of previous exposure to ionising radiation — especially external irradiation in childhood. Other suggestive features on examination include asymmetry, unusual location of the swelling, firmness, lymphadenopathy, a rapid painful increase in size, which may be caused by haemorrhage, hoarseness of the voice and fixation to skin and underlying tissues. The investigation of choice is a fine-needle aspiration (FNA) which allows immediate identification of cysts and microscopic examination of the aspirated cells. Ultrasonography is the most sensitive method available for delineating nodules and identifying cysts (7.72) but it will not distinguish benign from malignant. Radioiodine scanning may also give valuable information.

The prognosis and management of thyroid carcinomas varies according to the histological type:

- Most thyroid carcinomas are the **papillary** type, which may be multifocal and spread to regional lymph nodes and to lungs (4.27) and bone (3.122). Most occur in women aged less than 50 years with a tumour size less than 4 cm in diameter. Treatment is by total thyroidectomy; radioiodine ablation is needed post-operatively, as the metastases and any remaining thyroid take up iodine under TSH-drive after thyroidectomy. Thereafter the patients are treated with a sufficiently high dose of T4 to suppress TSH completely. Papillary carcinoma carries a good prognosis.
- **Follicular** carcinoma is more aggressive. It is usually unifocal and rarely spreads to lymph nodes, but spreads via the blood to lungs and bone. Treatment is similar to that for papillary carcinoma.
- **Medullary** carcinoma is derived from the parafollicular C cells of the thyroid. When sporadic it is usually unifocal; but when familial, it is typically bilateral and multicentric and may form part of the 'multiple endocrine neoplasia' syndrome (MEN). In MEN Type IIa, it is associated with phaeochromocytoma and parathyroid adenoma. In Type IIb, it is associated with a marfanoid habitus, mucosal neuromas of lips, eyelids and tongue, proximal myopathy and ganglioneuromatosis of the bowel. Medullary carcinoma metastasises as above and is treated in the same way, but it produces calcitonin which can be used as a tumour marker.
- **Anaplastic** carcinoma is very aggressive and may be inoperable at presentation.

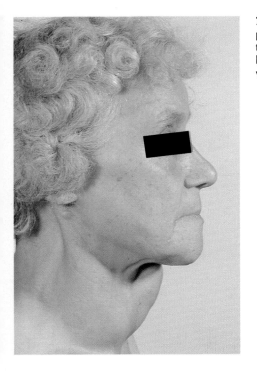

7.71 Multinodular goitre. The patient was euthyroid, but surgical treatment was ultimately required because of retrosternal extension with tracheal compression.

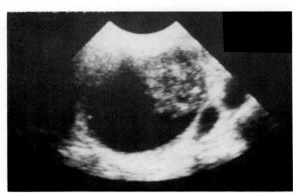

7.72

7.72 Ultrasound is the imaging technique of choice in the investigation of thyroid nodules. In this patient, one large and several smaller lesions are seen. Further investigation is indicated, and aspiration biopsy is likely to provide a definitive cellular diagnosis.

Parathyroid diseases

Hyperparathyroidism

For a discussion of hyperparathyroidism, *see* p. 154.

Hypoparathyroidism

Failure of parathyroid hormone (PTH) secretion is rare; the major causes are neonatal, post-surgical or idiopathic hypoparathyroidism. The clinical features are mainly caused by hypocalcaemia. They include tetany, which is characterised by carpopedal spasm (7.73) and paraesthesia. Idiopathic hypoparathyroidism may be sporadic or familial and is often associated with autoimmune diseases such as Addison's disease. Candidiasis, together with impaired nail and dental development is common. Cataracts and calcification of the basal ganglia are common, but parkinsonian features are rare.

Pseudohypoparathyroidism is caused by a defect at the PTH-receptor level. In addition to the characteristic biochemical profile of hypoparathyroidism (low serum calcium, raised inorganic phosphorus and usually normal alkaline phosphatase), these patients have a raised PTH and they exhibit somatic features. They have short stature, mental retardation, a round face and short neck, abnormal dentition and shortening of some of the metatarsals and metacarpals (usually the third, fourth and fifth, 7.74). A few families have these somatic features without the biochemical abnormalities; this condition is known as pseudohypoparathyroidism.

Treatment of tetany is with intravenous calcium and, as oral calcium is rarely adequate alone, an active metabolite of vitamin D is prescribed to normalise the serum calcium levels.

7.73

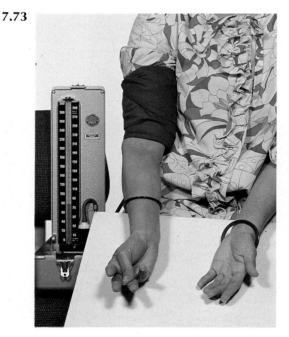

7.74

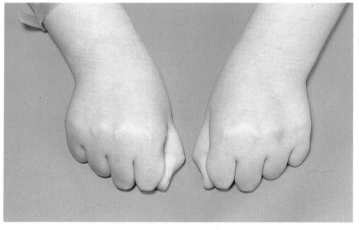

7.74 Pseudohypoparathyroidism is associated with characteristic somatic features including shortening of the metatarsals and metacarpals, in this patient especially in the fourth and fifth fingers. This shortening results in an apparent absence of the relevant knuckles on making a fist.

7.73 Carpopedal spasm (Trousseau's sign) is the most obvious manifestation of tetany in hypocalcaemia. Its onset can be provoked by inflating a sphygmomanometer cuff to just above systolic pressure for at least 2 minutes.

Gastrointestinal hormone abnormalities

A number of rare syndromes are associated with abnormalities in gastrointestinal hormones. These are summarised on p. 384.

Diabetes mellitus

Diabetes mellitus is a disease characterised by a chronically elevated blood glucose concentration, often accompanied by other clinical and biochemical abnormalities. The hyperglycaemia of diabetes results from an inadequate action of insulin, caused by low or absent insulin secretion, the presence of antagonists to the peripheral action of insulin or a combination of these factors.

The effects of the disease may be acute or chronic, involving many organs, including the eye, the kidney, peripheral nerves and large arteries. Primary diabetes mellitus is traditionally divided into either insulin dependent (IDDM or Type 1) or non-insulin dependent (NIDDM or Type 2). The classification is important because of the different genetic backgrounds, clinical presentations, metabolic effects, treatment and consequences of the two types. Diabetes may also be secondary to other disorders (**Table 7.5**).

Diabetes is defined biochemically by the following criteria:

- A fasting venous plasma glucose level greater than 7.8 mmol/l (140 mg /dl) on more than one occasion.

or

- A 2-hour (plus one other) venous plasma glucose level in excess of 11.1 mmol/l (200 mg/dl) in a formal 75 g oral glucose tolerance test (GTT).

Table 7.5 A classification of diabetes mellitus.

Impaired glucose tolerance without diabetes (IGT)

Primary diabetes mellitus
    Insulin dependent (IDDM; Type 1)
    Non-insulin dependent (NIDDM, Type 2)

Malnutrition-related diabetes mellitus (MRDM)

Secondary diabetes mellitus
    Pancreatic disease
    Endocrine disorders
    Drug therapy
    Inherited disorders

Impaired glucose tolerance (IGT)

IGT is often classified as 'chemical', 'borderline' or 'latent' diabetes. It is defined as the finding of a fasting venous plasma glucose level below 7.8 mmol/l, and a 2-hour sample, following oral GTT, with levels between 7.8 and 11.1 mmol/l. Annually, about 2–4% of these patients develop diabetes. IGT carries the same risk of atherosclerotic vascular complications as diabetes, although the risk of retinopathy 10 years after diagnosis is negligible. Management of patients with IGT should be aimed at diminishing the risk of metabolic and physical deterioration, by reducing obesity, hypertension, physical inactivity and hyperlipidaemia and by stopping smoking. In pregnancy, IGT should be taken seriously and treated as gestational diabetes.

Primary diabetes mellitus

Primary diabetes is either insulin dependent diabetes (IDDM or Type 1) or non-insulin dependent (NIDDM or Type 2). The prevalence of diabetes in industrialised countries is approximately 3–4% and about 10% have IDDM. Some communities, such as the Pima Indians, have a diabetes prevalence of over 30%, mainly obese NIDDM.

- **IDDM** patients are ketosis-prone and C-peptide negative. They have an absolute requirement for insulin from diagnosis. IDDM is believed to be an autoimmune condition, where environmental factors trigger the diabetogenic process via islet cell antibodies in genetically susceptible individuals.

Most patients presenting under the age of 25 years have IDDM.

- **NIDDM** generally occurs over the age of 40 years in patients with resistance to insulin and abnormal beta cell function. An underlying genetic susceptibility is even more important than in IDDM and most patients are obese. The onset of the disease is insidious and biochemical evidence of diabetes may be present for several years before symptoms or complications lead to the diagnosis. These patients are not dependent on insulin for treatment but may require it temporarily for glycaemic control under stress.

327

Malnutrition-related diabetes mellitus (MRDM)

The World Health Organisation has recognised malnutrition-related diabetes (MRDM) with two subtypes—fibrocalcaneous pancreatic diabetes (FCPD) and protein deficient pancreatic disease (PDPD). MRDM has a high prevalence in certain tropical developing countries, where it presents with severe symptoms but without ketosis in young people. Pancreatic calcification is common in the FCPD subtype.

Secondary diabetes mellitus

7.75

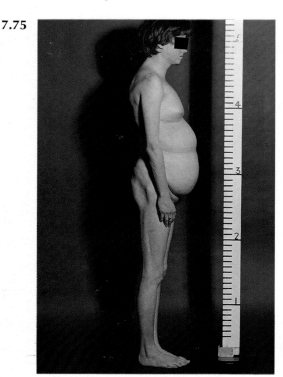

Diabetes may be secondary to pancreatic disease (e.g. haemochromatosis, chronic pancreatitis), other endocrine disorders (e.g. Cushing's syndrome, acromegaly, phaeochromocytoma), drug therapy (e.g. thiazides, steroids, phenothiazides), insulin receptor abnormalities (lipodystrophy, 7.75) and various inherited disorders (e.g. Type 1 collagen diseases, DIDMOAD syndrome, Prader–Willi syndrome).

7.75 Lipodystrophy is a rare cause of secondary diabetes. The atrophy of adipose tissue occurs throughout the body, and is well seen here, especially in the gluteal region. Non-ketotic insulin resistance is combined with severe hyperlipidaemia with subcutaneous xanthomas and hepatosplenomegaly.

Presenting features of diabetes

Patients with diabetes may be detected by a range of presentations which include:

- **Acute** — the typical presentation of the young patient with IDDM. Features include polyuria, polydipsia and weight loss of short duration, often associated with or apparently precipitated by a viral infection. When these symptoms have been neglected there may be visual disturbance or impairment of the conscious level associated with severe ketoacidosis.
- **Chronic** — the typical presentation of a patient with NIDDM. The symptoms have usually been present for some months and often include weight loss, thirst, excess urine volume, genital infection with *Candida albicans* and skin infections, often with *Staph. aureus*.
- **Coincidental discovery.** Routine screening for urine or blood glucose as part of a pre-employment medical, during pregnancy or in local campaigns.
- **Complications.** The patient may present with visual disturbance or overt retinopathy, neuropathy, nephropathy or after major thrombotic events such as premature stroke or myocardial infarction.
- **Drug-related diabetes** may develop in patients on long-term steroids or thiazide diuretics.
- **Disease-related** as in acromegaly, Cushing's syndrome, phaeochromocytoma, thyrotoxicosis, pancreatitis, haemochromatosis, cystic fibrosis, carcinoma or surgical removal of the pancreas.
- **Gestational**—pregnancy may unmask diabetes in a woman who is predisposed.

A full history and clinical examination are essential to detect any of the causative diseases and document the consequences.

Investigations

Investigations are required for screening, diagnosis, monitoring of control and the early detection of degenerative changes.

- **Urine testing for glucose** is still widely used, but glucose will be found in the urine only when it rises above the renal threshold (usually about 10 mmol/l). Urine tests are simple and cheap. Enzyme strip tests are specific for glucose.
- **Urine testing for ketone bodies** is also simple. The presence of ketones suggests loss of control.
- **Proteinuria** is a reflection of the development of renal complications and is an early indicator of diabetic renal disease.

Multiple test strips allow rapid testing for all these substances in urine (**6.7**).

- **Blood glucose** is the key to diagnosis in diabetes.(*see* p. 327) Careful attention to detail is required in skin preparation, blood collection and monitoring the reaction (**7.76–7.79**). The colour change may be recorded visually but is better recorded electronically, and meters are available for home use. If the patient is to read the strips visually it is important to check colour vision.

- **Glucose tolerance test** is of value where random blood glucose results are equivocal. It defines the response to a 75 g oral glucose load. Blood and urine are monitored before and for $2\frac{1}{2}$ hours after the glucose drink. The renal threshold for glucose can be determined as can the presence of diabetes (capillary glucose ≥11.1 mmol/l) or impaired glucose tolerance (IGT—capillary glucose 7.8–11.1 mmol/l).
- **Glycosylated haemoglobin** and other proteins — measurement of these proteins reflects the degree of diabetic control in the previous 4–6 weeks and is of value in long-term management and control.
- **Microalbuminuria** is a very sensitive marker of early and potentially reversible renal impairment. It is the term given to the presence of protein below the level of detection with the stick methods, i.e. 200 mg/l.
- **Serum electrolytes, blood gases, osmolality and anion gap** are all of value in metabolic crises where there is loss of water, sodium and potassium and where acidosis is developing, or where there is a hyperosmolar state.
- **Lipid profile.** Elevations in serum cholesterol are common, and elevation of serum triglycerides is a reflection of poor glycaemic control, which usually reverts to normal when euglycaemia is achieved.

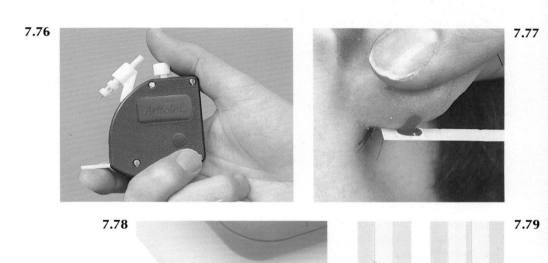

7.76 **7.77** **7.78** **7.79**

7.76–7.79 Capillary blood sugar measurement requires careful attention to technique. A clean disposable lancet or a spring-loaded stilette (**7.76**) should be used. Blood can be obtained from the ear lobe or from the side of the finger (**7.77**). No attempt should be made to collect the sample until the drop of blood has reached an adequate size. For strip testing, the drop should be an adequate size to wet the reagent thoroughly and enable the colour change to be easily seen (**7.78**, **7.79**). The result can be read visually or using a reflectance meter.

Principles of management

The aim of management is to control symptoms, prevent acute metabolic complications of ketoacidosis and hypoglycaemia, encourage self reliance and self care, prevent or treat complications early and prevent the increased morbidity and mortality associated with poorly managed diabetes.

In IDDM glycaemic control is achieved by subcutaneous insulin administration two or more times a day using modified insulins with differing absorption characteristics to provide an insulin profile that controls the glycaemia around meals and provides a background level for basic metabolic functions. Glycaemic control is best assessed by blood glucose monitoring. Dietary modification is essential, and involves eliminating simple sugars and eating a low-fat, high-fibre diet with 50% of the calories from carbohydrate, 30% from fats (mainly polyunsaturated) and 20% from protein.

In NIDDM the main form of treatment is dietary, with the emphasis on avoiding simple sugars and calorie restriction. Weight reduction is important in most patients with NIDDM, and only if this cannot be achieved and the patients are unacceptably hyperglycaemic, should oral hypoglycaemic agents be added. Sulphonylureas are first-line treatment treatment in non-obese NIDDM patients, while biguanides have a particular role in the obese diabetic.

Complications of diabetes

The most important **acute complications** of diabetes are metabolic: diabetic ketoacidosis (**7.80**), hypoglycaemia (**7.81**), lactic acidosis and non-ketotic hyperosmolar coma.

Other acute complications include insulin allergy, acute infections and acute neuropathy.

Insulin allergy (**7.82**) is becoming very rare with the increasing use of highly purified animal insulins or genetically engineered human insulin.

Acute infections may be the presenting complaint in NIDDM. They may include:

- Candidal infections, presenting in the genital region as balanitis or vulvitis (**1.171**), in the finger nails (**2.50**) or as intertrigo beneath the breasts (**2.49**).
- Carbuncles (**1.92**), boils (**2.37**) and other staphylococcal skin infections.
- Osteomyelitis, urinary infections, pneumonia, tuberculosis and other systemic bacterial infections.
- In the diagnosed diabetic, finger pulp infections following non-sterile finger pricks (**7.83**).

Acute motor or sensory neuropathy may be seen in various guises during or after a period of poor metabolic control. The most typical are mononeuritis multiplex, often affecting the third, sixth or seventh cranial nerves (**7.84**) and diabetic amyotrophy caused by a proximal radiculopathy. Pain and skin tenderness with weakness and wasting of the upper thigh muscles is the most common presentation of amyotrophy (**7.85**). With improved glycaemic control (often with insulin), these complications may resolve.

The **chronic complications** of diabetes are summarised in **Table 7.5**.

Insulin lipodystrophy results from frequent injections into the same injection sites, particularly in girls. Hypertrophy (**7.86**) is caused by hypertrophied fat cells, and fat cell atrophy may also occur (**7.87**).

Most chronic complications result from disease of either the large blood vessels (macroangiopathy) or the small blood vessels (microangiopathy).

7.80

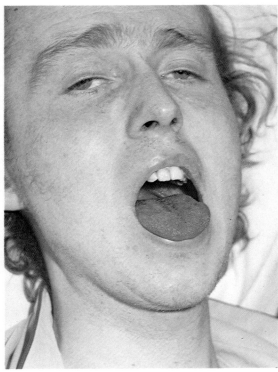

7.81

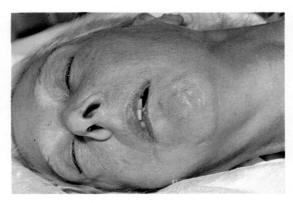

7.81 Hypoglycaemic coma in diabetes. Coma resulted from self-administration of an excessive insulin dose by an alcoholic patient who did not subsequently eat any food. Where the patient is comatose, hypoglycaemia is more immediately dangerous than hyperglycaemia. This patient died.

7.80 Diabetic ketoacidosis. There is evidence of marked dehydration, and the patient's eyeballs were lax to pressure. The patient was hyperventilating and confused, though not (yet) comatose. The smell of ketones on the breath allowed an instant probable diagnosis.

7.82

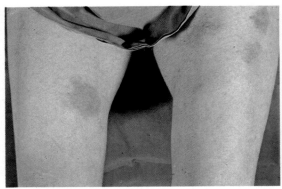

7.83

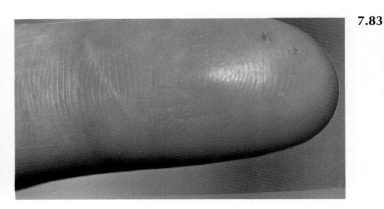

7.82 Local allergy to insulin injections is less common when purified preparations are used, but may still occur. The usual manifestations are erythema and sometimes urticaria at injection sites. The areas are itchy and hot to the touch.

7.83 Septic finger pulp in diabetes. This young diabetic girl had been using the finger-prick method to test her own blood sugar level, but the finger had become infected.

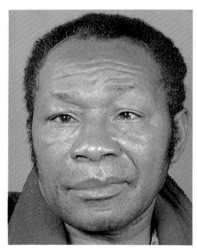

7.84 Mononeuritis multiplex in diabetes, affecting the right sixth and seventh facial nerves in a mild diabetic. The presenting symptoms were facial weakness and double vision. The right side of the face is palsied, as seen in this attempt to smile by the patient. He also had double vision on looking to the right, because a right sixth nerve palsy prevented lateral gaze in the right eye.

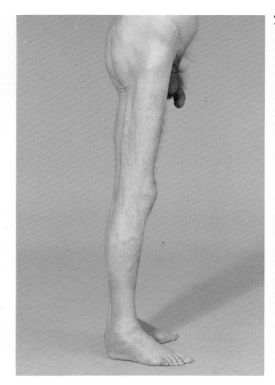

7.85 Diabetic amyotrophy, causing wasting of the thigh muscles. Adequate control of diabetes may lead to partial or total resolution of diabetic neuropathy.

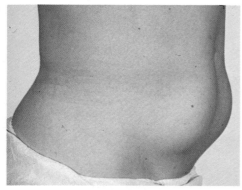

7.86 Lipohypertrophy at the site of repeated insulin injections in the lower abdomen in a young female diabetic.

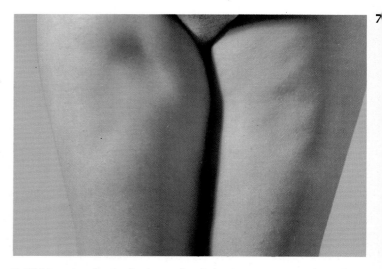

7.87 Lipoatrophy in the legs of a diabetic patient, resulting from repeated insulin injections in these sites.

Macroangiopathy is responsible for a high prevalence of coronary, peripheral and cerebral artery disease in diabetics. Accelerated atherosclerosis occurs at a young age and runs an aggressive course in diabetes, especially in women. It accounts for most deaths from diabetes, particularly in NIDDM.

Microangiopathy is a generalised microvascular (capillary) disorder that is specific to diabetes and clinically most apparent in the eyes, kidneys and nerves. It is characterised by capillary basement membrane thickening, endothelial cell dysfunction, platelet aggregation, impaired fibrinolysis and a pro-thrombotic tendency, and results in microvascular occlusion and tissue ischaemia. The sequence of events in microangiopathy is best seen in the retina (p. 336–339).

Diabetic renal disease is an important cause of morbidity and mortality, especially in IDDM. Its diagnosis and management are discussed on p. 291.

Chronic diabetic neuropathy may have a microvascular component in its etiology, but intraneural metabolic derangement caused by alternative pathways of glucose metabolism is also implicated.

- Sensory neuropathy usually presents in the feet as a painless trophic ulcer (7.88) or as a neuropathic arthropathy — a Charcot joint (7.89). Stiffness of the joints is a common feature best demonstrated by the 'prayer sign' (7.90).
- Motor neuropathy may lead to interosseous muscle wasting in the hands and feet (7.91).

- Autonomic neuropathy may cause postural hypotension, impaired cardiovascular reflexes, gastroparesis, atonic bladder, impotence and disturbance of sweating (7.92).

The diabetic foot. The common combination of neuropathy and peripheral vascular disease often results in peripheral gangrene (7.93). Sometimes patients have good peripheral pulses, the ischaemic damage being secondary to small vessel occlusion. Care of the feet is an important part of the management of diabetes. As in other peripheral vascular diseases (*see* p. 252), gangrene usually requires treatment by amputation.

Dermatological manifestations of diabetes include acanthosis nigricans (2.75), necrobiosis lipoidica (2.120), granuloma annulare (2.119) and candidal and staphylococcal infections (1.92, 2.49, 2.50). Xanthomata are common as a result of hyperlipidaemia (*see* p. 339).

Diabetes in pregnancy poses special problems, but the outlook for the fetus is greatly improved by good diabetic control. Even so, the typical baby born to a diabetic mother is overweight and prone to neonatal complications (7.94), which can however, usually be overcome by intensive care in the neonatal period. Congenital abnormalities are more common in babies born to diabetic mothers.

7.88

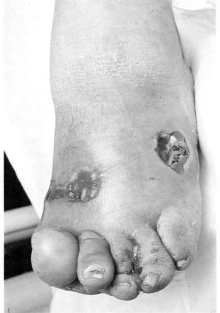

7.88 Painless trophic ulceration of the foot is a common presenting feature of sensory neuropathy in diabetes. Diabetic ulcers are commonly complicated by infection, and where peripheral vascular disease is present, gangrene may also develop.

7.89

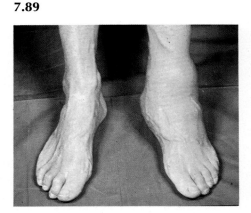

7.89 Charcot joint in diabetes. Sensory neuropathy has led to derangement of the left forefoot and ankle. Note the distortion and swelling. The derangement was painless, and there was little functional disability. On examination, the patient had loss of sensation and reflexes in the left ankle and foot.

7.90

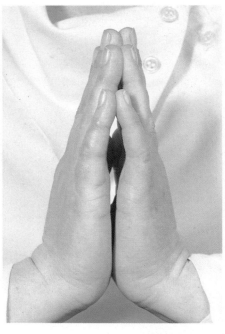

7.90 The 'prayer sign' in diabetes. Joint movement is limited, and the patient is unable to bring together the palms of the hands as in prayer. Note also the 'waxy' changes in the skin. Both these features are associated with diabetic microangiopathy.

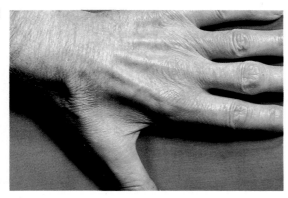

7.91 Ulnar mononeuropathy in a diabetic patient, causing wasting of the small muscles of the hand.

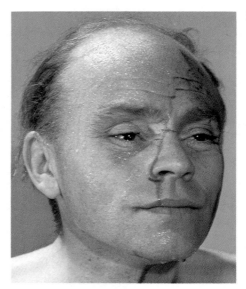

7.92 Autonomic neuropathy has led to gustatory sweating in this diabetic patient. Spicy food and cheese provokes sweating in an area on the right side of the head and trunk, as outlined with iodine in this picture. Autonomic neuropathy is an important and irreversible chronic complication of diabetes.

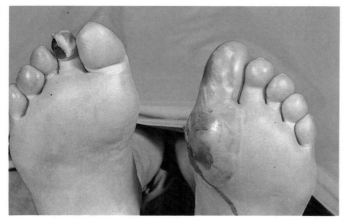

7.93 Gangrene of the foot is a common complication of chronic diabetes. In this patient 'wet' gangrene has developed in the hallux of the left foot, and dry gangrene in the second toe of the right foot. Ulceration and gangrene of the foot are commonly the result of a combination of diabetic neuropathy with large and/or small vessel disease.

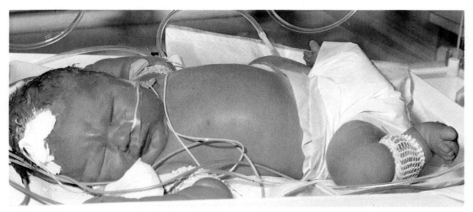

7.94 A baby born to a diabetic mother at 38 weeks' gestation. The baby was large, oedematous and plethoric. Management in a special-care baby unit is advisable to overcome the risks of respiratory distress, but the overall outcome is now much better than in the past.

Diabetes and the eye

Diabetes has numerous effects on all parts of the eye (**Table 7.6**). 'Senile' cataract (**7.95**) occurs at a younger age in diabetics than in other patients, and rarer conditions such as rubeosis iridis (**7.96**) may also affect the anterior parts of the eye.

Extreme hypertriglyceridaemia may be visible in the retinal vessels as lipaemia retinalis (**7.97**).

The major retinal changes in diabetes are a reflection of microangiopathy, and their progress gives valuable information on the likely effect of the diabetes on other organs (especially the kidney), as well as on the retina itself.

The characteristic early lesions are microaneurysms associated with exudates and venous dilatation (**7.98**). These early changes are best visualised by fluorescein angiograms (**7.99**) and are designated early background retinopathy (**7.100, 7.101**). They are common, occurring in 80% of patients who have had diabetes for 20 years. They do not always threaten sight and need no specific treatment, but must be monitored because exudates around the macula with associated oedema are a common cause of diabetic blindness (**7.102, 7.103**). Cotton wool spots (**7.104**) are retinal infarcts and are a bad prognostic sign, as the retina responds to ischaemia by capillary proliferation. The formation of new vessels (**7.105, 7.106**) is a serious form of retinopathy as they give rise to vitreous haemorrhages and blindness. New vessels may form on the disc (**7.106**) or in the periphery (**7.107**), and they tend to extend forward into the vitreous leading to haemorrhage (**7.107, 7.108**) and fibrosis.

Diabetic retinopathy may be complicated by the presence of hypertension (**7.109**) or by thrombosis in the retinal veins (**7.110**).

Proliferative retinopathy and maculopathy can often be treated by laser photocoagulation which may prevent blindness by producing an iatrogenic choroidoretinitis (**7.111**).

Table 7.6 The ocular manifestations of diabetes mellitus.

Eyelids:	xanthelasmata caused by hyperlipidaemia (**7.113**)
Conjunctiva:	microaneurysms, venous dilatation
Extra-ocular muscles:	palsy with diplopia caused by 3rd, 4th or 6th cranial nerve involvement (**7.84**)
Orbit:	mucormycosis—a potential complication of severe diabetic acidosis
Iris:	neovascularisation of the anterior surface (rubeosis iridis, **7.96**)
Glaucoma:	neovascular glaucoma, chronic open angle glaucoma
Pupil:	poor dilatation caused by rubeosis iridis, Argyll Robertson pupil (**11.8**)
Lens:	cataract (**7.95**), refractive errors
Vitreous body:	vitreous haemorrhage (**7.108**), asteroid hyalosis
Retina:	diabetic retinopathy (**7.98–7.111**), retinal vein occlusion (**7.110**), lipaemia retinalis (**7.97**)
Optic nerve:	ischaemic papillitis, optic atrophy

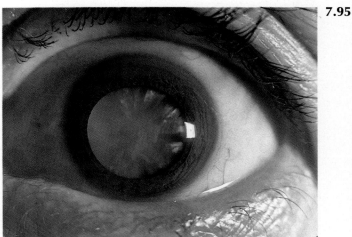

7.95

7.95 'Senile' cataract occurs at a younger age in diabetic patients than in the normal population. Reversible 'osmotic' cataracts may also form acutely in poorly controlled diabetics.

7.96

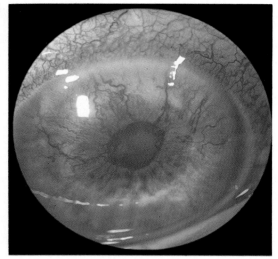

7.96 Rubeosis iridis. New vessels develop on the anterior surface of the iris in response to severe ocular ischaemia. Resulting obstruction to aqueous drainage may lead to glaucoma. Rubeosis iridis is most commonly a complication of diabetes, but may also occur in patients with carotid stenosis, long-standing retinal detachments, central retinal vein occlusion or ocular tumours.

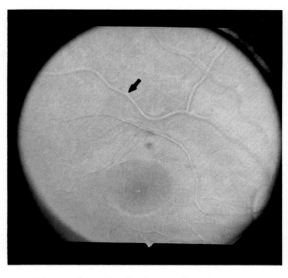

7.97 Lipaemia retinalis is a reflection of severe hypertriglyceridaemia. The retinal vessels appear white as a result of the 'milky' chylomicron-rich plasma within them. Lipaemia retinalis is commonly seen in acute uncontrolled diabetes.

7.98

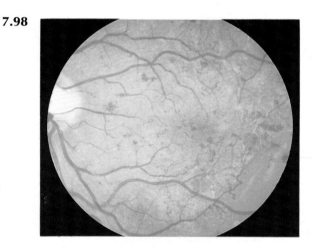

7.98 Background diabetic retinopathy. Note the presence of multiple microaneurysms and some small areas of haemorrhage.

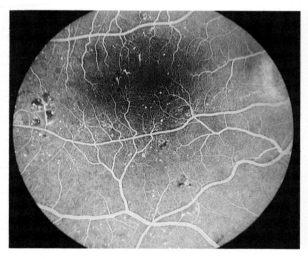

7.99 Fluorescein angiogram in background diabetic retinopathy, showing the presence of multiple microaneurysms.

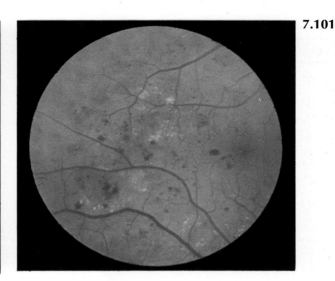

7.100 Background diabetic retinopathy. The arrow points to a soft exudate. This represents an area of retinal infarction. Small haemorrhages are also present, and there is evidence of deterioration in the retinal microcirculation.

7.101 Background diabetic retinopathy with microaneurysms (dots), retinal haemorrhages (blots) and hard yellow exudates. Despite the appearance, the patient's visual acuity is usually unaffected at this stage.

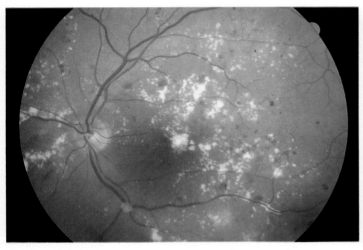

7.102 Macular involvement in diabetic retinopathy is a common cause of diabetic blindness. Note the presence of multiple exudates and the blurring caused by macular oedema—the most common cause of visual impairment in macular disease.

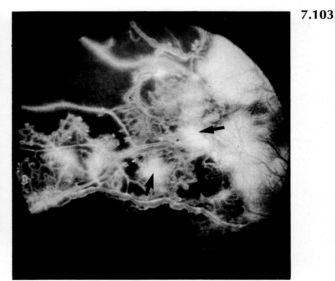

7.103 Fluorescein angiogram of diabetic retinopathy with macular involvement and blindness. Note the widespread capillary microaneurysms and the extensive capillary leakage in the two areas arrowed.

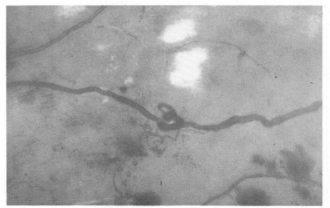

7.104 Cotton wool spots in diabetic retinopathy. These are retinal infarcts resulting from arterial occlusion. They are a bad prognostic sign, because they are likely to herald capillary proliferation.

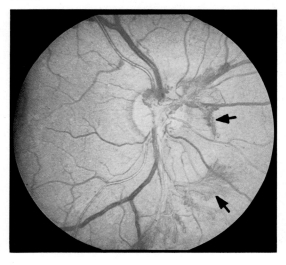

7.105 Proliferative diabetic retinopathy. Fronds of new vessels (arrowed) can be seen emerging from the disc and elsewhere.

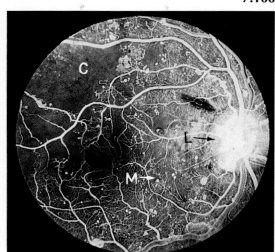

7.106 Fluorescein angiogram in diabetic retinopathy showing dark ischaemic areas in which capillaries are abnormally absent (C), micro-aneurysms (M) and leakage from new vessels on the optic disc (L).

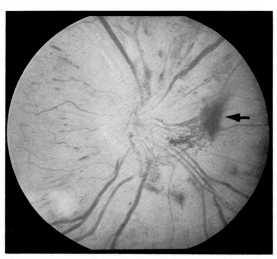

7.107 Proliferative diabetic retinopathy. Some new vessels have grown forwards into the vitreous, and haemorrhage has occurred into the retina and the vitreous (arrow).

7.108 Vitreous haemorrhage resulting from proliferative retinopathy in diabetes. These haemorrhages appear as a haze or a red or black reflex through the ophthalmoscope as in the curvilinear accumulation of blood seen here. This patient's proliferative retinopathy has been treated by laser photocoagulation, which has left typical circular scars.

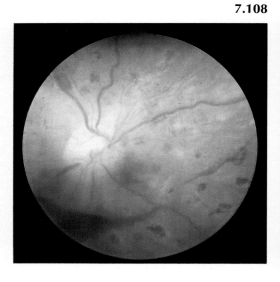

7.109

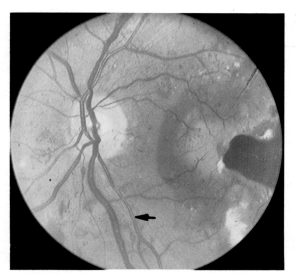

7.109 Diabetic retinopathy in a hypertensive patient. Note the presence of hypertensive vessel changes (silver-wiring—arrowed) and a macular subhyaloid haemorrhage. Hypertension adds to the risk of haemorrhage in diabetic retinopathy.

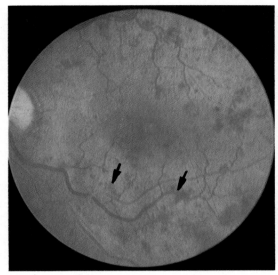

7.110 Retinal venous thrombosis occurring in a diabetic patient with background retinopathy. Pointers to the diagnosis include unilateral capillary engorgement and haemorrhage (arrowed) along the whole length of the vessel. Retinal venous thrombosis is more common in diabetics than in other patients, and may be unassociated with other features of diabetic retinal disease.

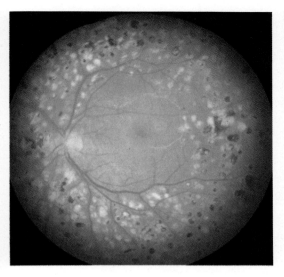

7.111 Photocoagulation is usually the treatment of choice for proliferative diabetic retinopathy. Here it has resulted in numerous typical scars in the peripheral retina, many of which reveal the black pigmentation of the choroid beneath the destroyed retinal cells.

Hyperlipidaemia

Hyperlipidaemia may be classified on the basis of laboratory findings, disease entities or genetic and genetic environmental causes. All such classifications are complex and potentially confusing.

The importance of hyperlipidaemia relates mainly to its association with atheromatous vascular disease. There is clear evidence that elevation of the level of cholesterol (and probably also of triglycerides) is important in the premature development of atheroma and thrombotic events, such as myocardial infarction, thrombotic stroke and peripheral gangrene. There is also evidence at population and individual patient levels, that a lowering in total blood cholesterol (specifically in the LDL fraction) leads to a decrease in the risk of cardiovascular morbidity and mortality.

In many patients, lipid abnormalities are now identified in screening programmes, but a number of clinical signs may give clues, especially in patients with gross hyperlipidaemia. These include:

- Premature arcus cornealis (7.112, 7.113, 8.2, 9.5)
- Xanthelasmata (7.113, 9.5, 9.36)
- Skin xanthomata (7.114, 7.115, 9.6)
- Tendon xanthomata (7.116, 7.117)
- Lipaemia retinalis (7.97)

The diagnosis of hyperlipidaemia is easily made on a fasting blood sample. In Western countries, counselling and treatment can often be based on cholesterol and triglyceride levels alone, but the measurement of LDL, and HDL, cholesterol may be useful in some patients. It is important to identify or exclude causes of secondary hyperlipidaemia (**Table 7.7**).

It is essential that any recommendations for dietary modification or drug therapy are made in the context of an overall assessment of the patient's cardiovascular risk profile. Other risk factors (smoking, hypertension, etc., *see* p. 222) should be identified and treated at the same time, and the patient's family history should be investigated so that other at-risk family members can be identified, especially where a familial disorder is suspected.

A number of international working parties have recommended levels at which treatment should be instigated for hyperlipidaemia, and a consensus view is summarised in **Table 7.8**. Treatment of hyperlipidaemia starts with a diet low in saturated fats, and rich in fibre, complex carbohydrates and in poly- or monounsaturated oils and fish. If this is unsuccessful over a 3- to 6-month period, a range of lipid lowering drugs is available, but drugs should usually be given only when diet has failed.

Therapy for hypercholesterolaemia may involve the use of a bile acid sequestrant resin, a fibrate, a nicotinic acid derivative or an HMG-CoA reductase inhibitor. A fibrate or nicotinic acid derivative can be used to lower triglyceride when diet has proved ineffective. Combinations of hypertriglyceridaemia and hypercholesterolaemia are usually treated by fibrates or nicotinic acid derivatives.

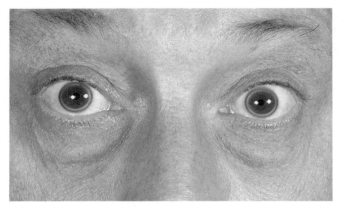

7.112 Corneal arcus is a normal phenomenon associated with ageing (arcus senilis), but its occurrence in patients under the age of 50 years suggests the possibility of underlying hyperlipidaemia. The ring represents deposits of phospholipid and cholesterol in the corneal stroma.

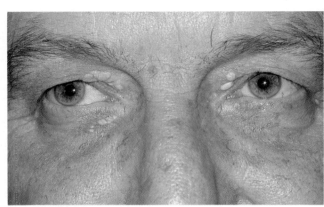

7.113 Corneal arcus and xanthelasmata in the same patient. This combination is strongly suggestive of an underlying hyperlipidaemia, and the presence of xanthelasmata alone is an indication for investigation of lipid status.

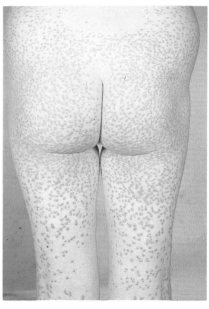

7.114 Eruptive xanthomas may be quite widespread in the skin, but they are most commonly found over the buttocks. They are strongly suggestive of an underlying hyper-lipidaemia.

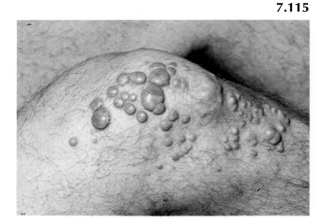

7.115 Tuberous xanthomata on the knee, occurring in a patient with familial hypercholesterolaemia. Massive xanthomata may sometimes require surgical removal.

7.117 Tendon xanthomata are characteristically found over the tendons and extensor surfaces of joints. They are particularly common over the patellar and Achilles tendons. This patient had familial hypercholesterolaemia.

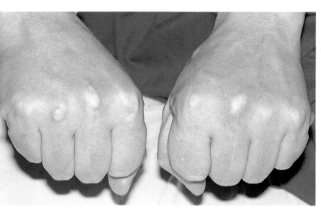

7.116 Tendon xanthomata were the first clue to the diagnosis in this patient with familial hypercholesterolaemia and premature coronary heart disease.

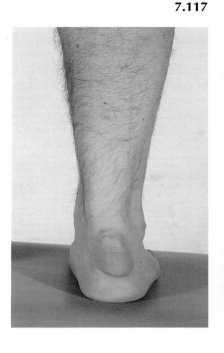

Table 7.7 Secondary causes of raised cholesterol and triglyceride.

Raised cholesterol
Diet
Hypothyroidism
Liver disease
Nephrotic syndrome
Porphyria

Raised triglyceride
Obesity
Poorly controlled diabetes
Alcohol excess
High-carbohydrate diet
Renal failure
Oestrogen therapy

Table 7.8 Action levels for treatment of hyperlipidaemia.

Cholesterol

<5.2 mmol/l	**Satisfactory:** No action.
5.2–6.5 mmol/l	**Moderately elevated:** Diet and counselling on other risk factors. Recheck in 3/12.
6.5–7.8 mmol/l	**High:** Diet first—consider drugs only if diet fails and other risk factors are present.
>7.8 mmol/l	**Very high:** Diet, assess other risk factors, other family members. If diet fails use drugs.

Triglyceride

<3.0 mmol/l	**Satisfactory:** No action.
3.0–6.0 mmol/l	**High:** Check HDL; lose weight; diet; counsel on other risk factors; consider drugs if diet fails, especially if HDL is <1.0 mmol/l.
>6.0 mmol/l	**Very high:** Check HDL; lose weight; diet; drugs are indicated to prevent CHD and pancreatitis.

Nutritional disorders

Obesity

Storage of lipids in excess of daily requirements results in obesity — an excess of adipose tissue that is associated with a health risk. Obesity is defined as a 20% excess over ideal body weight and in many Western populations, 30–40% of individuals are obese. Most obese individuals ingest excess calories that are then stored. The reasons for overeating are not clear, but they may involve psychosocial factors that modulate the activity of the satiety centre; and this may be coupled with reduced calorie expenditure resulting from a sedentary existence, or with alterations of thermogenesis. In a small number of cases, obesity is secondary to diseases such as hypothyroidism, Cushing's syndrome and extremely rare disorders such as insulinoma, Fröhlich's syndrome and the Prader–Willi syndrome.

The end result of excessive calorie intake is an increase in fat deposition around the internal organs, muscles and in subcutaneous sites, such as abdomen, buttocks, breasts, thighs, face and upper arms (7.118–7.120). Such obesity is associated with insulin resistance and glucose intolerance, hyperlipidaemia, hypertension and an increased incidence of thrombotic arterial and venous disease and of degenerative joint diseases.

Tables of desirable weights are available for age, sex and height. A more acceptable and accurate assessment method is to use the Body Mass Index (BMI), which is calculated as weight in kilograms divided by height in metres squared. Measurement of skin-fold thickness is valuable over the upper arm and back (7.121).

Treatment is by calorie restriction, which must be permanent and represent a real change in lifestyle. Patients should also be encouraged to exercise. Adherence to a diet providing 800–1200 calories per day results in weight loss. A waist cord may encourage the patient to maintain the lower weight (7.122).

Attempts may also be made to stop patients eating by wiring the jaws (7.123), using an inflated balloon to fill the stomach or by surgery to create a jejuno-ileal bypass. All these procedures may have major complications and are used only as a last resort.

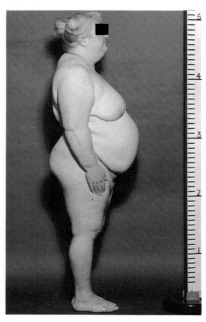

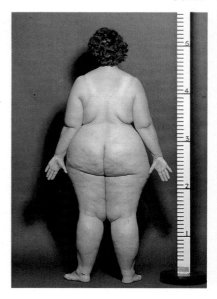

7.118, 7.119 Simple obesity in these women has led to excessive fat deposition in the upper arms, breasts, abdomen, buttocks and thighs. This distribution is typical.

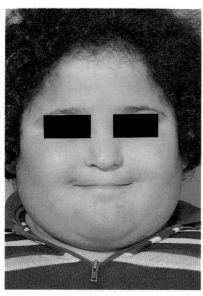

7.120 Simple obesity may lead to gross roundness and fatness of the face. It is important to differentiate this appearance from that of Cushing's syndrome (**7.26**).

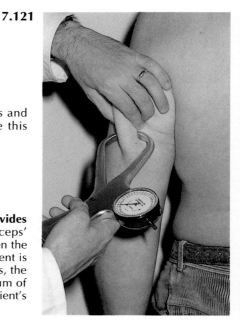

7.121 Skinfold thickness, using special calipers, provides an objective measure of body fat. Here, the 'triceps' skinfold thickness is being measured halfway between the acromial and olecranon processes. If this measurement is accompanied by other measurements over the biceps, the subscapular region and the suprailiac region, the sum of the four thicknesses can then be used to assess the patient's degree of obesity.

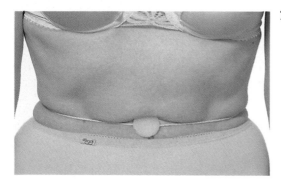

7.122 A waist cord may be useful in maintaining weight loss in the obese patient. Once the patient has lost weight, the cord is firmly fixed around the waist, and its ends are knotted and held within the plastic button. If the patient gains weight, the extra pressure of the tightened cord serves as a reminder to eat less.

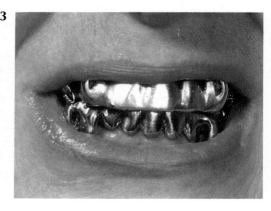

7.123 Jaw wiring is an extreme method of accomplishing rapid weight loss. A stainless-steel cast is made from a wax impression of the teeth and jaw, and this is then cemented to the teeth. The upper and lower casts are held together with wire loops which can be cut rapidly in an emergency. Liquid food is then taken via a straw inserted through a gap in the cast. This technique is hazardous if the patient vomits for any reason, as the vomit is likely to be inhaled. Nevertheless, some still use the technique, especially when an obese patient must lose weight before important surgery.

Protein-energy malnutrition

In protein-energy malnutrition (PEM) there is a loss of adipose tissue and lean body mass, usually as a result of deficient quantitative and qualitative food intake in the Third World, or of malabsorption or organic disease (usually malignancy) in the West. PEM is of insidious onset, and up to a quarter of the world's population lives on the verge of insufficiency of protein and calorie intake.

The group most commonly affected is children. Their growth is stunted, and they may show evidence of loss of muscle mass with spindly arms and legs, and with a bloated abdomen, caused partly by ascites. There is usually little or no subcutaneous fat. Most internal organs are also affected. There is a small heart with reduced cardiac output, atrophy of endocrine glands producing hypofunction, atrophy of the intestinal wall that may lead to rectal prolapse, atrophy of muscle and an increased risk of infection because of reduced immune function; the liver may be enlarged as a result of fatty infiltration. The terms 'kwashiorkor' and 'marasmus' are descriptive terms of the extent of the PEM. In marasmus, there is a deficiency in total food intake. The child is apathetic, withdrawn, and stunted in growth with spindly arms and legs. In kwashiorkor, the major deficiency is in protein intake. The child has a swollen abdomen with dependent oedema of the legs, often with skin and eye infections, a large fatty liver, and a reddish-yellow tinge to the hair, The two conditions are part of a spectrum and may co-exist in the same community (7.124).

In the adult, weight loss is the most common feature of the disease. Often these people are old, poor or reclusive; they may have alcoholism or psychiatric disease and take an extremely deficient diet. There may be evidence of chronic infections (e.g. tuberculosis), malignancy, previous surgery (particularly alimentary) or diseases of kidneys or liver. The appearances are typical, with obvious major weight loss so that the person looks skeletal with significant loss of adipose tissue, skin hanging in folds, wasted limbs, ascites, dependent oedema, dry flaky skin and depigmentation (7.125). The blood pressure is reduced, the pulse slow, and central core temperature may be reduced. The triceps skin fold thickness and muscle bulk are reduced. There may also be other features of vitamin or trace element deficiency.

The diagnosis is usually made clinically, but investigations show anaemia that may be caused by iron and/or folate deficiency; biochemistry shows the extent of the protein deficiency, with low serum albumin and transferrin. There may also be impairment of renal and liver function. Immunity is also depressed, with cutaneous energy and lymphopoenia. Death is often caused by infection.

Treatment is with a diet of normal calorie content and constituents. This should be implemented slowly and young children may require nasogastric feeding. Hypothermia and infections require treatment. Supplements of vitamins and minerals should also be given.

PEM is probably the most common cause of death worldwide. The mortality of severe cases is 50–75%, and there is a massive morbidity resulting from physical and mental stunting.

7.124

7.125

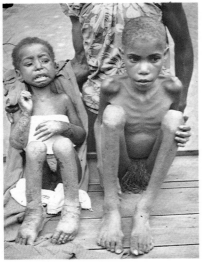

7.124 Kwashiorkor and marasmus in brothers. The younger brother, on the left, has kwashiorkor with generalised oedema, skin changes, pale reddish-yellow hair and a miserable expression. The older child, on the right, has marasmus, with generalised wasting, spindly arms and legs and an apathetic expression.

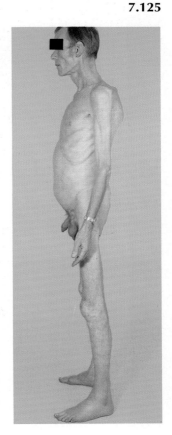

7.125 Malnutrition has resulted in severe weight loss. Underlying malignant disease, chronic infection or malabsorption is the most likely cause, but occasionally the condition may result simply from self-neglect and inadequate food intake.

Anorexia and bulimia nervosa

Anorexia nervosa usually occurs in white adolescent girls. It results in severe weight loss as a result of 'voluntary' starvation. There is often a history of obesity in childhood; there may have been psychological trauma with teasing at school, which has produced an intense desire to alter the body image; and there may be associated psychosexual problems. Patients often deny hunger or weight loss. They become devious about avoidance of eating and may vomit up a meal surreptitiously if they have been forced to eat. The clinical features include:

- Onset before age 25 years in a female.
- Loss of >25% of body weight — absence of body fat.
- Secondary amenorrhoea.
- Presence of lanugo hair over body.
- Preservation of breast tissue.
- Parotid enlargement.
- Dependent oedema.
- Low blood pressure with bradycardia.

The facial and bodily appearances are recognisable, but not in themselves diagnostic (7.126, 7.127).

There is no diagnostic laboratory test, but there may be anaemia and leucopenia, and the serum albumin may be low. There is often a disturbance of glucose tolerance. Many patients show disturbance of other endocrine function with reduction of LH/FSH secretion and reduced cortisol and thyroxine levels.

Treatment is often difficult, but includes psychological and physical support.

Bulimia nervosa is a related condition in which binge eating is associated with self-induced vomiting.

7.126

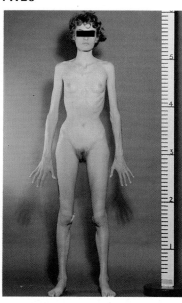

7.126 Anorexia nervosa in a 20-year-old woman. Note the low body weight and the preservation of breast tissue. Fine lanugo hair was present over the patient's back, and she had developed secondary amenorrhoea. Her blood pressure was 100/60 mmHg and her pulse 60/minute.

7.127 Lanugo hair in anorexia nervosa. Fine, downy body hair is characteristic of anorexia nervosa but may also occur in normal individuals.

7.127

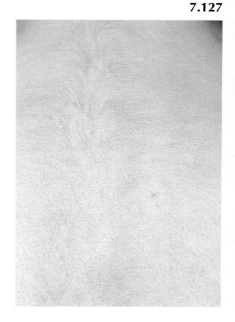

Vitamins and disease

Vitamin A (Retinol)

In the human diet, vitamin A is found mainly in dairy products (milk, butter, eggs and cheese) and in liver and is added to various foods, especially margarine, as ß-carotene, the immediate precursor. A normal balanced diet provides 750–1000µg per day — sufficient to maintain the liver stores of this vitamin.

Vitamin A is necessary for the normal function of most cell lines but particularly for function of the retinal cells (especially the rods), and for the integrity of the conjunctival epithelium and the skin generally. Dietary deficiency may be found worldwide, particularly amongst rice-eating populations and those suffering from protein-energy malnutrition. In the West it is found in patients with malabsorption, especially following surgical removal of portions of the small intestine.

Deficiency of vitamin A leads rapidly to night blindness because of failure of rhodopsin regeneration in the rods. Alterations to the conjunctival and corneal epithelium and the tear glands produce dryness and roughness with loss of sensation, followed by erosions and local inflammation (xerophthalmia). Bitot's spots are frothy waxy white accumulations of desquamated epithelium on the exposed conjunctiva at the corneal edge (7.128). The end result may be visual impairment and blindness as the erosions enlarge, become infected and allow prolapse of the iris and lens (keratomalacia).

The skin is also generally affected, with loss of sebaceous gland function as the glands become covered with keratin.

The diagnosis is clinical, but the plasma vitamin A may be measured, as may the visual fields in different light intensities. Fluorescein angiography is of value in defining the retinal changes.

Treatment is with vitamin A. This may require health education and dietary change for a community. Those with features of deficiency will readily respond to vitamin A given orally, or by injection where there is malabsorption.

Intoxication with vitamin A is rare and may present acutely with nausea, vomiting and headache as a result of a rise in intracranial pressure. Chronic overdosage results in changes in the skeleton as a result of painful periosteal proliferation. Hypercalcaemia may also be found. Stopping the excessive vitamin intake results in rapid healing of the lesions.

Excess ingestion of ß-carotene-containing foods, i.e. carrot juice, carrots, or dark green leafy vegetables, may lead to pigmentation of the skin (7.129).

7.129

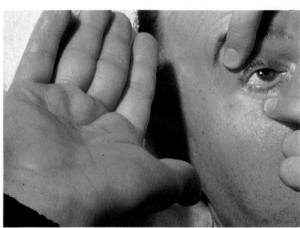

7.129 Carotenaemia has resulted in an orangy pigmentation of the skin in this patient. The condition can be distinguished from jaundice by examination of the sclerae, which remain white. This rare condition is usually the result of excessive ingestion of carrots or other carotene-containing foods. It is benign and usually subsides after withdrawal of the source.

7.128

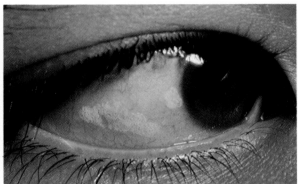

7.128 Bitot's spots in vitamin A deficiency. These may be single or, as here, multiple, and they represent areas of desquamated, keratinised conjunctival cells, together with lipid material. The patient also has dryness and inflammation of the scleral conjunctiva (xerophthalmia). This combination is typically seen in nutritional deficiency, especially where there is a lack of vitamin A.

Niacin

Niacin is the generic name for nicotinic acid and related compounds which are widely available in the diet and can be synthesised in the body from tryptophan. The daily requirement is of the order of 20 mg, and if absent from the diet, clinical features of deficiency (pellagra) appear in about a month. Pellagra is found particularly in populations who eat maize as their staple diet, as tryptophan is absent from maize proteins and niacin is present in an unavailable form. It may also be found in general malnutrition, as in chronic alcoholism or malabsorption syndrome, with low protein diets and in certain genetic disorders. Use of isoniazid for treatment of tuberculosis may induce deficiency.

The typical clinical presentation of pellagra is that of a chronic wasting disease associated with the triad of dermatitis, dementia and diarrhoea. The skin lesions are symmetrical, often, but not only, on skin exposed to sunlight (7.130). The features of dementia are associated with peripheral neuropathy. Diarrhoea is associated with mucosal changes that may also manifest as glossitis, proctitis and vaginitis.

Diagnosis is purely clinical and is confirmed by a rapid response to therapy with niacin or tryptophan.

7.130

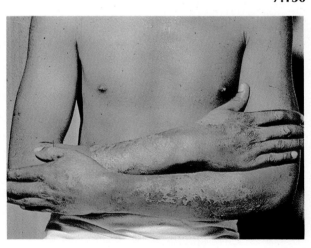

7.130 Pellagra. The skin changes begin as an erythema with pruritus and burning. Bullae may form and rupture. At the slightly later stage shown here, the skin becomes hard, rough, cracked, blackish and brittle; and with more severe involvement, extensive exfoliation may occur. Here only sun-exposed areas are affected, but any part of the body may become involved.

Thiamine

Thiamine is found extensively in vegetable products and in animal tissues. There may be major losses during preparation of food (e.g. machine milling of rice) and also during cooking above 100°C. The absorption and metabolism of thiamine are affected by factors such as pregnancy, alcoholism and co-incidental diarrhoeal disease. Storage in the body is minimal and deficiency develops rapidly on a diet containing under 1 mg per day. Two rather diferent syndromes may result:

- Wet beriberi is characterised by peripheral vasodilation with a hyperkinetic circulation, heart failure and retention of fluid, with oedema of the legs, ascites, hepatomegaly and pulmonary congestion (7.131). Peripheral neuropathy is a common accompaniment.
- Dry beriberi is manifest as peripheral neuropathy with symmetrical loss of sensation, and loss of motor function

(7.132), encephalopathy with cranial nerve palsies, ataxia, confusion, coma and death. The Wernicke–Korsakoff syndrome is usually associated with thiamine deficiency in alcoholic patients. It consists of retrograde amnesia and confusion in association with other features of dry beriberi.

The diagnosis is often made on clinical grounds, as there is usually evidence of cause (e.g. alcoholism, inadequate diet or famine). A range of biochemical tests is available in specialised laboratories, including blood thiamine, pyruvate, lactate and red cell transketolase. Clinical response to added thiamine can be dramatic, with reversal of heart failure, spontaneous diuresis and improvement of neurological signs, but only about half the patients with severe deficiencies recover full neurological function.

7.131

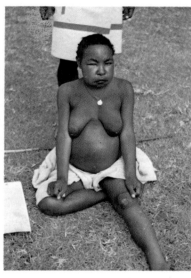

7.131 Wet beriberi. The patient has generalised oedema and signs of pulmonary congestion resulting from left heart failure. Peripheral neuropathy was also demonstrable.

7.132

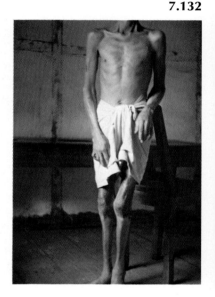

7.132 Dry beriberi. This patient has chronic polyneuritis, with wrist drop and foot drop. In dry beriberi, there is also: loss of tendon reflexes; joint position sense and vibration sense; tenderness in the calf muscles on pressure; anaesthesia of the skin, especially over the tibia; paraesthesia in the legs and arms; and motor weakness.

Riboflavin

7.133

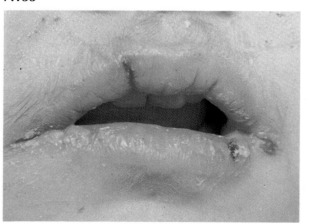

Riboflavin is found in vegetables and meat. The daily requirement is about 1.5 mg, and deficiency is most commonly seen in association with deficiencies of other vitamins and minerals. The clinical picture is that of muco-cutaneous changes which are known as the oro-oculo-genital syndrome. There are extensive changes in the mouth and pharynx with glossitis, cheilosis (7.133), angular stomatitis and oedema of the pharyngeal and oral mucosa. There may also be marrow depression with a normochromic normocytic anaemia and widespread seborrhoeic dermatitis involving the scrotum or perineum.

7.133 Cheilosis is one manifestation of riboflavin deficiency, and may also occur with deficiency of iron and other vitamins. It is characterised by vertical fissuring, which is later complicated by redness, swelling and ulceration of the lips. Angular stomatitis may also be present, as here; and many patients with riboflavin deficiency also have widespread seborrhoeic dermatitis involving the scrotum or perineum.

Pyridoxine (Vitamin B₆)

Pyridoxine and related vitamin B_6 molecules are found widely in meats, vegetables and grains and an intake of about 2 mg is required per day. Dietary deficiency is rare, but may be found as part of a more generalised deficiency in patients with malabsorption syndromes or chronic alcoholism. The most common presentation now results from B_6 antagonism by drug therapy with penicillamine, cycloserine or isoniazid.

The clinical features of deficiency are seborrhoeic dermatitis and glossitis (**9.35**). The diagnosis may be made by measurement of tryptophan metabolites, and deficiency rapidly responds to dietary supplementation with pyridoxine.

Also described are a range of pyridoxine-responsive disorders that include a genetic liability to epilepsy and brain damage, chronic anaemia with ringed sideroblasts, cystathioninuria and xanthenurenic aciduria.

Biotin

Biotin deficiency is exceptionally rare and is found only in food faddists. The clinical features may include dermatitis, fatigue, depression and mucosal changes in the mouth and intestine.

Vitamin E

Vitamin E deficiency is rare in man, but has been associated with haemolysis. Recent work suggests that the vitamin also has a role as an antioxidant and may prove to be of long-term value in the prevention of atheroma formation.

Other Vitamins

Diseases related to deficiencies or excess of other vitamins are included elsewhere in the book:

- Folic acid: pp. 368, 427.
- Vitamin B_{12}: pp. 368, 427.
- Ascorbic acid: **8.19**, p. 459.
- Vitamin D: pp. 153, 368.
- Vitamin K: **9.14**, pp. 368, 462.

Trace elements in nutrition

A large number of inorganic ions are essential for the maintenance of health. These include iron, iodine, copper, zinc, cobalt, selenium, chromium and tin. Deficiencies of iron and iodine are discussed on p. 424 and p. 323 respectively. Identifiable clinical syndromes have also been described in zinc and copper deficiency.

Deficiency of zinc in the diet may lead to retarded growth, retarded sexual development, hyperkeratotic dermatitis, loss of hair and anaemia. Supplementation of the diet with zinc produces a growth sprint and correction of anaemia.

Acrodermatitis enteropathica is an inherited disorder of zinc absorption which presents with chronic diarrhoea and growth retardation, weight loss, dermatitis, and perianal and perianal ulceration, often caused by candidal infections. It responds dramatically to zinc therapy.

Deficiency of copper in the diet is rare and is usually associated with other deficiencies, especially of protein and vitamins. Anaemia and leucopenia are the usual manifestations and these respond to normalisation of the diet. Menke's kinky hair syndrome results from an extremely rare disorder of intestinal copper absorption. Death results from central nervous system and arterial degeneration.

Inherited metabolic disorders

The porphyrias

The porphyrias are a heterogeneous group of inborn errors of metabolism in which there is an overproduction of various intermediate compounds (porphyrins) in the biosynthesis of haem. Their classification is summarised in **Table 7.9**.

Table 7.9 The classification of porphyrias.

	Hepatic	Erythropoietic
Acute:	Acute intermittent porphyria Variegate porphyria Hereditary coproporphyria	
Non-acute:	Porphyria cutanea tarda	Congenital porphyria Erythropoietic protoporphyria

Acute intermittent porphyria

Acute intermittent porphryia is an autosomal dominant condition. It presents acutely in early adulthood with fever, abdominal pain and vomiting, which may be mistaken for an acute abdomen, but is caused by autonomic neuropathy. There may also be a history of acute onset of peripheral neuropathy with limb paralysis and loss of sensation, often associated with depression or anxiety. The diagnosis is often missed, and the symptoms may be attributed to hysteria. The clues lie in a positive family history and in examination of the urine, which turns dark red-brown on standing. Attacks may be precipitated by alcohol or by drugs such as anticonvulsants and oral contraceptives, and they may be associated with a rise in pulse rate and blood pressure. Between attacks there may be no clinical features.

During the acute attacks, there may be a polymorphonuclear leucocytosis, which may be misinterpreted as an indicator of infection. There may also be hyponatraemia, hypomagnesaemia and uraemia. The best screening test is to find porphobilinogen in the urine: on standing, the urine darkens, as a result of the formation of uroporphyrin and porphobilin, and it fluoresces in ultraviolet light after treatment with Ehrlich's aldehyde.

Treatment is supportive, with avoidance of drugs known to precipitate the acute attack.

Variegate porphyria

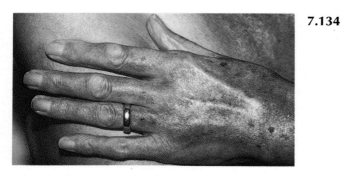

7.134

7.134 Variegate porphyria. Note the generalised pigmentation of the skin, associated with areas of atrophy and scarring. Bullae and hypertrichosis are also common in this condition, which is associated with chronic photosensitivity.

Variegate porphyria combines the acute features of acute intermittent porphyria with chronic skin sensitivity to sunlight and trauma. The inheritance is autosomal dominant. The clinical presentation is often similar to that of acute intermittent porphyria, but it occurs on a background of pigmentation of the skin, associated with bullae, ulceration, atrophy and hypertrichosis (7.134). The diagnosis is made by finding excess protoporphyrin in the urine at all times and a positive test for porphobilinogen during acute attacks. Important aspects of management include the avoidance of direct sunlight and the wearing of adequate protective clothing.

Porphyria cutanea tarda

Porphyria cutanea tarda is the most common type of porphyria and is characterised by chronic skin lesions and chronic liver disease, often associated with alcoholism and sometimes with hepatic siderosis. The clinical features are similar to the chronic features of variegate porphyria (7.135). The incidence of diabetes mellitus is increased and there is an association with a range of autoimmune diseases. As the disease is caused by an inherited deficiency of uroporphyrinogen decarboxylase, there is an increased excretion of uroporphyrin in the urine which may be pink or brown.

A similar clinical picture may be found in people poisoned with a range of polychlorinated hydrocarbons and with primary and secondary liver neoplasia.

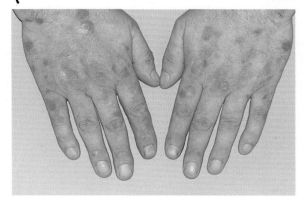

7.135 Porphyria cutanea tarda. Photosensitivity in this condition leads to blister formation and pigmented scarring.

7.136

Erythropoietic porphyria

This is a very rare genetic disorder of porphyrin metabolism in which the transmission is autosomal recessive. The usual clinical presentation is with solar urticaria without blistering, scarring or hyperpigmentation. Occasionally, patients may develop cirrhosis of the liver, splenomegaly, gallstones and anaemia. A characteristic feature is red pigmentation of the teeth (erythrodontia 7.136). The chemical defect is in the enzyme ferrochelatase which promotes the incorporation of ferrous iron into protoporphyrin. As a result, there is excessive protoporphyrin in many tissues, especially in haemopoietic cells, liver and skin. The diagnosis is made by demonstrating the red fluorescence of protoporphyrin in red cells in a blood film.

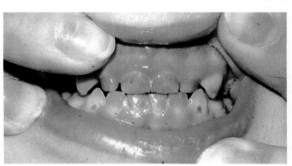

7.136 Erythropoietic porphyria leads to erythrodontia—reddish pigmentation of the teeth. Excessive protoporphyrin may also lead to abnormalities in the skin, liver, biliary tract, spleen and blood.

Disorders of amino acid metabolism

Phenylketonuria

This is an autosomal recessive disorder that produces deficiency of the enzyme (phenylalanine hydroxylase) responsible for the conversion of phenylalanine to tyrosine, with resultant high levels of phenylalanine and its metabolites in the blood and body tissues. This results in progressive mental retardation and epilepsy. There is usually fair, sparse hair and eczema. Neonatal screening is routinely available (the Guthrie test), and should enable most affected individuals to be detected early and dietary restrictions imposed.

7.137

Homocystinurias

The homocystinurias are transmitted as autosomal recessives and are caused by at least three enzyme defects which allow the accumulation of homocystine in the body. There is progressive mental impairment with epilepsy, subluxation of the lens (7.137), arachnodactyly and a likelihood of arterial and venous thrombosis.

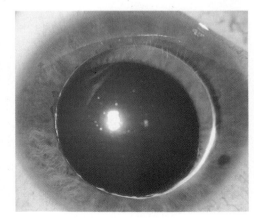

7.137 Subluxation of the lens is a common feature in homocystinuria. A familiar abnormality is a feature of Marfan's syndrome, but whereas the subluxation is usually downwards in homocystinuria, it is most commonly upwards in Marfan's syndrome. In this case, there is complete anterior dislocation of the lens.

Cystinosis

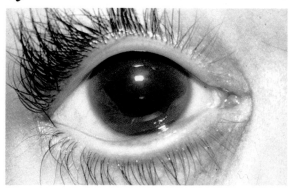

Cystinosis is an autosomal recessive disorder in which cystine accumulates in the tissues, especially the cornea, bone marrow, liver/spleen and kidneys. A range of disorders results: in childhood, the kidney is particularly affected and renal failure may develop (Fanconi syndrome); in the adult, the cornea is particularly affected (7.138). There are intermediate varieties. The diagnosis is made by finding typical cystine crystals in biopsy material or in the cornea by slit-lamp examination.

7.138 Cystinosis has led to the deposition of cystine in the cornea of this adult patient. The adult form of the disease is usually otherwise benign, though cystine also accumulates intracellularly in the reticuloendothelial cells.

Lysosomal storage diseases

Deficiencies of lysosomal enzymes may result in the accumulation of substrates or abnormal metabolites in all the tissues of the body. At least 30 separate enzyme deficiencies have been characterised and these produce different clinical syndromes of which only the most common are described here.

Lipoidoses

Gaucher's disease is an autosomal recessive disease, in which deficiency of the enzyme glucosylceramidase results in the accumulation of glucocerebroside in the body. The disease is found especially in Ashkenazi Jews, and presents in a wide variety of ways — especially with hepatosplenomegaly (7.139) with neurological involvement (epilepsy and mental retardation) in children, and involvement of liver and spleen, bone marrow, bone, lung and eye (7.140) in adults. The diagnosis is made by finding the characteristic Gaucher cell in biopsy tissue (e.g. bone marrow or spleen biopsy). There is no treatment.

Niemann–Pick disease is an autosomal recessive disease in which a deficiency of sphingomyelinase results in accumulation of sphingomyelin in the tissues, especially in the central nervous system, liver/spleen and bone marrow. The clinical presentation varies according to the sub-type of the disease. The common presentation in childhood is with mental retardation and hepatosplenomegaly. In Type A disease, there is often a cherry-red spot in the retina (7.141). The diagnosis is made by finding the characteristic lipid-laden sea-blue histiocyte in biopsy material. Adults with Type E disease present with hepatosplenomegaly but no neurological abnormalities.

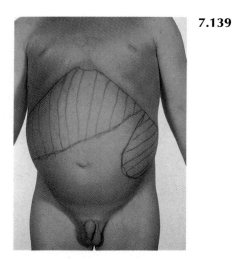

7.139

7.139 Gaucher's disease commonly presents with hepatosplenomegaly in all age groups. The grossly enlarged liver and spleen have been outlined in this boy with the juvenile form of the disease.

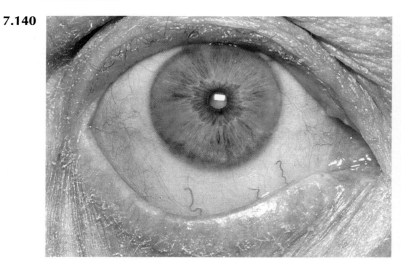

7.140

7.140 Pingueculae are commonly seen in adult patients with Gaucher's disease, though they may also be found in otherwise normal individuals. They are small areas of degenerative change in the conjunctiva. Although sometimes conspicuous, they require no treatment, and, in contrast to pterygia, they do not encroach on the cornea.

Tay–Sachs disease (familial amaurotic idiocy) is an autosomal recessive disorder in which a deficiency of hexosaminidase A and B results in the accumulation of GM2 gangliosides in the brain and peripheral nerves. The result is mental retardation and epilepsy. There is usually a cherry-red spot on the retina (7.141). Programmes of antenatal detection are available.

Fabry's disease is an X-linked recessive disease that is caused by deficiency of α-galactosidase A resulting in accumulation of a trihexoside in body tissues. Typical features include punctate angiomatous lesions on the skin, corneal dystrophy, progressive renal failure and liability to thrombotic arterial disease. There may also be mental retardation, epilepsy and peripheral neuropathy.

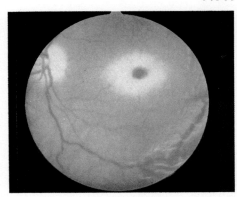

7.141 A cherry-red spot at the macula is commonly found in Type A Niemann–Pick disease and in Tay–Sachs disease.

Mucupolysaccharidoses

There are 7 disorders in this group of metabolic defects, with very similar presentations.

Hurler's syndrome is an autosomal recessive disorder caused by a defect in the breakdown of complex carbohydrates. The glycosaminoglycans chondroitin dermatan and heparan sulphate accumulate in subcutaneous tissues, bone, brain and liver leading to characteristic physical and mental changes. The appearances are typical with coarse facies (7.142), hepatosplenomegaly, corneal opacities and multiple bone abnormalities causing stunting of growth. There is severe mental retardation.

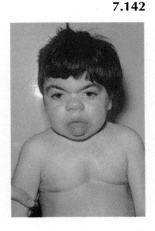

7.142 Hurler's syndrome is associated with characteristic facial features, including prominent supra-orbital ridges, thick eyebrows, a depressed nasal bridge, a broad bulbous nose, thick lips, a large protruding tongue and coarse hair. In an extreme form, the syndrome produces 'gargoylism'. Patients with other forms of mucopolysaccharidosis have a broadly similar appearance.

Laurence–Moon–Biedl syndrome

This is an autosomal recessive disorder which is associated with mental retardation, polydactyly (7.143), retinitis pigmentosa, hypogonadism and obesity.

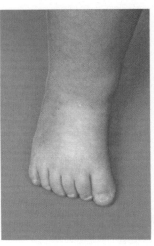

7.143 Polydactyly is a feature of the Laurence–Moon–Biedl syndrome, though it may occur in association with many other congenital abnormalities or as an isolated aberration.

Down's syndrome

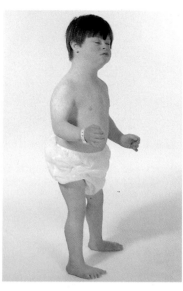

7.144

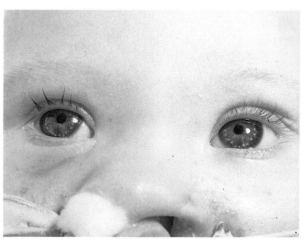

7.144 Down's syndrome in a child. This child is typically rather short, and he shows the characteristic appearance of a rather small head with a small nose and ears. Note the abnormal orientation of the fifth finger on each hand (clinodactyly).

Down's syndrome accounts for up to one-third of children in schools for the mentally retarded. The degree of disability ranges from mild to severe. The physical features are typical and include a small head with a flat occiput, up-slanting palpebral fissures, epicanthic folds, small nose with a poorly developed bridge and small ears (7.144–7.146). Grey-white areas of depigmentation are seen in the iris (Brushfield spots, 7.147); the mouth is often held open and the tongue protrudes. The hands are broad with a single transverse palmar crease (7.148), and the fifth finger shows clinodactyly (7.144). Congenital heart lesions are common (7.145). Adult stature tends to be small; and there is a significant incidence of leukaemia in the older patients.

As these children tend to be born to older mothers (over 35 years of age), it is important to offer amniocentesis to this group in pregnancy, to look for trisomy or translocation of chromosome 21.

7.145

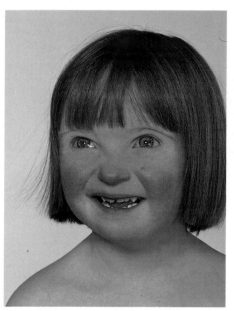

7.146

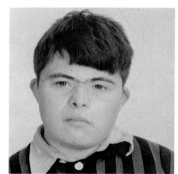

7.145 Down's syndrome is commonly associated with congenital heart disease, as in this girl who has Fallot's tetralogy (*see* p. 240). Her facies show the characteristic features of Down's syndrome, with prominent epicanthic folds and a small nose with a poorly developed bridge. Note that she also has a webbed neck. Her congenital heart disease has led to a prominent cyanosed facial flush.

7.146 Down's syndrome in a young adult showing the characteristic adult facies. Note the prominent epicanthic folds and the small nose and ears.

7.147

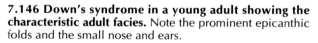

7.148

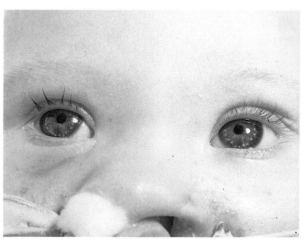

7.147 Brushfield spots are a common feature of Down's syndrome and may be seen in the newborn baby, as here. They are tiny, whitish areas of depigmentation on the iris.

7.148 Single palmar crease is a classic feature of Down's syndrome, but it is important to remember that it can occur with other chromosomal abnormalities, and as a normal variant. It is diagnostic of Down's syndrome only when associated with the other features of the condition.

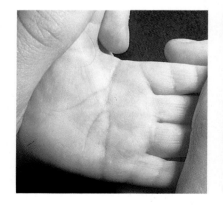

8. Gastrointestinal Disorders

History and examination

Patients with gastrointestinal disease present with a variety of symptoms (**Table 8.1**). These may indicate a specific disease, but patients often have alimentary disease without specific symptoms, so the clinician must be alert to clinical signs.

General inspection is of particular importance. Muscle wasting, as well as the more obvious depletion of fat stores, is indicative of malnutrition (**4.1, 7.125, 8.1**). Pallor of the mucous membranes is indicative of anaemia (p. 424 and **8.2, 10.2, 10.3**) and koilonychia is found with prolonged iron deficiency (**2.89, 10.4, 10.19**). Finger clubbing accompanies malabsorption, small intestinal disease and cirrhosis (**2.90, 2.91**). Palmar erythema occurs in chronic liver disease and such patients may also have jaundice, spider naevi, ascites, and, in male patients, gynaecomastia and testicular atrophy (*see* p. 386). Skin rashes such as erythema nodosum (**1.123, 2.40**) may accompany inflammatory bowel disease and these patients sometimes also suffer from arthritis. Inspection of the mouth and tongue may reveal evidence of candidiasis (**1.28, 1.169, 1.170**) or apthous ulcers (**8.3**) which may be associated with intestinal disease.

Examination of the regional lymph nodes is important: patients with gastric carcinoma sometimes have left-sided supraclavicular lymphadenopathy (**8.4**), and posterior cervical lymphadenopathy may occur in pharyngeal carcinoma. General lymphadenopathy is a feature of Whipple's disease. Abdominal examination may reveal enlargement of the spleen

Table 8.1 Common gastrointestinal symptoms.

Heartburn
Chest pain
Dysphagia
Anorexia
Abdominal pain
Vomiting
Constipation
Diarrhoea
Gastrointestinal bleeding
Anaemia
Malabsorption and weight loss
Jaundice
Ascites

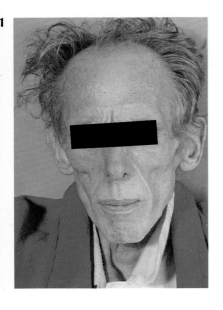

8.1 Malnutrition secondary to carcinoma of the stomach in a 61 year-old-man (*see* **8.43**). Note the wasting of the facial tissues, and the pallor of his lips—an indication of probable iron deficiency anaemia.

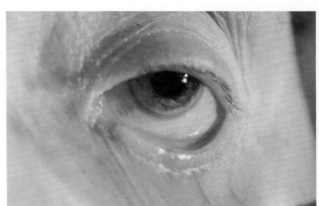

8.2 Pallor of the conjunctivae is suggestive of severe anaemia—in this case resulting from chronic gastrointestinal blood loss. Note the incidental finding of a corneal arcus.

or liver, or the liver may be small or craggy (*see* p. 386). Ascites (8.5, 9.12), detected by shifting dullness, most commonly reflects cirrhosis or malignancy. Abdominal masses suggest colonic or other malignancy, or an inflammatory disease of the bowel such as Crohn's disease or diverticulitis.

Rectal examination provides important clues. Perianal skin tags denote thrombosed haemorrhoids. In Crohn's colitis, they may be associated with fistula-in-ano (8.6, 8.7). Perianal condylomata (8.8) may be mistaken for anal carcinoma; they are most commonly found in homosexual males.

8.3

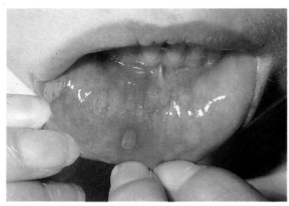

8.4

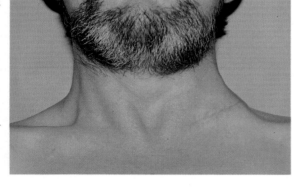

8.3 Aphthous ulcers commonly occur in isolation, but they may be an indication of an underlying intestinal disease, such as gluten enteropathy or inflammatory bowel disease.

8.4 Left-sided supraclavicular lymph-adenopathy (Virchow's node) may result from lymphatic spread of a gastric or pancreatic neoplasm via the thoracic duct. This may be the first sign of malignancy, as in this patient. The node mass was biopsied one month before this picture was taken, and has regrown since then. Histology revealed adeno-carcinoma cells. The primary tumour was in the stomach.

8.5 Gross ascites in a 68-year-old woman, who had no other symptoms on presentation. Note the development of stretch marks and eversion of the umbilicus. This patient had an inoperable leiomyosarcoma, but a similar clinical appearance may be seen in patients with other abdominal disorders and with cirrhosis.

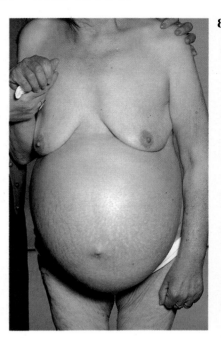

8.7

8.6

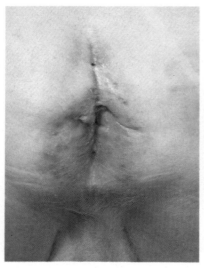

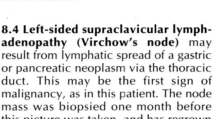

8.7 Multiple perianal fistulae resulted in the chronic, painful inflammatory reaction seen here in a patient with longstanding Crohn's disease.

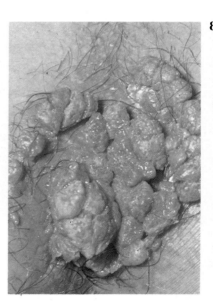

8.6 Fistulae-in-ano in a patient with Crohn's disease. A number of fistulae have developed between the skin and the rectum, as could be demonstrated by the insertion of a probe along the tracts. Although fistulae may be caused by chronic infection (e.g. tuberculosis) the most common cause is Crohn's disease affecting the rectum.

8.8 Perianal condylomata result from human papillomavirus infection. They are usually sexually transmitted and are most common in homosexual men (*see* p. 81).

Investigations

Investigations of both structure and function may be needed, including endoscopy, radiology, nuclear medicine, histopathology, tests on blood and stool, and manometry.

The **fibreoptic or video endoscope** allows direct inspection and biopsy of lesions as well as therapeutic intervention:

- *Upper alimentary endoscopy* with the forward viewing endoscope, performed in the fasting patient, usually under light sedation, facilitates the demonstration of oesophagitis (**8.9**), the dilatation of oesophageal strictures and the injection of oesophageal varices. Gastric ulcers and tumours (**8.10**) and duodenal ulcers (**8.11**) are readily seen and biopsied, and haemorrhage can be arrested by the use of a laser beam or heater probe, passed down the biopsy channel.

- *The side-vewing endoscope* placed in the second part of the duodenum, permits cannulation of the ampulla of Vater and retrograde examination of the pancreas and biliary tree (endoscopic retrograde cholangiopancreatography, ERCP—*see* p. 391).

- *The flexible sigmoidoscope and colonoscope* are used to examine the distal and entire colon. Sigmoidoscopy and/or colonoscopy are indicated for the diagnosis and staging of inflammatory bowel disease and for the investigation of colonic symptoms, particularly rectal bleeding. When polyps are found, they can be removed with a diathermy snare (**8.12**).

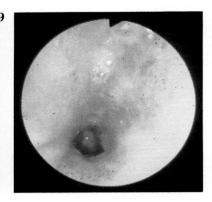

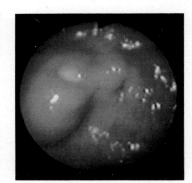

8.9 Upper alimentary endoscopy allows direct visualisation of the mucosa of the upper gastrointestinal tract. This endoscopic view shows a tight stricture of the lower oesophagus resulting from peptic oesophagitis, which is still active.

8.10 A chronic prepyloric gastric ulcer. The ulcer sits on the top of a raised area, which increases the possibility of malignancy. All gastric ulcers should be further investigated cytologically or histologically. In this case, the lesion was benign.

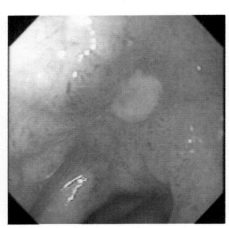

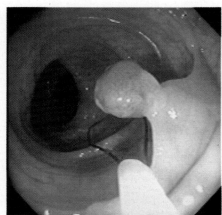

8.11 A typical duodenal ulcer, seen through a videoendoscope. Duodenal ulcers are almost invariably benign, so histological examination is not usually required to exclude malignancy. Antral biopsies may, however, be taken to investigate the possibility of infection with *Helicobacter pylori*.

8.12 Colonoscopic polypectomy. A wire snare has been introduced through the colonoscope. It will be looped over the pedunculated colonic polyp, tightened around its stalk, and diathermy will then be applied via the snare to sever the stalk without bleeding.

Radiological investigations are important. Endoscopy has reduced the need for the barium meal and the barium enema, but double-contrast techniques can still provide valuable information (**8.13**, **8.14**); and small bowel meals or enemas are still important for the identification of structural disease of the jejunum and ileum such as Crohn's disease (**8.15**). Plain abdominal radiographs are important for the recognition of toxic dilatation in colitis and to confirm clinical suspicions of intestinal obstruction (**8.16**).

Ultrasound and CT scanning are especially useful in the investigation of the liver, pancreas and biliary tract (*see* p. 391), but also have a useful role in generalised abdominal disease (**8.17**).

Nuclear medicine has been used extensively for structural imaging of the liver and biliary tract, and can also be applied to the assessment of intestinal function. Oesophageal dysmotility and gastric emptying can both be assessed by reference to the pattern and time of transit of swallowed isotope, measured by the gamma camera.

The glychocholate breath test utilises the ability of bacteria to deconjugate bile acids to investigate bacterial overgrowth in the small intestine. The patient is given ^{14}C-glycine glycocholic acid. Deconjugation leads to the rapid absorption of glycine, which is metabolised, and the measured exhaled $^{14}CO_2$ is a measure of the extent of deconjugation. A similar principle is applied to the measurement of fat malabsorption using the triglyceride glyceryl-^{14}C-triolein.

The absorption of vitamin B$_{12}$ can be investigated by measuring the urinary excretion of the labelled vitamin, which is administered by mouth after saturating the body stores with an intramuscular injection (*see* p. 420).

Histopathology is important for the confirmation and staging of tumours, the recognition of different types of bowel inflammation such as Crohn's disease, and the identification of small bowel disease such as gluten enteropathy and its response to a gluten-free diet. Biopsy samples may be obtained on endoscopy (**8.42**) or using a Crosby capsule (**8.55**).

Blood tests provide evidence of malabsorption (macrocytic or hypochromic microcytic anaemia), malnutrition (low transferrin, fibronectin and lymphocyte count) and liver dysfunction.

Faecal occult blood testing may point to intestinal blood loss, **Faecal fat measurement** aids the assessment of malabsorption.

Microbiological investigation of the stool is important. The need for microscopy of stool or jejunal aspirate to identify protozoa such as *Giardia* (**8.18**) is often overlooked.

Manometry is increasingly used to investigate motility disorders.

Laparoscopy has an increasing role in the investigation of intra-abdominal disease.

8.13

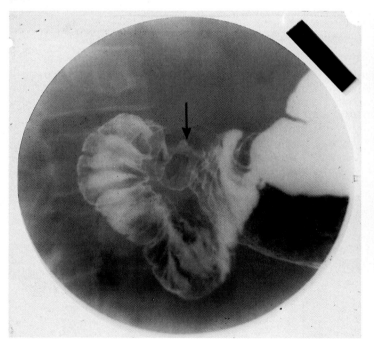

8.13 Double-contrast barium meal, showing a small duodenal ulcer crater (arrow). In expert hands, this technique has a diagnostic accuracy similar to that of endoscopy for many lesions of the stomach and duodenum; but, of course, biopsy is not possible with radiology alone and most lesions of the stomach require biopsy.

8.14

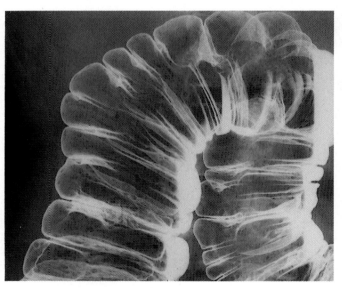

8.14 Double-contrast barium enema in a patient with familial polyposis coli. This close-up view shows multiple small, sessile colonic polyps, appearing as small, rounded, dark patches. The surface of polyps is poorly coated with barium, while their edges and the rest of the colonic wall retain more contrast medium. The radiological appearance of the polyps corresponds to their colonoscopic appearance (*see* **8.85**). Familial polyposis is a pre-malignant condition and prophylactic colectomy is usually advised.

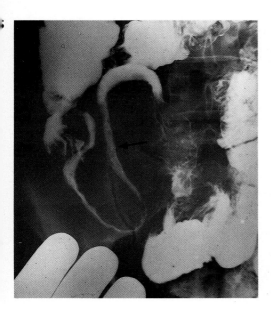

8.15 A small bowel meal demonstrates a typical feature of Crohn's disease—a long stricture of the terminal ileum. Strictures may also be caused by tuberculosis and lymphoma, but the 'cobblestone' appearance (arrow) is strongly suggestive of Crohn's disease.

8.16 Plain abdominal X-ray, taken in the erect position, demonstrating multiple fluid levels in the bowel. In combination with a supine film, this appearance shows apparent obstruction to the gut at the distal end of the small bowel. It is important to remember that similar appearances may occur in paralytic ileus, peritonitis, gastroenteritis and coeliac disease. The films must always be interpreted in their clinical context.

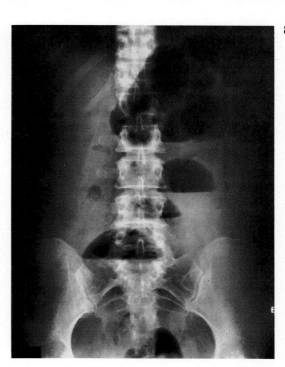

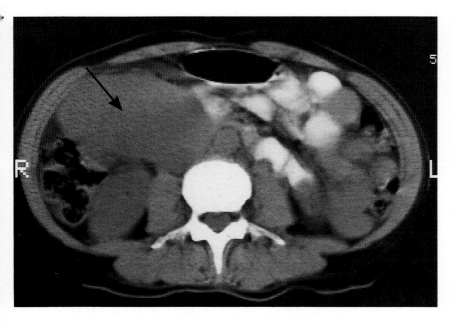

8.17 CT scan demonstrating a large abdominal tumour (arrowed). CT-guided biopsy showed this to be a leiomyosarcoma, which originated in the duodenum.

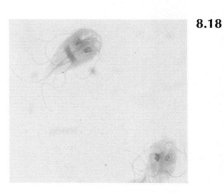

8.18 Microscopy of fresh stool or small bowel aspirate remains important in the diagnosis of intestinal infections. This jejunal aspirate, from a patient with chronic diarrhoea and weight loss, showed *Giardia lamblia* trophozoites.

Mouth and tongue

Important information may be gained from the inspection of the mouth:

- The lips and tongue are blue in conditions associated with central cyanosis (4.5).
- Angular stomatitis (7.133) is common in iron deficiency.
- Aphthous ulcers occur anywhere in the oral cavity (8.3). They may be found in otherwise healthy people, especially women, but are associated with poor dental hygiene, haematinic deficiency, gluten enteropathy and inflammatory bowel disease. Large deep ulcers are sometimes found as part of Behçet's syndrome (3.53).
- The gums may bleed where there is periodontal disease, and in patients with monocytic leukaemia or scurvy (8.19, 10.65).
- Hypertrophied gums are a feature of prolonged treatment with phenytoin (8.20).
- A blue line is found at the margin of the gum and teeth in lead poisoning (8.21).

- Yellow-brown staining of the teeth may occur where tetracycline was administered during childhood or fetal life (8.22).
- Candidal infection (1.28, 1.169, 1.170) is common in debilitated and immunosuppressed patients, and under ill-fitting dentures.
- The tongue may be smooth and sore in patients with haematinic- and B-vitamin deficiencies (9.35, 10.29); enlarged in patients with acromegaly (7.18), myxoedema and amyloidosis; and small and spastic in motor neurone disease. Inspection may reveal evidence of hereditary haemorrhagic telangiectasia (9.44, 10.6).
- Leukoplakia (2.112, 8.23) is a premalignant condition and can lead to carcinoma (8.24). Hairy leukoplakia may occur in patients with HIV infection (1.29).
- Conditions as varied as herpes simplex (1.71), lichen planus (2.59). Peutz–Jeghers syndrome (2.74) and scleroderma (3.79, 3.80) may present with oral or peri-oral lesions.

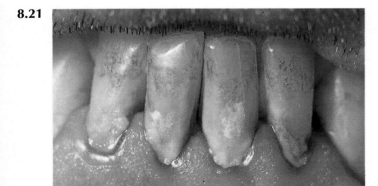

8.19 The gums in scurvy. Vitamin C deficiency characteristically leads to gingivitis. The gingival papillae are swollen and fragile, with a purplish colouration. In this patient, grossly neglected oral hygiene with resulting caries has compounded the problem.

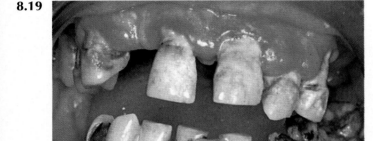

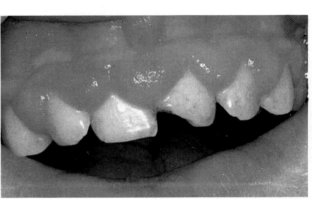

8.20 Hyperplastic gingivitis is a well-established complication of phenytoin therapy (for epilepsy). Careful attention to oral hygiene may minimise the extent of this complication.

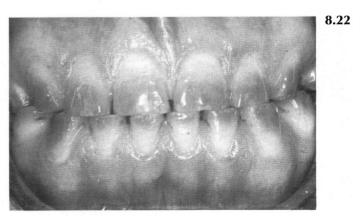

8.21 Lead poisoning produces a blue line at the margin of the gum and teeth. This patient's employment involved the dismantling of car batteries. He presented with colicky abdominal pain.

8.22 Tetracycline staining of the teeth occurs when tetracycline is administered during the period of tooth formation: via the mother in fetal life; or to the child up to the age of 12 years. In this patient, there is generalised staining without any hypoplasia of the tooth substance. Hypoplasia often occurs, but this may frequently result from the underlying condition for which the tetracycline was administered, rather than to the tetracycline itself. There are almost always satisfactory alternatives to tetracycline therapy during pregnancy and childhood.

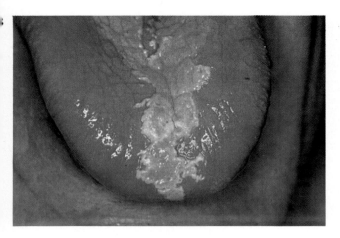

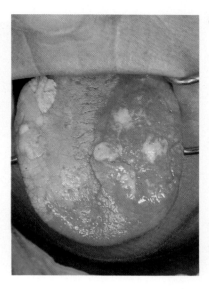

8.23 Leukoplakia of the tongue. The aetiology in this 83-year-old patient was unclear. Characteristically, leukoplakia cannot be wiped off, and it shows a non-specific histological appearance which excludes other diagnoses. Leukoplakia sometimes has no consequences, but should always be regarded as a potentially premalignant condition.

8.24 Carcinoma of the tongue. There is an extensive squamous cell carcinoma on the left side of the tongue. Note also the patch of leukoplakia on the right border of the tongue posteriorly.

Oesophagus

Peptic oesophagitis

A lax oesophageal sphincter permits the reflux of corrosive gastric contents, containing acid pepsin and sometimes bile acids, into the oesophagus. The tendency to gastro-oesophageal reflux may be compounded by the intrathoracic position of the gastro-oesophageal junction in patients with a hiatus hernia (**8.25, 8.26**), by increased abdominal pressure in the obese and pregnant, and by the consumption of fatty meals, alcohol, caffeine and tobacco, all of which relax the sphincter. The refluxed gastric content damages the squamous oesphageal mucosa and may impair the underlying muscle function leading to delayed oesophageal clearance which exacerbates the problem.

The patient complains of heartburn and acid reflux, which is worse after meals and at night when recumbent. The diagnosis of oesophagitis is confirmed by endoscopy (**8.28**).

Complications of oesophagitis include stricture formation (**8.9, 8.27**), which causes dysphagia; oesophageal ulcer, characterised by severe pain and dysphagia; and Barrett's syndrome, in which chronic reflux leads to the replacement of the squamous epithelium by metaplastic columnar epithelium, with a risk of ulceration and carcinoma. Aspiration pneumonia may occur.

Treatment depends on the severity of the symptoms and mucosal damage. For mild disease, advice about diet, i.e. losing excess weight and avoiding late, large and fatty meals, and coffee and alcohol; stopping smoking; and avoiding sleeping flat; together with symptomatic or regular use of a protective alginate preparation; may be sufficient. More severe disease requires acid suppression with an H_2 antagonist. Occasionally, total acid suppression with a proton pump inhibitor may be necessary. The efficacy of such treatment can be enhanced by pro-kinetic drugs, such as domperidone and cisapride, which increase gastric emptying and oesophageal sphincter tone.

Oesophageal stenosis is usually amenable to endoscopic dilatation using balloons or other dilators.

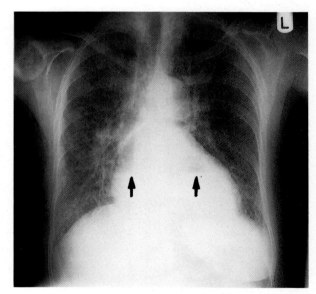

8.25 A hiatus hernia may first be revealed on chest X-ray, especially when chest pain is the presenting feature. The presence of a fluid level behind the heart (arrow) is virtually diagnostic. This patient has also had a previous right mastectomy for carcinoma of the breast and has an osteolytic secondary in the head of the humerus.

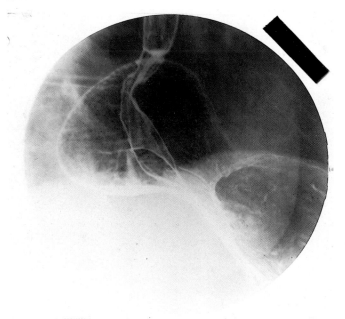

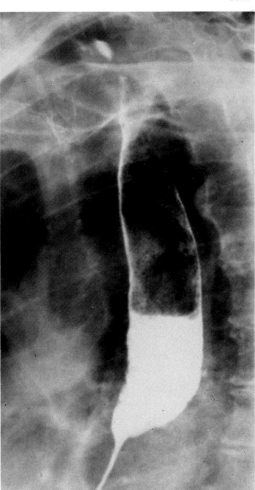

8.26 Rolling hiatus hernia on double-contrast barium meal. The fundus of the stomach has herniated into the thorax alongside the oesophagus. The constriction in the stomach marks the level of the diaphragm, and the gastroesophageal junction is still beneath it. By contrast, in a sliding hernia, the gastroesophageal junction (cardia) slides into the chest.

8.28

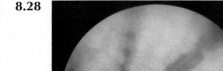

8.27 Benign oesophageal stricture, seen on barium swallow. The stricture is smooth with a tapering (or funnelling) upper end that narrows gradually from normal oesophagus. The most common cause of such a benign stricture is chronic reflux oesophagitis.

8.28 Haemorrhagic linear oesophagitis shown endoscopically. The patient had symptomatic gastroesophageal reflux.

Infective oesophagitis

8.29

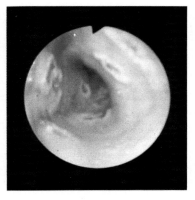

Oesophageal candidiasis occurs in debilitated patients who have received broad spectrum antibiotics. It is also found in patients infected with the HIV virus (in whom it is diagnostic of AIDS). The radiological appearances of oesophageal candidiasis are shown in **1.34**, and the diagnosis should be confirmed endoscopically. Patients without AIDS may respond to topical treatment with nystatin, but those with AIDS require a systemically active agent such as ketoconazole.

Patients with AIDS may also aquire oesophageal infections with herpes simplex (**8.29**) and cytomegalovirus, and HIV itself may cause oesophagitis.

8.29 Herpes simplex ulceration of the lower oesophagus in a patient with AIDS. Note the multiple shallow ulcers in the lower part of the oesophagus. Treatment with high-dose intravenous acyclovir may be helpful.

Oesophageal strictures

Oesophageal strictures may develop as a consequence of oesophagitis (8.27), following the ingestion of corrosives or after radiotherapy. Such strictures are usually benign, but may require dilatation or surgery to relieve dysphagia.

The Plummer–Vinson or Patterson–Brown–Kelly syndrome is the association of iron deficiency anaemia (with koilonychia) with angular stomatitis, glossitis and atrophy of the oesophageal mucosa in the postcricoid region, which forms an obstructing post-cricoid web (8.30 and p.424). Iron therapy may reverse the process, but there is a risk of malignant change.

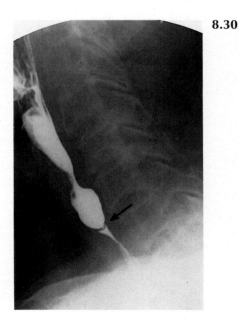

8.30 Oesophageal web in the Plummer–Vinson syndrome. The post-cricoid web is arrowed on this barium swallow, and the element of oesophageal obstruction is obvious. The patient was a post-menopausal woman, and she showed other signs of severe iron deficiency anaemia.

Oesophageal carcinoma

Oesophageal carcinoma presents with progressive dysphagia for solids, and subsequently for liquids as the luminal stenosis progresses. Weight loss may be obvious.

The diagnosis is confirmed by the typical radiological and endoscopic features (8.31, 8.32). Surgical resection offers the only curative treatment, but is frequently not feasible.

Palliation can be achieved by the endoscopic insertion of a prosthetic (Atkinson) tube, or by endoscopic laser therapy. Other tumours, including leiomyomas, lymphomas and Kaposi's sarcoma, may be found in the oesophagus, but are rare.

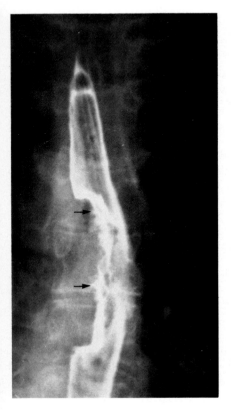

8.31 Oesophageal carcinoma. The patient had a 6-week history of dysphagia and weight loss. Note the abrupt change from normal oesophagus to the area of the tumour (cf. **8.27**). The barium spicules (arrows) represent areas of ulceration in the tumour. There is, as yet, no dilatation of the proximal oesophagus.

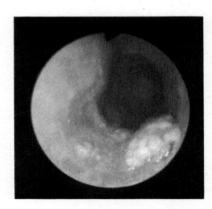

8.32 Carcinoma of the oesophagus seen endoscopically. There is a pale sessile polypoid lesion situated at four o'clock, just above the gastro-oesophageal junction. Biopsy confirmed that this was a carcinoma.

Oesophageal motility disorders

Achalasia is characterised by the failure of the lower oesophageal sphincter to relax, and impaired peristalsis of the oesophagus. This results in dysphagia and ultimately the retention of food debris in a dilated oesophagus (**8.33**). Aspiration pneumonia is a common complication (*see* p.187).

The diagnosis is confirmed by manometry. Treatment is by balloon dilatation or cardiomyotomy. Chagas' disease may produce a similar motility disorder (*see* p. 71).

Diffuse oesophageal spasm is another cause of chest pain and dysphagia, in which there are multiple high pressure incoordinate waves. Barium examination demonstrates abnormal contractions known as tertiary waves. This disorder may complicate gastro-oesophageal reflux. Other patients may suffer severe chest pain with no demonstrable radiological abnormality but manometric studies may show that occasional peristaltic waves generate very high pressures.

There is reduced oesophageal motility in patients with systemic sclerosis (**3.82**).

Coughing or retching, especially in alcoholic patients, may lead to an acute tear at the gastro-oesophageal junction (a Mallary–Weiss tear) with resulting upper gastrointestinal bleeding. Most patients heal spontaneously, but a few require surgery. Oesophageal varices are another cause of major lower oesophageal bleeding (*see* p. 394).

8.33

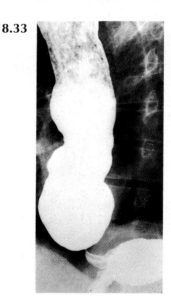

8.33 Achalasia of the oesophagus. The barium swallow shows that the dilated oesophagus narrows conically at the gastro-oesophageal junction (the cardia).

The stomach

Gastritis

Gastritis is a common problem and its incidence is increasing. It is best defined as 'an inflammatory response to gastric mucosal injury'. Various previous classifications have been superseded by the Sydney system (1990) which takes account of the aetiological role of *Helicobacter pylori* and integrates the clinical presentation, endoscopic findings, histological appearance and anatomical involvement of different regions of the stomach.

There is little association between symptoms, endoscopic abnormality, histological abnormality, anatomical distribution of any abnormalities found, and the presence or absence of *H. pylori* infection or other causative factors. Endoscopy alone is not diagnostic of any particular form of gastritis, though various abnormalities may be seen. Gastritis is now best classified as follows:

- **Acute gastritis caused by viruses or bacteria.** Vomiting is a common clinical presentation following infection with rotavirus, Norwalk agent and type-specific *E. coli*. Acute infection with *H. pylori* is associated with epigastric pain, nausea, vomiting and a feeling of fullness. *H. pylori* is easy to identify on biopsy samples, if they are examined properly.
- **Acute gastritis caused by drugs or chemicals.** Aspirin (and other NSAIDs) and alcohol are the most common agents to cause acute gastritis. They have a synergistic effect on the gastric mucosa. Aspirin inhibits local prostaglandin production and removes its cytoprotective effects, while alcohol produces local reduction of mucosal blood flow. The end result is acute erosions, which may bleed (**8.34, 8.35**).
- **Chronic gastritis.** This is found in an asymptomatic form in the elderly and is often associated with *H. pylori* infection. Other causes include drugs, alcohol and gastroduodenal reflux of bile.
- **Atrophic gastritis.** A few patients have autoimmune gastritis, with a positive test for parietal cell antibodies. These patients fail to secrete acid and intrinsic factor, and may eventually develop a deficiency of vitamin B_{12} (*see* p. 427).

H. pylori infection is commonly found in biopsies of the gastric antrum in patients with duodenal ulceration, even where the endoscopic appearance of the stomach is completely normal. In these circumstances, and with symptomatic gastritis, treatment of *H. pylori* infection is with triple therapy—a bismuth preparation, amoxycillin and metronidazole.

Ménétrièr's disease is a rare, possibly pre-malignant condition, in which there is thickening and enlargement of the gastric mucosal folds. It may affect the entire upper gut (**8.36**).

8.34

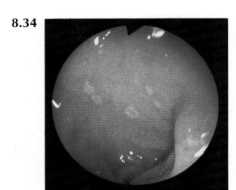

8.34 Gastric erosions. The patient had been taking aspirin, and was experiencing dyspeptic symptoms. Endoscopy revealed numerous small 'aphthous erosions', a common finding in patients taking aspirin and other non-steroidal anti-inflammatory drugs (NSAIDs).

8.35

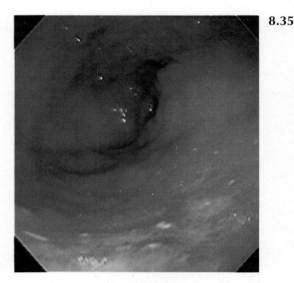

8.35 Haemorrhagic gastritis in a patient on NSAID therapy. The picture is dark because the patient was still actively bleeding, but multiple small erosions can be seen, and the mucosa bled when touched by the endoscope.

8.36

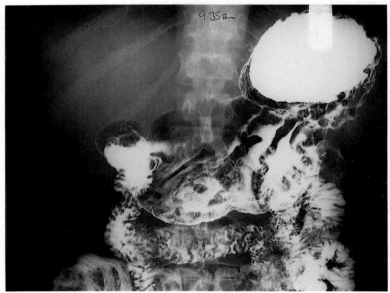

8.36 Ménétrièr's disease. The patient presented with epigastric pain and melaena. Barium meal and follow through revealed rugal hypertrophy in the stomach and similar changes throughout the small intestine.

Gastric ulcers

Gastric ulcers are most common in the elderly. NSAIDs are often an important factor in their genesis, and both acid and gastroduodenal bile reflux may also have a role.

Gastric ulcers present with epigastric pain and/or anaemia. Bleeding is usually chronic, but acute haemorrhage can occur; it is a major threat in elderly patients.

Gastric ulcers cannot be distinguished on clinical grounds from duodenal ulcers or gastric cancers. Barium studies may demonstrate an ulcer and give strong clues to its benign nature (**8.37**), but definitive diagnosis requires endoscopy with brush cytology and biopsy (**8.38–8.40**).

Gastric ulcers usually respond to H$_2$ receptor antagonists (though more slowly than duodenal ulcers), but a number of other drugs may also be used. Follow-up to confirm healing is wise.

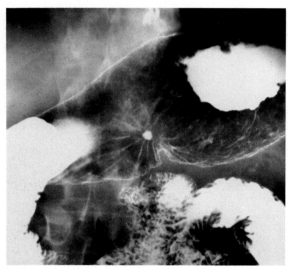

8.37

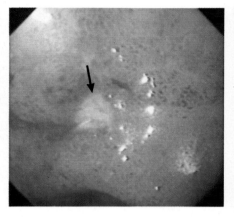

8.37 Benign gastric ulcer, as seen in a double-contrast barium meal. The ulcer heals by fibrosis and contraction, and this draws mucosal folds towards the base of the ulcer. These give rise to the streaks of barium which radiate from the ulcer crater in this view. Although these appearances are strongly suggestive of a healing benign gastric ulcer, endoscopy, brush cytology and biopsy are all wise precautions to exclude gastric carcinoma.

8.38 Benign gastric ulcer (arrow) seen on endoscopy. There is no sign of bleeding, and no evidence to suggest malignancy, but biopsy is essential to exclude this.

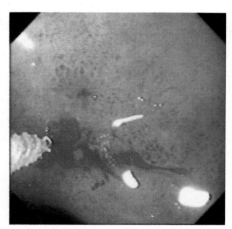

8.39

8.39 Brush cytology of the gastric ulcer seen in 8.38. In this simple technique, a small brush is passed through the operating channel of the endoscope. The brushings can be examined for malignant cells. Both malignant ulcers and gastric lymphomas may resemble benign ulcers even when viewed endoscopically, hence the need for further investigation.

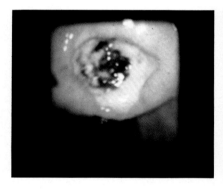

8.40 A bleeding gastric ulcer. The endoscopic view shows both the ulcer crater and the area of bleeding within it very clearly. Biopsy is essential to exclude malignancy, and the bleeding may be treatable endoscopically.

Gastric tumours

The most common gastric tumour is adenocarcinoma. There is a high incidence of this tumour in some parts of the world, especially Japan, but generally it is becoming less common in developed countries. Predisposing factors may include a high salt consumption, aflatoxins, and living in regions with a high nitrate content in the soil. There is an increased incidence in patients who have undergone gastric surgery, and those with atrophic gastritis. Factors which encourage bacterial overgrowth may favour nitrosation of luminal amines to form carcinogens.

Unfortunately, symptoms do not usually occur until the disease is advanced; then, patients complain of anorexia and weight loss. The tumour sometimes ulcerates, leading to dyspeptic symptoms and anaemia. Occlusion of the pylorus or cardia respectively may cause vomiting and dysphagia. Spread to the liver and lymph nodes is often present at diagnosis. Left-sided supraclavicular lymphadenopathy may be evident (**8.4**).

Diagnosis is best confirmed at endoscopy, which reveals a tumour mass or malignant ulcer (**8.41**) and permits biopsy and histological examination (**8.42**). Sometimes the size of the tumour and its extension are best appreciated by a barium meal examination (**8.43, 8.44**).

The only effective treatment is surgery. This can be curative in early gastric cancer when the 5-year survival is 90%, but by the time lymph node spread occurs this figure falls to 10%.

Other tumours that may be found in the stomach include leiomyoma (**8.45, 8.46**), leiomyosarcoma (**8.5**) lymphoma, and Kaposi's sarcoma.

8.41

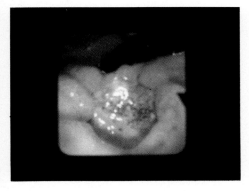

8.42

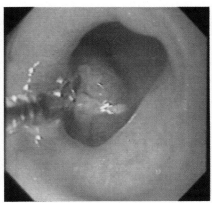

8.43

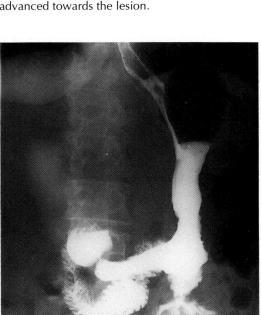

8.41 Malignant gastric ulcer. The bulging of the ulcer into the stomach is strongly suggestive of malignancy, and this was confirmed by biopsy.

8.42 Endoscopic biopsy of an ulcerating mass in the stomach wall. The forceps are being advanced towards the lesion.

8.43 Carcinoma of the stomach. The barium meal demonstrates a large fungating mass in the gastric fundus. The patient presented with severe weight loss and iron deficiency anaemia (**8.1**).

8.44 Linitis plastica of the stomach. In this form of gastric carcinoma, there is widespread submucosal invasion giving a rigid and immobile appearance on screening during the barium meal.

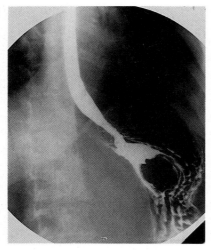

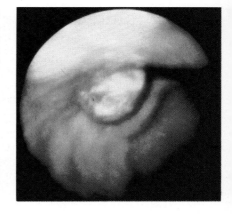

8.45 Gastric leiomyoma is a benign tumour of smooth muscle. In this patient, the barium meal shows a huge mass in the stomach. Patients with leiomyomas present with dyspeptic symptoms or with bleeding, which may be occult and lead to iron deficiency anaemia. Surgical resection is usually possible and curative.

8.46 Gastric leiomyoma. This endoscopic view shows a much smaller lesion than that seen in **8.45**, projecting into the stomach. Note the superficial ulceration and evidence of recent bleeding.

The duodenum

Duodenal ulceration

Duodenal ulceration is very common in the developed world, but the cause of duodenal ulcer diathesis remains unknown. Recent attention has focussed on the potential role of *Helicobacter pylori,* which is often found in mucus and on the surface of cells in gastric biopsies from patients with duodenal ulcers, many of whom have an associated antral gastritis. The organism splits urea and may increase the local pH, leading to the secretion of more gastrin and thus acid. NSAIDs may also play a role in some patients. Multiple and resistant ulcers should prompt consideration of a gastrinoma (*see* p. 384).

Intermittent epigastric pain that is relieved by food, with night waking and heartburn, is characteristic of peptic ulceration. Many patients, however, do not have symptoms, and become aware of their ulcers only when complications occur. Suspected ulcers are best investigated by endoscopy (**8.11**, **8.47**, **8.48**), although high-quality barium meal examination can still provide useful information (**8.13**, **8.49**,

8.50). Antral biopsy during endoscopy is necessary to confirm the presence or absence of *Helicobacter* infection.

Complications of duodenal ulceration include haemorrhage (**8.51**), pyloric stenosis caused by scarring, and perforation, leading to acute peritonitis and pneumoperitoneum (**8.52**).

Duodenal ulcers usually respond to treatment with H_2-receptor antagonists (e.g. cimetidine, ranitidine) or proton pump inhibitors (e.g. omeprazole). Other drugs including bismuth preparations may be used, and 'triple therapy' may be useful if *Helicobacter* is found (*see* p. 363). Maintenance therapy with an H_2-receptor antagonist may be required to prevent relapse.

Surgical treatment is rarely needed now for the management of ulcer disease, but patients who have previously undergone surgery may present with complications including stomal ulceration, diarrhoea, 'dumping syndrome' and nutritional deficiencies.

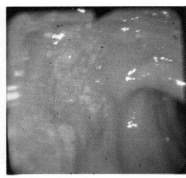

8.47 Duodenitis. Endoscopy shows superficial erosions of the duodenal mucosa on a background of inflammation, but no frank ulceration. Duodenitis may occur in isolation, or as a result of other inflammatory bowel diseases. It is often associated with peptic ulceration of the duodenum or stomach. If symptomatic, it usually responds to H$_2$-receptor antagonists.

8.48 Duodenal ulceration in the second part of the duodenum. This videoendoscopic view shows a linear ulcer (arrow) and a circular ulcer to the top right of the picture. Patients often prove to have more than one ulcer on endoscopy, but multiple ulcers should raise the suspicion of possible Zollinger–Ellison syndrome.

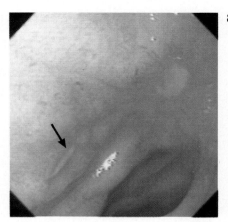

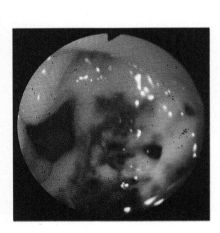

8.49 Duodenal ulcer. A deep crater in the second part of the duodenum (a post bulbar ulcer) is demonstrated on this tangential view in a double-contrast barium meal. Note the residual barium in the ulcer crater (arrow). This patient also has osteoarthritis of the spine and was taking a non-steroidal anti-inflammatory drug, which contributed to his presentation with haematemesis.

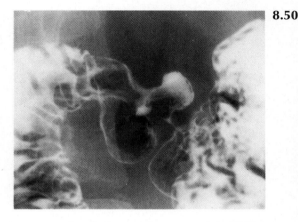

8.50 Duodenal ulcer with a scarred duodenal cap showing a 'clover leaf trefoil' deformity. Note the ulcer crater, and the radiating barium spicules representing folds in the scarred mucosa.

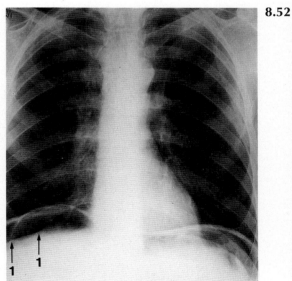

8.51 Haemorrhage is one of the commonest complications of peptic ulceration, and urgent endoscopy may yield a rather poor view, because of the presence of altered blood and food residues. This patient has fresh friable clot adherent to the base of a duodenal ulcer.

8.52 Pneumoperitoneum in a patient with a rigid abdomen caused by a perforated duodenal ulcer. The onset of his pain and rigidity was abrupt. Note the upper edge of the liver (1), and the air under both diaphragms.

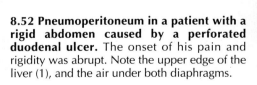

367

Peptic ulceration at other sites

Peptic ulceration may occur in the oesophagus (*see* p. 359), at or near the stoma following gastric surgery, or in the ectopic gastric mucosa in a Meckel's diverticulum.

Small intestine

Malabsorption

Malabsorption is the most common presenting symptom of small intestinal disease and is characterised by failure to digest and/or absorb nutrients from the intestinal tract. Important causes are summarised in **Table 8.2**.

Patients may present with pale offensive stools that float and are difficult to flush away, and they may exhibit features of nutrient deficiency (**8.1, 8.53, 8.54**) in addition to those that characterise the underlying disease process.

Investigations are undertaken with three objectives:

- To confirm impaired absorption, for example faecal fat collection and the Schilling test.

- To identify specific deficiencies, e.g. anthropometric measurements, blood count, iron, transferrin, folate, vitamin B_{12}, prothrombin and related vitamin K-dependent clotting factors, and vitamin D levels.

- To establish the mechanism and cause of malabsorption. This may include a search for bacterial overgrowth, testing pancreatic exocrine function, and aspiration or biopsy of the proximal small bowel (**8.55**) to look for evidence of giardiasis (**8.18**) or gluten enteropathy (**8.56, 8.57**).

8.53

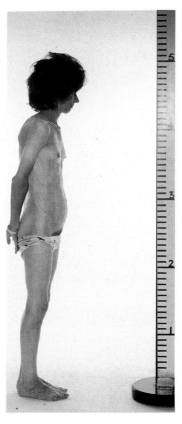

8.54

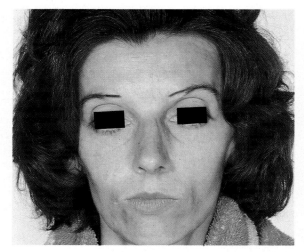

8.53, 8.54 Malabsorption in coeliac disease may remain undiagnosed for many years. This woman was diagnosed at the age of 32 years, but her height—5 feet (1.52 m)—was lower than all other members of her family, suggesting that her malabsorption dates from childhood. On presentation she weighed 40 kg (88 lbs), she had marked steatorrhoea and she was pale and anaemic. Small bowel biopsy showed villous atrophy. A gluten-free diet relieved her steatorrhoea and reversed the changes in her jejunal mucosa. She rapidly gained weight, but should probably remain on a gluten-free diet for life.

Table 8.2 Causes of malabsorption.

Gluten enteropathy
    Coeliac disease
    Dermatitis herpetiformis
Tropical sprue
Bacterial overgrowth
Intestinal resection
Whipple's disease
Radiation enteritis (*see p.* 374)
Parasite infestation. e.g. *Giardia lamblia* (*see* p. 379)
Pancreatic exocrine failure
    Chronic pancreatitis (*see* p. 413)
    Surgical resection
Chronic cholestasis

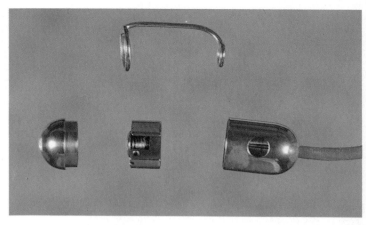

8.55 The Crosby capsule, seen here dismantled, is designed to obtain small samples of jejunal mucosa. After assembly it is swallowed by the paatient and it passes through the stomach and duodenum into the jejunum, where its position is checked radiologically. The application of suction to the tube leading to the capsule pulls a small piece of mucosa into the port of the capsule, and triggers the cutting mechanism, which slices off a thin mucosa sample. The capsule is then withdrawn through the mouth.

8.56   **8.57**

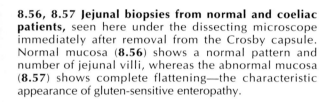

8.56, 8.57 Jejunal biopsies from normal and coeliac patients, seen here under the dissecting microscope immediately after removal from the Crosby capsule. Normal mucosa (**8.56**) shows a normal pattern and number of jejunal villi, whereas the abnormal mucosa (**8.57**) shows complete flattening—the characteristic appearance of gluten-sensitive enteropathy.

Gluten enteropathy (coeliac disease)

Some patients develop an immunological respose to gluten which damages the small intestinal mucosa, resulting in partial or subtotal villus atrophy. Gluten is a protein found predominantly in wheat, but also in rye, barley and (to a lesser extent) oats. The degradation of gluten in the intestinal lumen means that the proximal small intestine is maximally affected. Thus almost half of all patients are diagnosed through the incidental finding of iron or folate deficiency as a result of a blood count. Those who have more severe involvement develop steatorrhoea. This may arise not only as a consequence of damage, and resultant loss of surface area of the small intestinal mucosa, but also because impaired release of cholecystokinin from the diseased proximal small intestine impairs pancreatic secretion in response to meals. Presentation in infancy at the time of weaning is common, but gluten enteropathy can occur at any age.

The diagnosis is confirmed by proximal small bowel biopsy, either endoscopically or with the Crosby capsule (**8.56–8.59**); or by sequential biopsies with an improved and subsequently deteriorated appearance of the mucosa, on introduction of a gluten-free diet followed by a gluten challenge. Barium follow-through may also provide useful information (**8.60**).

A gluten-free diet relieves symptoms and reverses the biopsy appearances in most patients. Small intestinal lymphoma and carcinoma are more common in patients with coeliac disease than in the general population; extra-gastrointestinal cancers are also more common. The effect of a gluten-free diet on the risk of these complications is unclear.

In **dermatitis herpetiformis**, a gluten-sensitive enteropathy is accompanied by a bullous skin eruption (**2.61, 2.62**). Both may respond to a gluten-free diet, though treatment with dapsone may also be needed for the skin eruption.

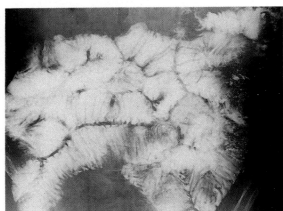

8.58, 8.59 Microscopic sections of jejunal biopsies from normal and coeliac patients. The sections correspond to the appearance seen in **8.56** and **8.57** respectively. The normal microscopic appearance of the jejunal mucosa is seen in **8.58**, whereas **8.59** shows the jejunum of a previously undiagnosed patient with gluten-sensitive enteropathy on a normal diet. The normal intestinal villi are absent, the mucosa is flattened and there is hyperplasia of the intestinal crypts. There is lymphocytic infiltration, and the surface mucosa is cuboidal rather than columnar.

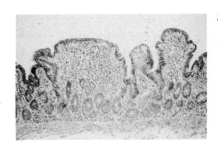

8.60

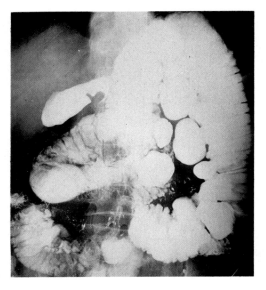

8.60 Barium follow-through in coeliac disease in a 26-year-old man. The film shows dilatation of the small bowel with 'simplification' of the mucosal pattern. The transverse folds are straight in appearance, rather than 'feathery' as they would be in a normal film. Flocculation of barium used to be described as a classic sign of coeliac disease, but the additives in modern barium prevent this sign from appearing. Nevertheless, the diagnosis is clearly suggested by the film.

Bacterial overgrowth

8.61

Small intestinal bacterial overgrowth commonly accompanies the reduction of gastric acidity by drugs or surgery, blind loops (**8.61**) and motility disorders. It is an important consideration in the elderly. Diagnosis is supported with a glycocholate or hydrogen breath test (*see* p. 356).

8.61 Multiple wide-mouthed jejunal diverticula are seen in this barium follow-through X-ray. The diverticula are sites of stasis; in this patient they were colonised by bacteria which created a malabsorption syndrome.

Tumours of the small intestine

Small intestinal tumours account for only 1% of gastrointestinal neoplasms. In descending order of frequency they comprise adenocarcinomas, carcinoids, lymphomas, and leiomyosarcomas. Kaposi's sarcoma of the intestine may occur in patients with HIV infection.

Adenocarcinomas may complicate Crohn's disease, particularly in a by-passed segment, and coeliac disease. Almost half occur in the duodenum. Presentation is with pain and vomiting, anaemia and, in the case of periampullary tumours, jaundice. Diagnosis is often made by a small bowel barium study (**8.62**).

Intestinal *lymphomas* also occur more commonly than expected in patients with coeliac disease (**8.63**). The lymphoma is often located in the distal small intestine, whereas the proximal intestine bears the brunt of the damage from gluten. Lymphomas also occur in patients who are immunosuppressed after organ transplantation or by HIV infection. Patients develop diarrhoea and pain, and lose weight.

Most small intestinal *carcinoid* tumours arise in the ileum. The clinical features are determined by local growth which can lead to intestinal obstruction, and by their secretion of humoral agents that become systemically active after metastases have developed in the liver. The characteristic syndrome of flushing (8.64) with diarrhoea, bronchospasm and congestive cardiac failure is well known. Patients may even develop pellagra caused by nicotinic acid deficiency as a result of disturbed tryptophan metabolism.

Tumours and vascular malformations may present with recurrent gastrointestinal bleeding of obscure cause. As with Meckel's diverticulum, the diagnosis may be made on mesenteric angiography, or—for slow bleeding—by a technetium-labelled red-cell scan.

8.62

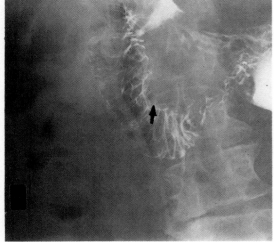

8.62 Carcinoma of the ampulla of Vater (arrowed), shown as a filling defect in the second part of the duodenum on this double-contrast barium meal. The patient presented with anaemia and mild jaundice.

8.63

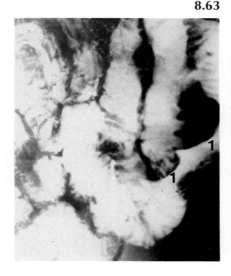

8.63 Intestinal lymphoma in a patient with coeliac disease that had been well controlled on a gluten-free diet for the past 13 years. An irregular shouldered stricture (1) is seen on barium follow-through. Radiologically, the appearance suggests lymphoma or carcinoma, and at operation a lymphoma was found. Even with surgery followed by radiotherapy or chemotherapy, the prognosis is poor.

8.64

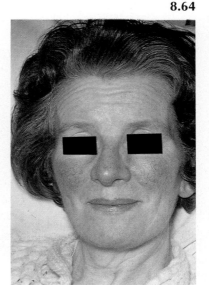

8.64 Facial flush in carcinoid. This is usually seen only when hepatic secondaries are present, although it may occur with primary tumours which drain directly into the systemic circulation (in the lung, testis or ovary). Other symptoms resulting from the release of vasoactive substances by these tumours may include abdominal pain, diarrhoea, bronchospasm and congestive cardiac failure.

Inflammatory bowel disease

Idiopathic inflammatory bowel disease is a term that encompasses two main conditions: ulcerative colitis and Crohn's disease.

Crohn's disease

Crohn's disease is a chronic granulomatous inflammatory disease of unknown cause, which is becoming more common. The terminal ileum and colon are principally involved, but the disease may affect any part of the intestinal tract, often with discontinuous patches of inflammation of all the bowel wall structures. Initially, aphthoid ulcers may be seen at endoscopic examination with macroscopically normal intervening mucosa (8.65). Subsequently, more severe inflammation leads to more extensive ulceration (8.66, 8.67) or even to a 'cobblestone' appearance of the mucosa; and ultimately fibrosis can cause bowel strictures (8.15, 8.68). Inflamed bowel may adhere to surrounding structures and matted loops of bowel are a cause of internal or external fistulae (8.69) and intestinal obstruction (8.16). Involvement of the perianal area in up to 80% of

patients leads to a characteristic appearance with skin tags, fissures and fistulae (8.6, 8.7). Less commonly, the lips and oral cavity are affected (8.3).

The clinical presentation is varied depending upon the region, extent, and manner of the intestinal involvement. Common features include diarrhoea, abdominal pain, anorexia, weight loss and pyrexia. Eventually the patient may suffer from intestinal obstruction and intestinal failure, with malnutrition or growth failure.

Patients with Crohn's disease may develop diarrhoea for numerous reasons. These include extensive intestinal inflammation, partial obstruction, small intestinal bacterial overgrowth, bile-acid malabsorption caused by terminal ileal disease or excision, entero-enteral fistulae, short-bowel syndrome, amyloidosis and intestinal infections. It is important that the true cause is identified and treated.

Extra-intestinal manifestations of Crohn's disease are similar to those experienced by patients with ulcerative colitis and may include sclerosing cholangitis (8.70), arthritis, uveitis and skin rashes such as pyoderma gangrenosum (2.118) and erythema nodosum (1.123, 2.40, 2.39). Most patients with Crohn's disease who develop pain and jaundice do not have sclerosing cholangitis, however. The majority have gall-stones.

Crohn's disease can be controlled in most patients with short-term courses of corticosteroids, and azathioprine is useful in resistant patients. Surgery is required for the relief of obstruction and the correction of fistulae. Nutritional support, either enteral or parenteral, corrects malnutrition thus making a major contribution to the patient's well-being.

8.65

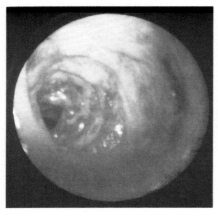

8.66

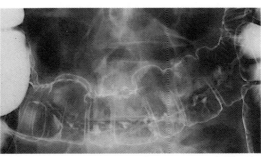

8.66 Crohn's colitis on double-contrast barium enema. Many ulcers can be seen in this view of the transverse colon, by their retention of barium, but the remaining mucosa appears normal.

8.67

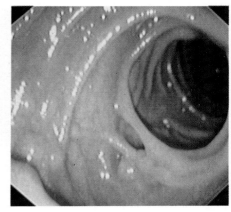

8.67 Crohn's disease in the duodenum. This videoendoscopic view shows 'bridging' lesions in the mucosa. Ulceration and healing leads to these isolated bridges of mucosa.

8.65 Crohn's colitis. In this colonoscopic view, there are multiple small ulcers with surrounding areas of inflammation. The adjacent mucosa looks normal. Similar patchy lesions were present throughout the colon.

8.68

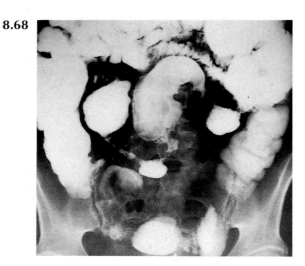

8.68 Crohn's disease of the small intestine revealed on barium follow-through X-ray. Four strictures of the small intestine are clearly seen, and the dilated segments of bowel appear between the strictures. These 'skip lesions' are characteristic of Crohn's disease, and similar appearances may be seen in the colon when there is colonic involvement.

8.69

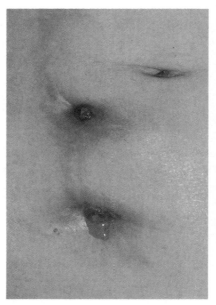

8.69 Enterocutaneous fistulae in Crohn's disease are most common, as here, in patients who have undergone bowel resection, but they may also occur in unoperated cases. Sinography may be used to demonstrate communication with the affected bowel.

8.70

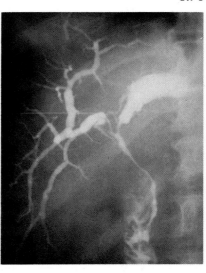

8.70 Primary sclerosing cholangitis may complicate inflammatory bowel disease. This percutaneous transhepatic cholangiogram shows typical appearances, with patchy dilation and stricturing of the biliary tree. Some of the contrast has passed into the duodenum in this view. ERCP examination is an alternative method of diagnosis, which will demonstrate the same radiological appearance.

Ulcerative colitis

Ulcerative colitis has an incidence and prevalence of 6 and 60 per 100,000 respectively in the UK. It is primarily a mucosal disease that extends for a variable distance and in a continuous fashion, around the colon from the rectum, which is always involved.

Symptoms depend on the extent and severity of colonic involvement. Patients in whom the disease is confined to the rectum experience rectal bleeding and tenesmus, but the stool is formed and constipation may be a problem. Diarrhoea is the predominant symptom with more extensive disease, and severe attacks are accompanied by pyrexia and tachycardia.

Endoscopy reveals an inflamed bleeding mucosa, barium enema shows characteristic findings (8.75, 8.76) and biopsies show (8.71–8.74) goblet cell depletion, crypt abscesses, distortion of the architecture with little submucosal inflammation and no granulomas (in contrast to Crohn's disease).

Extra-intestinal manifestations include skin rashes, erythema nodosum (1.123, 2.40) and pyoderma gangrenosum (2.118), hepatobiliary disease, especially sclerosing cholangitis (8.70) and arthritis. Inflammation involving the peripheral joints reflects the activity of the intestinal disease, but this does not apply where patients have sacro-iliitis or ankylosing spondylitis.

Complications of acute disease include colonic dilatation (8.77) which may lead to perforation and haemorrhage. Chronic disease may also produce anaemia, and carries a small but increasing risk of colonic carcinoma in patients with extensive disease of more than 10 years' duration (8.78). Colonoscopic surveillance facilitates the detection of premalignant dysplasia in the mucosa, allowing timely surgical intervention.

Medical treatment involves the control of disease activity with short courses of corticosteroids, the maintenance of remission with sulphasalazine or one of the newer preparations that are designed to deliver 5-aminosalicylic acid to the colon (mesalazine or olsalazine) and the correction of anaemia. Surgery is required if medical management fails, and to prevent acute and chronic complications such as perforation or carcinoma. Pan-proctocolectomy with a permanent ileostomy is usually necessary, although pouch procedures involving ileoanal anastomoses are currently fashionable.

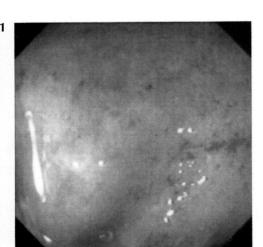

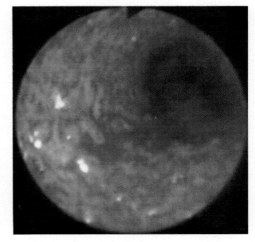

8.71 Ulcerative colitis. Early changes are seen in this colonoscopic view. These include swelling of the mucosa, loss of normal haustrations and friability of the mucosa with bleeding caused by the touch of the colonoscope.

8.72 Ulcerative colitis. More severe changes than in **8.71**. Ulceration has extended, and bleeding is more apparent. Some 'pseudopolyps' are visible. Endoscopy is hazardous in the acute phases of ulcerative colitis, due to the risk of perforation and/or bleeding.

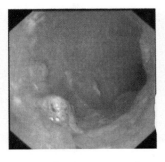

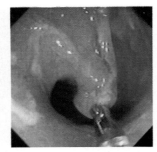

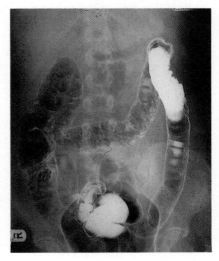

8.73 Inflammatory polyps (often known, rather confusingly, as 'pseudopolyps' are invariably found in the progression of ulcerative colitis. They are composed of granulomatous tissue, and, like any inflammatory reaction, they are highly vascular.

8.74 Biopsy of large inflammatory polyps in ulcerative colitis is sometimes advisable to exclude the possiblity of carcinoma, which is a major risk of chronic ulcerative colitis. (*see* **8.78**).

8.75 Ulcerative colitis. This double- contrast barium enema shows typical chronic changes throughout the colon. There is loss of the normal haustral pattern, giving the colon a smooth tubular appearance. Deep, penetrating ulcers can be seen, especially in the barium-filled splenic flexure, and there are many pseudopolyps, best seen in the transverse colon.

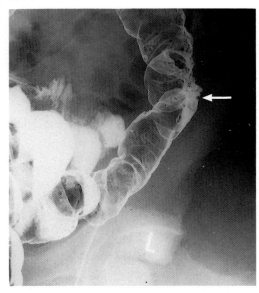

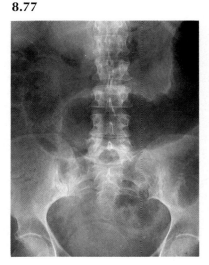

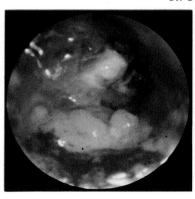

8.76 Ulcerative colitis with multiple inflammatory polyps ('pseudopolyps'). The double-contrast barium enema technique demonstrates the appearance well in the descending colon, and this correlates with the endoscopic view (**8.73**). Note the area of deep ulceration (arrow). On screening, this area showed a lack of movement which raised the suspicion of carcinomatous change.

8.77 Colonic dilatation in ulcerative colitis ('toxic megacolon').This complication of acute ulcerative colitis requires urgent intensive management, including fluid replacement and steroid therapy. The patient presents with a tender, swollen abdomen, which is tympanitic, due to the amount of gas in the colon. Fever and signs of shock are common accompaniments. It is important to auscultate the abdomen, as barrel sounds are usually absent.

8.78 Carcinoma of the colon has developed as a complication of long-standing ulcerative colitis in this patient with a 24-year history of the disease. Regular colonoscopic surveillance should allow identification of this complication at an earlier stage.

Drugs and the colon

Inflammation of the colon may occur as an indirect consequence of antibiotic administration (pseudomembranous colitis—*see* p. 379), or as the result of treatment with non-steroidal anti-inflammatory analgesics. Some, such as mefenamic acid, are particularly prone to cause diarrhoea with an associated colitis.

Other disorders affecting both small and large intestine

Radiation enterocolitis

Radiation enterocolitis is a sequel to radiotherapy for pelvic and abdominal malignancy. The safety margin between therapeutic effect and damage to surrounding structures is narrow and factors such as previous surgery may enhance intestinal damage by fixing loops of bowel within the field of exposure.

Early changes after exposure include increased crypt cell death and loss of villus height, and the extensive loss of intestinal function may lead to fluid and electrolyte imbalance. However, the initial clinical features of nausea, vomiting and diarrhoea, frequently with rectal bleeding, may settle.

Late complications develop from endarteritis obliterans, which leads to intestinal ischaemia. After a period that varies from a few months to many years, ischaemic strictures and fistulae may develop, and patients may suffer from subacute obstruction and chronic malabsorption (**8.79**). Sometimes, damage to the enteric nerves causes a pseudo-obstruction. The colonic symptoms can resemble idiopathic ulcerative colitis, but endoscopy reveals the typical picture of an atrophic mucosa with telangiectasia.

Medical therapy is limited in scope. Antibiotics are useful for the treatment of secondary bacterial overgrowth, cholestyramine may be helpful with bile acid malabsorbtion when the terminal ileum is affected, and topical steroids or mesalazine should be given to patients with proctitis. Some patients with intestinal failure need prolonged parenteral nutrition. Surgery is required for perforation, stricture and fistulae, but the morbidity of operative intervention is considerable.

8.79 Radiation enterocolitis. This 3¼-hour barium follow-through film shows narrowing of the terminal ileum, with gross thickening of the normal mùcosal folds. On screening, the ileum was seen to be matted together as an immobile mass. These changes were associated with a rapid transit time and malabsorption. This 55-year-old woman had been treated by radiotherapy for carcinoma of the cervix.

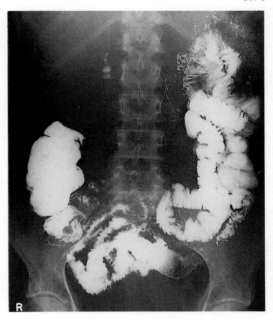

Ischaemic disorders

Intestinal ischaemia may be acute or chronic, and it may affect the small or large intestine:

- Acute mesenteric ischaemia usually occurs in patients with generalised atheroma, but it may be embolic. Rarely, it is caused by venous occlusion in patients who are taking oral contraceptives or who have antithrombin-III deficiency. The initial presentation with diarrhoea, vomiting and vague abdominal pain, is rapidly followed by increasing pain and shock. Early laparotomy and resection of the affected segment offers the only prospect of survival.
- Chronic mesenteric insufficiency causes intestinal angina, a postprandial abdominal pain that usually prompts an intitial search for peptic ulcer or biliary disease.
- Colonic ischaemia is more common than mesenteric ischaemia and usually effects the splenic flexure. The patient complains of abdominal pain and diarrhoea. After a few hours the diarrhoea contains fresh blood. At this stage, the diagnosis may be suspected from plain abdominal X-ray in which 'thumb-printing' is evident (**8.80**). Infection with *E.coli* 0157 may produce a similar clinical picture. Occasionally, the affected segment perforates, but usually the features subside. Fibrosis may lead to stenosis causing alteration of bowel habit or chronic intestinal obstruction (**8.81**).

8.80

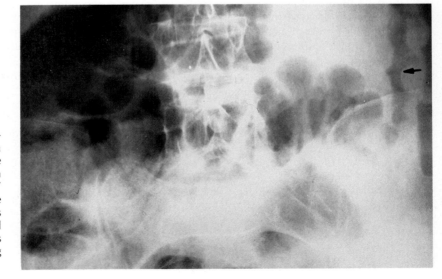

8.80 Acute ischaemic colitis. The patient was a 60-year-old woman who presented with acute bloody diarrhoea and left-sided abdominal pain. This plain X-ray of the abdomen in the supine position shows a narrowing in the bowel lumen and mucosal 'thumb-printing' (arrowed) in the descending colon. The narrowing of the colon is caused by spasm, and the thumb-printing is caused by a combination of sub-mucosal oedema and haemorrhage. Note that the proximal large bowel is somewhat distended—the ischaemic lesion is causing partial obstruction.

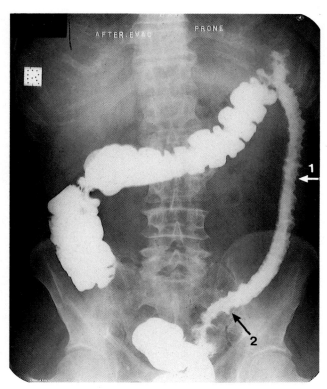

8.81 Colonic ischaemia This single contrast barium enema shows gross ischaemic changes throughout the descending colon. There is narrowing of the lumen, accompanied by typical 'rose-thorn' ulcers (1) and some 'thumb-printing' (2) in the sigmoid colon, where a partial stricture has formed. The apparent stricture at the hepatic flexure disappeared on screening. The patient also had symptomatic coronary heart disease and peripheral vascular disease.

The colon and rectum

Diverticular disease

Diverticula are acquired pouches of the colonic mucosa that have herniated through the muscular layers of the colon. They are present in about half of the population over the age of 65 in the developed world, and are often found by chance in barium enemas which have been carried out for other purposes. The most common site is the sigmoid colon, where they are usually multiple. The cause is unclear, but they may result from an increased pressure within the lumen in the sigmoid colon. They are most common in patients in whom dietary fibre intake is low.

Many patients have no symptoms, but some have recurrent lower abdominal pain, particularly in the left iliac fossa, associated with flatulence and constipation or, sometimes, diarrhoea. Pain follows a meal and is often relieved by passing gas or by defaecation. Bleeding and localised abscess formation (diverticulitis) may occur. Diverticulitis is associated with severe localised pain in the abdomen, fever and localised guarding. Septicaemia may result, and other complications include fistulae, colonic obstruction and generalised peritonitis.

The diagnosis is made on barium enema (**8.82**, **8.83**) or colonoscopy. Most symptoms settle with conservative treatment, and patients should be given a high-fibre diet. Surgery may be required for complications and anaemia may require iron therapy or blood transfusion.

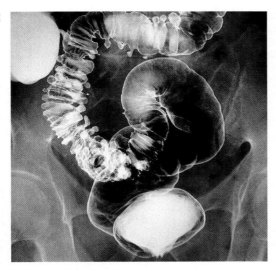

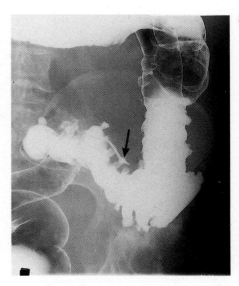

8.82 Diverticular disease of the colon. This barium enema shows typical changes, with multiple diverticula outlined by the double contrast technique. The patient presented with a change in bowel habit and abdominal pain, and although this could be caused by the diverticular disease itself, it is important to exclude the possibility of co-existent colonic carcinoma in these circumstances. This is best done by colonoscopy.

8.83 Diverticular disease of the colon with sinus formation. This patient with known diverticular disease was reinvestigated for right iliac fossa pain and tenderness. The barium enema shows the presence of multiple diverticula, and a communicating sinus is clearly seen (arrow). This appearance is diagnostic of local abscess formation.

Colonic and rectal cancer

Colorectal cancer is predominantly found in Western societies. It is the most common gastrointestinal malignancy in the UK, and is responsible for approximately 16,000 deaths each year. High-fat, low-fibre diets have been blamed for supporting bacterial flora that result in the formation of carcinogens from intestinal contents, including bile acids, an effect compounded by a delayed transit time.

Most cancers develop from benign adenomas. There is a low risk of malignancy in single polyps that are less than 1 cm in diameter, but a much higher risk when the diameter exceeds 2 cm (**8.12, 8.84**) or the polyps are multiple. The histological type is also important, as malignancy is much more common in villous (40%) than tubular (5%) adenomas.

Patients with *familial polyposis coli* (**8.14, 8.85**) almost invariably develop bowel cancer, so they are advised to undergo prophylactic colectomy. Patients at risk include the family members with familial polyposis, those who have previously developed polyps, patients over 40 years of age with first degree relatives with colonic cancer, those with long-standing extensive ulcerative colitis, and possibly patients who have undergone cholecystectomy.

Patients with colonic cancer may present with alteration of bowel habit, rectal bleeding, abdominal pain, anaemia or syptoms of disseminated disease.

The diagnosis is established by a barium enema examination (**8.86, 8.87**), which should be preceded by sigmoidoscopy. When the barium examination fails to provide conclusive information, or when polyps are found, colonoscopy is required to detect lesions missed on the barium films and to allow biopsy of suspect areas and the removal of polyps (**8.12, 8.78, 8.88**). Investigations are also needed to determine the effects of the disease, for example a blood count and film to look for iron deficiency, and a CT scan or ultrasound examination of the abdominal nodes and liver to search for metastatic disease (**9.18**).

Colonic cancer may be prevented by the identification and removal of polyps. The established tumour is treated by surgical resection, a right or left hemicolectomy or abdomino-perineal excision of lower rectal tumours. Rectal lesions may be palliated by laser treatment in patients unfit for surgery. The prognosis is influenced by the extent of spread and this is the basis of Duke's classification. Follow-up is mandatory, and should involve at least annual barium enemas or colonoscopy plus measurement of the tumour marker, carcinoembryonic antigen (CEA).

8.84

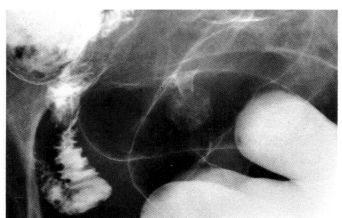

8.84 A single colonic polyp, beautifully revealed by double-contrast barium enema. Its pedunculated nature should mean that it can be successfully removed by snare diathermy performed through the colonoscope (*see* **8.12**). If the excision is histologically complete, no further treatment is required for this polyp; but the patient should have a full-length colonic examination at the time of colonoscopy and any further polyps should be similarly treated. Because of the risk of recurrence of the polyp at the same or a different site, follow up colonoscopy is usually recommended.

8.85

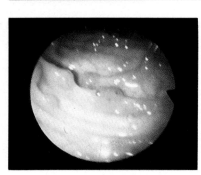

8.85 Familial polyposis coli. Multiple sessile polyps are seen in this colonoscopic view. Histologically, the lesions are adenomatous polyps, but there is a high risk of malignant change in this dominant condition, which usually presents in the second decade of life with diarrhoea, rectal bleeding and, sometimes, abdominal pain. Multiple polyps can usually also be seen on double-contrast barium enema examination (**8.14**) Prophylactic colectomy is usually advised.

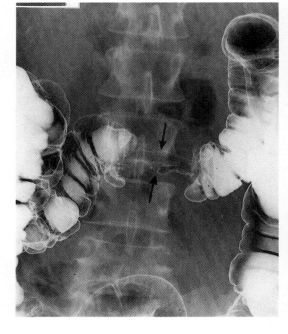

8.86 Colonic carcinoma in the transverse colon, revealed by double-contrast barium enema. This annular carcinoma has produced a characteristic apple-core appearance (arrow). This is strongly suggestive of the diagnosis, but it must be confirmed by biopsy via the colonoscope. This patient presented with chronic iron deficiency anaemia and was found to have a positive faecal occult blood test.

8.87

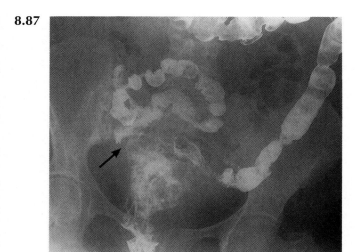

8.87 Entero-colic fistula (arrowed) in colonic carcinoma. This was an unexpected finding in a patient who presented with malabsorption and diarrhoea. A carcinoma of the sigmoid colon has formed a fistula with an adjacent loop of small intestine (identifiable by its typical mucosal pattern). Colonisation of the small bowel by colonic bacteria is the cause of the malabsorption in this condition.

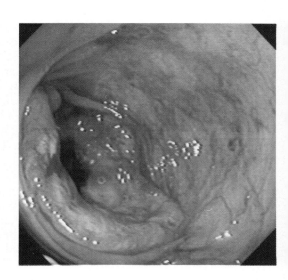

8.88 Colonic carcinoma seen through a video-colonoscope. This sessile lesion in the descending colon presented with frank bleeding. The lesion was ulcerating in places and bled readily when touched. It nearly encircled the colon. Tumours in this location are often resectable and carry a relatively good prognosis.

Gastrointestinal infections

Infection may occure at any level in the gut. Infection of the mouth and oesophagus are important causes of local symptoms (*see* pp. 65, 358 and 360). *Helicobacter pylori* infection plays a role in the genesis of gastritis and peptic ulceration (*see* pp. 362 and 366).

Intestinal tuberculosis is rare in the developed world but still relatively common elsewhere. It usually affects the terminal ileum, where it may produce symptoms and a barium X-ray appearance similar to those of Crohn's disease (**8.15**). Management is usually medical (*see* p. 46).

Gastroenteritis is a common problem throughout the world. The most common symptom is diarrhoea, and it is important to distinguish infective from other causes (**Table 8.3**).

Secretory diarrhoea may be caused by *Vibrio cholerae* (p. 52), *Campylobacter jejuni* and many strains of *E. coli* and *Salmonella*. Typically, there are copious fluid stools, and dehydration is the most important clinical problem.

Dysentery is a condition in which the stool contains pus, mucus and blood. This results from colonic mucosal invasion by organisms such as enteroinvasive *E. coli*, *Shigella*, *Campylobacter jejuni* and rotavirus. Other invasive organisms may cause a predominantly septicaemic illness. The most important example is *Salmonella typhi*: intestinal symptoms occur relatively late in the evolution of typhoid fever (*see p.* 51). Pseudomembranous colitis is a serious infection with *Clostridium difficile* that may follow treatment with broad-spectrum antibiotics (**8.89**).

Most acute infective diarrhoea is self-limiting, but oral or intravenous fluid replacement is always important where diarrhoea is profuse, and antibiotic treatment is indicated for some invasive infections.

Transmission of infection is usually by the faecal–oral route, and prevention is based on hygienic measures in food and water preparation.

Protozoal infections are another important cause of gastrointestinal symptoms.

Giardiasis is common. The organism infests the small intestine and may cause acute diarrhoea or chronic malabsorption. The cysts may be evident on stool microscopy, but small intestinal aspiration or biopsy is sometimes needed to confirm the diagnosis (**8.18**). Eradication is achieved with metronidazole.

Table 8.3 Common causes of diarrhoea.

Viral	Rotavirus
	Norwalk agent
	Adenoviruses
Bacterial toxin	*Escherichia coli* (enterotoxigenic)
	Vibrio cholerae
	Staphylococcus
	Clostridium perfringens
	Clostridium difficile
	Clostridium botulinum
	Bacillus cereus
Bacterial invasion	*Escherichia coli* (enteroinvasive)
	Shigella
	Salmonella
	Yersinia enterocolitica
	Vibrio parahaemolyticus
	Campylobacter jejuni
Parasites	*Giardia lamblia*
	Cryptosporidium
	Entamoeba histolytica
After infection	Lactase deficiency
	Bacterial overgrowth
Drugs	Laxatives
	Antacids with magnesium
Food toxins	Ciguatoxin, scombroid, pufferfish
Chronic gastrointestinal disorders	Inflammatory bowel disease
	Ischaemic colitis
	Malabsorption
	Irritable bowel syndrome
Metabolic disorders	Hyperthyroidism
	Adrenal insufficiency
	Hyperparathyroidism
	Diabetes mellitus

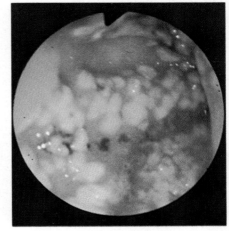

8.89

8.89 Pseudomembranous colitis may develop during, or up to 6 weeks after, treatment with antibiotics such as lincomycin, ampicillin and cephalosporins. The major symptom is diarrhoea, which may be bloody. Sigmoidoscopy or colonoscopy usually shows multiple yellow plaques and inflammatory changes and the diagnosis can be confirmed histologically. *Clostridium difficile* and its toxin are found in the stools. Patients with pseudomembranous colitis should be barrier-nursed, because there is a risk of cross infection. If the diarrhoea is severe, they may need intravenous fluid replacement, and treatment with vancomycin will eliminate the *Clostridium* infection.

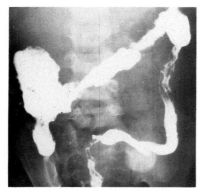

8.90 Amoebic colitis. This barium enema performed during the recovery phase of fulminating amoebic colitis shows extensive strictures and areas of mucosal damage in the colon. It is essential that these are not mis-diagnosed as inflammatory bowel disease or tumours. Stool examination, colonoscopy and biopsy may all be helpful in diagnosis.

Entamoeba histolytica invades the colonic mucosa (**8.90**) and the patient suffers from bloody diarrhoea. The possibility of amoebiasis must always be considered in a patient with this complaint who is in, or has returned from, a Third World country. An erroneous diagnosis of inflammatory bowel disease followed by corticosteroid treatment may be fatal. The management of amoebiasis and its complications is covered on p. 66.

Cryptosporidium has been widely recognised as a cause of diarrhoea in cattle, and is now known to produce a self-limiting diarrhoeal illness in man. In patients with AIDS, it may produce a catastrophic illness with extreme dehydration, shock and death.

Intestinal worm infestations

Roundworms

Threadworm infestation with *Enterobius vermicularis* is very common worldwide. It commonly causes pruritus ani, especially in children, but may be asymptomatic.

Infestation with *Ascaris lumbricoides* may also be asymptomatic, but some patients develop a cough and fever during the migration of the larvae to the lung after they penetrate the intestinal mucosa. After development, the worms are coughed up, swallowed and become established in the instestinal tract. Heavy infestation can lead to distal small intestinal obstruction and, rarely, migration can cause obstruction of the bile duct (**8.91**). Piperazine and mebendazole are effective treatments (**8.92**).

The whipworm, *Trichuris trichiura*, has a simple life cycle, and it does not migrate from the gut. Heavy infestation may lead to abdominal symptoms as a result of mucosal penetration or intestinal obstruction.

Hookworm larvae penetrate the skin and also migrate via the lungs. The adult worms such as *Ancylostoma duodenale* and *Necator americanus* are an important cause of anaemia in many underdeveloped countries (*see* p. 424, **10.18**).

Strongyloides stercoralis infestation resembles hookworm infestation in some respects, but the worms can have a free-living cycle in the soil. In man, the eggs hatch into larvae in the instestine; and the larvae can mature into filariform worms

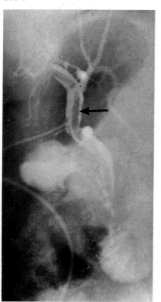

8.91 Partial common bile duct obstruction caused by a roundworm (arrow). The worm was revealed by T-tube cholangiography performed after cholecystectomy in this patient who had complained of right upper quadrant pain and dark urine. Gallstones were present, but her obstructive symptoms may well have been caused by the worm.

8.92 Massive *Ascaris* infection in a child has been successfully treated by anthelminthic treatment. This bolus of roundworms had caused obstructive symptoms.

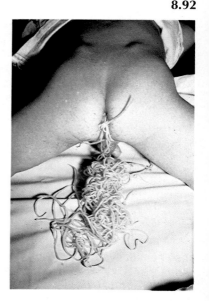

and cause autoinfection by direct penetration from the gut. Larva migrans may occur (**1.208**). Systemic invasion is of particular importance in immunosuppressed patients: in patients with AIDS, for example, hyperinfection by this route may result in severe disease of the lungs, heart, liver, kidneys and nervous system. Patients starting treatment with corticosteroids or other immunosuppressive drugs are also at risk of these complications. Thiabendazole and mebendazole are the drugs of choice in treatment.

Other roundworm infestations are covered on pp. 72–76.

Flatworms

Flatworm (Trematode) infestations include schistosomiasis (*see* p. 77) and paragonimiasis (*see* p. 78).

Fasciolopsis buski is the most important intestinal fluke. It occurs in the Far East, has an intermediate water-snail host, and is transmitted via metacercariae on edible water plants such as water chestnuts. Severe infestation may result in abdominal pain, malabsorption, diarrhoea and even obstruction as a result of the attachment of flukes to the intestinal mucosa. Preventive measures involve eradication of the intermediate host and education of affected populations. Treatment with praziquantel or niclosamide is usually effective.

Fasciola hepatica and other liver flukes are also transmitted via water-snails and edible water plants such as watercress. Infection occurs worldwide, mainly in sheep-rearing areas (sheep and cattle are the primary hosts). Ingested larvae migrate across the duodenal wall, and via the peritoneal cavity and the liver to the bile ducts. Here they may cause biliary obstruction, hepatitis and—in the long-term—portal cirrhosis.

Opisthorchis sinensis (the Chinese liver fluke) is transmitted via snails and freshwater fish, and may produce similar hepatic damage (**8.93**, **8.94**) and ultimately cholangiocarcinoma (*see* p. 408).

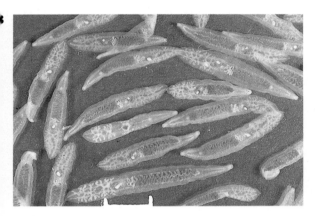

8.93 Adult *Opisthorchis sinensis*. The young worms migrate up the common bile duct to the liver. At maturity, they may reach 2 cm in length.

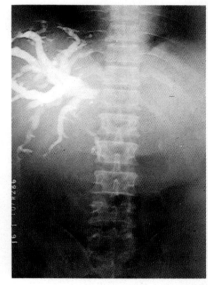

8.94

8.94 Chinese liver fluke infestation. This cholangiogram shows dilatation of the main bile ducts and disorganisation of the biliary tree, resulting from the presence of multiple adult *Opisthorchis sinensis*.

Tapeworms

Tapeworms include *Taenia saginata* from beef and *T. solium* from pork. Infestation occurs with the ingestion of infected and inadequately cooked meat containing viable cysts which develop in the human intestine. There may be no symptoms, but occasionally tapeworms may cause abdominal discomfort, diarrhoea or 'hunger pains'. The patient may notice proglottids in the faeces. Treatment with niclosamide or alternative drugs is effective (**8.95**).

T. solium is important because man can be affected by the larval stage. The larvae may penetrate the instestinal wall, enter the circulation and migrate to the brain, lungs, eyes, muscle and connective tissue to cause cysticercosis. Serious neurological symptoms may result where the brain is affected, and these may worsen when the cysticerci die and calcify. Radiology (**8.96**), CT scanning (**8.97**) and MRI are of value in locating cysts. Treatment with praziquantel may be helpful, but surgery may be needed and neurological or ophthalmological damage may be irreversible.

Diphyllobothrium latum, the fish tapeworm, is a rare cause of vitamin B_{12} deficiency, and may provoke pernicious anaemia in individuals who are genetically predisposed to the condition.

Man may act as an intermediate host for the dog tapeworm (*Echinococcus granulosus*) and develop cysts—hydatid disease (*see* p. 78). The intestinal tract is not affected in this 'dead-end' infestation.

Various other tapeworm species may occasionally infest man, and the larval forms of some may also invade directly, producing sparganosis (*see* p. 79).

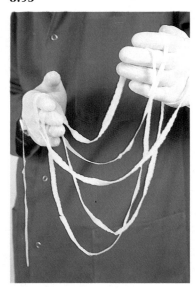

8.95 Adult *Taenia saginata* tapeworm. This is only part of a worm that was passed after treatment with niclosamide. *T. saginata* can grow to 10m or more in length.

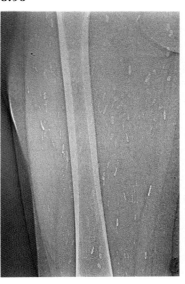

8.96 Calcified cysticerci in the soft tissues of the thigh were clearly seen on plain X-ray in this patient with cysticercosis.

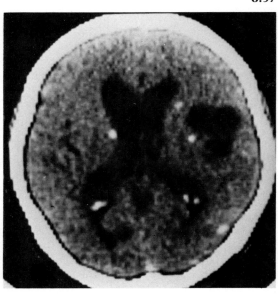

8.97 Cysticercosis of the brain revealed by CT scanning. This 'cut' shows multiple cysts (dark areas) and multiple calcifications (light areas). The calcifications represent dead cysticerci, while the cysts represent the earlier stages of cysticercosis.

Irritable bowel syndrome

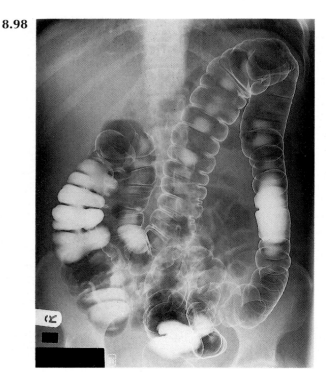

The irritable bowel syndrome (**IBS**) is probably the most common intestinal disease in clinical practicein the developed world, but it is one of the most poorly understood. It is a functional disease in which intestinal motility may be increased or decreased. The most common sympton is abdominal pain, and this is often accompanied by variable diarrhoea and/or constipation. The symptoms may be exaggerated during times of stress. The patient may gain symptomatic relief from passing gas and from defaecation. Despite this, he often feels his bowels have not emptied completely and may pass small motions many times a day. The stool is often compressed and ribbon-like. Patients with constipation often abuse purgatives, and may present with diarrhoea for this reason. Examination reveals very little except some vague lower abdominal tenderness. Rectal examination is normal. Colonoscopy and barium enema are not always required; when performed to exclude other pathology, they are normal (**8.98**). There is no specific treatment, but patients should be reassured and may benefit from a high-fibre diet and an antispasmodic.

8.98 A normal barium enema, as seen in the irritable bowel syndrome (IBS). The investigation is not always necessary, but may sometimes be needed to exclude other causes of abdominal symptoms or change in bowel habit. Colonoscopy also reveals no abnormal findings in IBS.

Food allergy and food intolerance

A number of symptoms and syndromes can be clearly related to food and food additives (**Table 8.4**). It is clear that both gastrointestinal and remote disorders may result from food intolerance in a number of ways, most of which do not directly involve allergic or immunological reactions (**Table 8.5**). Even where immunological abnormalities or allergic reactions have been demonstrated clearly—as, for example, in gluten-sensitive enteropathy—it is often not clear whether these are involved in the primary disease process, or whether they are simply a secondary consequence of other initiating factors. The patient will often suspect an association, but where the food is part of the everyday diet, the association may be less obvious. The possibility of food intolerance should be considered in all patients with:

- Urticaria and angioedema.
- Atopic eczema.
- Migraine.
- Asthma.
- Rhinitis.

In rhinitis with nasal polyps, intolerance to aspirin may also be present.

The manifestations of food intolerance may be immediate or delayed. Symptoms such as angioedema (swelling of lips and tongue—**8.99**), urticaria (**2.33**), vomiting, rhinorrhoea and asthma often develop within minutes as a result of an IgE-mediated reaction or a direct pharmacological effect. Late reactions may develop some hours or even days after ingestion of food, possibly as a result of a delayed immune response involving circulating immune complexes. Such late reactions pose a particularly difficult diagnostic problem, because:

- There are no reliable laboratory tests for food allergy or idiosyncrasy.
- Skin-prick testing with a few food extracts such as egg, fish, nuts and yeast gives results which correlate well with clinical symptoms, but positive results tend to persist even when clinical sensitivity has been lost.
- Serum IgE may be raised in an allergic response, but this does not demonstrate that the responsible antigen entered via the gut.
- Radioallergosorbent tests (RASTs) for specific IgE antibodies may sometimes demonstrate raised circulating antibody levels to specific foods, but for most of the food extracts used the correlation with symptoms is poor.
- 'Fringe' techniques, such as sublingual or cytotoxic food tests, hair analysis, etc., are widely advertised but valueless.

A diagnostic exclusion diet, followed by appropriate food challenge, is the mainstay of investigation, but the difficulty of adhering to and interpreting such a diet should be considered before embarking on this course. Appropriate exclusion diets are summarised in **Table 8.6**.

Table 8.4. Symptoms and syndromes which may be related to food.

Gastrointestinal symptoms	Swelling of lips or mouth
	Oral ulceration
	Vomiting
	Diarrhoea
	Abdominal pain
	Bloating
	Constipation
	Pruritus ani
Secondary syndromes	Steatorrhoea and 'coeliac-like' syndromes
	Protein-losing enteropathy
	Blood loss and anaemia (rare)
	Eosinophilic gastroenteritis
Remote effects	Anaphylaxis
	Rhinitis
	Nasal polyps
	Asthma
	Eczema
	Urticaria and angioedema
	Dermatitis herpetiformis
	Transitory joint pains
	Migraine
	Hyperactivity in children (food association very rare)
	Henoch–Schönlein purpura (rare)
	Nephrotic syndrome (rare)

Table 8.5. Causes of food intolerance.

Pharmacological
 Caffeine
 Tyramine—e.g. in cheese
 Histamine—e.g. in fish and canned foods
 Histamine liberators—e.g. egg white, strawberries
 Nitrates—e.g. in preserved meat

Toxic
 Irritants of the intestinal mucosa—e.g. peppers and spices
 Poisons—e.g. from tropical sea fish; acetanilide in rape-seed oil; aflatoxin in mouldy peanuts

Idiosyncracy
 Deficiency of enzymes, e.g. lactase (cow's milk intolerance) and possibly phenolsulphotransferase (some cases of dietary migraine)

Indirect associations
 Fat intolerance caused by gall bladder disease, cystic fibrosis or steatorrhoea
 Intolerance to fried or spiced foods in peptic ulceration
 Irritable bowel syndrome (possible effects of fermentation of unabsorbed food residues)

Food allergic disease
 IgE-mediated—usually associated with other allergies
 Other immunological abnormalities—e.g. coeliac disease, cow's milk and soya protein intolerance in infants

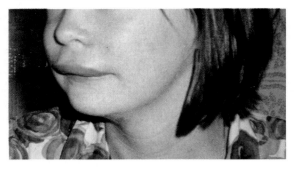

8.99 Angioedema resulting from sensitivity to tartrazine. This girl had recurrent, severe angioedema and urticaria, with episodes of life-threatening laryngeal oedema. An exclusion diet showed tartrazine (E102) to be the cause of her symptoms. This food colouring is widely used in many processed foods and drinks, so a rigorous maintenance exclusion diet is required to prevent symptoms. The mechanism of tartrazine sensitivity is unclear, and it may not have an allergic basis. Cross-sensitivity with other azo dyes, salicylates (including aspirin) and benzoates is common.

Table 8.6. Diagnostic exclusion diets appropriate for possibly food-related symptoms.*

Condition	Diagnostic diet
Urticaria or angioedema	Tartrazine, salicylate and benzoate free
Eczema	Cow's milk and egg free
Coeliac disease	Gluten free
Dermatitis herpetiformis	Gluten free
Cow's milk sensitive enteropathy	Cow's milk free
Asthma and rhinitis	Full exclusion
Migraine	Full exclusion
Irritable bowel syndrome	Full exclusion

* A full exclusion diet should be tried if a more specific diet is unsuccessful.

Gastrointestinal hormone-producing tumours

8.100

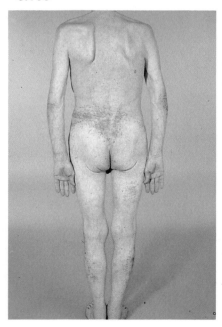

8.100 Glucagonoma syndrome is usually associated with a characteristic rash, the cause of which is obscure. The rash evolves through stages of erythema, blistering and crusting, and may ultimately be much more severe than in this patient. Note the accompanying weight loss.

The gastrointestinal tract contains the largest mass of endocrine cells in the body. The hormones produced in the gut and pancreas include gastrin, cholecystokinin (CCK), vasoactive intestinal polypeptide (VIP), somatostatin, enteroglucagon, secretin, insulin, glucagon, gastric inhibitory peptide, motilin, substance P, neurotensin, pancreatic polypeptide, enkephalin and endorphins, bombesin and other peptides.

Pancreatic endocrine tumours are rare. The Zollinger–Ellison syndrome is caused by a gastrin secreting tumour; 85% of these arise in the pancreas (*see* p. 416). Appropriately two-thirds are sporadic, while a third form part of the multiple endocrine neoplasia (MEN) Type 1 syndrome. The major symptoms are caused by hyperacidity, which causes multiple duodenal and even jejunal peptic ulceration. High gastrin levels and hypertrophied gastric folds suggest the diagnosis. Treatment with H_2-blockers or the H/K ATPase inhibitors is effective, but the tumours should ideally be removed, as 60% are malignant.

Verner–Morrison syndrome and VIPomas present with chronic profuse watery diarrhoea leading to hypokalaemia, hypochlorhydria, dehydration and flushing. Treatment of the symptoms by corticosteroids, metoclopramide, indomethacin and opiates has limited effects, whereas somatostatin analogues appear to be useful, particularly where the tumour is inoperable.

The glucagonoma syndrome is usually caused by a malignant pancreatic tumour, and patients have a characteristic rash. The skin lesions (necrolytic migratory erythema) start as erythematous areas that become raised with superficial central blistering and rupture to leave crusts (**8.100**). They tend to heal from the centre leaving increased pigmentation. Diagnosis is based on clinical suspicion in patients with the rash, weight loss, glucose intolerance and often thromboembolic complications, combined with a plasma glucagon level above 300 pmol/l. Treatment is by tumour removal and the rash may improve with oxytetracycline, steroids or zinc.

Somatostatinoma has been described in about 20 cases. Most were malignant pancreatic tumours occurring in patients with mild diabetes and gallbladder disease. Tumours secreting other gastrointestinal hormones have been described, particularly pancreatic polypeptide, but all are exceedingly rare, with the exception of insulinomas, which present with hypoglycaemia.

9. Disorders of the Liver and Pancreas

History

Some patients with liver disease have few symptoms, but acute liver disease may present dramatically with acute anorexia, nausea and vomiting. There may be intolerance to the sight and smell of food, to alcohol and to cigarette smoke. An intense itch may develop in the skin and this may precede the development of jaundice, which may be noticed by the family before the patient. As jaundice appears, other symptoms may disappear. The patient may now notice dark urine and pale stools. There may now be right-sided abdominal discomfort caused by an enlarged or inflamed liver, or by an obstructed biliary tree.

Complications of liver disease include liver cell failure and portal hypertension. Hepatic encephalopathy tends to develop insidiously as liver cells fail, and a history of mood change, confusion and somnolence is often obtained from the family. Portal hypertension may be associated with a history of abdominal swelling and peripheral oedema, but the patient may become aware of this only when he has difficulty in putting on his shoes or trousers. Gastrointestinal blood loss may indicate the presence of oesophageal varices or reflect a coagulation defect caused by liver disease or associated thrombocytopenia. Key symptoms in liver disease are summarised in **9.1**.

It is important in the history to ask about:

- Close contact with a jaundiced person or someone in a high-risk group.
- Recent eating of shellfish, salads, etc.
- Recent blood transfusion.
- Foreign travel.
- Sexual activity and proclivity.
- Occupation – health professional, etc.
- Habits—drink and drugs.
- Family history of liver disease.

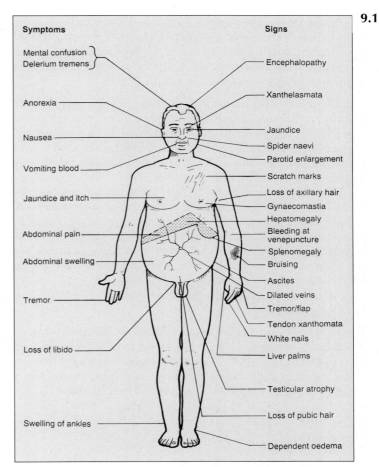

9.1

Symptoms: Mental confusion, Delerium tremens, Anorexia, Nausea, Vomiting blood, Jaundice and itch, Abdominal pain, Abdominal swelling, Tremor, Loss of libido, Swelling of ankles

Signs: Encephalopathy, Xanthelasmata, Jaundice, Spider naevi, Parotid enlargement, Scratch marks, Loss of axillary hair, Gynaecomastia, Hepatomegaly, Bleeding at venepuncture, Splenomegaly, Bruising, Ascites, Dilated veins, Tremor/flap, Tendon xanthomata, White nails, Liver palms, Testicular atrophy, Loss of pubic hair, Dependent oedema

9.1 Common symptoms and signs in liver disease.

Examination

The diversity of signs in liver disease (**9.1**) reflects the key role that the liver plays in homeostasis.

Jaundice is a frequent sign, and it can be detected clinically when the serum bilirubin level rises above 50 μmol/l:

- In haemolytic states the pigment circulates attached to albumin and does not appear in the urine—it usually imparts a pale yellow colour to the skin and sclerae (**9.2**).
- In hepatocellular and obstructive jaundice the conjugated bilirubin accumulates to very high levels and may give a much darker colour to the skin and sclerae, which may become orange or greenish in colour (**9.3–9.5**).

Other yellow pigmentation of skin, which may mimic jaundice, follows mepacrine ingestion or the excessive ingestion of carotenes (**7.129**), but these do not colour the sclerae. Pruritus may result from retained bile salts, and it may appear before the onset of frank jaundice. Scratch marks may be present in accessible skin areas (**9.4**, **9.6**).

In obstructive jaundice, the stool is pale in colour, because of the lack of bile pigments and the presence of steatorrhoea. In haemolytic jaundice, the stool is dark. The urine is dark in obstructive and hepatocellular jaundice, as a result of conjugated bile pigments; whereas in haemolytic jaundice, no bile pigment is present but there is an excess of urobilinogen which may darken on standing.

A variety of signs may result from the liver's failure to metabolise oestrogens:

- Spider naevi, which are usually found in the upper part of the body, above the nipple line, especially in areas exposed to sunlight (**9.7–9.9**). Healthy people, especially women during pregnancy, may have one or two spider naevi, but a larger number is strongly suggestive of liver disease.

- Gynaecomastia is commonly seen in males with chronic liver disease (**9.4**, **9.10**), though there are many other possible causes (**Table 9.1**). It is important to differentiate gynaecomastia from obesity by feeling for breast tissue around the nipple.
- Palmar erythema is a red flushing on the thenar and hypothenar eminences (**9.11**). This is common but not specific to liver disease. Similar changes may also be found in the soles of the feet.
- Loss of body hair, including pubic and axillary hair, and testicular atrophy are also common (**9.12**, **9.13**).

A range of other signs develops with long-standing liver dysfunction:

- Finger clubbing (**2.90**, **2.91**) is a common feature of liver disease and may also involve the toes. It is non-specific, being also found in respiratory, cardiac, alimentary and endocrine diseases.
- White nails (**2.88**): the cause is unknown but their whiteness mirrors the severity of the liver disease. White nails are also found in other conditions in which the serum albumin is low.
- Spontaneous bruising and excessive bleeding (**9.14**) are a reflection of the failure of the liver to synthesise coagulation factors II, VII, IX and X, often compounded by the failure to absorb vitamin K, as a result of retention of bile salts.
- Xanthelasmata (**7.113**, **9.5**, **9.36**) develop as a result of long-standing cholestasis and hyperlipidaemia, and are a common feature of chronic primary biliary cirrhosis. They develop in the soft tissues of the upper and lower lids. Xanthomas may also appear in other skin areas (**7.114**, **7.115**, **9.6**) and in tendons (**7.116**, **7.117**).

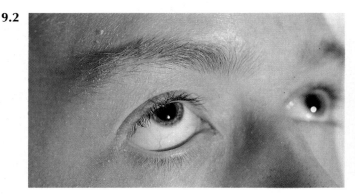

9.2 Haemolytic jaundice in a young man, who was subsequently found to have a lymphoma. The skin and sclerae have a pale lemon-yellow tinge, due to the elevation in unconjugated bilirubin.

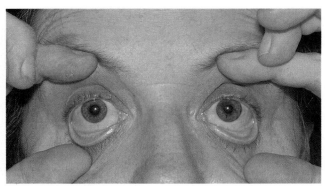

9.3 Jaundiced sclera in a patient with hepatitis A. Mild jaundice is often most evident in the sclerae, and may be unaccompanied by obvious jaundice in the skin.

- Hepatomegaly (**9.15**) is frequently found in liver diseases, particularly where the liver is infiltrated with carcinoma or fat, or replaced by fibrous tissue, and in some chronic infections (e.g. **1.211**) and metabolic disorders (e.g. **7.139**). The liver may be abnormally firm, and localised masses or nodules may be felt. The liver may also be tender, especially if the enlargement is caused by inflammation or venous congestion. It is important to be aware of the anatomical variants of the normal liver, especially of Riedel's lobe. The upper border of the liver may be pushed down into the abdomen by an extreme degree of emphysema, giving a misleading impression of hepatomegaly.
- Ascites, the accumulation of fluid in the peritoneal cavity (**8.5**, **9.12**), is often associated with liver cell failure and portal hypertension. The mechanism is complex: low serum albumin, prostaglandins, atrial natriuretic factor, secondary hyperaldosteronism and venous pressure all play a role. Ascites may also result from the presence of a primary or secondary malignancy. The diagnosis is usually obvious if the condition is gross, but it should be differentiated from other causes of abdominal swelling (fat, fluid, faeces, fetus, fibroids, etc.). Peripheral oedema is a common accompaniment of ascites and is gravitational. There may also be bilateral hydrothorax.
- Splenomegaly (**9.15**), often the result of a rise in portal venous pressure, may be associated with the primary liver pathology and may occur in haematological (**10.53**, **10.81**), infective (**1.185**, **1.188**, **1.211**) or metabolic (**7.139**)

Table 9.1 Causes of gynaecomastia.

Liver disease
Hyperthyroidism
Oestrogen-producing tumours
    (testis, adrenal)
HCG-producing tumours (testis, lung)
Starvation/refeeding
Carcinoma of breast
Drugs: Oestrogenic
              Oestrogens
              Digitalis
              Cannabis
              Diamorphine
          Anti-androgens
              Spironolactone
              Cimetidine
              Cyproterone
          Others
              Gonadotrophins
              Cytotoxics

Physiological: Neonatal
                 Pubertal
                 Old age

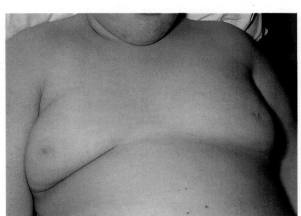

9.4 Jaundiced skin in a youth with chronic active hepatitis. The jaundice results from an elevated level of conjugated bilirubin, which produces a deeper yellow colour than unconjugated bilirubin. Note the associated gynaecomastia, and the scratch marks which result from pruritus due to the accumulation of bile salts.

9.4

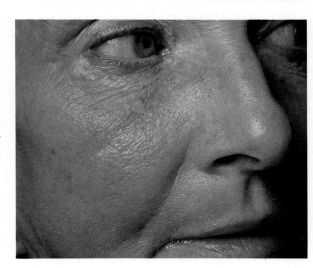

9.5 Severe cholestatic jaundice in a patient with primary biliary cirrhosis (PBC). The high level of conjugated bilirubin, maintained over a long period of time, gives a characteristic dark brown-orange pigmentation to the skin and sclerae. Patients with PBC usually develop large xanthelasmata and corneal arcus as a consequence of disordered lipid metabolism.

9.5

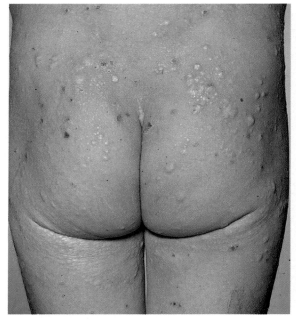

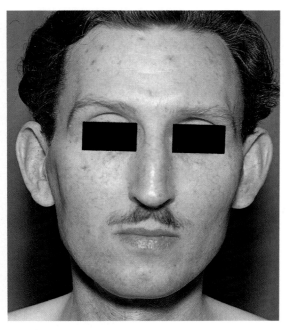

9.6 Scratch marks associated with severe pruritus, and eruptive xanthomas, in a child with intrahepatic cholestasis resulting from biliary atresia.

9.7 Spider naevi. This barman had alcoholic cirrhosis, accompanied by multiple spider naevi on the head and neck. The occurrence of a large number of spider naevi points strongly to underlying liver disease, though occasional solitary spiders may be found in normal people.

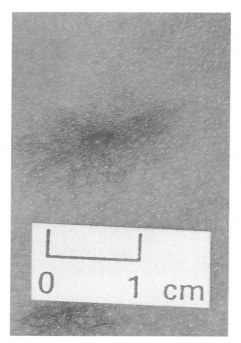

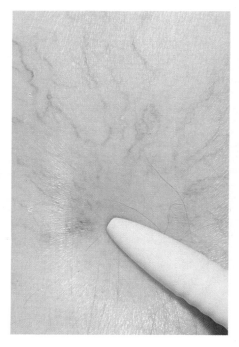

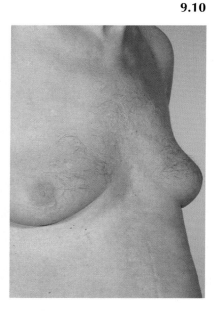

9.10 Gynaecomastia in a male patient. This patient had cirrhosis, and a hepatocellular carcinoma (hepatoma).

9.8 A typical spider naevus consists of a central spiral arteriole, which supplies a radiating group of small vessels. This spider naevus is of typical size, though larger and smaller examples may occur.

9.9 The spider naevus blanches if the central spiral arteriole is occluded by pressure, demonstrating that this is the single source of its blood supply.

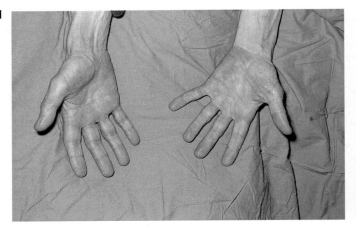

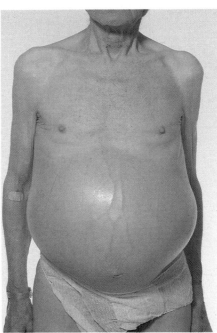

9.11 Palmar erythema is a common finding in chronic liver disease, but is also found in pregnancy, during oral contraceptive use, in rheumatoid arthritis and in thyrotoxicosis. It may also occur without apparent cause. It is usually particularly marked on the thenar and hypothenar eminences.

9.12 Severe ascites in a patient with hepatocellular carcinoma. The accumulation of fluid within the peritoneal cavity has led to gross abdominal distension with downward displacement and eversion of the umbilicus. Note the presence of distended veins in the abdominal wall. The flow in these veins was away from the umbilicus (*see also* **9.13**), and the underlying diagnosis was alcoholic cirrhosis. Note the absence of body hair in this patient—another sign of chronic liver disease.

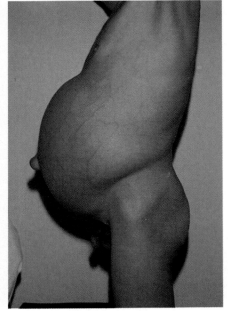

9.13 Superficial abdominal wall veins are obvious in this patient with alcoholic cirrhosis (and in the patient in **9.12**). These are a reflection of the extensive collateral circulation between the portal and sytemic venous systems. The direction of flow in portal hypertension uncomplicated by vena caval obstruction is away from the umbilicus. Note the reduced body hair – another feature of chronic liver disease.

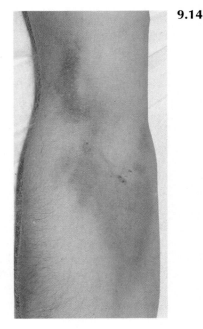

9.14 Abnormal bleeding and bruising at venepuncture sites may suggest a disturbance of coagulation mechanisms – a common problem in chronic liver disease. Clumsy venepuncture alone is unlikely to account for the appearance seen here, in a patient with severe acute hepatitis.

9.15

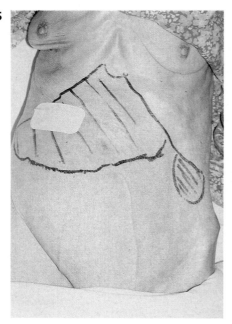

9.15 Hepatomegaly and splenomegaly commonly co-exist in chronic liver disease in the presence of portal hypertension, and hepatomegaly may also occur alone in many liver disorders,. This patient shows signs of weight loss, and has dilated abdominal veins. Her hepatomegaly has just been further investigated by CT-guided biopsy.

disorders (**Table 10.6**). The spleen must be differentiated from the left kidney by palpation and percussion.

- Superficial veins may often be seen on the abdominal wall surface. These may originate from the umbilicus, representing a communication from the portal to systemic circulations (caput medusae). The blood flow is from the umbilicus outwards (**9.12, 9.13**). Large veins may also be found running from the inguinal region to the chest wall. The blood flow is usually upwards, implying blockage of the inferior vena cava (**9.40**).
- Weight loss is common in patients with liver dysfunction. Limb size is often in stark contrast to the swollen abdomen.
- Encephalopathy is an acute or chronic neurological impairment that may result from liver cell failure associated with shunting of blood from the portal system. It is probably caused by to the failure of the liver to detoxify some as yet unidentified component in the portal blood. There is progressive impairment of higher cerebral function, with eventual coma and death. Early features suggesting encephalopathy include fetor hepaticus—a sweet apple-like smell on the breath, a coarse flapping tremor and an inability to draw or write accurately. A clinical test to monitor changes in status is the patient's signature (with date) on the casesheet.

Investigations

Investigations are of value in defining the cause of liver disease, the extent of damage and the effects of treatment. They should be used selectively.

- **Urinalysis**. In obstructive jaundice the urine is dark orange in colour and, as obstruction deepens, it may develop a greenish tinge; it gives a positive test for bile and a negative test for urobilinogen. In haemolytic jaundice, the urine may be normal in colour but darken on standing; tests for bile are negative and tests for urobilinogen are positive. In compensated cirrhosis, there is no bile in the urine, but tests for urobilinogen are usually positive because of failure of the liver cells to cope with the normally re-absorbed amount of urobilinogen.
- **Stools.** The pallor of the stools depends on the degree of

biliary obstruction and is associated with a degree of steatorrhoea as the bile salts are not excreted. The stool in haemolysis is dark in colour because of the increased levels of stercobilin. A positive faecal occult blood test is of value in detecting carcinoma of the ampulla of Vater and also primary alimentary lesions which may have produced hepatic secondaries.
- **Full blood count** is of value in detecting anaemia — often iron deficient because of a primary bowel lesion or bleeding from oesophageal varices. Macrocytosis is often found in liver disease with biliary obstruction and may not reflect vitamin B_{12} deficiency (B_{12} levels may be elevated if there is hepatic cell necrosis). Folate levels are often low, caused by a combination of malabsorption and poor dietary intake. Thrombocytopenia is often present, because of a

combination of factors that may include the direct effects of alcohol on the bone marrow, secondary hypersplenism, disseminated intravascular coagulation and marrow aplasia in acute fulminant hepatitis, and folate deficiency.

- **Coagulation abnormalities** are common and often complex, as the liver makes most coagulation factors and destroys others. Correct investigation often requires expert haematological advice. Tests should include the activated partial thromboplastin time (APPT), the prothrombin time (PT), the thrombin time (TT), whole blood platelet count and simple tests of fibrinolysis such as measurement of fibrinogen–fibrin degradation products (FDPs).
- **Routine biochemistry** is the keystone of diagnosis and assessment of progress. Tests should include total bilirubin, with direct and indirect values as necessary, alkaline phosphatase, the aminotransferases (especially alanine aminotransferase, ALT), γ–glutamyl transpeptidase, total proteins, albumin and γ-globulins. None of these tests is specific or diagnostic, but all are of value in combination and in following the course of the disease. Measurement of serum iron, total iron binding capacity, per cent saturation and ferritin level is of value when looking for haemochromatosis. A low serum iron and ferritin may be found in chronic blood loss states, such as following bleeding from oesophageal varices or neoplasia.
- The **α-fetoprotein level** is elevated in most primary hepatocellular carcinomas and is of value as a diagnostic and prognostic test.
- **Viral markers.** Levels of viral antigen and antibody are a pointer to infection, and sequential samples provide evidence of the course of the disease.
- **Autoantibodies.** Some immunological disorders are associated with liver disease. Primary biliary cirrhosis is associated with the presence of antimitochondrial antibodies. Diseases such as SLE (p. 142), rheumatoid arthritis (p. 126), dermatomyositis (p. 146) and CRST syndrome (p. 144) have specific immune abnormalities.

Imaging investigations are often useful in disorders of the liver, pancreas and biliary tract.

Plain X-rays of the right upper quadrant are of value when lesions are calcified or contain air. About 10% of gall stones are radio-opaque (**9.16**), cysts of liver and pancreas may calcify, there may be generalised pancreatic calcification (**9.56**), and the soft-tissue shadow of the spleen, or air in the biliary tree or under the diaphragm (**8.52**), may be seen. X-ray of the chest may show an elevated diaphragm caused by subphrenic pus or a paralysed diaphragm, or there may be a 'sympathetic' pleural effusion or empyema.

- Cholecystogram, intravenous cholangiography and T-tube cholangiography involve the administration of a contrast medium to outline the gall bladder, hepatic ducts, and the hepatic ducts after surgery.
- **Percutaneous transhepatic cholangiography** involves passing a cannula towards the hilum of the liver in patients who have obstructive jaundice. Bile reflux occurs if the intrahepatic ducts are dilated. Contrast medium is then injected to define the site(s) of obstruction (**9.48**).
- **Ultrasound** is the best, simplest and cheapest test for gallstones (**9.17**). It is also of value in detecting space-occupying lesions in the liver and pancreas. It may be used to locate the site for a needle biopsy.
- **Computed tomography** (CT, **9.18**) and **magnetic resonance imaging** (MRI) are of major value in detecting intrahepatic lesions, regional lymph nodes, associated tumours, abnormalities of the pancreas, and lesions in the porta hepatis. They can also be used to locate sites for biopsies.
- **Endscopic retrograde cholangiopancreatography** (ERCP) is an endoscopic technique in which the ampulla of Vater is cannulated and contrast medium is injected to outline the biliary tree and pancreatic ducts (**9.19, 9.38**). It is of value in detecting and removing stones impacted in the lower biliary tree. Pancreatitis and ascending cholangitis are complications.
- **Angiography and portal venography:** selective angiography of the hepatic artery may reveal vascular tumours. The portal venous system can be imaged by splenic venography (**9.20**) and by digital subtraction angiograms.
- **Isotope scans:** intravenous injection of ^{99m}Tc sulphur colloid results in diffuse uptake of the isotope by the RE cells of the liver. The technique may show abnormalities in the position of the liver and filling defects caused by space-occupying lesions (**9.45**).
- **Laparoscopy** allows direct visualisation of the liver, pancreas and gall bladder, and is of value in assessing the presence and the extent of disease (**9.21**). Biopsy under direct vision is possible, and surgery may be undertaken without laparotomy (keyhole surgery).

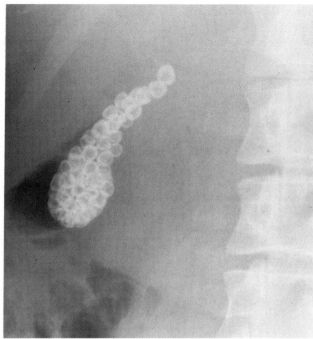

9.16 Calcified gallstones seen on plain X-ray. Only about 10% of gallstones contain enough calcium to be visible on the plain film. This patient had had remarkably few symptoms before the incidental discovery of her gallstones.

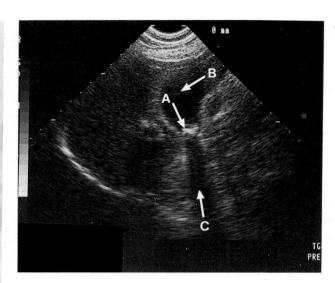

9.17 Ultrasound is the optimal initial investigation for gallstones. The scan shows a typical gallstone (A) in the gall bladder (B). The acoustic shadow (C) cast by the stone is typical.

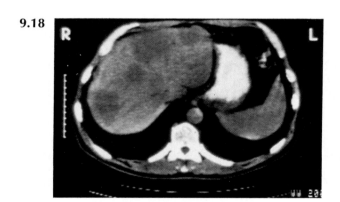

9.18 Computed tomography is of major value in the assessment of patients with many disorders of the liver and pancreas. This patient has multiple secondary tumour deposits throughout the liver, which have contributed to marked hepatomegaly. The primary tumour was in the colon.

- **Electroencephalography** (EEG) is of value in determining the presence and severity of encephalopathy.
- **Liver biopsy** will often give the tissue diagnosis of a lesion. It may be done blind when the disease is disseminated, as in cirrhosis or haemochromatosis, or it may be performed under ultrasound or CT guidance, or by direct vision on laparoscopy. A range of special stains helps to define the pathology.

Before undertaking liver biopsy, some safety precautions are necessary. These include:

- Measurement of prothrombin time (PT not greater than 3 seconds over control).
- Measurement of platelet count (platelet count should be above 100×10^9/l).
- Informed patient consent.
- There should be no evidence of dilated bile ducts or a major degree of ascites.
- The patient should be able to hold his breath for at least 20 seconds.

9.19 Endoscopic retrograde cholangiopancreatography (ERCP) is of great value in assessing and sometimes treating abnormalities in the biliary tree and pancreatic ducts. In this patient a cholangiocarcinoma is causing major obstruction of the common bile duct (arrowed). The biliary tree proximal to the obstruction is grossly dilated. The pancreatic duct is also filled with contrast medium.

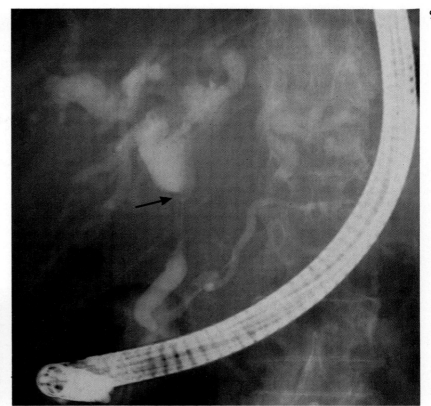

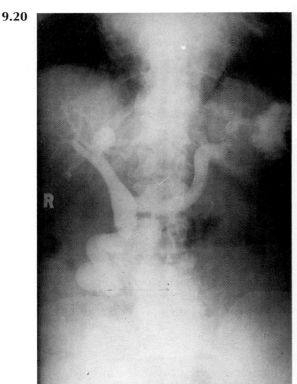

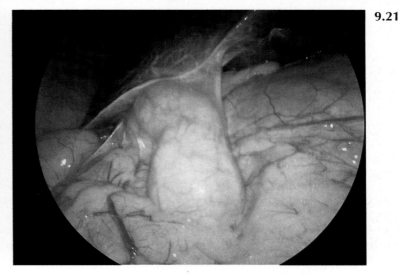

9.20 Splenic venography can be used to delineate the portal venous system in patients with portal hypertension. Contrast is injected via a needle inserted into the enlarged spleen (on the right of the picture). In this patient, with advanced cirrhosis, the technique demonstrates the extent of the collateral circulation. Note the dilated splenic and hepatic veins, which contrast with narrowed intrahepatic vessels, affected by the cirrhotic process. A tortuous, grossly dilated vein leads towards the umbilicus. The patient had a typical dilatation of the superficial abdominal veins (**9.12, 9.13**)

9.21 Laparoscopy is valuable in many disorders of the liver and biliary tract. This picture was taken immediately prior to laparoscopic cholecystectomy and shows an enlarged, turgid gallbladder. Above the gallbladder, the smooth lower border of a normal liver is clearly seen, and abnormalities in the liver can often be well visualised by this technique. Note also the loops of normal bowel to the right of the liver (left of picture) and the pylorus to its left.

Clinical presentations of liver disease

Cirrhosis

Cirrhosis is a descriptive term for a liver which has been largely replaced by fibrous tissue. This distorts the normal architecture, and is associated with regeneration of parenchymal nodules; both processes interfere with portal circulation, raising its pressure, opening up communications between the portal and systemic circulations and causing splenomegaly. Cirrhosis is the end result of a variety of pathological processes (**Table 9.2**), the most common causes being viral hepatitis, alcohol, chronic heart failure, immunological and metabolic diseases.

The clinical features of cirrhosis are a result of portal hypertension and liver cell failure, and at different stages of the disorder may include any of the symptoms and signs shown in **9.1**. Initially, the liver may be normal in size or even enlarged; as cirrhosis progresses it usually becomes contracted and shrunken. Primary liver cell cancer is a potential complication of cirrhosis.

Table 9.2 Causes of cirrhosis.

Alcohol
Chronic active hepatitis
Primary biliary cirrhosis
Haemochromatosis
Hepatic vein obstruction
Wilson's disease
Lupoid hepatitis
Drugs
α_1-antitrypsin deficiency
Cystic fibrosis
Galactosaemia/fructose intolerance
Veno-occlusive disease
Cardiac failure
Unknown

Portal hypertension

Portal hypertension may arise from obstruction in the portal vein before it reaches the liver (pre-hepatic), within the liver (intra-hepatic) or between the liver and the inferior vena cava (post-hepatic). A rise in pressure rapidly leads to the opening up of latent anastomoses between the systemic and portal venous systems, which are mainly to be found in the gastro-oesophageal region (**9.20**), in the rectum and at the umbilicus. Dilatation of these collaterals allows portal–systemic shunting and this may give rise to specific clinical problems. The spleen may be grossly enlarged.

Oesophageal varices lie in the submucosa of the lower oesophagus and are liable to rupture because of portal pressure and local trauma. Bleeding is also compounded by severe coagulation defects caused by liver cell failure. Haematemesis and melaena or chronic iron deficiency are the main presentations. Diagnosis is made by barium swallow or at endoscopy (**1.212**, **9.22**, **9.23**), and some endoscopic appearances are associated with a particularly high risk of bleeding. Treatment by balloon tamponade in an emergency or by sclerotherapy (**9.24**) may provide temporary relief, but definitive treatment is surgical. Porta-caval anastomosis may be curative if liver function is adequate; a preliminary investigation is portal venography (**9.20**).

Rectal anastomoses may become extremely large and bleed following bowel movements. Massive bleeding is extremely rare. Surgery is the treatment of choice.

Umbilical anastomoses are rarely clinically obvious. The anastomotic veins radiate from the umbilicus across the abdomen to join systemic veins, forming a 'caput medusae'. Lesser degrees of anastomosis are more common (**9.25**).

9.22 Oesophageal varices. A barium swallow, showing the typical appearance of multiple lower oesophageal varices, evident as barium-coated filling defects. In addition, gastric varices can be seen, along the lesser curvature of the stomach. These thin walled varices are easily damaged, and bleeding is a frequent complication.

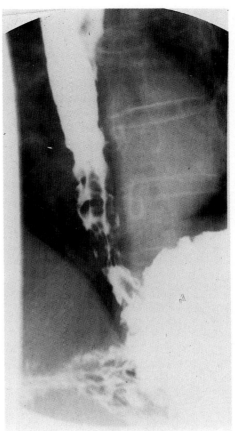

9.23 Oesophageal varices seen through the endoscope. 'White' varices like these have been shown to have a relatively low risk of immediate bleeding, because they are covered with a thick layer o f mucosa. The presence of red lines (red wale markings) or spots (cherry-red spots) is associated with a strong likelihood of bleeding

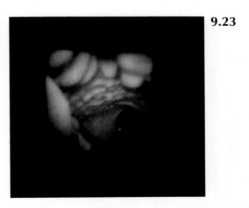

9.24 Oesophageal varices after treatment by scleropathy. The injection of a sclerosant via the endoscope results in local variceal thrombosis, followed by fibrosis and, often, mucosal ulceration. Definitive surgical treatment (porto-systemic anastomosis) may subsequently be necesssary.

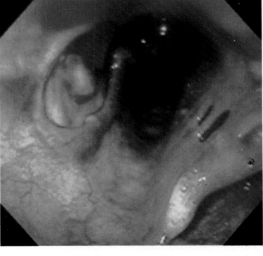

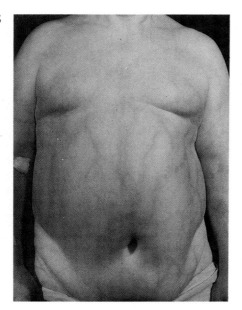

9.25 Umbilical anastomoses in portal hypertension, demonstrated by infra-red photography. The patient had ascites but the veins were not obvious clinically. An extensive network of veins radiating from the umbilicus becomes obvious. Note the co-existence of gynaecomastia.

Liver failure

9.26

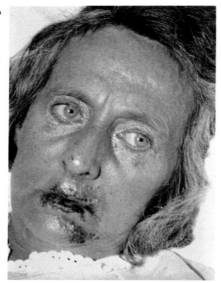

9.26 Liver failure with gastrointestinal bleeding and a high risk of encephalopathy. This patient has primary biliary cirrhosis. Note the severe jaundice and pigmentation resulting from this chronic disease. The blood around her mouth results from haematemesis from oesophageal varices, and the combination of chronic liver failure with recent haematemesis puts her at great risk of encephalopathy. Intensive management is required in these circumstances.

Liver failure can develop acutely in a previously normal liver (as in fulminant viral hepatitis or drug-induced hepatitis), or it may develop insidiously in a chronically damaged liver. Fluid retention is an early problem which presents with ankle and leg oedema, ascites and small pleural effusions. Bruising is seen spontaneously and following trauma, sometimes even from the pressure induced by a blood pressure cuff. This results from defective coagulation factor synthesis and from thrombocytopenia associated with splenomegaly. A bleeding tendency may also be shown by excessive bleeding at venepuncture sites (**9.14**). Nausea, vomiting, anorexia, drowsiness, tremor and confusion may lead on to encephalopathy: deep coma with fits and decerebrate posture (**9.26**).

Other metabolic disturbances, including hypoglycaemia, pancreatitis and renal failure are common.

Treatment requires co-operation between a variety of specialties. Bleeding requires the intravenous administration of vitamin K, and often fresh frozen plasma. Haemodialysis may be required for renal failure. Oesophageal varices must be identified and bleeding arrested. Blood and other proteins, which contribute to the encephalopathy, must be removed from the bowel.

Death is usually caused by cerebral oedema or gastro-intestinal bleeding.

Acute hepatitis

Acute hepatitis may result from a variety of causes, the most common of which are viruses and drugs (**Table 9.3**). The clinical features at onset are usually similar, but the course and ulitmate prognosis are different. Hepatitis may be so mild that the patient does not become jaundiced but has malaise and anorexia (especially for alcohol). In the more severe cases, jaundice appears after 10–14 days, often accompanied by flitting arthralgia, lymphadenopathy, a skin rash and hepatic discomfort (**9.27**). The urine is usually dark and the stools become pale. Usually the jaundice is mild and lasts only a few days with gradual recovery. In some patients, an intrahepatic cholestatic phase develops, with pruritus, deepening jaundice and increasing hepatomegaly. Investigations should include:

- **Biochemistry:** the first changes are rises in the levels of ALT and alkaline phosphatase, followed by a rise in serum bilirubin. Urine tests for urobilinogen are positive before jaundice occurs, and then bilirubin is found in the urine. Persistence of enzyme disturbance suggests the persistence of hepatitis.
- **Haematology:** there is often leucopenia.
- **Viral markers** can be detected in the blood.

Table 9.3 Causes of acute hepatitis.

Viruses:	Hepatitis virus A, B, C, D, E, nonA/nonB Epstein–Barr virus (*see* p. 32) Cytomegalovirus (*see* p. 31) Yellow fever virus (*see* p. 23) Ebola/Marburg (*see* p. 26, 27)
Bacteria:	*Leptospira icterohaemorrhagiae* (*see* p. 58) *Toxoplasma gondii* (*see* p. 67) *Coxiella burnetii*
Drugs:	alcohol paracetamol halothane erythromycin chlorpromazine aspirin isoniazid methyldopa rifampicin oral contraceptives anabolic steroids
Poisons:	carbon tetrachloride *Amanita phalloides*
Pregnancy	

9.27

9.27 Acute viral hepatitis. This boy had acute type A hepatitis, although the clinical picture is similar in all types of hepatitis. He had deep jaundice and a spider naevus, but made a full uncomplicated recovery.

Viral hepatitis

Hepatitis A is water- or food-borne, and occurs in vast epidemics, especially in countries with poor water and sewerage facilities (*see* 1.4). Prodromal symptoms last 10–14 days, and the icteric phase is associated with a lessening of symptoms. Jaundice usually disappears in a week and most patients recover rapidly. In a very small number of patients, liver necrosis ensues, followed by coma and death. The diagnosis of hepatitis A infection is established by demonstrating a rise in specific IgM. Treatment is supportive. Immunoglobin may be given to those at risk, and protection lasts three months.

Hepatitis B virus is found in most body fluids and tissues. It is usually transmitted by sexual activity, by transfusion of blood and blood fractions, on needles (by nurses and doctors pricking fingers, tattooing (9.28), intravenous drug abusers (1.10) and by aerosol during dental treatment. It may also be transmitted by medical and dental attendants who are carriers through open wounds. The Delta agent (hepatitis D) may also be transmitted in close association with the hepatitis B virus. The symptomatology and course are similar to the other viral hepatitides. The specific diagnosis is made by finding hepatitis B antigen and antibodies in serum. A small percentage of people get fulminant hepatitis and die, a small number develop chronic liver disease and a small number become carriers. People at risk may be actively vaccinated and emergency immunoglobulin cover may be given following exposure such as needle-stick injury. There is no specific treatment for carriers.

Hepatitis C virus is transmitted by blood and blood products, and also sexually. This type of hepatitis tends to be more serious than A or B, with neurological manifestations and bone marrow suppression. There is a high incidence of progression of the hepatitis to chronic disease (50%). The diagnosis is now made serologically.

Other types. Studies of the incubation period of acute hepatitis suggest that there are other strains of virus still to be described. The best characterised is a long incubation 'non-A, non-B type' virus which is transmitted by water or food. It is not associated with long-term liver impairment. Viral hepatitis may also be caused by Epstein–Barr virus (p. 32), cytomegalovirus (p. 31) and yellow fever virus (p. 23), and it is a component of many viral haemorrhagic fevers (pp. 26–27).

9.28 Tattooing is an important route of transmission for viral hepatitis. This patient developed acute hepatitis B after being tattooed in the Far East, and he subsequently became a long-term carrier of the hepatitis virus. The prevalence of tattoos always raises the possibility of the presence of transmissible infections, including viral hepatitis and HIV.

Drug-induced hepatitis

Drugs and chemicals may cause a range of hepatic damage, from acute and chronic hepatitis to cirrhosis and liver tumours. An acute hepatitis-like picture may be produced by a number of drugs (**Table 9.3, 9.29**). The most common of these in the UK is paracetamol, usually taken as an intentional overdose. Early features are nausea and vomiting. Most patients have few sequelae, but in some who have taken a larger dose, presented late or taken alcohol (which induces the hepatic microsomal enzymes), mild jaundice and liver tenderness appear on the third or fourth day. Despite treatment at this stage, there is progressive deepening of jaundice, increasing liver cell failure and death.

Halothane hepatitis is rare and usually follows multiple exposures to the gas for general anaesthesia. The clinical picture is of acute hepatitis that may be fatal.

An increasingly common cause of drug-induced liver dysfunction is anabolic steroid use for body-building (9.30). Poisoning with other toxins is rare. Epidemics of liver failure caused by exposure to *Amanita phalloides* occur when this fungus is mistaken for the edible mushroom.

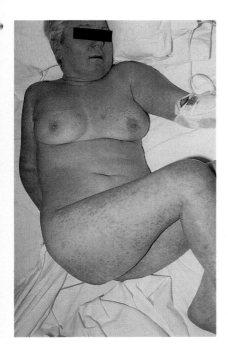

9.29 Drug-induced hepatitis. This patient developed severe hepatitis soon after phenytoin was added to the therapy she was receiving for epilepsy. She was clinically only mildy icteric, but her liver function was severely deranged. She made a full recovery after withdrawal of phenytoin.

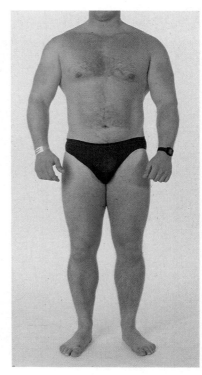

9.30 Anabolic steroid abuse is an increasingly common cause of liver dysfunction. This weight-lifter was taking a cocktail of non-prescribed drugs including stanozolol, bendrofluazide and thyroxine (a common combination, believed to enhance his muscle profile), and he developed mild jaundice with elevated liver enzymes.

Chronic liver disease

Chronic persistent hepatitis (CPH)

Hepatomegaly may persist after an attack of hepatitis. In CPH, liver biopsy shows continuing periportal inflammation, but there is normal liver architecture. Enzymes may remain persistently high but other biochemistry is normal. There are no long-term sequelae.

Chronic active hepatitis (CAH)

CAH may occur as a sequel to hepatitis B, D and C (**9.31**), but occasionally there has been no identifiable acute episode. CAH may also follow drug-induced hepatitis, and it may be seen in Wilson's disease and α_1-antitrypsin deficiency. Many patients present with evidence of advanced liver damage. Biochemistry shows raised bilirubin, AST, ALT and alkaline phosphatase. Markers for hepatitis B (with a positive e antigen) and for hepatitis C are present. Liver biopsy shows a plasma cell infiltrate with extensive parenchymal necrosis. Progression to cirrhosis is common, and this is associated with a high incidence of primary liver cell cancer. Treatment is unsatisfactory, but some patients respond to interferon.

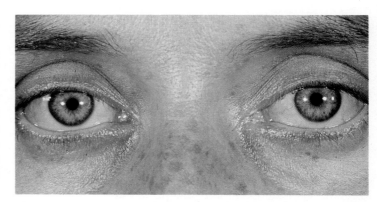

9.31 Chronic active hepatitis. This patient developed chronic active hepatitis as a sequel to hepatitis B infection, and developed the long-term complications associated with portal hypertension.

Lupoid hepatitis

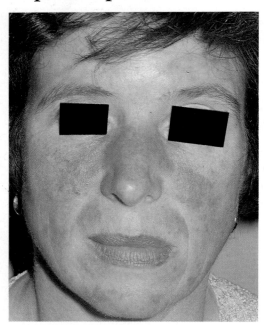

9.32

9.32 Lupoid hepatitis may be associated with a butterfly rash on the face, similar to that seen in systemic lupus erythematosus (SLE) **(3.72, 3.73)**, but the two syndromes are distinct, and patients with lupoid hepatitis do not develop all the features of SLE.

Lupoid hepatitis is associated with a variety of other autoimmune disorders, including pernicious anaemia and thyroid disease. A variety of immune markers is found in some patients:

- Lupus erythematosus (LE) cells.
- Hyperglobulinaemia.
- Antibodies against smooth muscle mitochondria.
- Impairment of T-cell function.

Clinical presentation usually suggests a multi-organ disease. Associated features may include acne, hirsutes, vitiligo, striae, fever, polyarthritis, acute glomerulonephritis, pleurisy, pneumonia, fibrosing alveolitis and hepatosplenomegaly. A 'lupoid' butterfly rash may be seen **(9.32)**. Investigations show disturbance of liver function with an obstructive jaundice, elevated alkaline phosphatase and high levels of AST and ALT. Liver biopsy shows the features of chronic active hepatitis. Treatment is with steroids and azathioprine.

Alcohol-induced liver disease

Excessive alcohol intake over a prolonged period may cause damage to almost every organ in the body—especially to the liver. Three separate conditions are recognised:

- Alcohol-induced fatty infiltration.
- Alcoholic hepatitis.
- Alcoholic cirrhosis.

Fat infiltration is common in the heavy drinker, and its only clinical feature is a large, palpable liver. Liver function tests, especially the liver enzymes (ALT and γ-GT), may be abnormal. With abstinence the liver can return to normal size and function.

Acute alcoholic hepatitis usually follows an acute bout of heavy drinking and may occur in the drinker with a fatty liver or in one who has already become cirrhotic. The usual presentation is with sudden-onset jaundice which becomes rapidly deeper **(9.33)** and the liver usually enlarges. If there is pre-existing cirrhosis, there may be an exacerbation of the signs of liver failure and portal hypertension. There may be persistent leucocytosis and fever, with dark urine and pale stools.

In the chronic alcoholic, the features of cirrhosis and its consequences are usually identical to those resulting from cirrhosis of other causes, but some features are suggestive of an alcoholic origin:

- Parotid enlargement.
- Dupuytren's contracture **(9.34)**.
- Red, sore, smooth tongue caused by associated vitamin deficiency **(9.35)**.
- Beri-beri (p. 346).
- Neuropathy.
- Cardiomyopathy.
- Acne rosacea.
- Associated chronic pancreatitis.
- Associated peptic ulceration.

The diagnosis is made on the basis of the history and clinical features. The extent of liver damage can be monitored by blood tests and by liver biopsy.

Treatment is by abstinence from alcohol and correction of associated vitamin deficiencies. Hepatic failure and portal hypertension may require treatment in their own right.

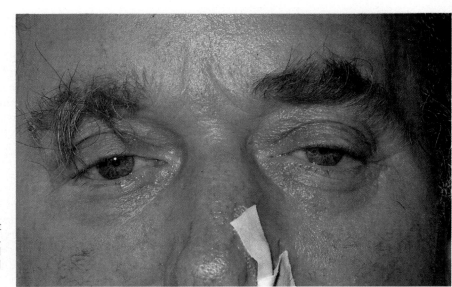

9.33 Acute alcoholic hepatitis. The patient presented with sudden-onset jaundice. At first sight, the condition might be confused with acute viral hepatitis, but the patient had a history of several previous admissions following alcoholic excess.

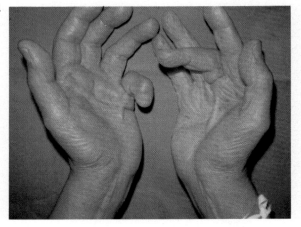

9.34 Dupuytren's contracture is commonly seen in association with alcoholic cirrhosis, though it may also occur as a completely independent abnormality. Contracture of the palmar fascial bands produces flexion contracture of the metacarpo-phalangeal and proximal inter-phalangeal joints, the flexor tendon apparatus and the skin itself. In this patient, the condition particularly affects the right middle finger and the left little finger. Surgical correction is usually possible.

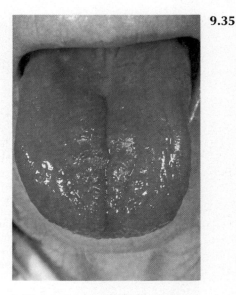

9.35 A red, sore, smooth tongue is commonly seen in patients with alcoholic cirrhosis as a result of associated vitamin deficiency. A similar appearance may occur in patients with nutritional deficiencies of other origins.

Primary biliary cirrhosis

Primary biliary cirrhosis is a slowly progressive disease of unknown etiology that affects women more commonly than men and usually occurs between the ages of 40 and 60 years. Many patients are diagnosed by chance observation of disturbed liver function tests measured for some unrelated problem. Clinical presentation often is with itching of the skin due to retention of bile salts or with increased pigmentation of skin, part of which is due to a progressive rise in bilirubin levels.Cholestatic jaundice appears later (9.5, 9.36, 9.37). Connective tissue disorders, including Sjögren's syndrome, Raynaud's phenomenon, rheumatoid arthritis, dermatomyositis and scleroderma, are sometimes an associated feature. During the course of the illness, the patient becomes more icteric and pigmented, usually with marked periocular xanthelasmata (9.5, 9.36) and hepatosplenomegaly. Patches of vitiligo may be present. The patient may complain of persistent steatorrhoea, weight loss and metabolic bone disease. The end result of the disease is liver failure, encephalopathy, and bleeding from oesophageal varices.

Serum anti-mitochondrial antibodies are present in over 90% of patients. Liver function tests are abnormal, with elevated bilirubin and alkaline phosphatase. Serum cholesterol is usually high. Coagulation tests are grossly abnormal, because of a combination of loss of functioning hepatocytes and malabsorption of vitamin K. Liver biopsy shows an acute inflammatory reaction in the portal tracts with the formation of fibrous septae and granulomas.

Ultrasound and, if necessary, ERCP should be carried out (9.38) to ensure the patient does not have obstruction of the larger biliary ducts, as stone formation is a common association.

There is no specific treatment for the disease, but the hyperlipidaemia and the malabsorption can be treated. Persistent pruritus may respond to the use of cholestyramine.

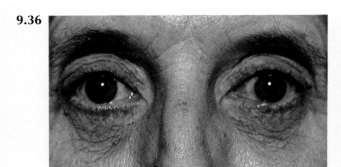

9.36

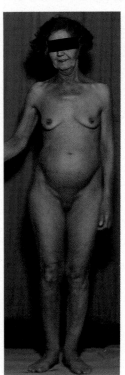

9.37

9.36, 9.37 Primary biliary cirrhosis. This 55-year-old woman presented originally with severe pruritus, and jaundice developed slowly over the next three years. When these photographs were taken, she had deep jaundice, typical brown pigmentation, spider naevi, xanthelasmata around both eyes, enlargement of the liver and spleen, and ascites. The deepening jaundice and ascites are poor prognostic signs, and are usually followed by encephalopathy and death within weeks or months.

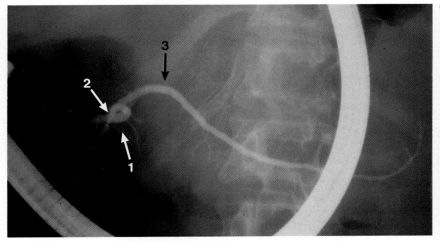

9.38 Primary biliary cirrhosis in its early stages is usually associated with a normal endoscopic retrograde cholangiogram (ERCP), as here. The intrahepatic bile ducts (1), the common bile duct (2), and pancreatic duct (3) are normal. The ERCP becomes abnormal when the cirrhotic process is advanced or, as commonly, when gallstones have formed.

Haemochromatosis and haemosiderosis

Haemochromatosis is an inherited condition in which excess iron is absorbed and stored in the body tissues. It typically presents in middle-aged men. It is rarer in women and presents much later in life, because of iron loss at menstruation and in child-bearing.

There is a wide spectrum of clinical features at presentation. Asymptomatic patients showing biochemical abnormalities alone may be found by screening families of known patients, while others present with the later effects, including hepatic cirrhosis, pancreatic insufficiency with diabetes mellitus and pigmentation of the skin (bronze diabetes). Skin pigmentation is usually slatey-grey in colour (**9.39**) and results from the deposition of a combination of melanin and iron. Many patients also develop a pyrophosphate arthropathy in which chondrocalcinosis involves the articular cartilages (*see* p. 141). This particularly involves the first and second metacarpophalangeal joints and the knees.

Excess iron deposition is also found in the pituitary, where it reduces hormone production, and in the testes. The end result is gonadal atrophy. Cardiac involvement is also common and arrhythmias and heart failure are the presenting features.

The main organ involved is the liver, which is often cirrhotic at the time of presentation, and the patient may have the additional features associated with hepatic failure and portal hypertension. Primary liver cell cancer is a common complication and is often associated with a significant decline in liver function.

The diagnosis is made by finding a high serum iron with a very high saturation of iron-binding protein. Serum ferritin is also high and there may be disturbance of the profile of liver function tests. Excess iron is found in most tissues; and on liver biopsy, iron stains show iron in the parenchyma and in the Kupffer cells. There is also a coarse macronodular cirrhosis.

Treatment usually involves long-term repeated venesection. Chelating agents are rarely used, because of their expense, the difficulty of administration and poor results.

Haemosiderosis occurs where there is excess tissue iron but no subsequent damage. This is usually seen in patients with chronic haemolytic states who have been treated with repeated blood transfusions, e.g. sickle cell anaemia, thalassaemia (*see* p. 434–438). Very occasionally, the iron overload in these patients may give rise to a picture similar to primary haemochromatosis.

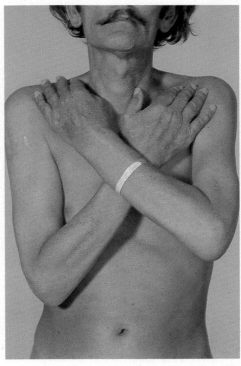

9.39

9.39 Haemochromatosis. The slatey-grey colour of this Caucasian patient's skin, most obvious in his hands, results from the deposition of a combination of melanin and iron. This patient had cirrhosis and pyrophosphate arthropathy at the time of presentation with the disease. Note also the absence of body hair, which was associated with hypogonadism.

Vascular disease of liver

The **Budd–Chiari syndrome** is a rare disorder that results from a large number of pathologies which ultimately obstruct the flow of blood from the hepatic veins into the inferior vena cava. These include congenital webs in the vena cava, thrombosis in the hepatic veins or adjacent vena cava as a result of thrombophilic states or use of oral contraceptives, infiltration by tumours, and alcoholic hepatitis. The signs depend on how acutely the syndrome develops. Usually this is gradual and the patient presents with an enlarged, sometimes tender, liver. There may be associated jaundice, ascites, peripheral oedema and splenomegaly. A characteristic of the disease is the development of masses of dilated veins on the

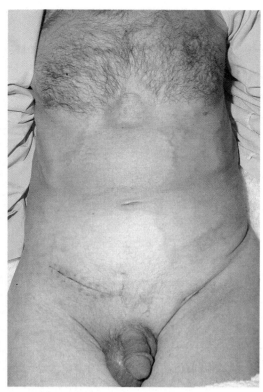

abdominal wall, the flow being upwards (**9.40**). The diagnosis may be surmised by the finding of centrilobular necrosis in the liver biopsy, and is established by CT scanning or by failure to catheterise the hepatic veins. Inferior vena-cavography may also be of value. The usual treatment is porta-caval shunting, but liver transplantation has been used in severe cases where the inferior vena cava is normal.

Veno-occlusive disease of the liver is a small-vessel variant of the Budd–Chiari syndrome which involves the hepatic venules.

It develops in people who drink medicinal teas containing pyrolozidine alkaloids from *Senecio* and *Crotalaria* plants, and rarely following bone marrow transplantation and the use of anti-mitotic therapy. It has also been reported following chronic alcoholism.

9.40 The Budd–Chiari syndrome (hepatic venous obstruction). Note the grossly dilated veins in the abdominal wall, in which the flow of blood was upwards. The patient had continued to work as a builder's labourer without symptoms, until he was admitted with coincidental appendicitis. The cause of his hepatic venous obstruction was unclear.

Wilson's disease (Hepato-lenticular degeneration)

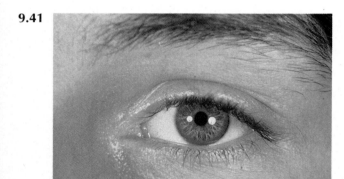

9.41 Wilson's disease. The clinical features of impaired liver function and neurological disorder are usually accompanied by Kayser–Fleischer rings in the corneae. The rings show as a rim of brown pigment, and are more clearly seen in patients with blue eyes.

Wilson's disease is caused by a defective autosomal recessive gene on chromosone 13. There is an abnormality in the handling of copper, which accumulates in various tissues especially the liver, basal ganglia, bones, renal tubules and cornea. The clinical presentation is usually with a combination of liver function impairment and enlargement and neurological features from loss of function of the basal ganglia (Parkinsonian tremor, expressionless facies, athetoid movements and dysarthria). A Kayser–Fleischer ring may be found in the cornea—this is most easily seen in blue-eyed patients as a brown ring (**9.41**). In brown-eyed patients slit-lamp examination is usually necessary. The diagnosis is made on finding a low caeruloplasmin level, an increased 24-hour urinary copper excretion and liver biopsy evidence of cirrhosis with excess copper in the liver cells. Treatment is with long-term penicillamine to chelate the excess copper.

Fibropolycystic diseases

There are a number of rare, congenital fibropolycystic hepato-biliary diseases, including adult polycystic liver, congenital hepatic fibrosis, congenital intrahepatic biliary dilatation and choledochal cysts. There is a high association with similar renal disorders and with malignant change. Diagnosis is made on ultrasound, CT scan (9.42) or angiography. Liver transplantation is a treatment option if there is serious liver decompensation or portal hypertension.

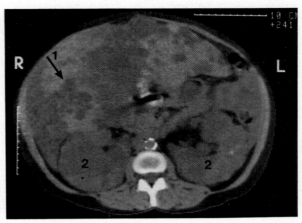

9.42 Polycystic liver disease, as seen on CT scanning. The patient has massive hepatomegaly, and a typical example of the many cysts in the liver is arrowed (1). She also had bilateral polycystic kidneys (2) (*see also* p. 296).

Other forms of cirrhosis

Metabolic causes of chronic liver disease that may lead to cirrhosis include α_1-antitrypsin deficiency, glycogen storage disorders (9.43), galactosaemia, fructose intolerance and the Fanconi syndrome. All of these are rare disorders.

α_1-antitrypsin deficiency is associated with neonatal hepatitis and cirrhosis in childhood. The aetiology is unknown, but liver biopsy shows the hepatocytes to contain granules of α_1-AT. The diagnosis is made by finding a low serum α_1 antitrypsin.

Cardiac cirrhosis is a rare complication of long-standing right heart failure, seen in patients with cor pulmonale, tricuspid incompetence, cardiomyopathy and constrictive pericarditis. The clinical features are those described in right heart failure (p. 216). Ultrasound may show dilatation of the inferior vena cava and the hepatic veins, and histology shows centrilobular necrosis resulting from chronic venous congestion.

Drugs are rarely implicated in the generation of cirrhosis. The most common is methotrexate if used for a prolonged period, e.g. in chronic psoriasis.

Hereditary haemorrhagic telangiectasia (9.44, 10.6, 10.92) has been associated with cirrhosis. This may be caused by hepatitis viruses transmitted in blood transfusions used for the treatment of long-term anaemia.

Ulcerative colitis and Crohn's disease are associated with a variety of liver pathologies. These include fatty infiltration of the liver, granulomas, cirrhosis, pericholangitis, primary sclerosing cholangitis (8.70) and carcinoma of bile ducts (*see also* pp. 371–374, p. 408).

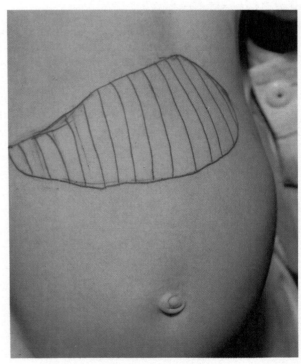

9.43 Gross hepatomegaly in glycogen storage disease. This 3-year-old child presented with a typical appearance—hepatomegaly (7cm below the costal margin in the mid-clavicular line), but no enlargement of the spleen.

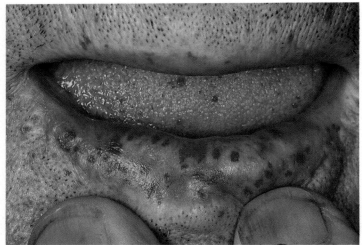

9.44 Hereditary haemorrhagic telangiectasia (HHT) is a rare association with cirrhosis. This patient had received multiple blood transfusions over many years because of HHT-associated gastrointestinal blood loss, and his cirrhosis was associated with hepatitis B antigen positivity.

Liver abscess

Pyogenic infection may result from biliary tract obstruction (ascending cholangitis), from infection carried in the portal vein (portal pyaemia) or, more rarely, from the hepatic artery in the course of generalised septicaemia.

Liver abscess is now uncommon as a result of better surgical management of intra-abdominal sepsis, but intra-abdominal pus may still occur with ruptured appendix, a perforated viscus (duodenal ulcer, diverticulitis, etc.), cholecystitis and cholangitis, infiltrating carcinomas and perinephric abscess. Often, the origin of intra-abdominal sepsis is unclear.

A wide range of bowel origin Gram-negative organisms may be involved. The commonly found organisms include *E. coli*, *Streptococci*, *Clostridia* (mainly *welchii*), *Klebsiella* and *Bacteroides*. Early administration of antibiotics often results in failure to culture the infecting organisms.

Patients with liver abscess are usually acutely unwell, and present with a high swinging fever, rigors, malaise, nausea, vomiting and, later, liver tenderness. There may be associated features of Gram-negative septicaemia with hypotension, peripheral vasoconstriction and oliguria. There may be associated icterus, caused by related biliary pathology or by a forming abscess. In addition, there may be a right-sided pleural effusion, especially if there is pus in the subphrenic space.

Investigations usually show a leucocytosis, elevation of the ESR and disturbance of liver function tests (elevation of bilirubin, alkaline phosphatase and ALT). Blood cultures are positive in half to three-quarters of patients who have not been treated with antibiotics. Chest X-ray often shows elevation of the right hemi-diaphragm and a reactive pleural effusion. Ultrasound (9.45), CT scan or isotope scanning will localise the site and size of the abscess and treatment is usually surgical evacuation under appropriate antibiotic cover. The pus collected should be sent for culture, and the antibiotic regimen finalised.

Amoebic liver abscess is a frequent complication of patients

9.45 Multiple liver abscesses revealed by liver scanning following ^{99m}Tc sulphur colloid administration. The patient developed the abscesses following peritonitis associated with acute appendicitis, and ultimately responded to intensive antimicrobial therapy. The scan appearance alone does not confirm liver abscesses. Similar appearances can result from secondary tumour deposits or multiple cysts.

with enteric amoebic infection, but may occur in the absence of a clinical episode of dysentery (*see* p. 66). The organism is carried to the liver in the portal vein, usually forming multiple abscesses that coalesce and may rupture into the peritoneal cavity or into the pleural space. Amoebic abscesses may also be revealed by ultrasound or CT scan (**1.175**). Diagnostic aspiration (**1.176**, **1.177**) produces reddish-brown pus (anchovy or chocolate sauce), which may contain motile amoebae. Small single abscesses may not require drainage and will respond to metronidazole alone. Larger, multiple abscesses, and abscesses in the left lobe of the liver may require drainage under ultrasound guidance.

Other infections of the liver

Schistosomiasis is a common cause of liver infection in the developing world, and is usually found in patients who also have disease in the colon or bladder. Migration of ova via the portal vein to the liver causes multiple granulomas and a generalised fibrotic reaction that results in portal hypertension and splenomegaly (*see* p. 77 and **1.211**, **1.212**).

Liver fluke infestation may lead to cholangitis, cirrhosis and cholangiocarcinoma (*see* p. 381).

Hydatid disease may result in multiple cysts in the liver and in many other organs (*see* p. 78). The cysts are often multiple and have daughter cysts. They act as space-occupying lesions and may produce pressure on the hepatic ducts. Eosinophilia is usual. Many of the cysts calcify and may be seen on plain X-rays. Diagnosis is made by ultrasound or by CT scan (**1.218**).

Liver tumours

Secondary tumours

Secondary spread from many primary carcinomas of the lung, breast, colon, stomach, kidney and pancreas frequently involves the liver. The resulting liver enlargement is often found in patients who have presented with vague symptoms, such as weight loss or anaemia. The liver is usually non-tender but firm and irregular. There may be few other signs, but a careful search for lymph node and skin metastases is required. Liver function tests may show only an elevation of alkaline phosphatase, occasionally with slight elevation of ALT or bilirubin. The diagnosis is made by ultrasound (**9.46**), CT scan (**9.18**) or isotope scan (**9.45**), which usually show multiple filling defects. Diagnostic biopsy guided by ultrasound or on laparoscopy may be of value to obtain a tissue-diagnosis. Multiple metastases are usually a poor prognostic sign.

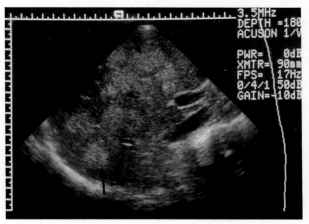

9.46

9.46 Secondary hepatic deposits demonstrated by ultrasound in a patient with primary carcinoma of the breast. The scan shows multiple well-defined hyper-echoic lesions (two examples are arrowed) and the appearances are typical of metastases.

Primary tumours

Primary hepatocellular carcinoma (primary liver cancer) is one of the most common cancers in West Africa and the Far East, but is relatively rare in the West. It is associated with chronic carriage of hepatitis B and related viruses, cirrhosis of any cause, haemochromatosis, use of some androgenic steroids, previous exposure to thorotrast, and aflatoxin from decayed food. The lesions are often multifocal and aggressively invasive. The patient often has pre-existing hepatomegaly and there is right upper quadrant pain with localised enlargement. There may also be weight loss, ascites and occasionally features of hypoglycaemia. Jaundice usually occurs only when the tumour is hilar in site. The diagnosis is confirmed by the finding of a raised circulating level of γ-fetoprotein (AFP), mild disturbance of the liver function tests and single or multiple defects on ultrasound or CT scanning (**9.47**). Arteriography may be helpful. Histological diagnosis is made on guided ultrasound or laparoscopic biopsy. A solitary lesion may be treatable by surgical resection of a liver lobe.

Cholangiocarcinoma is the second most common primary malignant tumour of liver and may be intrahepatic or extra-hepatic. Intrahepatic tumours have a similar clinical presentation to hepatocellular carcinoma; extrahepatic tumours commonly present with obstructive jaundice (**9.48**). Chinese liver fluke infestation is an underlying factor in the Far East (*see* p. 381).

Haemangiosarcoma is a rare, highly malignant tumour of liver that may result from occupational exposure to vinyl chloride monomers. Hepatic enlargement, local pain and blood-stained ascites develop rapidly, and a bruit may be heard over the tumour.

Benign tumours of the liver include:

- Liver adenomas, which may be associated with prolonged use of high-oestrogen oral contraceptives. They are highly vascular and may cause intraperitoneal bleeding.
- Cystadenomas, derived from bile ducts or from paren-chymal cells.
- Haemangiomas, which may be diagonosed by hearing a vascular hum over the liver. They are liable to rupture.

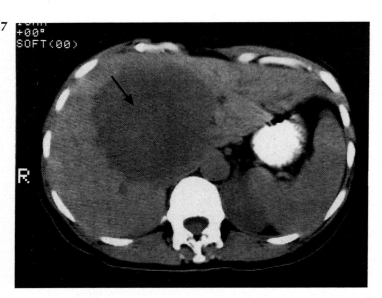

9.47 Primary hepatocellular carcinoma on CT scan. The massive tumour is obvious (arrow). The liver and spleen are both enlarged. This patient had a long history of chronic active hepatitis associated with hepatitis B antigen positivity, and signs of portal hypertension.

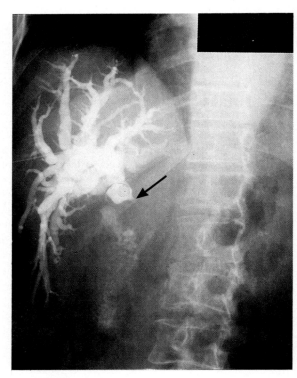

9.48 Cholangiocarcinoma causing a stricture in the hepatic duct (arrow), as shown by a percutaneous cholangiogram. The patient presented with deepening jaundice. No aetiological factor was apparent.

Diseases of the gall-bladder

Gallstones

There are three types of gallstones:

- **Pigment stones** are usually multiple and green-black in colour. They account for about 10–15% of all stones and are the result of bilirubin precipitation, caused by overproduction in chronic haemolytic states. They are later associated with recurrent ascending cholangitis.
- **Cholesterol stones** are often solitary. They form in bile in which cholesterol is in excess relative to bile salts, and are found in about 10% of patients with stones. They are common in women who have had many children or who have taken oral contraceptives.
- **Mixed stones** are by far the most common, are usually multiple and are a mixture of cholesterol, pigment, calcium carbonate and phosphate (**9.49**). They are found in people who are obese, who have taken oestrogen or who have lived on a diet rich in unrefined carbohydrate and high in calories.

In most patients stones form and remain in the gall bladder without causing symptoms, but they may produce a range of symptoms, including intolerance to fatty foods, with nausea, vomiting, flatulence and epigastric pain. Migration of stones may lead to additional symptoms such as colicky right hypochondrial pain, obstructive jaundice and recurrent bouts of ascending cholangitis and/or acute pancreatitis. Chronic cholecystitis may lead to adhesion of the gall bladder to surrounding organs, e.g. the small bowel, colon or stomach, with subsequent erosion of a stone which may then pass along the bowel and even cause intestinal obstruction if very large. The presence of a fistula leads to recurrent ascending infections in the biliary tree. Chronic cholecystitis with calcification may lead to carcinoma of the gall bladder.

9.49

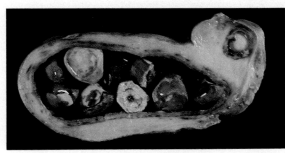

9.49 Multiple mixed gallstones in a surgically removed gall bladder with chronic cholecystitis. The gall bladder was non-functioning, and its wall was grossly thickened with oedema, fibrosis and chronic inflammation. Note the variation in size, shape and colour of the stones.

Acute cholecystitis

In acute cholecystitis, there is acute inflammation of the gall bladder, caused by migration of stone(s) and impaction either in the cystic duct or in Hartman's pouch. This leads to painful distension of the gall bladder. The swelling and inflammation may resolve, leaving the gall bladder full of mucus (hydrops or mucocele), with a risk of recurrence of pain and inflammation. Often by the time the patient seeks medical advice, little is to be found. Occasionally, the mucus becomes infected (usually with *E. coli* or other gut flora) and the inflammatory process continues with local pain and peritonitis. The gall bladder may be palpable at this time as it is distended with pus (empyema of gall bladder). There is usually an associated fever with rigors. The pain radiates to the lower rib cage at the back and to the right shoulder tip. The patient may be jaundiced if a stone has migrated into the common bile duct. The key sign is Murphy's sign, which is elicited by placing the hand under the rib cage and asking the patient to breath deeply. As the inflamed gall bladder descends and contacts the palpating hand, pain is elicited and the breath is held. In acute cholecystitis, the patient has a fever and a polymorph leucocytosis. Liver function tests are often normal. Plain X-ray may show a stone (**9.16**) and sometimes also a soft-tissue shadow of a distended gall bladder. The diagnosis is made on ultrasound which shows a distended gall bladder and cystic duct and single or multiple stones (**9.17**, **9.50**). ^{99m}TcHIDA scans may also be of value, but oral cholecystograms (**9.51**) have been largely replaced by ultrasound.

Treatment consists of intravenous fluids, analgesics and a broad spectrum antibiotic. Patients usually settle rapidly and cholecystectomy may be performed electively after 6 months.

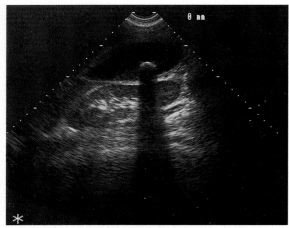

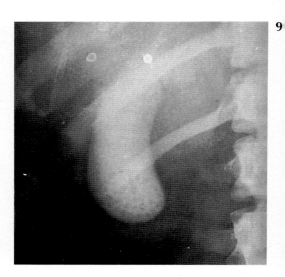

9.50 Ultrasound scanning of the gall bladder is now the preferred first investigation for gallstones. This scan shows the gall bladder containing one large stone, which casts a typical acoustic shadow (*see* **9.17**), together with many much smaller stones.

9.51 Multiple gallstones in the gall bladder as seen on oral cholecystography. This technique used to be the principal method of confirming a diagnosis of gallstones, but it has been largely superseded by ultrasound.

Chronic cholecystitis

Multiple episodes of acute disease lead to chronic cholecystitis, in which the wall of the gall bladder becomes thickened and fibrous (**9.49**), and does not usually distend when obstructed. Repeated infections also lead to the formation of mixed stones, which are small and have a greater chance of migrating into the common bile ducts and obstructing further down the system.

Common bile duct stones

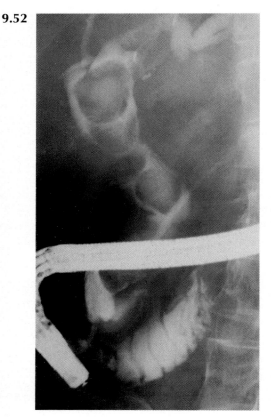

Bile duct obstruction is often with multiple mixed stones, which may lodge at the ampulla of Vater or just above. Colicky pain in the right upper quadrant is usually associated with obstructive jaundice, fever, rigors, acute nausea and vomiting. Ascending cholangitis may occur and lead to septicaemia. The features of obstructive jaundice may progress over several days and the patient develops pale stools with progressive darkening of the urine. The gall bladder is not usually felt, as it cannot distend because of progressive fibrosis from previous attacks of acute cholecystitis; there may however be some degree of hepatomegaly.

The patient usually has a fever with a brisk polymorphonuclear leucocytosis. Liver function tests are grossly deranged with a high conjugated bilirubin and alkaline phosphatase; the ALT may also be raised if there is ascending cholangitis. Tests of coagulation become abnormal, especially the prothrombin time, which is very sensitive to vitamin K malabsorption. Plain X-ray

9.52 Gallstones in the common bile duct, revealed by ERCP. Four stones are clearly seen, but, despite their size, there is little evidence of major biliary obstruction, as the hepatic ducts are not grossly dilated. Obstruction of the pancreatic duct by gallstones is not evident here, but may sometimes be demonstrated by this technique in patients with acute pancreatitis.

may show a stone, but the diagnosis is usually made by ultrasound which may show the stone and also shows the dilated bile ducts. Often the diagnosis requires an ERCP to define the position of the stone(s) more accurately (9.52) and also to remove them. Plain X-ray of the area may show gas in the biliary tree if infection is with a gas-producing organism (e.g. *C. welchii*). A percutaneous cholangiogram may provide important additional information.

Reflux of bile into the pancreatic duct, as a result of the obstruction, may produce acute pancreatitis, as may the ERCP itself.

Treatment is with fluids, bed rest, control of nausea and vomiting, and pain control. Elective surgery is necessary to remove the gall bladder, but ERCP is valuable to remove the impacted stones in the acute phase.

Acute cholangitis

Acute cholangitis is an ascending infection that results from any obstruction to the flow of bile, e.g. gallstones, carcinoma of the ducts, biliary stricture. The symptoms are identical to those already described for stones in the common duct. Treatment is supportive until elective surgery is possible to relieve the blockage.

Carcinoma of the gall bladder

Carcinoma of the gall bladder is an uncommon primary tumour which may be associated with the presence of gallstones and chronic cholecystitis. The presenting feature is a mass in the right upper quadrant. Jaundice occurs only when the liver is invaded. Treatment is surgical.

Pancreatic disease

Presentation and investigation

Clinical features of pancreatic disease may be extremely late in appearing, partly because of the deep position of the organ. Acute inflammation of the pancreas may present with epigastric pain, nausea and vomiting and occasionally hypotension. A pancreatic pseudocyst may present as a large abdominal mass. Chronic pancreatitis presents with epigastric pain, weight loss and steatorrhoea. Many patients have diabetes mellitus. There may be other signs to suggest the role of alcohol in the disease process (*see* p. 400).

Investigations in pancreatic disease include:

- Serum amylase (amylase is released from inflamed parenchymal cells).
- Stimulation tests of exocrine function with measurement of bicarbonate and enzymes (trypsin and lipases).
- Faecal fat estimation.
- ^{14}C breath tests.
- ERCP.
- Plain X-ray of the abdomen to show calcification.
- Ultrasound/CT scans.
- Exfoliative cytology by ERCP.

Acute pancreatitis

The major causes of acute pancreatitis are shown in **Table 9.4**. These stimuli trigger the release of pancreatic enzymes which then autodigest the pancreas. There is a wide spectrum of severity of the disease with mild to major autolytic digestion of the pancreas—often with haemorrhage.

The clinical presentation is usually with recurrent attacks of continuous epigastric pain which eventually localises to the back. There is usually fever, nausea and vomiting that does not relieve the pain. Examination shows the patient to be shocked and hypoxic (65% of acute deaths are caused by respiratory failure). Spontaneous bruising may be present as a result of inactivation of the coagulation mechanism by absorbed activated pancreatic enzymes. Bleeding may also track in the tissue planes of the body via the falciform ligament to the umbilicus (the umbilical black eye or Cullen's sign) and to the flanks (Grey Turner's sign **9.53**). The abdomen is rigid, with guarding on palpation. After some days, an abdominal mass may be felt.

The diagnosis is usually confirmed by an elevated serum or urine amylase. There may also be hyperglycaemia, hypocalcaemia, hypoalbuminaemia, raised levels of liver enzymes and renal impairment. Methaemalbumin may also form, as a result of intravascular haemolysis. Elevation of bilirubin and of alkaline phosphatase may occur as the bile duct is obstructed during passage through the oedematous pancreas. Ultrasound and CT scanning of the pancreas may show extreme swelling of the gland, an obstructing gall stone, a pancreatic abscess or pseudocyst formation (**9.54**). An obstructing gallstone may be shown on ERCP (**9.52**).

Over 70% of cases recover fully within a few days of treatment with intravenous fluids, nasogastric suction and analgesia. The rest have more severe disease and require intensive therapy—especially to prevent or support the patient through renal and respiratory failure. Surgery is occasionally required for abscess or pseudocyst formation.

Table 9.4 Causative factors in acute pancreatitis.

Gallstones and common bile duct obstruction

Excessive alcohol intake

Viral infections, e.g. mumps (p. 25)

Trauma—post-ERCP and other instrumentation
　　　　—major abdominal injury

Metabolic—hyperlipidaemia, hyperparathyroidism

Drug-associated—corticosteroids, azathioprine, thiazide diuretics

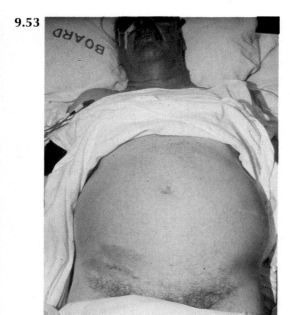

9.53 Grey Turner's sign in acute pancreatitis. This patient with severe acute pancreatitis presented with severe abdominal pain, distension and vomiting. Within 2 days of his admission, he developed characteristic discoloration in both flanks, which spread forwards to the iliac fossae. A general bleeding diathesis is demonstrated by the haemorrhage in the right arm. Grey Turner's sign results from the tracking of blood from the pancreatic area of the retroperitoneum.

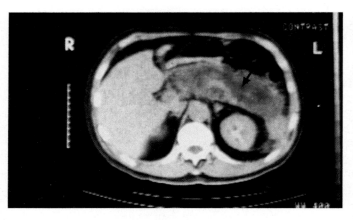

9.54 Acute pancreatitis. A pseudocyst in evolution can be seen in the pancreas (arrow). Autodigestion of the pancreatic tissue gives characteristic cystic appearance, and ultimately the cysts will coalesce to form one large pseudocyst, which may become palpable (*see* **9.56**).

Chronic pancreatitis

Most cases of chronic pancreatitis are associated with alcoholism, a few have had prior episodes of acute pancreatitis, often associated with gallstones and alcohol and in a few cases no cause is evident. In the Third World, protein-energy malnutrition (PEM) is a common association. The most common presentation is with chronic abdominal pain, usually in the epigastrium or left upper quadrant, which radiates through the back. Weight loss is common, caused by a combination of anorexia and steatorrhoea (9.55). Calcification of the pancreas is also common, and may be associated with diabetes. Measurement of faecal fat confirms steatorrhoea. Plain X-ray may show diffuse pancreatic calcification, and the extent of the pancreatic disease is apparent on CT scan.

Functional pancreatic tests are also of value and show a low bicarbonate and enzyme output. ERCP allows direct cannulation of the pancreatic duct for radiology (9.19) and pancreatic duct cytology.

Treatment of chronic pancreatitis is difficult and total abstinence from alcohol is essential. Pain is the major symptom that needs control, but care must be taken to avoid addiction to analgesics. Surgical resection and drainage may sometimes be helpful. Malabsorption is treated with pancreatic extract taken with food and supplemented with vitamins. Diabetes mellitus requires insulin, but care should be taken to prevent hypoglycaemia as the glucagon response is absent.

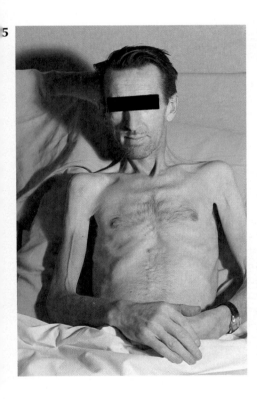

9.55 Chronic pancreatitis. The patient had a history of recurrent episodes of abdominal pain, resulting from acute pancreatitis, and leading to laparotomy on one occasion. Over the previous 2 years he developed steatorrhea and weight loss, associated with pancreatic exocrine dysfunction.

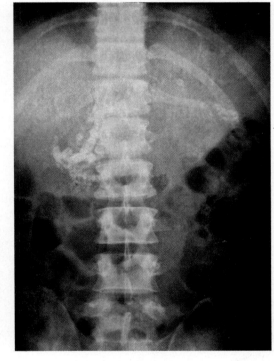

9.56 Chronic pancreatitis. The plain X-ray shows calcification throughout the pancreas, especially evident in the head. This patient was a chronic alcoholic. Pancreatic calcification is relatively unusual in the developed world, but commonly occurs in malnutrition-associated chronic pancreatitis, as seen in many parts of the developing world – often in association with diabetes..

Pancreatic pseudocysts

Pseudocysts are a common complication of acute and chronic pancreatitis, as shown by repeated ultrasound examination. Most are small and asymptomatic and will resolve if the pancreatitis is treated. Occasionally, very large cysts appear and produce local pain and palpable swelling in the epigastrium (9.57). Their extent may be revealed on CT scan (9.54) or barium meal (9.58) and they may need to be treated by repeated aspiration under ultrasound control or by marsupialisation.

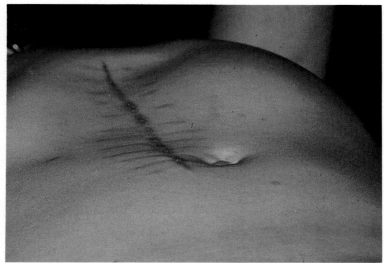

9.57 Pancreatic pseudocysts may become large enough to be visible on abdominal examination, as in this patient who underwent laparotomy at the time of presentation, and has subsequently developed an enlarging pseudocyst. Continued elevation of the serum amylase supports the diagnosis, which can be confirmed by imaging techniques (**9.54** and **9.58**).

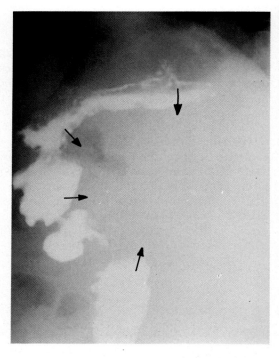

9.58 A massive pancreatic pseudocyst (arrowed) is evident in this left oblique view on barium meal. It has compressed the stomach, and pushed both the stomach and the duodenum forward.

Carcinoma of pancreas

Carcinoma of the pancreas is increasing in frequency and is the sixth most common cause of death from cancer in the USA. The disease presents late because of the anatomical position of the pancreas, and only 5% are suitable for surgical resection. The incidence of cancer is twice as high in smokers as in non-smokers and twice as great in diabetics as in non-diabetics. Over 70% occur in the head of the pancreas and patients often present with progressive obstructive jaundice caused by obstruction of the common bile duct (**9.59**). Pain may also be a feature, starting with epigastric discomfort and becoming a severe, constant pain that radiates to the back. Steatorrhoea is accompanied by severe weight loss. Secondaries form in the liver, which may be enlarged. The gall bladder is often easily felt but non-tender (Courvoisier's sign). Ascites is often a prominent feature. There is a significantly increased incidence of superficial thrombophlebitis and deep vein thrombosis (**9.60**).

Carcinoma of the body and tail of the pancreas presents with deep epigastric pain radiating to the back, associated with weight loss. Thirty per cent of patients also have frank diabetes or glucose intolerance.

Liver function tests in pancreatic carcinoma usually show an obstructive pattern with a high alkaline phosphatase and bilirubin. Serum amylase and carcinoembryonic antigen (CEA) may also be elevated.

The diagnosis of pancreatic carcinoma is made by ultrasound (**9.61**), CT scanning or ERCP. ERCP or percutaneous transhepatic cholangiography may show narrowing in the main duct (**9.62**) and also allows the collection of pancreatic juice for cytology. Barium meal examination may first suggest the diagnosis (**9.63**); and laparoscopy may provide supportive findings. Treatment options are limited, but surgery may help in palliation of the obstructive jaundice.

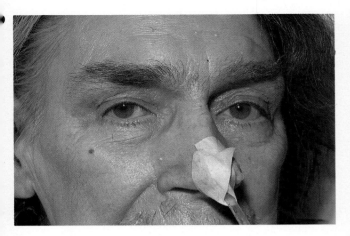

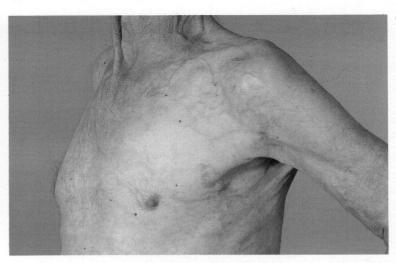

9.59 Carcinoma of the pancreas typically presents late in the course of the disease, as in this patient who is obviously jaundiced and has lost a considerable amount of weight. She presented with the painless onset of jaundice just 2 weeks before this photograph was taken, although her weight loss had occurred over several months. Pain is not always a feature of carcinoma of the pancreas—painless onset of jaundice is a common presentation of carcinoma of the head of the pancreas.

9.60 Thrombophlebitis in superficial or deep veins is relatively common in many forms of malignant disease, but it is particularly associated with carcinoma of the pancreas, and it is sometimes the presenting feature. Recurrent episodes of thrombophlebitis ('thrombophlebitis migrans') may precede the diagnosis of pancreatic carcinoma by many months, and their occurrence in an otherwise apparently fit patient should lead to a search for underlying malignancy—especially in the pancreas.

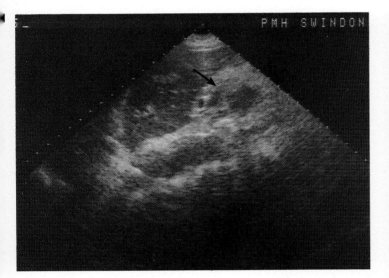

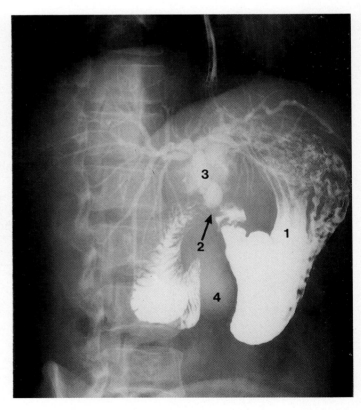

9.61 Pancreatic carcinoma. This ultrasound scan shows a mass in the head of the pancreas (arrow), containing several areas of decreased echogenicity, an appearance typical of carcinoma.

9.62 Pancreatic carcinoma, revealed by combined barium meal and percutaneous transhepatic cholangiography (PTC). The pancreatic tumour is compressing the stomach (1), obstructing the common bile duct as it passes through the head of the pancreas (2), leading to dilatation of the common bile duct and hepatic ducts (3), and leading to distension of the gallbladder (4), which was easily palpable.

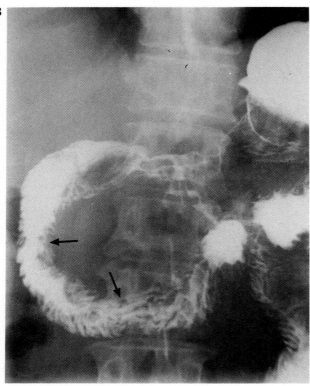

9.63

9.63 Pancreatic carcinoma may be diagnosed first when a barium meal is performed for undiagnosed gastrointestinal symptoms. In this patient, a large carcinoma in the head of the pancreas has led to a characteristic widening of the duodenal loop with compression of the second and third parts of the duodenum (arrows). This compression may lead to symptoms of intestinal obstruction, which may require palliative by-pass surgery.

Other pancreatic tumours

A variety of other rare endocrine tumours is found in association with the pancreas. Each may present with a specific set of symptoms and diagnosis is by measurement of tumour-specific peptides. Localisation of these tumours may be very difficult even with selective arteriography.

Primary carcinoid can occur in the pancreas—the symptoms arise from hepatic metastases, and diagnosis rests on urinary excretion of 5-HIAA—a 5HT metabolite. Treatment may be surgical, but recently somatostatin analogue has been successfully used.

The other pancreatic tumours all arise from a single cell line—APUD cells (amine precursor uptake and decarboxylation). They are classified by the main peptide produced, but they often produce more than one and the predominant peptide secreted can alter. The major tumour types are summarised on p. 384.

10. Disorders of the Blood

History and examination

Symptoms often develop late in the course of disorders of the blood and lymphoid system. In their early stages, anaemias, chronic leukaemias and other myeloproliferative disorders may be completely asymptomatic, or they may be associated with only vague symptoms, many of which are common in the general population, including fatigue, headaches, faintness, shortness of breath, palpitations, angina pectoris, intermittent claudication and recurrent minor infections.

Acute leukaemia commonly presents with a short history of more definite symptoms, which may include—in addition to the symptoms of anaemia—mouth ulceration, sore throat and other signs of infection; enlarged lymph nodes; bruising and bleeding; bone pain; and symptoms caused by tissue infiltration. Thrombocytopenias present with characteristic skin changes, and other major bleeding disorders also present with obvious symptoms; but more minor degrees of bleeding disorder may be subclinical and thus asymptomatic.

Thrombotic disorders usually present with symptoms and signs related to arterial or venous thrombosis; but disseminated intravascular coagulation may present with haemostatic failure and is usually seen in severely ill patients, who are likely to have multiple symptomatology from the underlying cause of the condition.

Patients with lymphomas often present with lymphadenopathy, fever or symptoms resulting from tissue infiltration or compression by the lymphomatous process, with failure of the immune system, or with a haemorrhagic or haemolytic disorder; but even here, some patients remain asymptomatic and are diagnosed largely by chance.

Because of the absence of specific diagnostic symptoms in many disorders of the blood, clinical examination of the patient is of great importance. Clinical signs in haematology may result from abnormalities of red cells, white cells, platelets, plasma globulins or coagulation factors.

Excess or lack of red cells in the circulation is often obvious on examination. Polycythaemia is associated with plethora, especially of the face, which may show a bluish, cyanotic tinge because of the high levels of unsaturated haemoglobin. Comparison with a normal skin is helpful (**4.6, 10.1**).

Anaemia is often suggested by pallor of the face, lips, tongue (**10.2, 10.3**), conjunctivae (**8.2**), nailbeds (**10.4**) and palms (**10.5**). Examination of the mouth, lips and tongue may give a clue to the etiology of the anaemia, e.g. iron deficiency is associated with atrophy of mucosa, especially on the tongue and often with the presence of angular stomatitis (**7.133, 10.2**). Lack of vitamin B_{12} and other B vitamins produces a tongue that is red and 'beefy' (**9.35, 10.29**). The finger nails may show evidence of tissue iron deficiency with 'spooning' (koilonychia, **2.89, 10.4, 10.19**).

Excessive breakdown of red cells results in changes in urine colour: if the red cell destruction has occurred in the intravascular compartment, the urine passed is black to brown in colour (blackwater, **1.184**); in extravascular haemolysis, it becomes dark and orange on standing because of the presence of excess urobilinogen, which is converted to urobilin.

Haemolysis usually imparts a pale lemon-yellow colour to the skin and conjunctivae, such as is seen in pernicious anaemia (**9.2, 10.28, 10.29**), or a deeper yellow to orange colour in more active haemolytic anaemias (**10.37**).

General examination may also show the cause of anaemia, as in the perioral black-brown pigmentation in Peutz–Jeghers syndrome (**2.74**), the telangiectasia in hereditary haemorrhagic telangiectasia (**9.44, 10.6, 10.92**), or the skin purpura or ecchymosis of a bleeding disorder (**2.116, 7.23, 9.14**). The associated neurological features of a vitamin B_{12} deficiency anaemia include combined deficiencies in the posterior and lateral column function of the cord.

If anaemia develops quickly, it can lead to rapid cardiac decompensation and presents with acute left ventricular failure (*see* p. 216). However, if it develops insidiously, there are compensatory mechanisms with tachycardia, tachypnoea and gradual onset of heart failure.

Bone and soft-tissue changes may result from extreme erythroid hyperplasia in chronic anaemia such as thalassaemia.

Deficient production of mature normal white cells leads to neutropenia (below $1.5 \times 10^9/l$), which increases the chances of infection—patients often present with bacterial, viral, fungal or protozoal invasion of the skin, gums, throat or lungs. In conditions with excessive white cell production, the skin, liver, spleen, lymph nodes, tongue, testes and ovaries may be infiltrated and enlarge. High white cell turnover may be associated with elevation of the serum uric acid, and occasionally with acute and chronic gout (*see* p. 140).

Increased production of collagen in the marrow cavity in myelofibrosis or myelosclerosis leads to haemopoiesis elsewhere, especially in the liver and spleen which become massively enlarged. Similar enlargement of the liver, spleen and lymph nodes (**10.7**) may be found in lymphomas and in chronic leukaemias.

Reduction of platelet number below about $40 \times 10^9/l$, or defects in platelet function, result in purpura and haemorrhages into the skin (**10.8**) and mucous membranes and may be associated with overt external or internal bleeding. Platelet number increases to over $1,000 \times 10^9/l$ results in a likelihood of thrombosis, usually in the periphery, with gangrene of the fingers or toes, but also occlusion in the cerebral or coronary arteries.

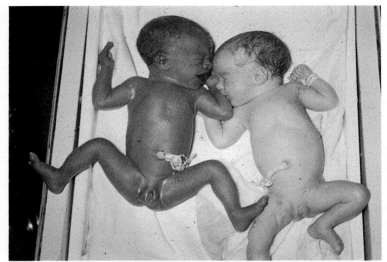

10.1 Polycythaemia and anaemia in identical newborn twins. The cause of this unusual condition was an arteriovenous fistula in the placenta; the picture is included here because it clearly exemplifies the difference in the appearance of polycythaemia (the twin on the left) from anaemia (the twin on the right). For a comparison of a polycythaemic adult with her normal sister *see* **4.6**.

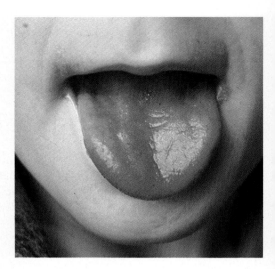

10.2 Iron deficiency anaemia commonly leads to pallor of the face, lips and tongue, and—when chronic—to atrophic glossitis and angular stomatitis. All these appearances are seen in this young woman whose iron deficiency anaemia resulted from excessive menstrual bleeding. She responded to oral iron supplementation.

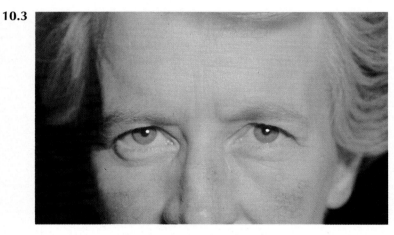

10.3 Severe anaemia commonly leads to generalised pallor, which is particularly obvious in the face. This patient had iron deficiency anaemia. Her haemoglobin was 5.0g/dl.

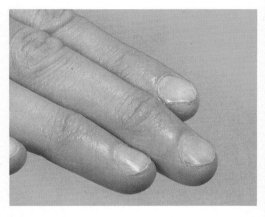

10.4 Pallor of the nailbeds is another sign in anaemia. This patient had iron deficiency anaemia associated with menorrhagia. Pallor of the nailbeds is best assessed by comparison with a normal hand. Note that this patient also has early koilonychia.

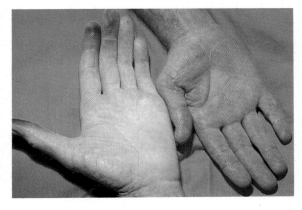

10.5 Pallor of the hand in anaemia is obvious in this patient, especially when compared with the physician's hand on the right. The patient's haemoglobin was 7 g/dl. The hand also shows that he was a heavy smoker. His anaemia resulted from chronic blood loss from a carcinoma in the oesophagus—a site where the risk of carcinoma is increased in smokers.

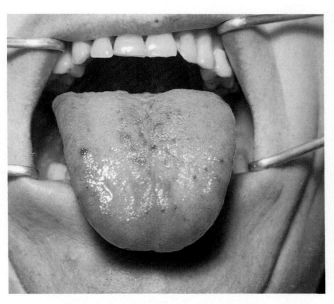

10.6 Hereditary haemorrhagic telangiectasia (HHT) is a condition in which occult blood loss in the gut may lead to severe iron deficiency anaemia. The diagnosis is usually clear from a careful clinical examination, although the telangiectasia are not always as obvious as in this patient with multiple lesions on the face, lips and tongue. This patient shows generalised pallor resulting from his iron deficiency anaemia.

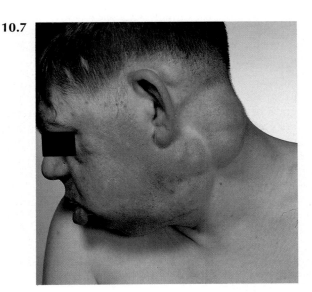

10.7 Gross enlargement of the cervical lymph nodes in a patient with Hodgkin's disease. The cervical lymph nodes are a common presenting site for lymphomas of all types, and for leukaemia— especially chronic lymphatic leukaemia.

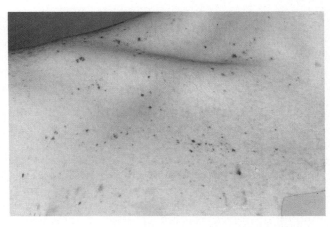

10.8 Purpura—in this case thrombocytopenic purpura (TP). The patient was a 15-year-old boy whose anti-epileptic treatment regimen had recently been modified to include sodium valproate. This is just one of a number of drugs that may induce TP (*see* p. 456) and **Table 10.9**), but the disorder is almost always reversible if the drug therapy is stopped.

Investigations

The **full blood count** (FBC) (**Table 10.1**) is easily measured using automated blood cell counters and is a routine hospital investigation (**10.9**). Preparation and staining of a **blood film** allows microscopic examination (**10.10**), particularly where the FBC shows an abnormality or where a haematological disorder is suspected for other reasons. This may reveal morphological changes characteristic of particular systemic diseases, e.g. eosinophilia in worm infestations and allergy (**1.17**), atypical lymphocytes in infectious mononucleosis (**1.88**), malaria parasites (**1.187**), trypanosomes (**1.18**) or other parasites (**1.198**); or of particular haematological disorders; e.g. the misshapen red cells of hereditary elliptocytosis (**10.41**), or leukaemic cells (**10.70, 10.71, 10.73, 10.74, 10.76**). More commonly, a general abnormality is suggested, e.g. anaemia or infection, and this may require more detailed investigation.

In the investigation of anaemia, the **reticulocyte count** (**10.11**), provides an assessment of effective red cell production. Reticulocytes are young red cells that still contain ribosomal RNA and a residual capacity to synthesise haemoglobin. The RNA is lost within about a day of their release from the bone marrow and, since the red cell lifespan is approximately 120 days, the 'normal' proportion of reticulocytes is about 1%. In anaemic patients, hypoxia stimulates increased production of erythropoietin by the kidneys, and the reticulocyte count should thus markedly increase. The absence of an appropriate increase suggests anaemia caused by disordered red cell production (either because of inadequate numbers of red cell precursors—hypoplasia; or as a result of their premature death within the marrow—ineffective erythropoiesis) rather than increased red cell destruction (haemolysis) or blood loss.

Red cell size and colour are important. Decreased production related to impaired haemoglobin synthesis, whether of haem (e.g. in iron deficiency) or globin (in thalassaemias), tends to give rise to hypochromic, poorly haemoglobinised, often small (microcytic) red cells. In contrast, the larger, well-haemoglobinised (macrocytic) cells are associated with disordered nuclear maturation (e.g. in megaloblastic anaemias). In many anaemias secondary to systemic disorders, the red cells are of normal size and haemoglobin content (normocytic, normochromic). The red cell mean cell volume (MCV) and mean cell haemoglobin (MCH) can thus be helpful, with the reticulocyte count, in the initial classification of the cause of anaemia. Precise diagnosis in haemolytic anaemias may then require extensive further immunological, cell membrane, haemoglobin or red cell enzyme studies.

A **bone marrow examination** may be indicated where the cause of anaemia is obscure or where an abnormality of production of one or more of the blood cell lines is suspected, or where there is other evidence of a malignancy that commonly involves the bone marrow (e.g. lymphoma). Marrow smears from a needle aspirate of sternal or posterior ilium marrow cavities are taken for detailed morphological studies of haemopoietic cells (**10.12**). A marrow aspirate can also provide cells for cytogenetic studies, detailed immunological studies of cellular antigens (cell-marker studies) or molecular analysis of DNA, all of which may help in defining the precise cell type of abnormal cells (e.g. in leukaemia or lymphoma). Histology of a trephine biopsy may be needed where marrow is scanty (**10.13, 10.14**). It provides less information about individual cells, but retains the marrow architectural relationships, gives a better guide to overall cellularity, and may identify focal lesions (e.g. tumour infiltration) which are absent in the aspirate.

Biochemical studies are of value in further defining the causes of anaemia:

- Serum iron with total iron binding capacity (TIBC) gives information about iron transport and is complemented by the ferritin level, which more accurately reflects body status.
- Serum levels of vitamin B_{12} and folate give a clue to the presence or absence of essential components for red cell haemoglobin synthesis. Low levels of vitamin B_{12} necessitate a two-stage Schilling test, which may indicate whether malabsorption of B_{12} is caused by lack of intrinsic factor or by intestinal disease.
- Excessive breakdown of haemoglobin can be monitored by measurement of indirect bilirubin, urobilinogen in the urine and stercobilinogen. Occasionally, in intravascular breakdown, haemoglobin will appear in the urine and there is depletion of haptoglobins and appearance of methaemalbumin.

The cause of haemolysis may become obvious from examination of the blood film (e.g. parasites), from the presence of antibodies coating the red cells, or from the presence of abnormal haemoglobins on electrophoresis or abnormal enzymes within the red cells.

Abnormalities of blood coagulation and related systems require the expertise of highly specialised laboratories and physicians.

Initial bedside investigations are still sometimes helpful (**10.15–10.17**), but laboratory studies are usually needed.

The basic screening tests should include a platelet count, the activated partial thromboplastin time (APTT), the prothrombin time (PT), the thrombin time and a test for fibrin degradation products (the D Dimer test). These indicate which part of the coagulation cascade is likely to be defective. Acquired haemostatic deficiencies (e.g. DIC, hepatic disease) may be the result of multiple deficiency in the coagulation and platelet system. Examination of the quality of the fibrin clot is worthwhile and it may also be incubated to see if there is active fibrinolysis present. These tests also may form the basis of control of anticoagulant therapy, but generally purpose-designed tests are more accurate. It is probable that the biggest group of patients with haemostatic defects are those on oral anticoagulant therapy or prophylaxis.

Table 10.1 Normal values for the full blood count (FBC).

	Men	Women	Units
Haemoglobin	13.5–17.5	11.5–15.5	g/dl
Red cells	4.5-6.0	3.8–5.2	$\times 10^{12}$/l
PCV (haematocrit)	40–52	37–47	%
MCV (mean cell volume)*	80–96		fl
MCH (mean cell haemoglobin)	27–32		pg
MCHC (mean cell haemoglobin concentration)	31–36		g/dl
Reticulocytes†	0.5–2.0		%
WBC (white blood cells)*	4–11		$\times 10^{9}$/l
Neutrophils	2.0–7.5		$\times 10^{9}$/l
Lymphocytes	1.5–4.0		$\times 10^{9}$/l
Monocytes	0.2–0.8		$\times 10^{9}$/l
Eosinophils	0.04–0.40		$\times 10^{9}$/l
Basophils	<0.1		$\times 10^{9}$/l
Platelets	150–400		$\times 10^{9}$/l

* In the neonate Hb and MCV are normally higher, and in children below 12 years of age lower, than these adult values. Children also have higher lymphocyte counts.

† Reticulocytes are best reported as absolute number since the red cell count may vary very considerably.

10.9

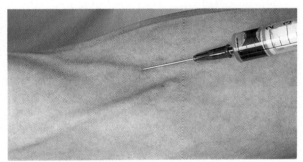

10.9 Venous blood sampling is a routine procedure, but it is important that it is carried out correctly for haematological and biochemical investigations to be accurate. In particular, it is essential that blood is not drawn up rapidly through a narrow-gauge needle, as this may cause artefactual haemolysis. The minimum possible degree of venous occlusion should be used for sampling, as stasis can affect the results of both biochemical and haematological investigations. It is essential that the blood sample is drawn up or immediately transferred into the appropriate container for the investigation required, and that the blood is processed rapidly.

10.10

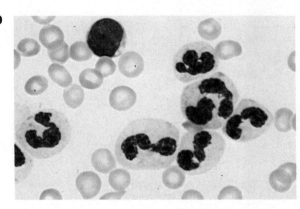

10.10 A blood film can often aid the interpretation of the full blood count. This patient had an elevated white cell count, and the film showed that most of the cells were neutrophils. Some of the neutrophils contain small blue-staining areas in the cytoplasm. These are known as Dohle bodies. They are a non-specific finding, but are commonly found in patients with infections.

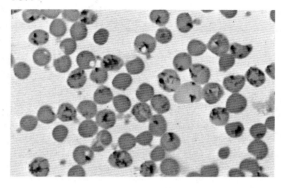

10.11 The reticulocyte count shows gross reticulocytosis in this patient. Up to 80% of the red cells in the peripheral blood film are reticulocytes, as shown by supravital staining for RNA. This patient had haemolytic anaemia caused by congenital pyruvate-kinase (PK) deficiency.

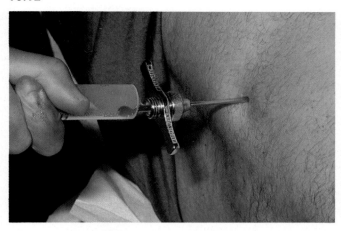

10.12 Bone marrow aspiration is most commonly and conveniently carried out from the sternum. Local anaesthetic is injected in the skin and down to the level of the periosteum, and an aspiration needle—often a Jamshidi needle, as used here—is pushed through the anterior table of the sternum into the marrow cavity. Marrow can then be aspirated into the syringe. A relatively small amount of marrow is required for investigation, but an inadequate or dry tap may be an indication for trephine bone biopsy.

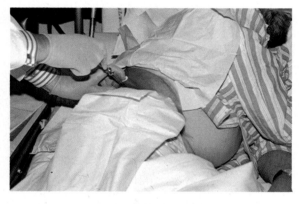

10.13 Trephine bone biopsy is most commonly carried out from the ilium, near the iliac crest. Again, local anaesthesia is used before the bone trephine (**10.14**) is pushed forcefully into the ilium.

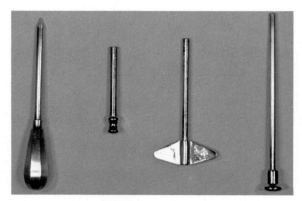

10.14 The components of the bone trephine used for iliac crest biopsy. The technique is useful in metabolic bone disease as well as a range of haematological disorders.

10.15

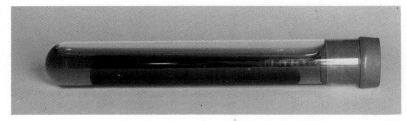

10.15 Blood clotting time can be measured simply by placing a sample of venous blood in a plain glass tube and measuring the time taken to form a clot. The normal range is 4–8 minutes. A prolonged blood clotting time implies a deficiency in coagulation factors.

10.16

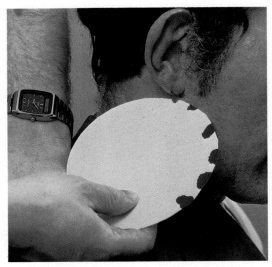

10.16 Bleeding time. This can be measured by pricking the ear, and removing the escaping blood every 15 seconds with the edge of a filter paper. The frequent blotting prevents the formation of a surface blood clot, and in these circumstances the arrest of bleeding depends largely on capillary contraction and platelet adhesion and aggregation. The normal bleeding time is 3–5 minutes; it is prolonged where capillary contractility is impaired, in thrombocytopenia or in platelet function defects.

10.17

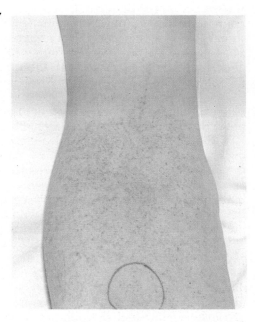

10.17 A positive capillary resistance test (Hess test). A circle is drawn on the surface of the forearm, and the skin blemishes within it are counted. A sphygmomanometer cuff is applied to the upper arm and inflated to a pressure midway between systolic and diastolic blood pressure for 5 minutes. The cuff is then deflated, and the skin within the circle is examined. Normally not more than two or three tiny haemorrhagic spots are to be seen, but where there is abnormal capillary fragility—as in this patient—a large crop of small haemorrhagic spots is found. The level of the bottom of the cuff is obvious.

Anaemias

Anaemia is defined as a condition where the blood has a deficient concentration of haemoglobin, which reduces its ability to transport oxygen. The most common form of anaemia worldwide, which affects over 500 million people, is that caused by iron deficiency. In hospital practice secondary 'anaemia of chronic disorders' predominates.

Iron deficiency anaemia

A normal diet containing green vegetables, red meat, eggs and milk should contain 15–20 mg of iron of which about 5–15% is absorbed in the duodenum and jejunum. Iron deficiency commonly arises from a combination of reduced dietary intake of iron (especially from vegetarian diets) with a physiological increase in iron requirement (e.g. in pregnancy, and in pre-menopausal women). Occult blood loss, usually into the gut, and more rarely malabsorption (e.g. in coeliac disease or after gastrectomy) can also give rise to negative iron balance. The most common form of blood loss worldwide is hookworm infection (**10.18** and *see* p. 380).

It is important to take a detailed dietary history extending over the past year or so, and enquiry should be made about intake of meats, liver, green vegetables, eggs and milk. In Asians who eat chapattis, iron deficiency may result from iron binding by phytate in the gut. Strict vegetarians may eat iron in a non-absorbable form. Babies who are breast fed for a prolonged time may become iron deficient.

A history of obvious blood loss should be sought, as in women who have had multiple pregnancies or in whom there has been excess loss at menstruation. It is important to ask directly about the frequency and heaviness of the periods (i.e. number of days between the periods, their duration, the presence of clots and the number of towels and tampons used). Obvious blood loss may also occur in patients with haemorrhoids and questions should be asked about blood on the stools or toilet tissue. If bleeding occurs higher up in the alimentary tract, the red colour of haemoglobin is converted to give the stool the black colour of acid haematin (melaena). Occult alimentary bleeding may occur in patients taking aspirin or related non-steroidal anti-inflammatory drugs (**3.9, 8.34, 8.35**), duodenal and gastric ulceration and from carcinomas and polyps in the bowel. Right-sided colonic carcinoma is particularly likely to present as unexplained anaemia. A history of previous alimentary surgery is important, especially if this has involved the removal of part of the acid-secreting portion of the stomach or the creation of a bypass. Evidence of malabsorption should also be sought (*see* p. 368).

The patient should be examined for the signs of anaemia (**10.1–10.5**), especially for those which point to iron deficiency, such as koilonychia (**2.89, 10.4, 10.19**); and for pointers to possible underlying blood loss such as telangiectasia (**10.6**) and haemorrhoids (**10.20**).

In iron deficiency, iron stores are first mobilised (reflected by a falling serum ferritin concentration—10–100 nmol/l), and only when these have been exhausted does the iron supply to the tissues, assessed by the serum iron (15–25 μmol/l) and transferrin saturation (55–70 μmol/l), begin to decline, eventually giving rise to frank anaemia. Iron is essential for maturation and function of all cells and non-haemopoietic effects of deficiency include koilonychia and oral changes. The underlying cause of the negative iron balance must always be sought, paying particular attention to possible gastrointestinal blood loss. Investigations should include:

- Full blood count and film. This shows a reduction in red cell numbers and haematocrit. The red cell size (MCV) is reduced (<75 fl) and may be as low as 60 fl. The cells have a reduced mean corpuscular haemoglobin (MCH) which is below 25 pg. The film confirms that the cells are microcytic, hypochromic and have variations in size and shape (**3.9, 10.21**). There may be early forms present. The platelet count may be raised, and white cells are usually normal. If the cause of anaemia is hookworm infection, eosinophilia is often present (**1.17**).
- Faecal occult blood measurement is of value, but the results must be interpreted with caution because of the possibility of false positive results from dietary causes.
- Serum ferritin is low, reflecting reduction of tissue iron; and a low serum iron and a high transferrin with a low percentage saturation is a reflection of deficient transport.
- Bone marrow aspiration shows a hyperplastic marrow dominated by active red cell series proliferation (**10.22**). Staining for iron with Prussian Blue shows reduced or absent iron staining (**10.23**).
- Endoscopy of the upper and lower alimentary tract may define bleeding lesions (e.g. **8.35, 8.71, 8.72, 8.88**).
- Barium series of the upper and lower alimentary tract may show associated changes of iron deficiency, e.g. the Plummer–Vinson or Paterson–Brown–Kelly syndrome (**8.30**) or a lesion that may have bled (**8.86**).
- Occasionally, mesenteric arteriography or nuclear medicine studies may help to reveal obscure sources of blood loss in the gut.

Treatment is usually with simple oral iron salts (ferrous sulphate or fumarate), and any adverse effects (e.g. constipation) may be ameliorated by reducing the dose or by changing to a preparation that contains less available iron in each tablet (e.g. ferrous gluconate). Failure of response is most commonly caused by lack of compliance, but should lead to re-assessment of the diagnosis since other causes of hypochromic anaemia include alpha- or beta-thalassaemia trait and sideroblastic anaemias, which may be associated with excessive iron absorption and thus with a risk of damage from iron overload with prolonged oral iron therapy.

10.18

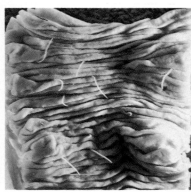

10.18 Hookworm infection is the most common cause of iron deficiency anaemia worldwide. The worms are seen attached by their buccal capsules to the villi of the small intestine, where they feed by sucking blood (up to 0.2 ml per day per worm). In gross hookworm infection, severe iron deficiency anaemia may result.

10.19

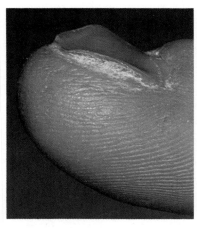

10.19 Koilonychia or 'spooning' of the nails is a result of a non-haemopoietic effect of iron deficiency. For another view of koilonychia *see* **2.89**, **10.4**.

10.20

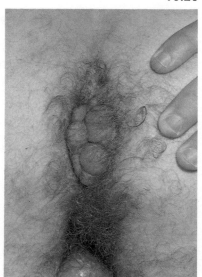

10.20 Haemorrhoids are a common cause of rectal bleeding. Intero-external piles—as seen here—commonly bleed on defaecation, and over a period of time this blood loss can lead to iron deficiency.

10.21

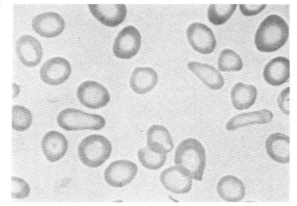

10.21 Blood film in iron deficiency showing hypochromia, anisocytosis and poikilocytosis. All the red cells show marked hypochromic central pallor. A few also show distortions in shape, but this is not a marked feature of simple iron deficiency.

10.22

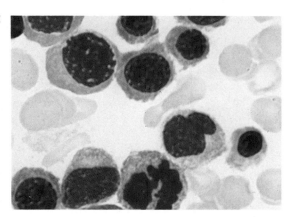

10.22 Bone marrow in iron deficiency anaemia. Erythropoiesis is normoblastic, but the normoblasts tend to be small, with ragged outlines and defective haemoglobinisation.

10.23

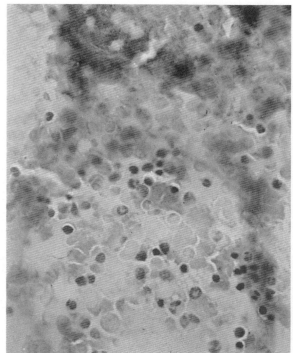

10.23 Bone marrow smear in iron deficiency anaemia, stained for free iron by the Prussian Blue method. Iron stores are completely absent in this marrow. Free iron would stain bright blue (*see* **10.25**).

Sideroblastic anaemia

Sideroblastic anaemias are a rare group of hypochromic anaemias in which the serum iron levels are high and the transferrin is saturated. A variety of acquired and inherited defects in porphyrin biosynthesis lead to diminished synthesis of haem which in turn results in increased cellular iron uptake. The key diagnostic feature is the presence of the ringed sideroblast in the marrow aspirate. This is a normoblast, containing ferritin-aggregates in the mitochondria which have a perinuclear distribution (**10.24**, **10.25**). The common acquired causes are alcoholism, drugs such as isoniazid, lead poisoning and myeloproliferative disease. Patients should abstain from alcohol and possibly causative drugs should be withdrawn. Lead poisoning may require treatment with chelating agents. Transfusion should be used as infrequently as possible in these patients, because of the dangers of iron overload. Some patients may respond to large doses of vitamin B_6 and rarely to androgens.

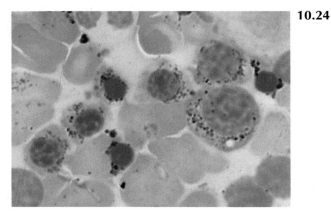

10.24

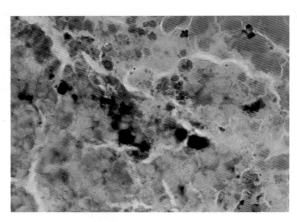

10.25

10.24 Bone marrow in sideroblastic anaemia. The marrow has been stained for free iron, thus revealing ringed sideroblasts. These are erythroblasts with free iron granules arranged as a nearly continuous ring around the nucleus. This iron is chiefly concentrated in mitochondria.

10.25 Bone marrow smear in sideroblastic anaemia. In this case, the bone marrow has been stained with Prussian Blue (the same method as used in **10.23**) revealing increased (blue) iron stores. Normal subjects have stainable free iron amounts midway between the appearance seen here and that in **10.23**.

Anaemia of chronic disease

The main differential diagnosis for early iron deficiency anaemia is the anaemia associated with many chronic disorders, e.g. chronic arthritis, chronic infections, renal and liver failure, neoplasia and endocrine disorders (**10.26**). This anaemia, at least initially, is normocytic and normochromic and is multifactorial in origin, with a slight reduction in red cell survival, inappropriately low production of erythropoietin, and a disturbance of iron delivery to the developing erythroblasts, which in time can give rise to a degree of hypochromia and microcytosis of the red cells (**10.27**). In contrast to uncomplicated iron deficiency, the iron stores in this form of anaemia tend to be normal or increased (high serum ferritin); increased storage by macrophages of the iron released from destroyed red cells results in impaired release of iron to circulating transferrin and thus reduced delivery of iron to the bone marrow (low serum iron and low transferrin).

Iron deficiency anaemia and the anaemia of chronic disease may co-exist (e.g. in a patient with active rheumatoid arthritis who also has occult gastrointestinal blood loss induced by non-steroidal anti-inflammatory drugs). Under such circumstances, a bone marrow examination is the best way to determine whether iron stores are reduced (*see* **10.23**, **10.25**).

The 'anaemia of chronic disease' improves only with treatment of the underlying disease and does not respond to iron therapy or other haematinics. Though a response to recombinant human erythropoietin (rEPO) has been seen in some patients, this is by no means established, in contrast to the proven value of this growth factor in the hypoplastic anaemia associated with chronic renal failure.

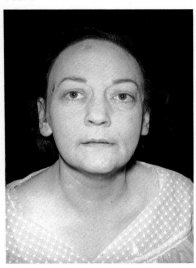

10.26 Anaemia of chronic disease, manifest as severe pallor in a diabetic patient with severe uraemia. Her haemoglobin was 6.5 g/dl, but the blood film demonstrated that the anaemia remained normochromic and normocytic.

10.27 Anaemia of chronic disease. The anaemia is normocytic, but some hypochromia is obvious. In addition, there is prominent rouleaux formation—red cells are grouped together in piles or stacks. In a properly prepared smear, rouleaux formation suggests the same range of abnormalities that are revealed by a high erythrocyte sedimentation rate, so rouleaux formation may be found in any chronic inflammatory process or malignancy and, especially, in multiple myeloma and other monoclonal gammopathies.

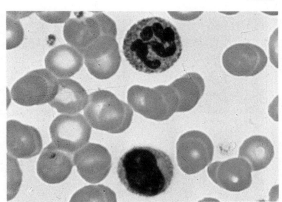

Macrocytic anaemia

Macrocytic red cells are most commonly seen in association with liver disease (where there may be excessive lipid deposition in the red cell membrane), as a result of regular alcohol intake or in haemolysis. They may also occur in hypothyroidism and in haemolytic anaemias where there is an increase in reticulocytes (which are larger than mature red cells). Macrocytosis also occurs as a result of an underlying nuclear maturation defect affecting blood cell precursors in the bone marrow and giving rise to a megaloblastic marrow. This is commonly caused by either vitamin B_{12} or folic acid deficiency, though cytotoxic chemotherapy and other intrinsic marrow disorders may give rise to a similar picture. Folic acid is required for the synthesis of the pyrimidines and purines of DNA, and vitamin B_{12} maintains the intracellular folate in an active form.

Causes of B_{12} deficiency are summarised in **Table 10.2**; causes of folate deficiency are summarised in **Table 10.3**.

Deficiencies in folate or B_{12} give rise to an anaemia of insidious onset, which is often very severe at the time of presentation. The usual presentation is with non-specific features of anaemia such as lethargy, tiredness and weight loss. Clinically, patients are pale, and the combination of pallor with mild icterus related to intra-medullary premature death of erythroblasts typically gives rise to a lemon-yellow skin colour (**10.28**). Glossitis may occur (**9.35, 10.29**). Bruising and purpura may suggest coexistent thrombocytopenia, and fundal haemorrhages may occur, as in any severe anaemia. There may be hepatosplenomegaly and signs of heart failure.

Subacute combined degeneration of the cord in vitamin B_{12}

Table 10.2 Causes of vitamin B_{12} deficiency.

Decreased intake
   Nutritional deficiency
      Vegan diet
      Alcoholism
      Severe protein-calorie malnutrition
   Competition by gut microflora or fish tapeworm
   Malabsorption
      Intrinsic factor deficiency
      Diseased terminal ileum
      Pancreatic failure
      Drugs — biguanides, K^+ supplements

Increased requirement
   Pregnancy
   Haemolytic states

Table 10.3 Causes of folate deficiency.

Decreased intake
   Nutritional deficiency
      Elderly
      Alcoholism
      Milk-fed premature infants
   Malabsorption
      Coeliac disease
      Tropical sprue
      Post-gastrectomy
      Crohn's disease
      Drugs — phenytoin

Increased requirement
   Physiological
      Pregnancy
      Lactation
      Prematurity
      Growth in childhood
   Pathological
      Haemolytic states
      Myeloproliferative disorders
      Severe inflammatory states
      Dialysis

Impaired folate utilisation
   Cytotoxic drugs — methotrexate
   Trimethoprim
   Anticonvulsants — phenytoin, phenobarbitone
   Alcohol

10.28

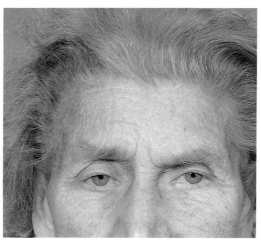

10.28 Pernicious anaemia often gives rise to characteristic pallor with a lemon-yellow tinge. The pallor relates directly to the haemoglobin level, while the mild jaundice is the result of the premature breakdown of erythroblasts—a form of haemolysis. Typically, patients with pernicious anaemia have blue eyes and (often prematurely) grey hair.

10.29 Pernicious anaemia. This patient shows similar skin coloration to that seen in **10.28**. In addition, she has a 'raw beef' tongue. The surface is smooth, with an absence of filiform papillae. Similar changes may be seen as a result of deficiency in other B-group vitamins.

10.29

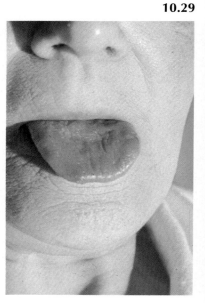

deficiency presents with symmetrical paraesthesiae of hands and feet, and impairment of proprioception and vibration sense (**10.30**) leads to ataxia. Higher cerebral function is also frequently impaired and dementia appears.

A dietary history may suggest B_{12} deficiency (especially in strict vegetarians or vegans) or folate deficiency (absence of fresh fruit and vegetables). Neurological signs, particularly posterior column signs, may point to deficiency of vitamin B_{12}, and a personal or family history of other autoimmune disorders (e.g. thyroid disease, diabetes, Addison's disease, rheumatoid arthritis or vitiligo, 2.75) may suggest pernicious anaemia.

Defective maturation of all proliferating cell lines means that a pancytopenia with reduction in neutrophils and platelets may be present. There may be nucleated megaloblasts in the circulation (**10.31**), but bone marrow examination is usually needed to confirm a megaloblastic basis for the macrocytosis of the circulating red cells (**10.32**). Serum B_{12} and folate assays and red cell folate assay help to identify the underlying deficiency.

In vitamin B_{12} deficiency, it is essential to demonstrate that impaired absorption of the vitamin is corrected by the addition of oral intrinsic factor, before making a diagnosis of classical pernicious anaemia, since other gut pathology (e.g. Crohn's ileitis) may also impair vitamin B_{12} absorption from the terminal ileum. This can be done using the Schilling test, where urinary B_{12} is measured after oral administration, or by whole-body counting of orally administered radio-labelled B_{12}.

There is often elevation of the indirect bilirubin and this is also reflected in the finding of excess urobilinogen in the urine. The serum iron is often elevated and the percentage saturation increased, except in the case of malabsorption (*see* p. 368), when the serum iron, B_{12} and folate levels are all low and a dimorphic blood picture may be present.

In pernicious anaemia, virtually all patients have circulating gastric parietal cell antibodies; 50% also have antibodies to intrinsic factor, and a small percentage have a range of other circulating autoantibodies.

Treatment is with oral replacement of folate and vitamin B_{12} where the cause is dietary. In classical pernicious anaemia, after gastrectomy, and with other uncorrectable gut pathologies, regular injections of hydroxocobalamin are required. Treatment results in a rapid rise in the reticulocyte count, which can be monitored (**10.33**) and precedes the rise in haemoglobin levels. There may also be a fall in the serum iron and a need for supplemental iron therapy. Hydroxocobalamin therapy may reverse early neurological changes in pernicious anaemia; progression of later changes may also be arrested by this therapy. Folate treatment should not be given in megaloblastic anaemia until B_{12} deficiency is ruled out, as folate administration may precipitate neurological changes in patients with B_{12} deficiency.

10.30

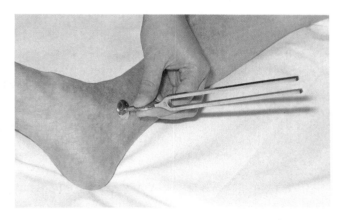

10.30 Loss of vibration sense is often an early sign of subacute combined degeneration of the cord in pernicious anaemia. Higher cerebral function is also frequently affected. The response of these early manifestations of neurological involvement to B_{12} therapy may be good; at later stages, arrest of progression may be the most that can be achieved.

10.31

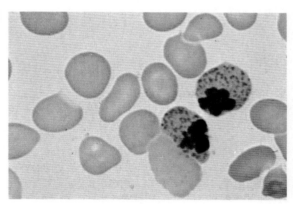

10.31 Peripheral blood in macrocytic anaemia caused by B_{12} deficiency. Note the presence of two late megaloblasts with nuclear rosette formation and basophil stippling. The red cells show macrocytosis, anisocytosis and poikilocytosis.

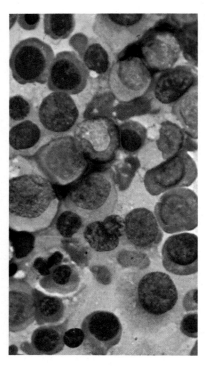

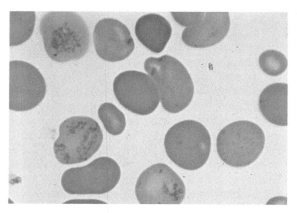

10.33 The 'reticulocyte response' to treatment of megaloblastic anaemia caused by B$_{12}$ or folate deficiency can be very dramatic. This peripheral blood film has been stained for reticulocytes, and it shows a strong response 5 days after the start of hydroxocobalamin therapy in a patient with pernicious anaemia. The rapid increase in erthryopoiesis on treatment may put the patient at risk of developing iron deficiency.

10.32 Marrow smear in pernicious anaemia. Erythroblasts predominate, and erythropoiesis is megaloblastic.

Aplastic anaemia

Marrow aplasia is a rare condition in which there is a peripheral pancytopenia resulting from failure of the stem cells of the bone marrow to continue to produce all cell lines. The marrow architecture remains normal, but fat replaces the normal haemopoietic cells. The result is anaemia and a fall in the white cell and platelet counts. Rarely, only one cell line may be initially affected—as in agranulocytosis—but this usually progresses to total aplasia.

Aplasia is the end result of a variety of processes that include autoimmunity, drugs, toxins, viral infections and radiation. Rarely, there may be a genetic component, and in many cases a cause is not found. In clinical practice the most common causes are drugs (**Table 10.4**), some of which may damage one cell line more than another. Often the drug therapy is being given as part of a treatment regimen for neoplasia or immunosuppression. In these cases the aplasia is usually reversible. There is also an association of aplastic anaemia with the later development of acute lymphocytic leukaemia in childhood; and in adults exposed to benzene or radiation there is a significant incidence of acute myeloid leukaemia after many years.

Clinical symptoms and presentation in aplastic anaemia relate to the lack of functional cells in the peripheral blood. There is an insidious onset of the symptoms of anaemia, with recurrent infections as the white cell count falls, and bleeding from multiple sites as a result of thrombocytopenia. Clinical examination usually shows purpura and ecchymoses (**10.34**), and there may also be internal bleeding especially from the gums and alimentary tract and into the eye. There may be infection in the mouth (**10.35**), or skin. There is rarely any splenic enlargement, and this helps to distinguish aplastic anaemia from pancytopenias associated with hypersplenism (*see* p. 443).

The diagnosis is made on finding pancytopenia in the peripheral blood. Bone marrow aspirate may yield little available marrow and a trephine bone biopsy may be required for histological section (**10.36**). Treatment should be initially directed at the cause. Androgens and corticosteroids are of value in some patients. Supportive treatment with red cell, platelet and white cell transfusions may be necessary. Bone marrow transplantation is successful in about 70% of patients with aplastic anaemia, but a matched donor is not always available. Anti-lymphocyte globulin (ALG) or other immunosuppressive therapy is sometimes helpful where marrow transplant is not possible. Recently, growth factors produced by recombinant DNA technology have been shown to be of value.

Table 10.4 Drugs that may cause marrow aplasia.

Antimitotics	methotrexate, cytosine arabinoside, busulphan, cyclophosphamide, 6-mercaptopurine
Antibiotics	chloramphenicol, methicillin, penicillin, tetracyclines, sulphonamides
Anti-rheumatics	gold salts, penicillamine, indomethacin, colchicine
Anticonvulsants	phenytoin, carbamazepine
Anti-diabetic	chlorpropamide, tolbutamide
Anti-thyroid	carbimazole, thiouracil, potassium perchlorate
Tranquillizers	chlorpromazine, chlordiazepoxide, meprobamate, promazine

10.34

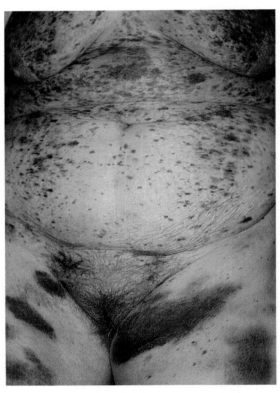

10.35

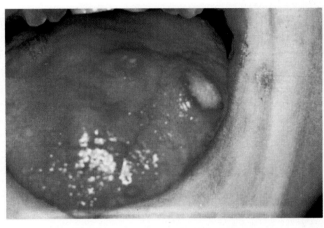

10.35 Aplastic anaemia. This patient initially developed agranulocytosis, manifest as severe, intractable mouth ulcers and respiratory tract infection. The cause was unclear, but he progressed to develop pancytopenia and true aplastic anaemia.

10.36

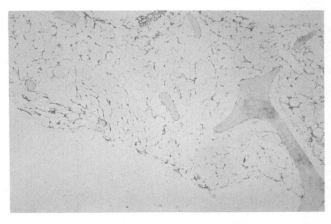

10.34 Aplastic anaemia developed when this 76-year-old woman was treated with co-trimoxazole for a urinary tract infection. Thrombocytopenia is responsible for her widespread purpura and ecchymoses, and she also had a severe throat infection as a result of her low white cell count.

10.36 Aplastic anaemia can be confirmed by trephine biopsy of iliac crest marrow. This low-power view of a trephine biopsy from a young woman with drug-induced severe aplastic anaemia, showed loss of virtually all haemopoietic cells, with only a few residual lymphocytes and no inflammatory response. This marrow picture usually carries a grave prognosis.

Haemolytic anaemias

Haemolysis is suggested by evidence of both increased red cell production (reticulocytosis) and increased red cell destruction. The destruction may be intravascular (giving rise acutely to haemoglobinuria, or chronically to haemosiderinuria) and a reduced concentration of serum haptoglobin (haemoglobin-binding protein), or extravascular (mediated by macrophages), and associated with increased unconjugated bilirubin in the blood. Clinically, the combination of pallor, jaundice (9.2, 10.37) and splenomegaly (9.19) should suggest haemolysis, and, in chronic cases, there may be symptoms or signs of pigment gallstones (*see* p. 409), or signs of iron overload (10.38). A blood film may sometimes show red cell abnormalities that are diagnostic of particular causes of haemolysis; but it may show only a non-specific polychromasia associated with the reticulocytosis.

Haemolysis may result from intrinsic, nearly always inherited, defects of the red cell, or from acquired disorders, usually related to extracorpuscular changes:

- **Intrinsic disorders** include those of the cell membrane (e.g. hereditary spherocytosis, hereditary elliptocytosis), of haemoglobin synthesis (e.g. sickle cell disease) and of cell metabolism (e.g. pyruvate kinase or glucose-6-phosphate dehydrogenase deficiencies).
- **Extrinsic causes of haemolysis** include chronic renal failure and liver disease, but the shortening of red cell survival in these conditions is usually only modest. Excepting these, the most common acquired haemolytic anaemias are immune in origin: iso-immune—as in haemolytic disease of the newborn or haemolytic blood transfusion reactions; auto-immune with antibodies directed against red cell antigens and giving rise to positive direct antiglobulin (Coombs') test; or drug-induced, where the effect may result from auto-antibodies or neo-antigens involving the drug as a hapten. Non-antibody-mediated haemolytic anaemia may also be acquired, as in paroxysmal nocturnal haemoglobinuria and in some drug-induced haemolysis.
- Fragmentation haemolysis may be seen in association with disseminated intravascular coagulation (microangiopathic haemolysis, 10.107), in patients with artificial heart valves and in malaria.
- Hypersplenism with haemolysis may be a feature of a variety of disorders associated with splenomegaly.

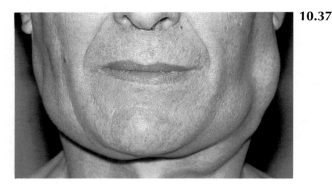

10.37

10.37 Haemolytic anaemia may lead to a characteristic lemon-yellow jaundice, as in this man who developed warm auto-immune haemolysis in association with chronic lymphocytic leukaemia (*see* pp. 439 and 447). Note his 'bull neck' appearance, which results from gross cervical lymphadenopathy.

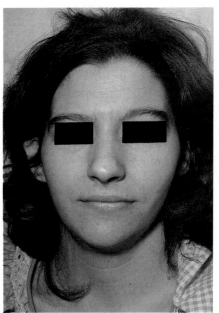

10.38

10.38 Secondary haemochromatosis, giving a characteristic skin pigmentation, may be a long-term consequence of the iron overload associated with chronic haemolytic anaemia. This 19-year-old patient had α-thalassaemia. Note the combination of pigmentation and pallor.

Red cell membrane defects

A variety of chemical and physical defects have been described in the red cell membrane. The most common and most important is **hereditary spherocytosis**, which is found in 1–2 per 10,000 of the population, and is usually transmitted as an autosomal dominant. The biochemical defect, which may be quantitative or qualitative, is in the production of the protein spectrin; the result is the production of spherical red cells which have an altered permeability and a significantly shortened half life. Clinically there is a wide spectrum of severity, even within families, but the picture usually includes haemolytic anaemia, acholuric jaundice and splenomegaly (**10.39**). Most patients can lead a normal life, even when slightly anaemic. However, at times (e.g. in acute infections) an acute haemolytic crisis may occur, which requires blood transfusion. Aplastic crises may also occur during *Parvovirus* and other infections in these patients, especially in young children (*see* p. 27). The erythroid hyperplasia leads to an increased need for folic acid, which should be given prophylactically. The chronic haemolytic state is associated with pigment gall stones in most adults and patients may present with a confusing mixed haemolytic and obstructive jaundice. Other cells require spectrin for normal function and associated abnormalities have been described in neurological and cardiac cell function.

The diagnosis is confirmed by finding evidence of chronic haemolysis and a typical blood film with microspherocytosis of red cells and reticulocytosis (**10.40**). The red cells are osmotically fragile and this provides a useful screening test. Assay of spectrin is possible in some laboratories. It is important to screen all available family members for the condition. The treatment of choice is splenectomy, which must be followed by appropriate vaccination against the pneumococcus, meningococcus and *H. influenzae* and by long-term prophylactic penicillin therapy. It is important at surgery to ensure that there are no accessory splenunculae as these will hypertrophy if not removed and haemolysis will continue.

Hereditary elliptocytosis is caused by a variety of molecular defects and is usually asymptomatic. The diagnosis is made on the typical appearances of the blood film (**10.41**), but only a few patients have significant anaemia or any evidence of haemolysis.

10.39

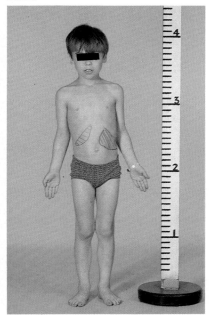

10.40

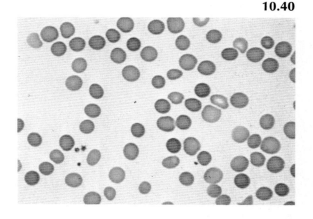

10.39 Hereditary spherocytosis. This 9-year-old boy shows typical mild pallor. He has marked splenomegaly and mild heptomegaly.

10.40 Hereditary spherocytosis. This low-power view of a peripheral blood film shows that approximately half the red cells are small and very deeply stained. These cells have the characteristic appearance of spherocytes, though the other cells in the film are within the normal range. Often, only a proportion of the red cells are affected in spherocytosis. Supravital staining revealed a reticulocyte count of 60% in this patient.

10.41

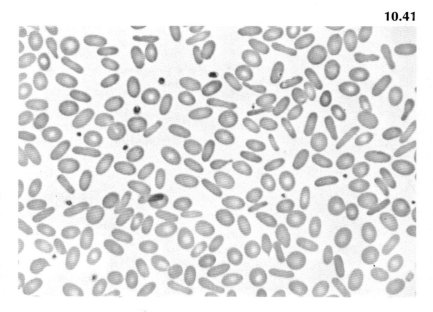

10.41 Hereditary elliptocytosis. This inherited anomaly of red cells leads to their assuming an oval or cigar shape. As in hereditary spherocytosis, some normal red cells are also usually present—in this case, about 50%. Pseudo-elliptocytosis may occur as a result of bad technique when a blood smear is prepared; but when this occurs, the 'elliptocytes' are usually found only at one end of the smear, and the long axes of the cells are roughly parallel.

Enzyme deficiencies in red cells

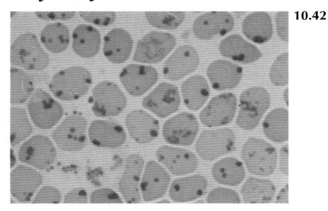

10.42

10.42 Glucose-6-phosphate dehydrogenase deficiency leads to the formation of Heinz bodies in the erythrocytes. Here, the bodies have been stained with methyl violet. They represent precipitates of denatured haemoglobin, resulting from the lack of reducing enzymes.

Normal function of red cells depends on the integrity of two enzyme systems to provide energy from glucose as the substrate. These are the Embden–Myerhof pathway and the hexose–monophosphate shunt. Many enzyme defects have been described, but only two are common:

- **Glucose-6-phosphate dehydrogenase (G6PD) deficiency** results in inability of the red cell to resist oxidants that may result from infections or from drug administration. As a result, haemoglobin is oxidised to methaemoglobin, which is functionless in terms of oxygen carriage, is relatively insoluble and precipitates in the red cells as Heinz bodies (**10.42**). The red cells are then vulnerable to destruction in the spleen. A large number of variants of enzyme activity have now been identified, accounting for a wide spectrum of disease activity. The disorder usually presents with acute intravascular haemolysis—jaundice, haemoglobinuria, anaemia and methaemoglobinaemia. A large number of drugs and foods have been implicated in precipitating the acute episodes. Offending substances should be avoided or withdrawn. Blood transfusion may be life-saving during acute attacks.
- **Pyruvate kinase deficiency** is the most common of the many enzyme defects of the glycolytic pathway. The disease is inherited as an autosomal recessive, and it is only the homozygotes that haemolyse. The enzyme-deficient cells have a significantly shortened life span, and the haemolysis is chronic and not related to infections, drugs or foods. Splenomegaly is usually found. The definitive diagnosis is made by measurement of enzyme activity, and homozygous patients are usually clinically anaemic with a reticulocytosis (**10.11**). Secondary haemochromatosis may occur (**10.38**).

Sickle cell syndromes

A single amino acid substitution (valine for glutamic acid) at position 6 of the β-chain of globin, results in a haemoglobin with abnormal physical and chemical properties. Haemoglobin S (HbS) can be found in the homozygous state (Hb SS, sickle cell disease), in the heterozygous state (Hb AS, sickle cell trait), or in association with all the other globin chain variants including haemoglobin C, D, F and β-thalassaemia. The abnormal gene has a worldwide distribution, but is most common in those of African origin. It may confer a biological advantage against infection with falciparum malaria and have increased in this ethnic group by natural selection.

Disease results from polymerisation of HbS molecules within the red cells. This causes chronic haemolytic states, chronic organ damage from vascular occlusion and acute crises with haemolysis, vascular occlusion and tissue death. Polymerisation occurs only when HbS is in the deoxy form, and the subsequent crystallisation results in cells that become rigid and sickle shaped and are unable to deform to pass through capillaries. This physical alteration is reversible when the molecules are again oxygenated, unless the red cell membrane is severely damaged.

People heterozygous for HbS (sickle cell trait) are usually asymptomatic unless exposed to lowered oxygen tensions (as in unpressurised aircraft, at high altitude, or sometimes during anaesthesia). Renal microinfarcts occur in heterozygotes, however, and patients may complain of haematuria and eventually develop renal impairment.

People who are homozygous for HbS (sickle cell disease) suffer from chronic haemolysis, which is usually adequately compensated. Their haemoglobin level runs at 5–10 g/dl, with a reticulocyte count of 10–30%. There is usually mild jaundice resulting from elevation of the unconjugated bilirubin fraction. Acute haemolytic crises may be precipitated by infections, pregnancy, drugs, surgery and anaesthesia, which may also precipitate acute vascular occlusion in the microcirculation with tissue death. Sickle cell crises are associated with fever, malaise and pain, which may be severe, and can occur in most parts of the body. Organs affected include bone (**10.43–10.45**), muscle, brain, eye (**10.46**), lung, spleen, liver, kidney and skin. Infection often occurs in the infarcted tissue, and chronic infection frequently complicates bone and joint ischaemia (**3.119, 10.47**). Pigment gall stones are common as a result of the chronic haemolysis. The disease carries a high mortality in young children, and death usually results from renal failure, overwhelming infection or vascular occlusion.

The diagnosis is confirmed by a positive sickling test (10.48, 10.49) and by haemoglobin electrophoresis (10.50). Pre-natal and cord-blood screening programmes should aid early diagnosis, and subsequent medical supervision may prevent long-term sequelae.

Management should be aimed at the prevention of infections and other situations that cause acute haemolytic and vascular crises. Acute crises require adequate oxygenation, rehydration, antibiotics and adequate pain control. Anaemia may be treated by blood transfusion, but in the long term, this may result in haemosiderosis/secondary haemochromatosis.

10.43

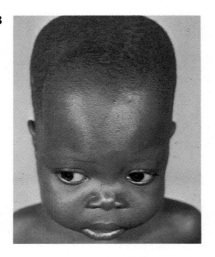

10.43 Bossing of the skull caused by hyperplasia of the bone marrow is common in sickle cell disease, and similar appearances may be seen in thalassaemia and other severe, congenital haemolytic anaemias.

10.44

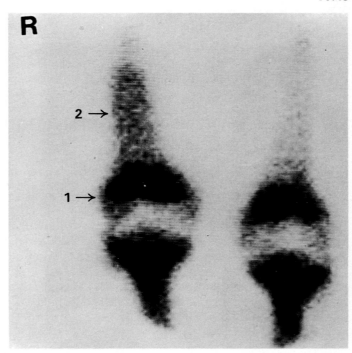

10.44 A 'hair on end' appearance of the skull on X-ray is commonly associated with frontal bossing in sickle cell disease. As with bossing, this appearance may also be seen in thalassaemia and other severe congenital haemolytic anaemias.

10.45

10.45 A bone scan in a patient with sickle cell disease. There is increased activity in both epiphyseal growth plates (1) and an area of abnormal isotope uptake in the lower right femur. This abnormality reflects recurrent episodes of avascular necrosis with repair, but this process also renders the bone especially susceptible to osteomyelitis caused by *Salmonella* or other organisms.

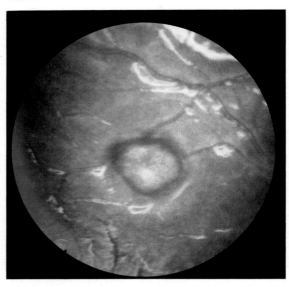

10.46 Sickle cell retinopathy. Intermittent occlusion of small blood vessels by inflexible sickle-shaped cells commonly leads to characteristic 'salmon-patch' haemorrhages in the retina. These may evolve into pigmented retinal scars. The retinal vessels are also tortuous. At a later stage, proliferative retinopathy may also occur. Similar changes may be seen in other severe haemolytic anaemias, including thalassaemia.

10.47 Severe dactylitis (inflammation of the fingers) is a common presentation of sickle cell disease in children, and similar changes may occur in the feet. The painful swelling of the fingers commonly results from destructive changes in the small bones resulting from multiple infarctions, and sometimes complicated by osteomyelitis.

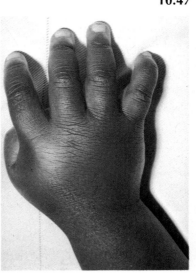

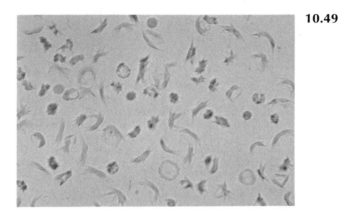

10.48

10.48 A fresh blood smear from a patient with sickle cell disease shows few elongated or sickled cells, but anisocytosis, poikilocytosis and target cells are all seen.

10.49

10.49 Sickle cells can be formed by exposing red cells from a patient with sickle cell disease to the reducing action of sodium metabisulphite under a sealed coverslip. As the reduced HbS crystallises within the cells, they all come to assume the distorted, elongated sickle shape.

10.50

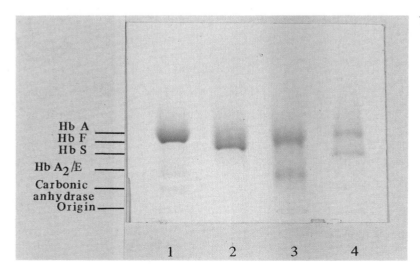

Hb A
Hb F
Hb S
Hb A$_2$/E
Carbonic anhydrase
Origin

1   2   3   4

10.50 Haemoglobin electrophoresis. Haemoglobins containing variant globin chains may have different electrophoretic mobility. Cellulose acetate electrophoresis at alkaline pH is commonly used as an initial screen. Lane 1, normal adult (predominantly HbA, $\alpha_2 \beta_2$); lane 2, neonatal cord blood (predominantly HbF, $\alpha_2 \gamma_2$), lane 3, heterozygous HbE (containing both HBA and HbE, $\alpha2 \beta^E_2$); lane 4, HbS heterozygote (sickle cell trait containing both HbA and HbS, $\alpha \beta^S_2$).

Thalassaemia

Thalassaemia is the name given to a group of haemoglobinopathies that result from genetic mutations affecting synthesis of normal globins. The two major types are α and β thalassaemia, which are caused by defective synthesis of the α and β globin polypeptides. This results in failure of normal haemoglobin synthesis and the production of abnormal red cells that are hypochromic and microcytic.

Thalassaemia trait

The most common abnormality is thalassaemia trait (or thalassaemia minor), which is the heterozygous form of α or β thalassaemia. This is usually associated with very mild defects in the red cells with microcytosis (MCV 55–75) and hypochromia (MCH 20–22) and sometimes with a chronic very mild anaemia with a haematocrit of about 30 and a slightly raised red cell count (10.51). The condition is common in certain parts of the world and affects up to 20% of people from parts of Africa, Asia and the Mediterranean. There are many variants of thalassaemia minor associated with a range of other minor abnormal haemoglobins. Thalassaemia trait probably confers protection against falciparum malaria and this selective advantage accounts for the high gene frequency in areas where malaria is evident.

No treatment is required for thalassaemia minor, but it is important to exclude iron-deficiency which may compound the anaemia: routine measurement of ferritin and serum iron is necessary. Detection of the condition before reproductive age allows appropriate genetic counselling.

10.51

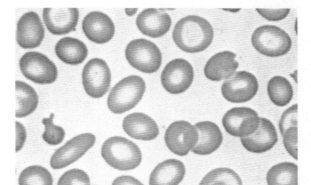

10.51 Blood film in ß-thalassaemia minor. The red cells are hypochromic, there are prominent target cells, and the film shows anisocytosis and poikilocytosis. Several thin, flat cells (leptocytes) and elliptocytes are also present. Some patients with thalassaemia minor show little more than microcytosis and hypochromia.

Severe β-thalassaemia (Cooley's anaemia)

People homozygous for β-thalassaemia (in whom both genes are defective) have a marked defect in β-globin synthesis, while α-globin synthesis continues normally. This results in the accumulation in red cells of excessive α-globin chains, which are relatively insoluble when uncombined with β-globin chains and thus form large intracellular inclusions. The red cells have a high incidence of failure of maturation within the marrow (ineffective haemopoiesis), and those that are released have a short life-span because of splenic trapping. The resultant severe anaemia stimulates production of excess erythropoietin which stimulates further erythroblast proliferation, extension of marrow production to most bones and increased absorption of iron. The process is so active that osteoporosis and pathological fractures may occur, and some bones may become extremely hyperplastic (10.43, 10.44, 10.52). Compression of the cord may result from vertebral growth, and alteration of the facies may result from overgrowth of the bones of the face ('chipmunk facies'). Retinal changes may occur, as in sickle cell disease (10.46). In severe anaemia (thalassaemia major), there is an absolute need for repeated blood transfusion (which results in iron overload) to maintain oxygenation. In less severe forms (thalassaemia intermedia), the patient is able to maintain a reasonable haemoglobin level (6–8 g/dl) without recourse to blood transfusion, and these patients survive into adult life.

In thalassaemia major, the clinical picture emerges in the first year of life with severe anaemia, failure to thrive and retardation of growth. Examination shows evidence of both spleen and liver enlargement (10.53). Laboratory tests show typical red cell appearances (10.54), and examination of the parents' blood shows the presence of thalassaemia trait. The diagnosis is confirmed by haemoglobin electrophoresis (10.50) and demonstration of defective β-globin synthesis by the reticulocytes.

There is a high morbidity and mortality unless the infants are regularly transfused with blood to suppress their own haemopoiesis. This can reduce the disease manifestations and allow normal growth and bone development. Repeated transfusion produces problems of iron overload with secondary haemochromatosis, and also a risk of viral infections (especially with hepatitis viruses and HIV). Cardiac disease is also common, with heart failure, myocarditis and pericarditis.

Iron overload can be treated with desferrioxamine infusions and there is evidence that this will prolong life, but it must be given by intravenous infusion, is difficult to administer to large numbers of patients and is expensive. Vitamin C may also be given to enhance iron chelation. Splenectomy should be considered, in an attempt to increase the life-span of red cells. If neutropenia and thrombocytopenia are present, this is good evidence that there is hypersplenism. After splenectomy, it is important to vaccinate the child against infection—especially with the pneumococcus—and to administer long-term prophylaxis with penicillin. Bone marrow transplantation should be considered in selected cases.

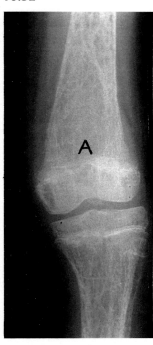

10.52 Thalassaemia major is usually associated with widespread bone changes resulting from marrow hyperplasia. The distal femur in this patient is expanded, giving a 'flask shaped' appearance. The bones are generally osteopenic (A), with a sparse, coarse, dense travecular pattern. This appearance is not in itself diagnostic of thalassaemia; similar appearances may occur in other haemolytic anaemias, especially sickle cell disease.

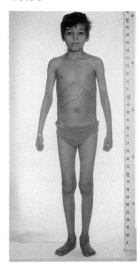

10.53 ß-thalassaemia major. Hepatosplenomegaly is usual, as in this young patient.

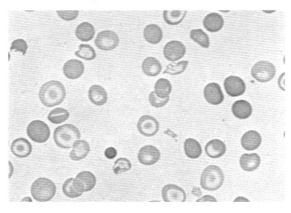

10.54

10.54 Severe ß-thalassaemia. The blood film shows much more severe changes than those seen in **10.51**, with hypochromia, target cells, macrocytes, spherocytes, schistocytes—including helmet cells—and small cell fragments.

Thalassaemia intermedia

Some patients with thalassaemia are able to maintain their haemoglobin levels adequately without recourse to blood transfusion. However, iron accumulation occurs because of increased intestinal absorption and eventually causes secondary haemochromatosis with all the effects already described. Osteoporosis, bone overgrowth and arthritis are frequent and produce disfiguring skeletal abnormalities.

α-Thalassaemia

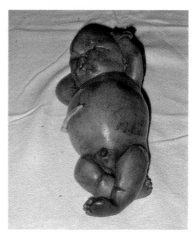

10.55

10.55 Hydrops fetalis in severe α-thalassaemia. The most severe form of the disease is incompatible with life, and the fetus usually dies in utero.

Various gene mutations or deletions may lead to defects in the synthesis of α-globin chains, and a spectrum of red cell abnormalities in which the red cells are hypochromic, microcytic and easily fragmented. The defective α chains may be accompanied by the production of abnormal β chain polymers, which are unstable and lead to rapid haemolysis.

From 1 to 4 genes may be involved, resulting in:

- No detectable disease (1 or 2 gene defect).
- Moderately severe haemolysis (3 gene defect – haemoglobin H disease).
- Fetal death – hydrops fetalis (**10.55**) (4 gene defect).

In haemoglobin H disease, splenomegaly is frequent, and the spleen may require removal if there is evidence of hypersplenism. Folic acid and occasional blood transfusion may be required.

Acquired haemolytic anaemias

The most common type of acquired haemolytic anaemia results from the presence of auto-antibodies, which attach to the red cells and reduce their survival by enhancing their phagocytosis by reticuloendothelial cells. This condition is diagnosed by finding a positive Coombs' test. The antibodies may be 'warm antibodies', most active at 37°C (usually IgG), or in 'cold antibodies', most active at lower temperatures (usually IgM). Both types of anaemia may be idiopathic, but underlying causes may be found:

- **Warm autoimmune haemolysis** may be associated with lymphoma, chronic lymphatic leukaemia (**10.37**), systemic lupus erythematosus, AIDS or hypogammaglobulinaemia. It gives rise to red cell spherocytosis, which can be morphologically indistinguishable from that of congenital spherocytosis

(**10.39**): treatment with prednisolone may produce a remission, but splenectomy needs to be considered where this is ineffective or requires an unacceptably high steroid dose.

- **Cold autoimmune haemolysis** (**10.56, 10.57**) may be transient in association with infectious mononucleosis (*see* p. 32) or mycoplasma pneumonia (*see* p. 60, 187), may be seen in malaria (*see* p. 68), and may occur with a monoclonal IgM paraprotein in idiopathic cold haemagglutinin disease (CHAD) and with lymphoma: avoidance of the cold is the main line of treatment to avoid precipitating intravascular haemolysis or exacerbating the Raynaud's phenomenon that is common in this disorder (*see* p. 255). Cold antibodies often do not cause haemolysis; they may then be suspected from the presence of a strikingly raised ESR.

10.56 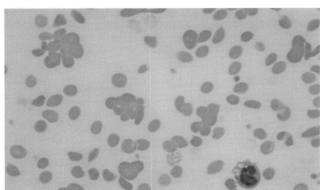 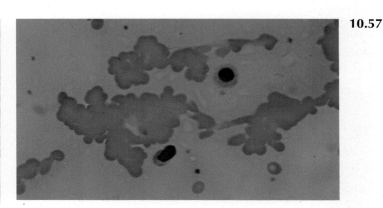 **10.57**

10.56, 10.57 Cold auto-immune haemolysis. A blood film from the patient viewed at 37°C (**10.56**) is essentially normal, though slight clumping of the red cells is seen in places. By contrast, in a film made at room temperature (**10.57**), extreme agglutination of the cells has occurred.

Drug-induced immune haemolysis

Drugs may induce haemolysis in three ways:

- **Acute intravascular haemolysis** may occur when a drug stimulates antibody formation and the resulting immune complex is absorbed on to the red cell where it fixes complement. Haemolysis occurs on a second exposure. Drugs such as chlorpropamide and quinine are involved.
- **Slow-onset haemolysis** may occur when a drug becomes attached to the red cell membrane and acts as a hapten. IgG antibody against the drug attaches to the cell and leads to extravascular destruction of the coated cell. This type of

reaction is seen with penicillins and cephalosporins.

- **Auto-immune haemolysis** may be seen after some months of therapy with methyldopa, L-dopa, mefenamic acid and flufenamic acid. The mechanism is not well understood. In up to 20% of patients on methyldopa, there is IgG coating of red cells, but only a small percentage of these patients (5–10%) show evidence of haemolysis.

Stopping the drug usually leads to rapid resolution, but a short course of prednisolone may be necessary in the auto-immune haemolysis caused by methyldopa.

Haemolytic disease of the newborn

In haemolytic disease of the newborn, maternal IgG antibodies to fetal red cell antigens cross the placenta and affect the fetal red cells, leading to iso-immune haemolysis. Antibodies are usually against the Rhesus-group antigens, usually Rh(D), and they develop where the mother is Rh(D) negative; but they may also be against ABO and other rarer blood groups. Sensitisation in a Rh(D)-negative mother occurs after a first pregnancy with a Rh(D)-positive fetus, usually as a result of leakage of fetal red cells into the maternal circulation at parturition; it may also result from a previous blood transfusion. Subsequent pregnancies may be affected with increasing severity, depending on the antibody levels that result. Severe haemolytic anaemia may appear in the fetus at the end of the first trimester or in the second trimester, and may result in fetal death (hydrops fetalis, **10.55**). In less severe cases, icterus may be apparent at birth and may lead to kernicterus, the deposition of indirect bilirubin in the basal ganglia of the neonate brain (**10.59**).

All mothers should have their blood tested for anti-Rh(D) antibodies at the initial booking visit to the antenatal clinic. A rising titre of antibody is an indication for fetal blood transfusion and careful fetal monitoring. Early delivery may be required, in which case prematurity with its complications must be weighed against the risks of anaemia.

If the presentation is at birth, the cord blood sample will show anemia with a positive Coombs' test, an elevated indirect bilirubin and normoblasts and a high reticulocyte count on the blood film. Exchange transfusion is urgently indicated.

The incidence of this disease has fallen dramatically as a result of the administration within 72 hours of delivery of human anti-D IgG to all Rh(D)-negative mothers who have their first Rh(D)-positive child and who are not already sensitised. This attaches to fetal red cells in the maternal circulation and neutralises their sensitising effect. Fetal cells can be detected in the maternal circulation using the Kleihauer technique (**10.58**); if they are still present after treatment, further anti-D may be needed. Occasional cases of haemolytic disease of the newborn still occur because of ABO blood group antibodies or because of Rh(D) sensitisation at earlier stages in pregnancy.

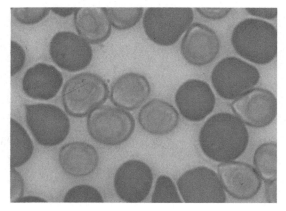 10.58

10.59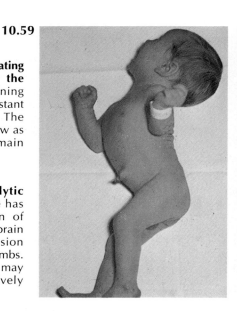

10.58 The Kleihauer reaction, demonstrating the presence of fetal red cells in the maternal circulation. The HbF-containing fetal cells are more acid and alkali resistant than the HbA-containing adult cells. The adult cells are lysed in the test and show as pale 'ghosts', while the fetal cells remain unlysed in this film.

10.59 Kernicterus in severe haemolytic disease of the newborn. The neonate has severe jaundice, and the deposition of bilirubin in the basal ganglia results in brain damage, manifest as neck hyperextension and hypertonic extensor spasm of the limbs. Severe motor and intellectual disability may result if neonatal jaundice is not actively managed.

Non-immune haemolytic anaemia

Paroxysmal nocturnal haemoglobinuria (PNH) is a clonal change in red cells and is part of the myeloproliferative spectrum of disorders. The red cell lacks a factor which destroys the complement which normally accumulates on red cells. This results in an intermittent type of acute intravascular haemolysis. PNH may complicate aplastic anaemia. Acute attacks of intravascular haemolysis are precipitated by infection, surgery and anaesthesia and the patient passes dark red-brown urine, often first thing in the morning. There is an association with acute thrombotic episodes caused by platelet and white cell activation and there may be a sequel of acute myeloid leukaemia or aplastic anaemia.

Myeloproliferative disorders

Polycythaemia

Polycythaemia refers to a group of disorders in which there is elevation of the haemoglobin, packed cell volume and the red cell count (**Table 10.5**). In true polycythaemia there is an absolute increase in the red cell mass, while in apparent or relative polycythaemias, the red cell mass is normal and the rise in packed cell volume is secondary to a reduced plasma volume. The clinical significance of these disorders is their significant association with thrombotic disorders, e.g. myocardial infarction, stroke, peripheral vascular disease and deep vein thrombosis. This results from the increase in whole blood viscosity, which leads to reduced blood flow.

The most important disease is **primary proliferative polycythaemia** (polycythaemia rubra vera), which, like myelofibrosis and essential thrombocythaemia, is a myeloproliferative disorder. The defect seems to be clonal and originate in a stem cell that produces defects in the erythroid, granulocyte and megakaryocyte components of the marrow.

Often, the diagnosis is reached by chance, with the finding of an elevated haemoglobin on a routine blood sample, or the chance finding of splenomegaly on clinical examination; or it may be recognised only after an acute thrombotic event. The major clinical clues are facial plethora (**10.60**), conjunctival suffusion and splenomegaly, present in 70% of patients. Other associated features are acne rosacea (*see* p. 106), urticaria (*see* p. 96), leg ulcers, retinal changes (**10.61**) and loss of vision because of retinal haemorrhage. The liver is enlarged in up to 50% of patients, and hypertension is present in about 20%.

Evidence should be sought of previous stroke, peripheral vascular disease or deep vein thrombosis. Itch is found in about 15% of patients, and there may be signs of chronic excoriation. The condition is also associated with peptic ulcer and acute gout (*see* p. 140).

The diagnosis is suspected from the full blood count and confirmed by the measurement of red cell mass. There may be associated elevation of the white cell count and platelets. The bone marrow shows gross erythroid hyperplasia with normoblastic erythropoiesis. There may be associated iron deficiency, seen on staining the marrow with Prussian Blue. The leucocyte alkaline phosphatase score is high, which is the opposite of that found in chronic myeloid leukaemia. The uric acid levels are characteristically elevated. About 60% of patients die of thrombotic events, about 20% progress to myelofibrosis and a small number (<10%) progress to acute myeloid leukaemia. Treatment is required to lower the haemoglobin and this is done with repeated venesection or with ^{32}P. Because radiophosphorus is associated with a tenfold increase in the risk of leukaemia, its use is best reserved for elderly patients. Allopurinol should be routinely administered to patients with hyperuricaemia to prevent gout.

Secondary polycythaemia (4.6) is not associated with such a large risk of thrombotic events. Treatment should be directed at the cause, but often this is not amenable to change. A reduction in haematocrit may be achieved by continuous oxygen therapy. Patients must stop smoking.

Table 10.5 Polycythaemia.

True
- Primary proliferative polycythaemia
- Secondary
  - (a) Hypoxic:
    - Altitude
    - Chronic lung disease
    - Cyanotic congenital heart disease
    - Smoking
  - (b) Excess erythropoietin:
    - Polycystic kidneys
    - Renal carcinoma
    - Renal cysts
    - Chronic glomerulonephritis
    - Chronic liver disease
    - Hepatocellular carcinoma
    - Ovarian carcinoma
    - Bronchial carcinoma
  - (c) Overtransfusion

Apparent
- Acute fluid loss
- 'Gaisbock's syndrome'

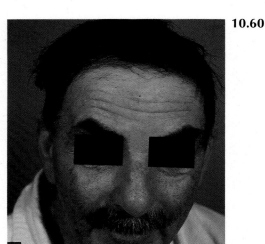

10.60 Primary proliferative polycythaemia (polycythaemia rubra vera). The patient has a generalised plethoric appearance, most obvious on, but not confined to, the face.

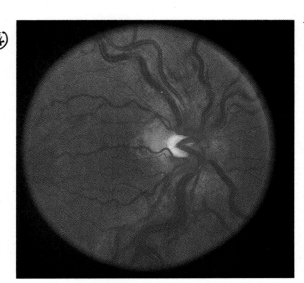

10.61 The fundus in polycythaemia of any cause usually shows engorged and tortuous vessels. Other causes of blood hyperviscosity, including multiple myeloma, may lead to a similar retinal appearance. Thrombosis in the retinal vessels and retinal haemorrhages may occur in patients with hyperviscosity of any cause.

Myelofibrosis

In myelofibrosis increased fibrous tissue is formed within the marrow cavity, normal haemopoiesis is disturbed and there is extramedullary haemopoiesis in spleen and liver. It is in the same group of myeloproliferative disorders as polycythaemia, chronic myeloid leukaemia and essential thombocythaemia and it may be a consequence of these disorders, the fibrous tissue being reactive to the other events in the bone marrow.

In many patients the disease is asymptomatic and the diagnosis is made by finding hepatosplenomegaly on routine clinical examination for some other reason. Alternatively, blood examination for some other purpose may show a leucoerythroblastic state. Some patients present with anaemia or with progressive abdominal swelling (caused by the hepatosplenomegaly) and some with splenic infarction as the enlarging spleen outgrows its blood supply. Portal hypertension may also develop in some patients, with ascites and even bleeding from oesophageal varices compounding the anaemia. Purpura and bleeding may result from thrombocytopenia as a result of hypersplenism, and also from coagulation abnormalities caused by liver disease. Gout may occur, as a result of the hyperuricamia.

In a typical patient, there is usually evidence of weight loss with thin spindly legs and arms that contrast with the obvious abdominal distension. The spleen is usually grossly, and the liver moderately, enlarged (as in other conditions, *see* **1.185, 1.188**). There may be some ascites. Lymph nodes may also be large but non-tender. Bruises and purpura may be present.

Characteristic changes in routine blood tests include a low haemoglobin, which may partly result from blood loss with iron deficiency, folate deficiency and dilution from an increased plasma volume. Normoblasts may be present in great numbers in peripheral blood (this may interfere with automated white cell counters) showing a leucoerythroblastic state (**10.62**). The platelet count and white cell count may be low. The leucocyte alkaline phosphatase is high, as in primary proliferative polycythaemia, and this allows differentiation from chronic myeloid leukaemia. Attempts to aspirate bone marrow often result in a 'dry tap' because of the amount of fibrous tissue. Trephine biopsy shows a hypercellular marrow with an increase in fibrous tissue, a decrease in fat and haemopoietic tissue, but often an excess of megakaryocytes. It is important to remember other causes of marrow fibrosis, including carcinomatous infiltration (especially from breast and prostate), previous radiation exposure, infections such as tuberculosis and osteomyelitis, and Paget's disease. Using cyclotron-produced iron-52 it is possible to identify the sites of active erythropoiesis, which will include the liver, spleen and lymph nodes (extramedullary haemopoiesis). X-ray of bones will show an increase in bone density, particularly in the vertebrae.

Treatment is supportive and symptomatic. Iron and folate deficiency should be corrected and gout treated with allopurinol. Blood transfusion may be necessary for severe anaemia. In some situations splenectomy should be considered to reduce haemolysis, remove an infarcted spleen, or when there is severe abdominal discomfort or swelling. Unfortunately, this may often lead to rapid enlargement of the liver. Splenic size may also be controlled with radiotherapy.

Death usually occurs from progressive marrow failure, with bleeding from thrombocytopenia, leucopenia and overwhelming infection, and persistent anaemia. Transformation to acute myeloid leukaemia sometimes occurs.

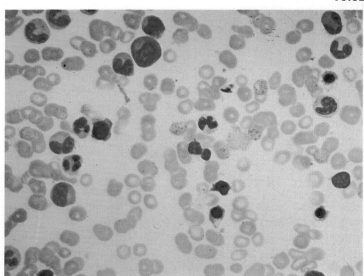

10.62 Leucoerythroblastic peripheral blood film in myelofibrosis. A leucoerythroblastic state is characterised by the presence of abnormally immature white cells and nucleated red cells, and the appearance commonly reflects severe marrow dysfunction. The appearance is not in itself diagnostic of myelofibrosis; it may be seen in chronic infection, malignancy, metabolic disorders that affect bone and in acute severe haemolytic anaemia. This blood picture is usually an indication for marrow aspiration or trephine biopsy.

Essential thrombocythaemia

Essential thrombocythaemia is part of the myeloproliferative spectrum in which there is proliferation of the megakaryocyte series with the production of excessive numbers of platelets, which may be functionally impaired. Patients present with some of the features of the associated disorders (polycythaemia, chronic myeloid leukaemia and myelofibrosis), including spontaneous bruising, epistaxis, gastrointestinal, vaginal or respiratory tract bleeding. Thrombotic occlusion of arteries, leading to myocardial infarction, stroke, gangrene or intestinal infarction, is common.

Clinical examination may show evidence of bleeding or of thrombosis. The spleen and liver are often felt, although in the later stages splenic atrophy is common.

The diagnosis is made on the finding of platelet counts of 1000–2000 $\times 10^9$/l. The red cell and white cell counts may also be high. The bleeding time may be prolonged and platelet function studies are often abnormal. Megakaryocytes are increased in the marrow. Straight X-ray of the abdomen may show an atrophic calcified spleen.

Treatment is aimed at reduction of the platelet count either by platelet pheresis or by use of ^{32}P or a cytotoxic agent such as busulphan or cyclophosphamide.

Hypersplenism

Any pathological condition that causes splenomegaly (**Table 10.6**) may result in peripheral blood cytopenia caused by:

- Pooling of cells within the spleen and their subsequent destruction.
- Increased plasma volume with dilution of cell numbers.

The diagnosis is usually obvious from the findings of peripheral cytopenia, a hypercellular marrow and splenomegaly. The diagnosis may be confirmed by ^{51}Cr-red cell labelling with surface counting over the spleen.

Splenectomy results in a rapid reversal of these abnormalities. Acutely, there is a transient thrombocytosis and neutrophil leucocytosis. In the long term in the red cells there may be nuclear remnants (Howell–Jolly bodies), siderocytes, target cells and occasional normoblasts. After splenectomy there is a risk of overwhelming infection: vaccination with polyvalent pneumococcal vaccine is mandatory and children should receive long-term prophylactic penicillin.

Table 10.6 Causes of splenomegaly.

Infections	
Viral:	Infectious mononucleosis
	Hepatitis
Bacterial:	Septicaemia
	Bacterial endocarditis
	Tuberculosis
	Typhoid
Protozoal:	Malaria
	Visceral leishmaniasis
Helminths:	Schistosomiasis
Sarcoidosis	
Connective tissue disorders	
Rheumatoid arthritis	
Systemic lupus erythematosus	
Metabolic disorders	
Glycogen storage disease	
Gaucher's disease	
Mucopolysaccharidoses	
Congestive disorders	
Portal hypertension	
Chronic congestive cardiac failure	
Hepatic or portal vein thrombosis	
Haematological disorders	
Haemolytic anaemias	
Myeloproliferative disorders	
Lymphoproliferative disorders	

Leukaemias

The leukaemias result from the clonal proliferation of cells derived from a single early haemopoietic progenitor cell that has undergone somatic mutation. In the **acute leukaemias**, this results in the accumulation of early myeloid or lymphoid precursors ('blast' cells) in the bone marrow, blood and other tissues; marrow failure rapidly follows as normal blood cell production ceases. In the **chronic leukaemias**, either the malignant clone allows differentiation to functional end cells (as in chronic myeloid leukaemia), or the malignant proliferation progresses over a slower time course (as in chronic lymphocytic leukaemia).

Acute leukaemia

Acute leukaemias have an incidence of between 5–10 cases per 100,000 of the population, and this is increasing. Acute lymphoblastic leukaemia (ALL) is found mainly in young children (peak incidence 3–5 years). In adults, acute myeloblastic leukaemia (AML) is more common. The aetiology of acute leukaemia is unknown, but may include viruses, chemicals and radiation; it is sometimes a sequel to the administration of chemotherapy or radiotherapy for previous cancers. Acute leukaemia presents with infection, bleeding or anaemia—all the result of bone marrow failure—and occasionally with bone pain. There may also be organ infiltration with lymphadenopathy, splenomegaly or central nervous system involvement. The peripheral blood may contain blast cells, or occasionally the leukaemic infiltration is discovered on bone marrow examination carried out to determine the cause of a pancytopenia. No clinical features absolutely distinguish between AML and ALL.

The clinical presentation is often with pallor and tiredness resulting from **anaemia**. Other signs of anaemia include dyspnoea, tachycardia and occasionally pulmonary oedema. The cause of the anaemia is usually ineffective erythropoiesis which may be complicated by an element of haemolysis.

Fever is also usually present and is often related to **infection**, especially when the white cell count falls below $1 \times 10^9/l$ (**10.64, 10.65**). **Bleeding** is usually due to thrombocytopenia and skin purpura is a frequent finding, especially when the platelet count falls below $20 \times 10^9/l$. There may also be a qualitative platelet defect and occasionally disseminated intravascular coagulation (DIC). The skin and gums are common sites of bleeding, but bleeding may occur from any site (**10.64, 10.65**).

Leukaemic infiltration is common and multiple small purple papular lesions can be found in the skin in a quarter of cases (**10.64, 10.66, 10.67**). There may also be gingival infiltration (**10.65**), often with involvement of the tongue and tonsils. The eye may also be affected and infiltrates may be visible in the retina and choroid (**10.68**). The testicle is involved in about 10% of cases, usually causing a painless swelling. Involvement of the testicles or ovaries and of the meninges (found on CSF examination) may be an important source of cells that cause relapse and this requires special consideration in treatment planning. Liver, spleen and bone marrow involvement are found in 40% of cases. Bone and joint involvements are rare at presentation, but become more common as the disease advances (**10.69**). **Bone pain** is often present at the sites of major marrow production, especially over the sternum. Periosteal elevation may be seen on X-ray, and bone infarction may occur.

The distinction of the types of leukaemia depends upon the morphology of the blasts and on detailed cytochemical and monoclonal antibody cell marker studies (**10.70, 10.71**).

Management should be carried out in specialised units. Chemotherapy may include combinations of steroids, viscristine, asparaginase, methotrexate, daunorubicin and cytosine arabinoside, and other combinations are currently under trial. Treatment with intensive cytotoxic chemotherapy exacerbates immunosuppression in the short term and isolation nursing and supportive therapy with broad-spectrum antibiotics sometimes including antifungal agents, and blood products, particularly red cells and platelets, are almost invariably required. In addition fluids are often needed to correct dehydration, and allopurinol to correct hyperuricaemia. In childhood ALL, around two-thirds of patients will enter long-term remission, and the inclusion of prophylactic treatment to the central nervous system largely prevents meningeal relapse. Similarly, testicular and ovarian radiotherapy may be of value. In adults with either AML or ALL, the outlook is much less good with chemotherapy alone; where the patient is less than approximately 40 years old and has an HLA-compatible sibling, allogeneic bone marrow transplantation would now be recommended after achieving a first remission.

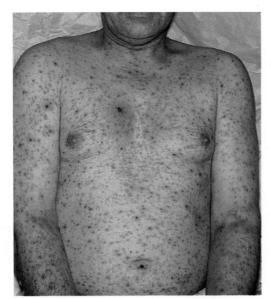

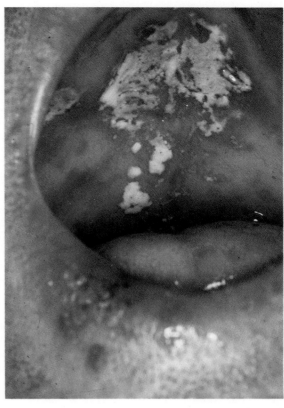

10.63 Chickenpox in an adult patient with acute myeloblastic leukaemia. Varicella zoster infection is a common complication of acute leukaemia, though it often presents with shingles rather than disseminated chickenpox (*see* **1.31, 1.79**).

10.64 Oral candidiasis is a common complication of acute leukaemia, as in other conditions associated with immunodeficiency. This patient also has multiple petechiae on the palate, tongue and lips; and some small nodules of leukaemic infiltrate can also be seen near the lower lip.

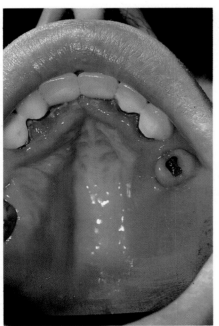

10.65 Infiltration of the gums is a common feature of acute leukaemia, and may be very marked. Secondary infection often exacerbates the swelling, and bleeding is a common complication.

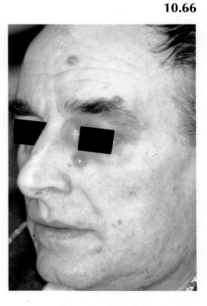

10.66 Leukaemic skin deposits in a patient with acute myeloblastic leukaemia. Similar small deposits may occur in patients with lymphomas or carcinomas; if the deposits are an isolated finding, biopsy is essential for diagnosis.

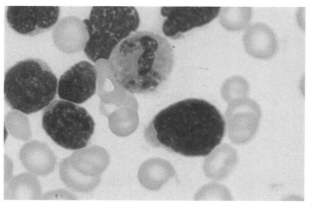

10.67 Extensive leukaemic infiltration of the skin may sometimes occur—most commonly, as here, in patients with acute myeloblastic leukaemia.

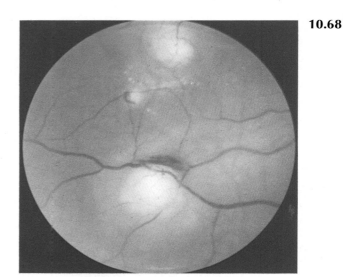

10.68 Leukaemic retinal infiltrates are often seen in acute leukaemia, as in this patient with acute lymphoblastic leukaemia. Retinal haemorrhage is often also seen but is probably a consequence of the thrombocytopenia that accompanies the leukaemia, rather than a manfestation of the leukaemic process itself. Similar haemorrhages are seen in patients with thrombocytopenic purpura.

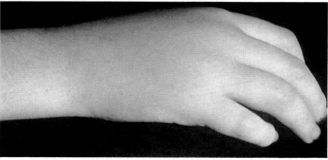

10.69 Acute, painful swelling of the hand was the presenting feature of acute lymphoblastic leukaemia in this 10-year-old child. Radiological examination confirmed leukaemic infiltration at the bases of the metacarpals and extensive periostitis.

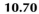

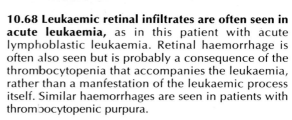

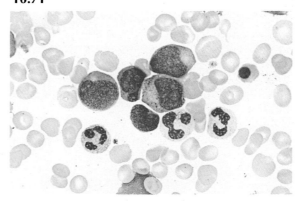

10.70, 10.71 Peripheral blood films often provide initial diagnostic information in acute leukaemia. 10.70 shows a film containing many lymphoblasts, while **10.71** shows a film with myeloblasts and polymorphs. Detailed typing of the leukaemia is dependent on cytochemical and cell-marker studies on peripheral blood and marrow aspirates. Classification of the leukaemia has important therapeutic implications, and a detailed diagnosis cannot be made on blood film alone.

Chronic leukaemias

In chronic leukaemias, there is an accumulation of abnormal white cells in the marrow with resultant disruption of normal marrow function and progressive infiltration into other tissues. Chronic leukaemias differ from the acute forms in that the time course is longer and the onset is more insidious, the cells are more mature and the treatments required are less intense. The classification depends on the cell type involved.

Chronic lymphocytic leukaemia (CLL)

CLL is the most common leukaemia in Europe and the USA and accounts for 30% of leukaemic deaths. It is a disease predominantly of the elderly, with a mean age at diagnosis of 60 years. In CLL, there is neoplastic proliferation of moderately mature lymphocytes—primarily in the marrow and blood, but also in the lymph nodes, spleen and liver. It is the result of a monoclonal transformation, usually of B lymphocytes (only 5% show a T-cell phenotype). The monoclonal nature of the disorder is confirmed by the finding of surface and cytoplasmic (and sometimes serum) immunoglobulins restricted to one light and heavy chain class.

CLL may present with lymphadenopathy, or increased numbers of small lymphocytes may be found coincidentally when a blood count is carried out for another reason (in about 25% of cases). Weight loss, night sweats, anorexia and lymph node enlargement in the superficial lymph nodes (10.37, 10.72), mediastinum and mesenteric nodes are common. On examination of the patient, there is usually moderate splenomegaly and sometimes hepatomegaly. Jaundice may develop as a result of lymphocytic infiltration of the liver or haemolysis (10.37). Later in the disease there may be extreme weight loss, pressure effects caused by lymph node involvement and skin infiltration which may be compounded by local infections with bacteria, viruses or fungi. Shingles is common (p. 30). Generalised infections are also common, as immunosuppression is related to a combination of hypogammaglobulinaemia, lymphocyte dysfunction and, in more advanced disease, neutropenia. The abnormal lymphocytes are usually monoclonal B cells, though a T-cell variant occurs. Related disorders with a different phenotype and prognosis have been recognised, including hairy cell leukaemia and prolymphocytic leukaemia, both typically associated with more pronounced splenomegaly and less lymphadenopathy than CLL.

The diagnosis depends on finding a persistent lymphocytosis of >15 × 10⁹/l lymphocytes, with a total white cell count that can range up to 200 × 10⁹/l (85–95% of the white cells are lymphocytes; neutrophil count reduced). Peripheral blood films show typical CLL lymphocytes (10.73, 10.74) with characteristic staining. Anaemia becomes more marked as the disease advances and is usually normochromic and normocytic. There is often a haemolytic component because of the presence of warm antibodies (10.37 and *see*

p 439). Marrow aspirate or trephine biopsy shows a reduction in normal marrow elements with a lymphocytic infiltrate (10.75). Serum immunoglobulin measurement and electrophoresis reveals hypogammaglobulinaemia and a monoclonal paraprotein spike. Lymph node histology shows a similar picture to that in well-differentiated lymphocytic lymphoma (*see* p. 454). X-ray of the chest may show marked mediastinal enlargement caused by bilateral lymphadenopathy.

Combinations of these clinical and laboratory criteria form the basis of a variety of staging techniques which may be used to plan treatment or as prognostic indicators. Complete remission is defined as disappearance of the abnormal lymphocytes from blood and marrow, and the normalisation of blood counts, immunoglobulins and light chains. A partial response is defined as a 50% reduction in lymphocytosis and a 50% reduction in adenopathy and splenomegaly, with haemoglobin >11 g/dl and platelets >100 × 10⁹/l.

Asymptomatic CLL usually requires no treatment, but more advanced cases with bone marrow failure, tissue infiltration or severe lymphadenopathy are treated with single alkylating agents (e.g. chlorambucil or cyclophosphamide) or local radiotherapy. Chemotherapy with a single agent can induce partial remission in 50–60% of cases and complete remission in 10–15%. Addition of corticosteroids increases the number of partial remissions to 70–80%, but also increases the chances of infectious complications. Resistant or advanced cases may require the use of vincristine, melphalan, and doxorubicin. All these agents may be associated with side-effects such as nausea, vomiting, anorexia and weight loss. Myelosuppression is inevitable, but improves when therapy is stopped or the dosage reduced. There is a significant incidence of acute myeloid leukaemia (10%) after 5–10 years of treatment. In the case of the prolymphocytic leukaemic variant, the very high white cell number requires reduction by leukopheresis for chemotherapy to be effective. In hairy cell leukaemia α-interferon is of value.

All patients require general supportive measures, often including the supportive treatment of anaemia with blood or red cell transfusions, treatment of thrombocytopenia with platelet concentrates and treatment of infections with antibiotics and gammaglobulin. Prevention of hyperuricaemia with allopurinol is usually required, and the patient must be adequately hydrated throughout treatment.

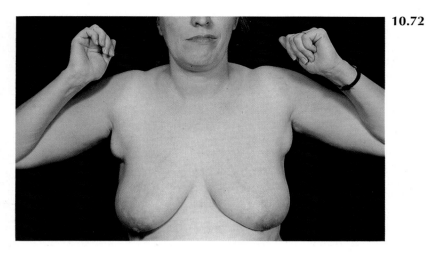

10.72 Chronic lymphocytic leukaemia commonly presents with widespread lymph node enlargement. Often these are first noted in the neck (*see* **10.37**), but in this patient the presenting feature was bilateral axillary lymphadenopathy.

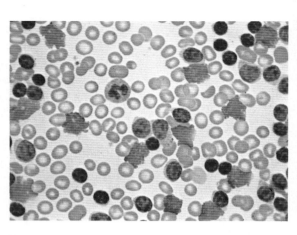

10.73 Chronic lymphocytic leukaemia. The intact white cells on the peripheral blood film are nearly all lymphocytes. A few precursor cells can be seen, and there are numerous smeared disrupted cells—a typical finding in this disease.

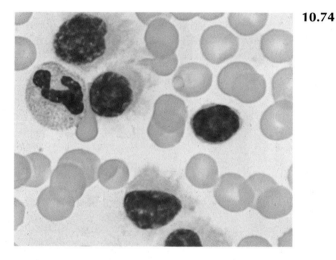

10.74 Hairy cell leukaemia. The peripheral blood film shows cells containing a typical eccentric nucleus and fine surface projections or hairs. The distinction between chronic lymphocytic leukaemia and hairy cell leukaemia has therapeutic importance.

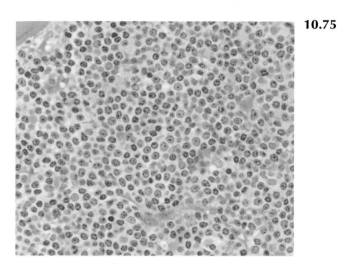

10.75 Chronic lymphocytic leukaemia. This high-power view of a trephine biopsy of bone marrow shows overwhelming, diffuse, uniform infiltration by lymphocytes—a picture found typically at advanced stages of the disease, and commonly associated with marked anaemia and thrombocytopenia.

Chronic myeloid leukaemia (CML)

CML accounts for 15% of leukaemias and is a disorder predominantly of middle life (median age at diagnosis is 45 years). The malignant clone of haemopoietic cells that spill into the peripheral blood is marked by the presence of the Philadelphia chromosome in about 95% of cases. In the minority of cases in which this is absent, there may be differences in the course of the disease and in the response to treatment. The most common cell type involved is the granulocyte series, but rare cases of eosinophilic, basophilic and neutrophilic leukaemia occur. CML in the young behaves like a different disease.

The clinical course of chronic myeloid leukaemia is insidious with overgrowth of cells, predominantly those of the myeloid series but also those of the erythroid and megakaryocytic series. This often results in a leucoerythoblastic picture (10.62) which may terminate after several years in an acute leukaemia relatively resistant to therapy, or in myelofibrosis.

Clinical features on presentation include those caused by anaemia, weight loss, abdominal distension from massive splenomegaly (*see* 1.188) and bone tenderness from periosteal infiltration. Purpura and bleeding from other sites as a result of thrombocytopenia may occur. Hyperviscosity syndromes may result in retinal haemorrhages, priapism and neurological deficit. Gouty arthropathy is rare despite the presence of hyperuricaemia.

The diagnosis is suspected when a white cell count in excess of $50 \times 10^9/l$ is found which is composed of myelocytes, metamyelocytes and blast cells in the peripheral blood film (10.76). There is also usually a normochromic normocytic anaemia, with a haemoglobin in the region of 9 g/dl. There may also be thrombocytosis with giant platelets and other fragments of megakaryocytes.

Bone marrow aspirate (10.77) or trephine biopsy shows a generalised increase in cellularity, with loss of fat spaces caused by the myeloid hyperplasia. The leukocyte alkaline phosphatase is greatly reduced in CML, and this allows its differentiation from the neutrophils resulting from infection and from other myeloproliferative disorders. The Philadelphia chromosome is of diagnostic and prognostic importance (10.78).

Treatment is by control of the hyperproliferation using busulphan or hydroxyurea, but after a median of 2–3 years the disease becomes more difficult to control, with increasing marrow fibrosis and/or a sudden transformation to acute leukaemia.

In patients with a hyperviscosity syndrome caused by the presence of excess white cells, leukophoresis is of value. During initial treatment, a high fluid intake and allopurinol are important in the control of hyperuricaemia. Splenic irradiation or splenectomy have little place in modern management.

Allogeneic bone marrow transplantation is of value in the chronic phase for younger patients who have a compatible donor, and this represents the best chance for cure. For the best chance, this should be carried out within the first year of treatment.

10.76

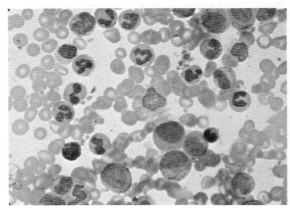

10.76 Chronic myeloid leukaemia. This low-power view of peripheral blood shows granulocytes at all stages of maturation. A peripheral blood smear with as many leucocytes of different stages of maturity as shown here is virtually diagnostic of chronic myeloid leukaemia.

10.77

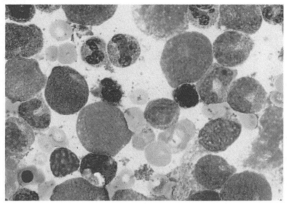

10.77 Bone marrow smear in chronic myeloid leukaemia (low-power view). There is a preponderance of neutrophil granulocytes, with all stages of development represented. Some erythroblasts and a pro-erythroblast can also be seen.

10.78

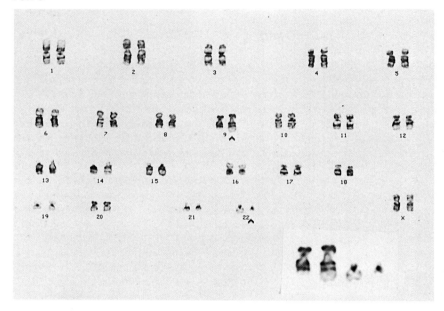

10.78 Philadelphia chromosome in chronic myeloid leukaemia. The Ph is a chromosome number 22 from which the long arms are deleted (22q-) and is found in nearly all patients with chronic myeloid leukaemia. It is part of a reciprocal translocation usually involving chromosome 9 (9q+). In this karyotype, the arrows indicate the truncated Ph chromosome 22 and the extended chromosome 9 in a Giemsa-banded metaphase from bone marrow cells of a patient with chronic myeloid leukaemia: the inset (lower right) shows the affected chromosomes and their normal partners in more detail. The reciprocal translocation results in the formation of a chimaeric gene, formed from part of the chromosome 22 and the c-abl gene from chromosome 9; this transcribes a novel mRNA to produce a protein with enhanced tyrosine kinase activity thought to be the metabolic basis of this leukaemia.

Myelodysplastic syndromes

The myelodysplastic syndromes are a heterogeneous group of disorders, characterised by the liability to develop acute myeloid leukaemia, which present with multiple cytopenias in the presence of a hypercellular marrow. The range of abnormalities includes refractory anaemia—which may be associated with excessive marrow or with ringed sideroblasts in the marrow—and chronic myelomonocytic leukaemia. These disorders occur particularly in the elderly, and clinical presentation is often caused by failure of the marrow, with signs of bleeding or with infection. Up to 20% of patients have splenomegaly. Occasionally signs of chronic myelomonocytic leukaemia are present.

Laboratory investigation usually shows that all three cell lines are involved. The red cells often show macrocytosis, ovalocytosis and poikilocytosis with 'tear-drop' forms. Circulating normoblasts may be seen. Anaemia is usually present. The white cells are often functionally defective, with defects in their granules and loss of peroxidase activity, are poorly lobulated and show nuclear and cytoplasmic anomalies. There may be abnormalities of T-cell function. Platelet function is often abnormal, with qualitative and quantitative abnormalities and prolongation of the bleeding time. The bone marrow is often hypercellular with granulopoiesis shifted to the left. Erythropoiesis is often megaloblastic with abnormal sideroblasts. Giant megakaryocytes are present and these show fragmented nuclei.

The prognosis is generally poor because of the patient's age, increasing anaemia, infection resulting from granulocytopenia and bleeding from thrombocytopenia. The median survival is of the order of 30 months.

Treatment consists of supportive care, with correction of anaemia with blood transfusion, and appropriate treatment of infections and bleeding.

Lymphoma

The lymphomas are a group of malignant disorders originating in one of the lymph nodes or other lymphatic tissues of the body and disrupting the normal lymphoid architecture. The disorders are divided into Hodgkin's disease (in which the origin of the abnormal Reed–Sternberg cell is still a matter of debate), and the non-Hodgkin's lymphomas (which can be shown to be of clonal B- or T-cell origin).

Hodgkin's disease

Hodgkin's disease is the most common of the lymphomas. It occurs more frequently in males than in females and has bimodal peaks of increased incidence in early adult life and after 45 years of age. The tumour is unusual in that the putative malignant cell (the Reed–Sternberg cell) forms a tiny proportion of the cells in the tumour, the remaining tissue being thought to be 'reactive'. It presents in 70% of cases with isolated painless swelling of a lymph node in the neck, axilla or groin, and spreads to adjacent groups of lymph nodes (10.7, 10.79).

In advanced cases there may be hepatosplenomegaly. Skin lesions may develop at a late stage (10.80).

Investigations show a variety of non-specific features, usually including a normochromic normocytic anaemia and elevation of the ESR (especially in the presence of 'B' grading). Lymphopenia is present in about one-third of cases, and there may also be neutrophilia, eosinophilia and monocytosis. There may rarely be auto-immune thrombocytopenia or haemolytic anaemia. The diagnosis is made on lymph node or tissue biopsy, which should be conventionally fixed and stained and also examined immunohistochemically.

The extent of the disease (and its prognosis) is determined by staging procedures (Table 10.7), including bone marrow examination, CT scan of the abdomen (10.81), ultrasound and/or lymphangiography (10.82). Bone marrow or iliac crest trephine biopsy has a low return—only about 5% will show involvement. Laparotomy with lymph node biopsy, liver biopsy and splenectomy is now considered unnecessary for staging. Chest X-ray (10.83) or CT scan (10.84) may reveal large mediastinal masses, especially when the patient has systemic symptoms.

Systemic symptoms (B-stage) including fever with sweats, especially at night (Pel–Ebstein pattern), and weight loss are characteristic of more advanced disease.

Hodgkin's disease is associated with impaired cell-mediated immunity and an increased risk of infections, including herpes zoster (see p. 30, 10.85).

Treatment of localised disease is by radiotherapy, especially where the disease is above the diaphragm, when the cervical, axillary, mediastinal and para-aortic nodes can be irradiated ('the mantle'). The prospects for cure are of the order of 80–90% over 5 years. For more advanced disease (Stage IIIB and IV) treatment is with a combination of chemotherapeutic agents which include mustine, vincristine, procarbazine and prednisolone (MOPP), and sometimes also chlorambucil, vinblastine, adriamycin and bleomycin. Such combinations must be given in specialised units and can give an 80% remission rate. Relapse is common; different drugs are then required and may be given in combination with radiotherapy.

Cytotoxic therapy compounds the existing defect in cell-mediated immunity and makes infective complications likely, e.g. disseminated tuberculosis, herpes zoster, and other bacterial, viral, fungal and protozoal infections.

10.79

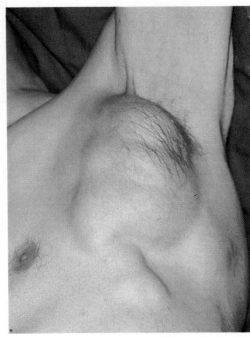

10.79 Gross, painless, rubbery lymph node enlargement is the common presenting feature of Hodgkin's disease. This patient had generalised lymphadenopathy, but his left axillary nodes were particularly prominent.

Table 10.7 Ann Arbor staging in Hodgkin's disease.

Stage I   Involvement of lymph nodes in a single region (I) or infiltration of a single extralymphatic site (IE)

Stage II Involvement of lymph nodes in two distinct regions on the same side of the diaphragm (II) which may also include spleen (IIs), localised extralymphatic involvement (IIE) or both (IIsE)

Stage III Involvement of lymph nodes on both sides of the diaphragm (III) which may include the spleen (IIIs), localised extralymphatic involvement (IIIE) or both (IIIsE)

Stage IV Diffuse or disseminated involvement of extralymphatic sites (e.g. bone marrow, liver and lung)

In addition, the suffix letters A and B are used to denote the absence (A) or presence (B) of any of the additional systemic features of fever, night sweats and loss of 10% of body weight in the previous 6 months.

10.80

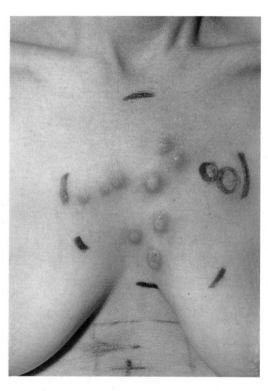

10.80 Skin deposits of tumour may occur in advanced Hodgkin's disease. This patient had multiple skin nodules, and their nature was confirmed by biopsy. Palliative radiotherapy is about to be started.

10.8

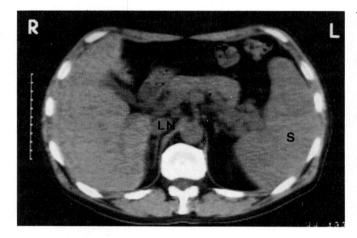

10.81 Hodgkin's disease. This CT scan of the abdomen shows gross enlargement of the spleen (S) and enlarged para-aortic lymph nodes (LN).

452

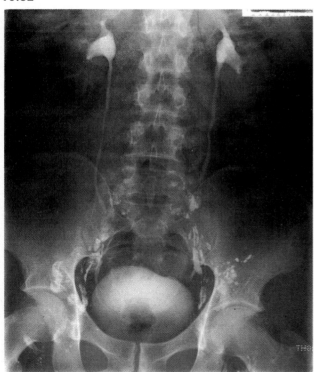

10.82 A lymphangiogram in Hodgkin's disease, performed by cannulating lymphatics in the feet. Markedly enlarged lymph nodes can be seen alongside the aorta. Intravenous contrast medium has been used to perform a simultaneous IVU, which reveals that the ureters are displaced laterally by the abnormal para-aortic nodes.

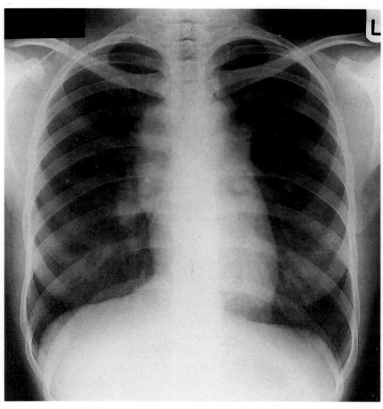

10.83 Chest X-ray in a patient with Hodgkin's disease, showing bilaterally enlarged mediastinal lymph nodes.

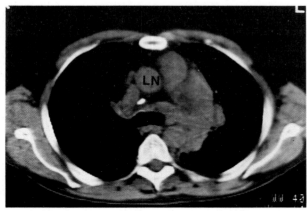

10.84 Thoracic CT scan in Hodgkin's disease, demonstrating enlarged mediastinal lymph nodes (LN).

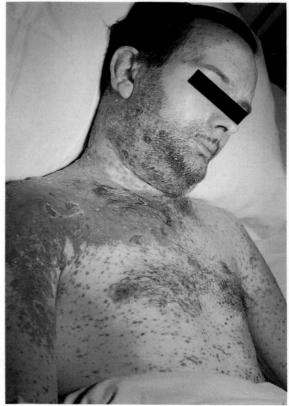

10.85 Widespread herpes zoster infection in a 38-year-old man with advanced Hodgkin's disease. Note that he has also developed a generalised chickenpox rash over the unaffected segments.

Non-Hodgkin's lymphomas

Non-Hodgkin's lymphomas are a heterogeneous group of neoplasms of the immune system. They differ in cell type, natural history and outcome from Hodgkin's disease. Non-Hodgkin's lymphoma may present in exactly the same way as Hodgkin's disease, with the diagnosis being made at lymph node biopsy (**1.42, 10.86**). However, the range of presentations and course of disease is highly variable, and extra-nodal tissue involvement, including the bone marrow and organs as varied as the tongue and the testis (**10.87**), is much more common. Histological classification of the non-Hodgkin's lymphomas has been difficult but has been improved by immunophenotyping. In general, tumours showing a diffuse (rather than follicular) pattern and larger 'blastic' cells (rather than small lymphoid cells) have a more aggressive course and are regarded as 'high-grade' rather than 'low-grade' lymphomas. Paradoxically, 'high-grade' lymphomas, which include B lymphoblastic (Burkitt's) lymphoma (p. 33), are curable in a proportion of cases with intensive cytotoxic chemotherapy combined with radiotherapy to 'bulky' areas of disease; whereas the 'low-grade' lymphomas, although compatible with long survival, are not currently curable, though they may be controlled by intermittent 'gentle' chemotherapy with alkylating agents, or with local radiotherapy. The cytotoxic drug of choice is chlorambucil, with or without steroids. Combination chemotherapy may be required in the presence of marrow impairment. Splenectomy may be required if there is hypersplenism.

The majority of non-Hodgkin's lymphomas are B-cell in origin and present in middle age with some of the features of CLL. Tumours of small lymphocytes or lymphoplasmacytoid cells may be associated with the production of paraproteins, and an IgM paraprotein may give rise to hyperviscosity problems (Waldenström's macroglobulinaemia, *see* p. 467).

The rarer T-cell lymphomas tend to be more aggressive. They include mycosis fungoides, a chronic skin lymphoma that progresses from psoriasiform lesions and skin plaques (**2.108**), sometimes associated with generalised erythroderma, to more generalised lymph node involvement and the appearance of typical convoluted lymphocytes (Sézary cells) in the blood. When the disease is localised to the skin it may run a benign course and be amenable to local therapy with ultraviolet light, radiotherapy or to local or generalised nitrogen mustard. Once it has spread to local lymph nodes the prognosis is bleak, with a median survival time of only 2 years despite intensive combination therapy.

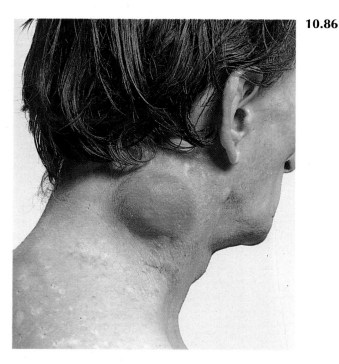

10.86

10.86 Non-Hodgkin's lymphoma may present in a similar way to Hodgkin's disease, as in this patient who developed lymphoma as a component of AIDS (the lymphoma of AIDS is usually of non-Hodgkin's type). Despite the redness of the skin over the enlarged lymph node in this patient, the lesion was completely painless.

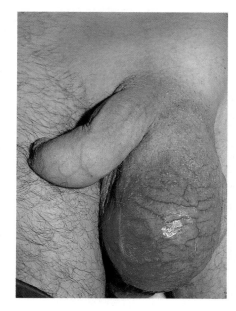

10.87

10.87 Lymphoma of the testis is the most common testicular neoplasm in the elderly. It usually presents with swelling of the testis and cord up into the abdomen, as here. It is commonly associated with lymphoma in the para-aortic nodes and elsewhere, and the prognosis is poor.

Platelet defects

Defects in either the number or the function of platelets may produce easy bruising, epistaxis and intestinal bleeding. Purpura is usually seen only when there is a fall in circulating platelets to around $10-20 \times 10^9/l$ from the normal of $200-300 \times 10^9/l$. Bleeding may occur at a level of up to $50 \times 10^9/l$ if there has been major surgery or extensive trauma. The causes of thrombocytopenia are numerous and are summarised in **Table 10.8**.

There is usually a history of spontaneous bruising and bleeding, especially recurrent bilateral nose bleeds, mucous membrane bleeding in the mouth, persistent menorrhagia, intestinal and joint bleeds. It is important to ask about recent drug therapy. Careful examination is required to identify a basic disease process such as infection, malignancy, liver disease or a connective tissue disorder. The age of the purpuric lesions may give a clue to the duration of the disease. Evidence of splenic enlargement should be sought. Investigations include a full blood count, platelet count, coagulation screen, bone marrow aspirate, bleeding time and assessment of platelet survival.

Table 10.8 Causes of thrombocytopenia

Infections	Malaria
	Many other infections
Immune	Acute/chronic ITP
Marrow disorders	Hypoplasia
	Infiltration – Leukaemia
	Carcinoma
	Myelofibrosis
	Myeloma
	B_{12}/folate/iron deficiency
Haemolytic anaemias	Microangiopathic
Hypersplenism	Lymphoma
	Infection
	Congestion
	Storage
Excess consumption	Massive blood transfusion
	Disseminated intravascular coagulation
	Trauma and burns
	Extracorporeal circulation

Idiopathic thrombocytopenic purpura (ITP)

ITP is caused by accelerated removal by cells of the reticulo-endothelial system of platelets coated by antibody. These antibodies may result from infections auto-immune disorders or lymphoproliferative disorders, or be associated with drug therapy. The likelihood of haemorrhage is related to the degree of thrombocytopenia or interference with normal function. Clinically, ITP can be classified as acute or chronic.

In acute ITP, purpura (**10.8, 10.88**), bruises and bleeding appear abruptly, usually in children or young adults. There is often a history of an upper respiratory infection in the preceding 2 weeks. Occasionally, there may have been an obvious viral disease such as measles, mumps or infectious mononucleosis. The blood film is usually normal, but may show some atypical lymphocytes. The platelet count is significantly reduced and some platelets may be larger than normal. Bone marrow examination shows an increase in megakaryocytes (**10.89**). Most children have a spontaneous remission in a week or so and few have any serious haemorrhage. If frank bleeding occurs, steroids should be given in a short course. Failure to remit spontaneously or with steroids should lead to re-evaluation for an alternative cause and/or to consideration of splenectomy.

Chronic ITP is a disease of adults which affects women more often than men. The usual presentation is with progressive purpura, ecchymoses and mucocutaneous bleeding. There may be a history of multiple episodes over many years, or of a concomitant systemic illness, especially an auto-immune disease or lymphoproliferation. Examination shows purpura and ecchymoses, and lesions may also be found in the mouth (**10.90**) and eye (**10.68**). The spleen is palpable in only 5% of patients.

The peripheral blood is usually normal unless blood loss has produced anaemia. The platelet count may vary over the years from $10-50 \times 10^9/l$; the level correlates well with episodes of bleeding. Bone marrow aspirate shows normal erythroid and myeloid cell lines with a normal or increased number of megakaryocytes. There may be evidence of increased platelet-associated immunoglobulin with reduced platelet survival. Other diseases should be excluded by appropriate investigations.

Treatment is with steroids, or sometimes cytotoxic immunosuppressive drugs. Splenectomy may be necessary. Temporary remissions to allow surgery can sometimes be gained using high doses of human IgG.

In pregnancy the chief danger is to the fetus, which may be thrombocytopenic as a result of transplacental passage of anti-platelet IgG and thus at risk of cerebral haemorrhage at delivery.

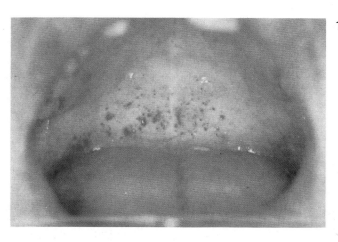

10.88

10.88 Acute idiopathic thrombocytopenic purpura (ITP) commonly presents with purpuric lesions of this kind, though they may often be more widespread by the time the patient seeks medical attention. It is important to remember that purpura of identical appearance may result from many other causes (**Table 10.5**).

10.89

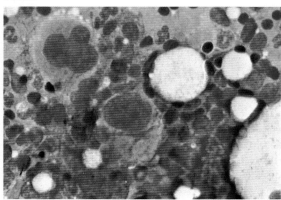

10.89 The bone marrow in idiopathic thrombocytopenic purpura shows numerous megakaryocytes, but few or no platelets are seen on the peripheral blood film.

10.90

10.90 Petechiae on the soft palate may be a sign of thrombocytopenic purpura, as in this patient (but it is important to remember that similar transient appearances may occur harmlessly during the course of the common cold or other viral throat infections).

Drug-induced immune thrombocytopenia

Many drugs may be associated with antibody-mediated thrombocytopenia (**10.8**). There are probably two principal mechanisms:

- The drug may bind to the platelet to produce a neo-antigen that stimulates an auto-antibody.
- The drug binds to a plasma protein which is antigenic and the resultant antibody produces an immune complex that binds to the normal platelet F_c receptor.

Drugs that have been implicated in immune-mediated thrombocytopenia are listed in **Table 10.9**. Bleeding may range from mild to life-threatening. Stopping the drug usually results in the cessation of signs. Steroids may aid the return of the platelet count to normal.

When this condition is associated with the use of heparin, the bleeding may be extremely severe because of the existing state of anticoagulation of the patient. Protamine sulphate should be given to reverse the action of the heparin, along with steroids to raise the platelet count.

Table 10.9 Drugs that may cause immune-mediated thrombocytopenia.

Thiazide diuretics	Quinine
Gold salts	Rifampicin
Heparin	Valproate
Carbamazepine	Sulphonamides
Phenothiazines	Penicillins

Vascular and non-thrombocytopenic purpura

Integrity of the endothelium is essential to maintain blood within the vascular tree. Abnormalities of the endothelium may be primary or secondary (**Table 10.10**) and depending on their nature, extent and site can give rise to a variety of clinical syndromes.

It is important to elicit any history of easy bruising or bleeding in the family, of epistaxis in childhood or of excessive bleeding after dental extraction, after surgery or during menstruation. Careful examination of the skin is necessary for petechiae, purpura or bruises. Tests of vascular function may be required and biopsy of lesions may give a diagnosis. Often the cause of the defect is not apparent.

Table 10.10 Causes of vascular and non-thrombocytopenic purpura.

Primary
Senile purpura
Hereditary haemorrhagic telangiectasia
Giant cavernous haemangioma (**10.105**)
Connective tissue disorders, e.g.
       Ehlers–Danlos syndrome (*see* p. 151)
       Marfan's syndrome (*see* p. 318)

Secondary
Henoch–Schönlein purpura
Metabolic: scurvy
           Cushing's syndrome and steroid use (*see* **7.23**)
           uraemia
           liver disease
Dysproteinaemia
Purpura fulminans
Embolic purpura
Mechanical purpura

Primary abnormalities

Senile purpura

This is a benign disease of the elderly, in which the characteristic lesions develop on the extensor surfaces of the hands (**10.91**), forearms and face and neck. The defect is loss of collagen support of dermal capillaries, associated with thinning of the skin. The purple spots tend to stay the same colour over many months before they fade to a brownish colour. They are often called 'age spots'. They are of no significance and are of only cosmetic importance. No treatment is available.

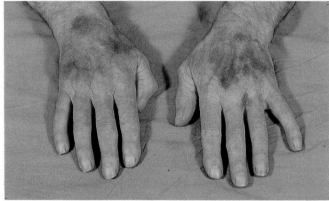

10.91

10.91 Senile purpura is a common and benign condition that results from impaired collagen production and capillary fragility in the elderly. In the absence of other signs of disease, no investigation is necessary.

Hereditary haemorrhagic telangiectasia

This disorder (also known as the Rendu–Osler–Weber syndrome or HHT) is transmitted as an autosomal dominant trait so both sexes are equally affected. The lesions consist of dilated arterioles and capillaries which are superficial, easily traumatised and likely to ooze (**9.44, 10.6**). They blanch on pressure with a glass slide. The most common site is the nasal mucosa, and epistaxis in childhood may be a presenting feature, although the disorder does not usually present until middle age. In the adult, lesions are to be found on the lips, mouth, tongue, face, hands (**10.92**), oesophagus, stomach and rectum; and more rarely in the eyes, bronchi, and gynaecological and urinary tracts. Bleeding may occur from any of these sites; a common presentation is with recurrent iron-deficient anaemia associated with occult intestinal bleeding. There is an association of this disease with pulmonary arteriovenous fistulae, cirrhosis of the liver, hepatomas and splenomegaly. There may also be abnormalities of coagulation factors and platelet function which compound the bleeding tendency.

Treatment is difficult because of the diffuse nature of the lesions. If individual lesions can be identified as the source of bleeding, they may be cauterised. Oestrogens may help to prevent epistaxis.

10.92

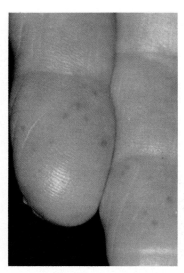

10.92 Hereditary haemorrhagic telangiectasia (HHT) commonly presents with lesions on or close to mucous membranes (*see* **9.44, 10.6**), but the telangiectasia may occur anywhere on the body, as in this patient whose fingers were affected. The lesions are dilated capillaries, and they blanch if pressure is applied with a glass slide.

Secondary abnormalities

Henoch–Schönlein purpura

This is an immunological disease in which the vascular endothelium is damaged by the deposition of immune complexes. It may result from reactions to drugs, food, insect bites or bacterial or viral infections. Bleeding may occur into the joints or into the bowel and there is often a generalised skin rash of a diffuse macular type which then becomes purpuric (**2.116**). Lesions may also be found in the brain and renal tract. The disorder is most common in children, and it usually resolves without complications, but about one-third of patients have an associated glomerulonephritis (*see* p. 287) and there may be an associated pleurisy, pericarditis or pneumonia.

Scurvy

Scurvy results from deficiency of vitamin C (ascorbic acid) in the diet—from a lack of fresh fruit or vegetables or from their prolonged cooking. It is rarely seen in the Western world except in groups with special problems, such as the isolated elderly, the demented, the alcoholic and food faddists. Deficiency results in failure to synthesise a normal quantity and quality of collagen fibres. Bleeding occurs from the resulting capillary wall weakness.

In babies, subperiosteal bleeding is a common presentation and is usually associated with anaemia. In adults, there may be gingival bleeding (**8.19**), purpura and perifollicular haemorrhages. Severe deficiency in the adult may result in gastrointestinal and brain haemorrhages. The diagnosis is essentially clinical, and confirmation is obtained by observing the response to added ascorbic acid. Measurement of ascorbate levels in platelets and white cells is possible in specialised laboratories.

Cushing's syndrome and steroid use (see also *p. 310*)

Excessive corticosteroids produce thin, friable, easily-bruised skin which also contains purpuric spots and ecchymoses (**7.22, 7.23**). This is a result of the loss of collagen that supports the dermal capillaries. Treatment of Cushing's syndrome or cessation of steroid therapy results in healing of the lesions.

Mechanical and factitious purpura

Sudden increase in venous pressure from coughing, vomiting, asphyxia or during an epileptic fit may cause leakage of blood even from normal capillaries (**1.146, 10.93, 10.94**). A similar situation may occur as the result of skin suction, social or professional, or as an attempt deliberately to deceive the doctor by a disturbed patient.

10.93   **10.94**

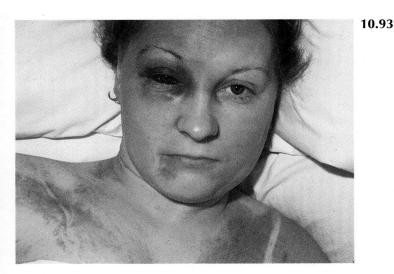

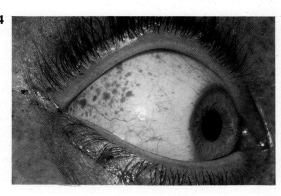

10.94 Petechiae of the sclera and cyanosis of the eyelids developed in another patient with traumatic asphyxia. Similar appearances may develop in children with whooping cough (*see* **1.146**).

10.93 Traumatic asphyxia may produce severe petechiae and frank haemorrhage. This woman was crushed in a crowd, and on admission was unconscious as a result of cerebral petechiae and oedema. She was treated with steroids and oxygen, but retained widespread skin petechiae and a right subconjunctival haemorrhage when this photograph was taken.

Disorders of blood coagulation

Blood coagulates by a complex series of reactions (a 'cascade') which involves the sequential activation of otherwise inert factors (pro-enzymes) in the plasma. A platelet thrombus forms first and is the main component of primary haemostasis; this is stabilised by the fibrin clot that results from the coagulation cascade.

Coagulation factor defects

Inborn defects (quantitative or qualitative) have been described in all known coagulation factors, but the clinical presentations tend to be very similar. The most common defects result in **haemophilia** and **Christmas disease** (factor VIII and factor IX deficiency respectively). Both are transmitted as sex-linked recessive characteristics and, using gene probes, the unaffected female carriers may be identified and counselled. There is a wide range of clinical severity.

Surprisingly, there is little bleeding at birth, though excessive cord bleeding may be noted, and the signs of excess bruising and internal bleeding usually start to manifest themselves at 6–9 months when the toddler starts to move around and fall. Bleeding may occur in every tissue of the body (**10.95–10.97**) but the most common bleeding site is into the joints. Acute haemarthrosis causes a sudden onset of acute pain and swelling, associated with signs that are similar to those of acute inflammation—hotness, redness, swelling and pain (**10.98**). The joint is usually held in a rigid semi-flexed position and movement (and examination) is resisted by the patient. Recurrent episodes of bleeding lead to chronic degenerative joint disease which may cause chronic pain in the affected joint, with severe deformity and limitation of movement (**10.99–10.101**). There is usually atrophy of the surrounding muscle cuff. Compression neuropathy is also common if bleeding occurs around a nerve, e.g. femoral nerve compression commonly follows bleeding into the iliopsoas muscle. The most common cause of death from bleeding is cerebral haemorrhage, which produces a range of neurological deficits.

Intrarenal bleeding often produces renal pelvic or ureteric obstruction, which causes colicky abdominal pain associated with haematuria. Bleeding into the bowel wall may produce intestinal obstruction.

Investigation shows a prolongation of the activated partial thromboplastin time (APTT); this finding should be followed up by measurement of the individual factor levels.

Treatment and management of these bleeding defects is best carried out in specialised haemophilia units. The deficient plasma factors are infused intravenously until bleeding stops. Surgery or trauma necessitate the use of appropriate plasma factor cover.

As a result of contamination of the source plasma, many patients with these disorders have been infected with HIV and many have developed AIDS. This resembles AIDS in other groups, but Kaposi's sarcoma is a rarity in the profile of HIV disorders in haemophilia. In addition, many patients have chronic active hepatitis following transmitted viral hepatitis.

Von Willebrand's syndrome is a group of similar types of bleeding disorders to haemophilia but is wholly transmitted by an autosomal recessive route and thus affects both men and women. There is a greater range of severity from symptomless to severe. The disease involves defects of the vessels, a platelet defect and low levels of factor VIII which may also be qualitatively abnormal. Clinical presentation is mainly with bleeding, usually from mucosal sites, especially from the genital, renal and alimentary tracts. Severely affected patients can also bleed internally into the joints and brain, but bleeding into joints is unusual. Diagnosis is made by finding prolongation of the skin bleeding time, a platelet functional defect and a low level of factor VIII.

Minor degrees of bleeding may be controllable with tranexamic acid or vasopressin preparations, but more serious bleeding requires treatment with cryoprecipitate or plasma.

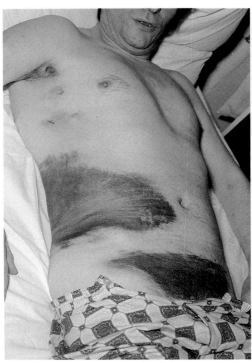

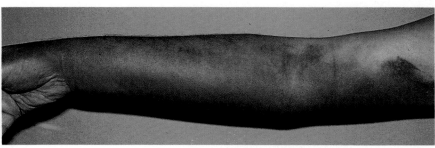

10.96 Massive haematoma of the arm in a patient with haemophilia. A major bleed resulted from very minor trauma. Again, other disorders of blood coagulation can produce a similar appearance.

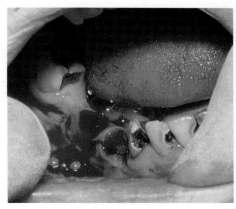

10.95 Massive haematomas in a patient with haemophilia. In the absence of major trauma, haematomas of this size always indicate a severe coagulation abnormality. Possible causes include haemophilia, Christmas disease, von Willebrand's disease and uncontrolled anticoagulant therapy. Internal bleeding is a common accompaniment, and patients require urgent investigation and treatment.

10.97 Severe haemorrhage following dental extraction is often the first clue to more minor degrees of coagulation disorder and is a common problem in haemophilia, Christmas disease and von Willebrand's disease.

10.99 Severe chronic arthritis may occur in patients with haemophilia and Christmas disease as a result of recurrent episodes of haemorrhage into joints. The knee is the most commonly affected joint. Both knees are severely deranged in this patient. Note that he is unable to stand with both feet flat on the floor.

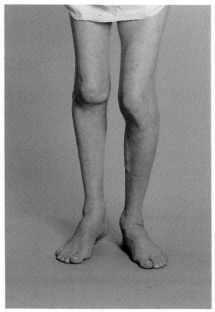

10.98 Acute haemarthrosis of the knee is a common complication of haemophilia. It may be confused with acute infection unless the patient's coagulation disorder is known, because the knee is hot, red, swollen and painful.

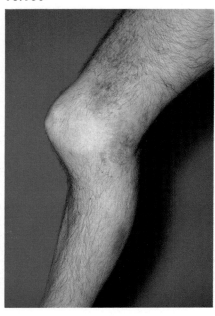

10.100

10.100 Genu recurvatum is a severe deformity of the knee which results from destruction of the joint by recurrent haemarthrosis. Note also the presence of acute skin haemorrhage in this haemophiliac patient.

10.101

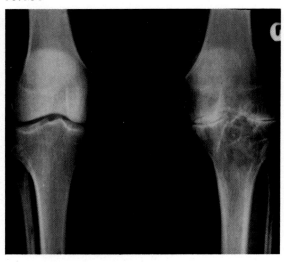

10.101 X-ray of the knees in a patient with haemophilia. The left knee joint has been severely damaged by recurrent haemarthrosis. Note the narrowing of the joint space, the presence of irregular erosions, and the evidence of cyst formation in the tibial head.

Deficiency of vitamin K

Lack of vitamin K in the diet, its malabsorption or the presence of anticoagulant drugs of the coumarin group leads to deficient hepatic synthesis of the plasma clotting factors, prothrombin, and factors VII, IX and X. Vitamin K is the co-factor necessary for the carboxylation of glutamic acid, which is necessary for the biological activity of the molecule. Deficiency from any of these causes can result in a bleeding tendency which may be seen in:

- Haemorrhagic disease of the newborn.
- Intestinal malabsorption, e.g. Crohn's disease, coeliac disease.
- Hepatobiliary disease, e.g. hepatic failure, obstructive jaundice.
- Dietary deficiency.
- Oral anticoagulant usage.

Haemorrhagic disease of the newborn
In the premature or immature infant there is defective synthesis of the vitamin K-dependent factors which are significantly lower than those in adult life. Bleeding results on the third or fourth day of life, usually into the skin or internal organs. It is usual to give vitamin K parenterally at birth to prevent bleeding, but this policy is currently under review.

Malabsorption and dietary deficiency
These are extremely common and result from a range of disorders of the gut (*see* p. 368) and pancreas, and from obstructive biliary tract disease. They are usually part of a mixed clinical picture and other features often dominate. The problem is often picked up on routine screening, e.g. before liver biopsy, or by excessive bleeding following a minor surgical procedure. Very occasionally, severe bleeding may occur from the skin, mucous membranes and the gastrointestinal tract, and in this situation it is common to find coincidental deficiency of vitamin C. Vitamin K by injection will reverse the biochemical lesion in malabsorption, but where there is serious liver cell necrosis it may not be effective.

Use of oral anticoagulants

Oral anticoagulant drugs (coumarins) such as warfarin, inhibit the action of vitamin K and result in the production of defective molecules of factors II, VII, IX and X which lack clotting activity. The higher the dose of warfarin used and the longer it is given the greater the clotting defect. For normal therapeutic purposes, this depression of coagulation is maintained by testing the patient's plasma using a modification of the prothrombin time. It is usual to extend this to 2–3 times that of a normal control. Only when this value is exceeded is bleeding likely to occur, and this may be from or into any tissue of the body. Patients who have been stabilised on a particular dose of warfarin often bleed because other drugs have been taken that interfere with the coagulation mechanism (e.g. aspirin interferes with platelets), displace warfarin from its binding site on the albumin molecule (e.g. mefenamic acid), or decrease its metabolism (e.g. cimetidine). Bleeding often occurs early in the skin (**10.95, 10.96, 10.102**), bowel or urinary tract and patients must be instructed to maintain careful observation and seek advice if signs of bleeding appear. Always consider the possibility of undeclared anticoagulant therapy in a bleeding patient.

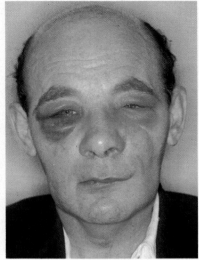

10.102

10.102 Spontaneous black eye in a patient on poorly controlled anticoagulant therapy. He reported no trauma to his eye, and his prothrombin time was grossly elevated. More massive bleeding may also result from uncontrolled anticoagulant therapy (see **10.95, 10.96**).

Parenchymal liver disease

Necrosis of liver cells as a result of hepatitis or alcohol or other toxins results in failure of coagulation factor synthesis, and severe bruising or bleeding may result (**9.14**). The defect is usually complex and may be associated with thrombocytopenia (*see* p. 455) and disseminated intravascular coagulation (*see below*). Defects of the vitamin K-dependent factors may not respond to the injection of vitamin K in this situation.

Disseminated intravascular coagulation (DIC)

DIC (also known as consumptive coagulopathy) occurs when the coagulation cascade is activated by a stimulus that results in the widespread deposition of fibrin-platelet thrombi in the arterial and venous tree. This in turn stimulates secondary fibrinolysis and, as the two processes continue in parallel, the end result is depletion of platelets, consumption of clotting factors, loss of haemostasis and excessive bleeding. A large number of conditions may be the stimulus to production of acute or chronic DIC (**10.103–10.105** and *see* **Table 10.11**).

Acute DIC presents as a dramatic illness with haemorrhagic manifestations. The patient is usually severely ill, with fever, acidosis, and hypoxia and hypotension caused by severe blood loss. There may be extensive petechiae or frank bleeding into the skin (**1.56, 1.106, 10.103**), especially at sites of trauma, e.g. wounds, venepuncture sites or under a blood-pressure cuff. There may also be bleeding in the eyes (**1.105, 1.183**) and the alimentary, respiratory, genital or renal tract. On occasions, thrombosis may dominate the initial picture, and there may be gangrene of skin and digits (**10.106**), with signs of ischaemia of heart, brain, kidneys and lungs.

Laboratory investigations require a specialist haematology laboratory to look for evidence of platelet activation, coagulation consumption and fibrinolysis. A routine blood film may show fragmentation of red cells (a microangiopathic haemolytic blood picture–**10.107**) which results from cell damage by strands of fibrin thrombus. Simple screening tests for DIC include: the platelet count, which is reduced; the partial thromboplastin time (PTT), which is prolonged; and the presence of fibrinogen-fibrin degradation products which have resulted from fibrin digestion. The cause of the process (**Table 10.11**), should be identified and treated whenever possible. The other keystones of treatment are:

- General intensive support of the patient.
- Restoration and maintenance of the peripheral circulation.
- Replacement therapy with plasma or plasma products.

Control of the thrombotic component with heparin. is often useful, but is complicated by the effects of some heparins on platelets.

Chronic DIC occurs in some patients with chronic inflammatory or malignant disorders, and is characterised by a combination of features relating to thrombosis as well as bleeding. On investigation, fibrinogen, cryofibrinogen and FDP levels are all high.

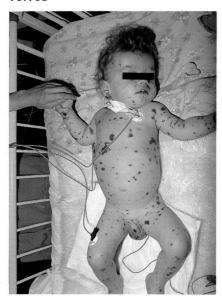

10.103 Disseminated intravascular coagulation (DIC) is often a consequence of severe infection. In this infant, meningococcal septicaemia was the underlying cause, and his widespread skin haemorrhages were accompanied by mucosal bleeding. Such devastating DIC is often fatal.

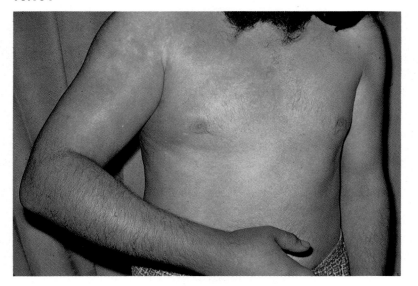

10.104 Snakebites and other venomous bites and stings are a potent cause of DIC. Adder bites rarely cause more than the severe local swelling experienced by this man, but envenomation by many other snakes and animals commonly causes DIC.

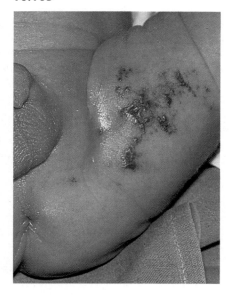

10.105 Cavernous haemangiomas may be associated with DIC (the Kasabach–Merritt syndrome). The damaged subendothelial surface of the neoplasm leads to excessive consumption of circulating platelets and clotting factors, which may result in the full clinical picture of DIC. Occasional diagnostic difficulty results from the presence of a visceral haemangioma with similar properties. Surgical excision or radiotherapy may be successful in eliminating the lesion and the consumptive coagulopathy.

Table 10.11 Causes of DIC.

• **Infections/infectious diseases:**	haemorrhagic fevers (*see* pp. 23, 27), meningococcal septicaemia (*see* p. 40), malaria (*see* p. 68), etc.
• **Obstetric causes:**	amniotic fluid embolism, pre-eclampsia, abruptio placentae, dead fetus syndrome
• **Malignant disease:**	especially lung, pancreas, ovary, prostate, acute leukaemias
• **Shock:**	traumatic, cardiac arrest, blood loss, extensive burns
• **Intravascular haemolysis/massive blood transfusion**	
• **Envenomation**	
• **Vasculitis:**	e.g. haemolytic uraemic syndrome (HUS), thrombotic thrombocytopenic purpura (TTP)
• **Extracorporeal circulation:**	e.g. cardiopulmonary bypass, artificial heart, dialysis
• **Cavernous haemangiomas**	

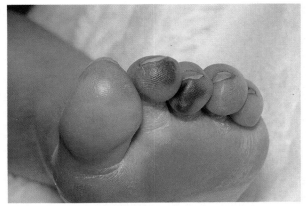

10.106 Peripheral gangrene can be a feature of DIC, as the balance between thrombosis and haemorrhage will vary from one part of the body to another and from time to time. This patient has meningococcal septicaemia, and despite his gangrenous toes he had haemorrhagic manifestations elsewhere in his body (*see* **1.105, 1.106, 10.103**).

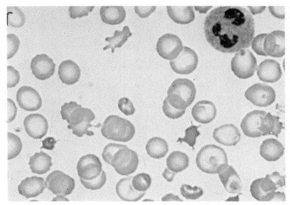

10.107 The peripheral blood film in DIC usually shows a microangiopathic haemolytic picture. Abnormal red cells, including burr cells, acanthocytes with multiple sharp projections and schistocytes of irregular fragmented shape, result from physical damage to the cells caused by their passage between strands of fibrin. The platelet count is reduced.

Multiple myeloma and related paraproteinaemias

The paraproteinaemias are a group of disorders in which there is proliferation of B cells leading to excessive production of immunoglobulins. Of these conditions, multiple myeloma is the most common and results from the neoplastic proliferation of mature and immature plasma cells. It is usually a disease of the middle-aged and elderly. The clinical features result from the uncontrolled growth of plasma cells in the marrow and the production of an abnormal paraprotein—usually an IgG, but sometimes IgA or light chains and rarely IgD, IgM or other group—to give:

- Lytic bone lesions resulting from local infiltration of bone, associated with hypercalcaemia (*see* p. 154) and painful pathological bone fractures.
- Bone marrow failure from infiltration, leading to anaemia, leucopenia and thrombocytopenia.
- Suppression of normal immunoglobulin synthesis, with resultant susceptibility to infections.
- Hyperviscosity syndromes caused by the physical properties of the paraprotein (M-protein). These are most common with IgG paraprotein and result in tissue ischaemia with overt arterial and venous thrombosis predominantly in the eye (**10.61**), heart, brain and kidneys.
- Renal impairment, which is common and is a critical factor in life-expectancy (p. 293). The kidney is damaged by hypercalcaemia, infection, deposition of amyloid, the deposition of light-chain fractions in the proximal tubules and hyperuricaemia.
- Neurological involvement, which results from ischaemia associated with hyperviscosity and from amyloid deposition.

Patients present with infections (70%), bleeding defects (10%) or renal failure (50%). Bone pain develops in all patients as the disease progresses.

Suggestive features of myeloma include a very high ESR (usually over 100 mm in the first hour), a normochromic normocytic anaemia with rouleaux formation (**10.27**), and often neutropenia and thrombocytopenia. The serum calcium levels are usually elevated.

The diagnosis can be made by finding evidence of two factors out of the following three: paraproteinaemia, bone marrow plasmacytosis and lytic lesions of bones.

- Paraprotein may be found in serum or urine (Bence–Jones protein **10.108**).
- Bone marrow aspiration or trephine shows sheets of plasma cells (**10.109**).
- Plain X-rays of the skeleton show 'punched out' areas, especially in skull (**10.110**), ribs, pelvis and long bones (**10.111**). There may also be pathological fractures.

A range of other investigations aid prognosis (*see* **Table 10.12**).

Treatment of patients with multiple myeloma is supportive with antibiotics for infection, analgesics for bone pain, a high fluid intake and effective management of hypercalcaemia. Hyperviscosity and cryoglobulinaemia may be managed by plasma exchange until the tumour mass can be controlled with either melphalan or cyclophosphamide or with radiotherapy for local lesions.

10.108

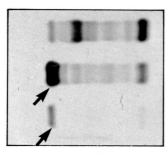

serum

urine ×25

urine neat

IgA myeloma

10.108 Serum and urine electrophoresis in multiple myeloma provide evidence of the presence of a paraprotein in serum and urine. In this case, the patient had IgA myeloma; the paraprotein band shows clearly in the urine (arrows) and a corresponding band is present in the serum.

10.109 Bone marrow trephine biopsy in myeloma. Note the predominance of neoplastic plasma cells; characteristically, these are large cells with an eccentric nucleus and a perinuclear halo. Note that there is erosion and cellular infiltration of the trabecular bone (top left).

10.109

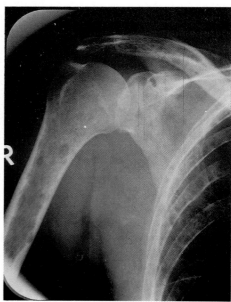

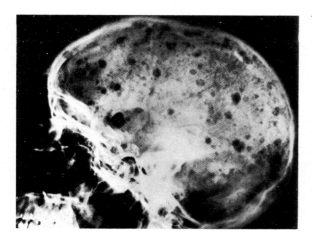

10.110 **10.111**

10.110 Myeloma lesions in bones show up as characteristic 'punched out' lesions without surrounding sclerosis. Secondary deposits from other tumours may occasionally give a similar appearance, but this appearance on skull X-ray is strongly suggestive of multiple myeloma.

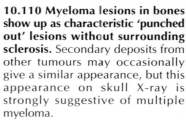

Table 10.12 Adverse prognostic factors in myeloma.

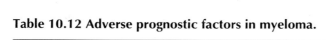

- Severe anaemia
- Low serum albumin
- Renal impairment
- High serum calcium
- High levels of light chains
- Extensive osteolytic lesions
- High monoclonal component
- High β_2-microglobulin levels
- Expression of CD10 antigen on the cells
- Active mitosis of plasma cells

10.111 Myeloma in the humerus, scapula, clavicle and ribs. The lesions have the same 'punched out' appearance as those seen in the skull. Myeloma lesions are also commonly seen in other long bones, in the ribs and in the pelvis. Pathological fractures may occur, and hypercalcaemia is common.

Solitary plasmacytomas

In a small number of cases of paraproteinaemia (7%) there is a localised plasma cell proliferation and the marrow elsewhere is normal. Such local plasmacytomas may arise in bone or in soft tissues and may grow to a large size before being diagnosed. Diagnosis is made by finding a solitary lytic lesion of bone, with an abnormal M-protein on electrophoresis, histological evidence of plasma cell tumour on biopsy and a normal marrow at a distant site. Surgical removal or radiotherapy produces a cure with a rapid disappearance of the M-proteins.

Waldenström's macroglobulinaemia

Waldenström's macroglobulinaemia is a condition characterised by the presence of monoclonal IgM in association with excessive numbers of tissue lymphocytes and plasma cells (lymphocytic lymphoma with plasmacytoid differentiation).

This is a disease of the elderly with a male preponderance of 2:1. The common presentation is with fever, anaemia, weight loss, weakness and fatigue. Bleeding may occur as a result of qualitative platelet defects and usually manifests as epistaxis, skin petechiae and gastrointestinal haemorrhage. Hyperviscosity features may dominate the picture and result in strokes, myocardial infarction, loss of vision and Raynaud's phenomenon.

Bence–Jones protein may be found in the urine and amyloid may develop. The lymphocytic infiltrate may cause hepatomegaly and splenomegaly, but can occur in any other body tissue. Osteolytic lesions are rare.

Investigations show a normochromic normocytic anaemia with rouleaux formation on the blood film (**10.27**). There may be leucopenia but more usually there is an atypical lymphocytosis. The ESR is characteristically elevated to above 100 mm in the first hour. Bone marrow shows a generalised diffuse lympho-plasmacytoid infiltrate with excess eosinophils. Such appearances may also be found in the peripheral lymph nodes. Examination of the serum shows an abnormal M-protein, cryoglobulin, and cold-reacting antibodies.

Treatment should be aimed at the hyperviscosity which dominates the clinical picture. This may be altered by haemodilution or plasmaphoresis. Chemotherapy with chlorambucil, cyclophosphamide or melphalan may be helpful. Supportive management is required for haemorrhage, anaemia, infections and cold-precipitation syndromes.

Benign monoclonal gammopathy

A monoclonal paraprotein sometimes appears in the absence of a detectable B-cell tumour. Some patients develop this paraprotein transiently in response to an infection such as viral hepatitis or leptospirosis, in an autoimmune disease such as rheumatoid arthritis, and occasionally in non-B-cell tumours. In other patients there is a stable benign paraproteinaemia which remains unchanged for many years, except in a small number who develop an overtly malignant plasma-cell myeloma.

Investigations should be directed at the underlying cause: non-B-cell malignancy, infection or autoimmune disease.

Bence–Jones proteins and M-band proteins are present. A level of paraprotein below 10 g/l usually indicates a benign cause. There is no marrow infiltration or immunosuppression, and no lytic bone lesions. Patients should be followed-up carefully over many years, as 10% develop overt myeloma. No specific treatment is necessary initially. Because the outcome is now realised not to be always 'benign', the term monoclonal gammopathy of undetermined significance (MGUS) is now being used.

Blood transfusion

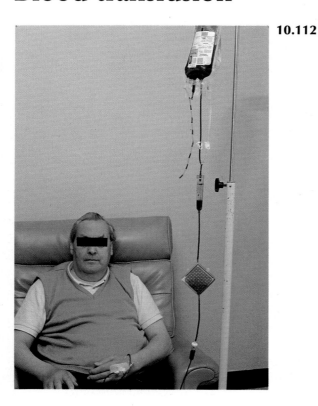

10.112 Blood transfusion. This patient receives regular monthly blood transfusions for refractory sideroblastic anaemia. Multiple transfusions may lead to sensitisation to the white cell (HLA) antigens, with resulting febrile transfusion reactions. These can be greatly ameliorated by passing the blood through a white cell filter such as the Sepacell filter shown 'in line' here. This patient was also receiving regular overnight subcutaneous infusions of desferrioxamine to deal with the iron overload inevitable with a chronic blood transfusion regimen.

The availability of blood components for transfusion underpins the management of many medical emergencies as well as the supportive therapy necessary in marrow failure.

Red cell grouping and crossmatching before transfusion is essential. Selection of red cells of the correct ABO group is the prime concern, since an ABO mismatched transfusion can result in a catastrophic immediate transfusion reaction with intravascular haemolysis, consumptive coagulopathy (DIC) and renal failure. Delayed haemolytic transfusion reactions, with extravascular haemolysis, are more common with antibodies to other red cell antigens, including Rh antigens, and give rise to jaundice and anaemia over several days.

Febrile transfusion reactions are common especially after multiple transfusions. They are often related to the development of antibodies to HLA antigens present on white cells and platelets, and can be largely avoided by removing white cells, e.g. by using in-line white cell filters at the time of transfusion (**10.112**).

Routine screening of donors now means that the risk of transmission of known viruses such as HIV and hepatitis B is negligible. However, chronic non-A non-B hepatitis is still a hazard, and this serves as a reminder that blood products should be used only with good reason: red cell transfusions for chronic anaemias which can be treated, albeit more slowly, with haematinics, should be avoided unless the patient is clinically compromised.

11. Disorders of Nerve and Muscle

History

Important facets of the history in a patient with neurological symptoms include the time course of the following:

- Higher cerebral dysfunction — dementia, confusional states and coma are common features and are the end results of a large number of acute and chronic neurological diseases.
- Fits — a wide range of epileptic phenomena may result from neurological diseases. These include generalised or partial seizures and are often best described by family or friends rather than the patient.
- Headache is one of the most common presenting symptoms and its causes include tension, stress, migraine and cranial arteritis. Space-occupying lesions cause headache that is often worse on waking and on coughing or bending. There may be associated vomiting. It is particularly important to define site of pain, exacerbating factors, radiation of pain and duration.
- Loss of power results from abnormalities of the upper or lower motor neuron in the brain or cord as well as disorders of the neuromuscular junction and muscle. Loss of power may be of acute or gradual onset. Lower motor neuron lesions result in localised muscle atrophy. Upper motor neuron lesions result in spasticity which produces a typical jerky gait.

- Vertigo is the feeling that the surroundings are moving. It reflects disease of the labyrinth or vestibular connections. Dizziness is a common symptom — the patient usually implies unsteadiness or lightheadedness.
- Abnormal movements — a variety of tremors may suggest a diagnosis, e.g. the typical 'pill rolling' tremor of Parkinson's disease, or the coarse flapping tremor associated with liver, respiratory or renal failure. In contrast are the coarse movements of chorea, athetosis and hemiballismus. These are the result of extrapyramidal lesions.
- Cerebellar ataxia may produce a loss of fine control of movement which results in dysmetria, dysynergia and a broad based gait, with a tendency to fall to the side of the lesion if it is unilateral. There are usually other symptoms and signs of the cerebellar lesion, including diplopia, dysarthria and hypotonia. Sensory ataxia results from lesions of the sensory pathways in the peripheral nerves or spinal cord and produces a stamping gait. There is compensation from visual stimuli and when the eyes are closed the problem is exacerbated.
- General medical, occupational, social and family history—all of which may point to underlying causes for neurological symptoms.

Examination

A pre-existing detailed knowledge of the anatomy and physiology of the brain, spinal cord and peripheral and autonomic nervous system is essential before embarking on CNS examination.

Appropriate tests must be planned and carried out with care, in an attempt to localise any focal lesions and assess possible causes.

General assessment

It is important to observe the patient and his movements. His posture and gait may reveal abnormalities (11.1–11.3); he may show signs of personal neglect or psychiatric disorder; there may be signs of systemic disease, or of local abnormalities.

11.1

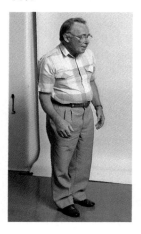

11.2

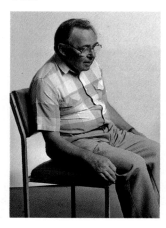

11.3

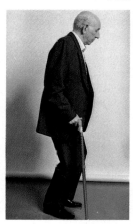

11.1–11.3 Posture and gait can provide important clues to neurological diagnosis. Both these patients have Parkinson's disease. The patient in **11.1** and **11.2** demonstrated rigidity and poverty of movement. Note his stooped posture and the typical position of his arms, which are held slightly flexed at the sides. The patient in **11.3** has a typical parkinsonian gait. He finds it difficult to initiate movement and walks with small shuffling steps. To stop himself falling forward he flexes his knees, and the forward movement on the forepart of the foot gives rise to a characteristic 'festinant' gait.

Higher cerebral function

Aspects of higher cerebral function often become obvious from the history, but the examination should include observations on conscious level, orientation in time and space, general level of intelligence, mental state, general attitude, speech and memory. Most of these functions can be quantified when necessary, using rating scales. Apraxia (11.4) and agnosia (11.5) may be revealed by appropriate tests. Cognitive function can be rapidly screened using the mini-mental state examination and other rating scales, prior to a more detailed assessment.

11.4

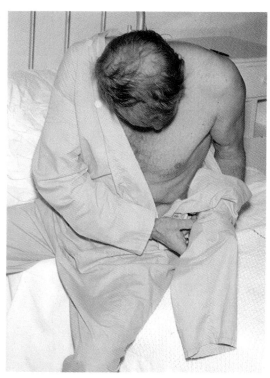

11.4 Apraxia is the inability to perform a familiar action which cannot be attributed to physical disability, incomprehension or agnosia (see **11.5**). This patient has dressing apraxia, associated with bilateral subdural haematomas. Apraxia results from higher cerebral dysfunction.

11.5 Visuo-spatial agnosia is an inability to recognise part of the environment despite normal sensation. In this patient a right (non-dominant) parieto-occipital lobe lesion has led to an inability to write on the left side of a sheet of paper. Patients with severe agnosia may even deny the ownership of limbs and neglect the affected side of the body and the environment.

11

Systematic examination

The upper and lower limbs and trunk must be examined systematically to assess motor power, sensation, the extrapyramidal system and the cerebellum. In each muscle group, assess:

- Muscle bulk, and look carefully for trophic changes and involuntary movements.
- Tone — spastic (clasp knife) or plastic (lead pipe).
- Power.
- Reflexes: superficial and tendon.
- Coordination.

In any abnormality it must be decided whether the upper or lower motor neuron is involved. Upper motor neuron lesions produce weakness of arm extensors and leg flexors (a 'pyramidal' pattern). Lower motor neuron lesions produce a deficit in a root or nerve distribution. Polyneuropathies usually present with distal weakness. Abnormal movements suggest probable extrapyramidal involvement.

Lesions of the cerebellum result in loss of tone, in coordination, altered posture, speech defects and nystagmus.

If patients have sensory symptoms the following sensory modalities must be tested carefully. The functions to be tested include:

- Tactile sensation and discrimination.
- Pain and deep pain.
- Temperature.
- Vibration (**10.30**).
- Proprioception.
- Two point discrimination, stereognosis, and graphaesthesia if cortical lesions are suspected.

Cranial nerves

I. Olfactory nerve

Chemoreceptors are present in the mucosa on the roof of the nose and pass through the cribriform plate in the ethmoid to synapse in the olfactory bulb. Secondary fibres then pass via the olfactory tract to the olfactory cortex on the anteromedial temporal lobe. Loss of smell (anosmia) may result from lesions of the:

- mucosa, e.g. the common cold;
- cribriform plate, e.g. fracture;

- olfactory tract, e.g. space-occupying lesions;
- rarely, temporal lobe, e.g. space-occupying lesions, haematoma, or trauma.

The nerve is tested by asking the patient to smell a scent. Lesions may be unilateral or bilateral. Parosmia is a distorted sense of smell.

II. Optic nerve

From an inverted image on the light-sensitive cells of the retina, the impulses pass via the optic nerves to the optic chiasma; at the decussation, fibres from the nasal side of the retina cross to the contralateral optic tract, while the temporal retinal fibres remain uncrossed. The optic tracts then pass to the lateral geniculate body where they synapse. The optic radiation fibres sweep posteriorly through the temporal and parietal lobes to the occipital cortex. The left half of the field of vision is represented in the cortex of the right hemisphere and vice versa. Some fibres from the optic tract do *not* synapse at the lateral geniculate body but pass directly to the midbrain as the afferent limb of the pupillary light reflex.

Full examination of the second nerves should include examination of the eyes (**11.6**), including the retina, and an assessment of:

- Visual acuity—using Jaeger or Faculty of Ophthalmologists' charts for near vision or Snellen test type for distance vision.
- Fields of vision by confrontation and perimetry (**7.1, 11.7**).
- Colour vision by Ishihara plates is required for individuals in many occupations.
- Pupillary reflexes — to light and accommodation.

The **Argyll Robertson** pupil (**11.8**) is the hallmark of neurosyphilis and is now very rare. The pupil is small, irregular and reacts to accommodation but not to light directly or consensually. The abnormality is present bilaterally.

The **Holmes–Adie pupil** (**11.9**) is characterised by a delayed or absent response to light and to accommodation. Once constricted it dilates only very slowly. The lesion may be unilateral and it may be associated with bilateral absent or diminished tendon reflexes.

Horner's syndrome (**4.128, 11.10**) results from paralysis of the cervical sympathetic nerve. Sympathetic supply to the pupil leaves the CNS in the lower cervical and upper thoracic portions of the cord, emerges in the first thoracic nerve root and runs via the sympathetic chain and along the internal carotid artery to the cavernous plexus and then via the ophthalmic division of the trigeminal nerve to the eye.

Any disorder that interferes with the integrity of the pathway causes Horner's syndrome, which comprises ptosis, pupillary constriction (miosis), enophthalmos and loss of sweating on half of the face and neck (anhidrosis). The common causes of Horner's syndrome are shown in **Table 11.1**.

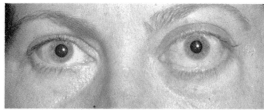

11.6

11.6 Unilateral proptosis resulted from a meningioma on the sheath of the optic nerve in this patient. A similar appearance may develop in Graves' disease (*see* p. 321), but exophthalmos is usually bilateral in that condition.

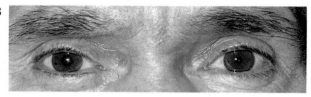

11.8

11.8 Argyll Robertson pupils are a feature of tertiary neurosyphilis. They are usually bilateral, but the abnormality was more marked in this patient's left eye. Argyll Robertson pupils are small, irregular and unresponsive to light, but they show an intact near response if the patient's visual acuity is adequate (i.e. they react normally on accommodation). They may also be found in patients with diabetes mellitus.

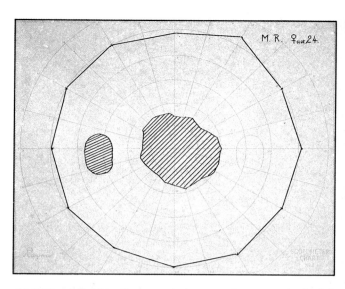

1

11.7 Visual field testing revealed a central scotoma in the left eye of a 24-year-old woman. This resulted from optic neuritis. She made a complete recovery from this condition, but has a 50% chance of developing other features of multiple sclerosis within the next 4 years.

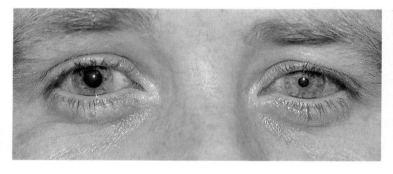

11

11.9 Holmes–Adie pupil in the right eye of a young woman. The affected pupil is 'tonic', i.e. it responds slowly to light and accommodation, but on rapid testing will appear unresponsive. The site of the lesion is usually obscure, but the condition is benign. There may be associated areflexia.

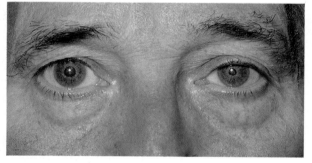

11.10

11.10 Horner's syndrome. Note the characteristic ptosis of the left eye, associated with constriction of the pupil (miosis). This patient had syringomyelia, but Horner's syndrome has many possible causes (**Table 11.1**).

Table 11.1 Disorders causing Horner's syndrome.

Pancoast tumour
Cervical rib
Carotid aneurysm
Carotid body tumour
Syringomyelia
Ponto-medullary CVA or tumour
Trauma

III, IV and VI. Oculomotor, trochlear and abducens

These three nerves together control the muscles of ocular movement.

Lower motor neuron lesions may lead to defective movements, squint, diplopia and pupillary abnormalities:

- Oculomotor lesions — ptosis is present, the eyeball is rotated downwards and outwards, and the pupil is dilated and fixed (**3.77, 11.11, 11.12**). Unilateral pupillary dilatation may be the sole manifestation of an early lesion.
- Trochlear lesions cause impaired downward movement — diplopia occurs on looking down (**11.13**).
- Abducens lesions cause convergent squint with inability to move the eye outwards and diplopia on trying to look outwards (**7.6, 7.84, 11.14**).

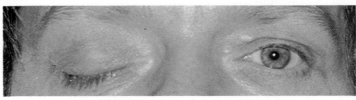

11.11

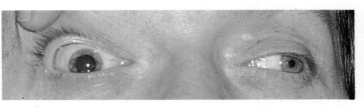

11.12

11.11, 11.12 Third nerve palsy. Note the complete ptosis and the fixed, dilated right pupil. In the resting position, the right eye was rotated laterally and downwards, but in **11.12** the patient is looking to the left, and the right eye has rotated to the mid position, demonstrating that the trochlear (fourth) nerve is intact. This patient's third nerve palsy was the result of compression by an aneurysm of the posterior communicating artery.

11.13

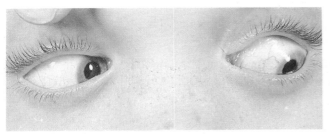

11.13 Right fourth nerve palsy. The patient is attempting to look down and to the left, but this movement is impaired in the right eye. The patient presented with diplopia, especially when reading, and difficulty in walking downstairs.

11.14

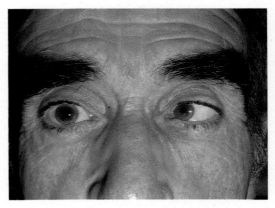

11.14 Right sixth nerve palsy. Failure of the right eye to abduct on lateral gaze. The lid, the pupil and other ocular movements are normal.

V. Trigeminal nerve

Lesions of the trigeminal nerve lead to loss of sensation in the skin of the face and crown of the head (**11.15**), the conjunctivae and the nasopharynx. The angle of the jaw is spared as this is supplied by the second cervical nerve. There is also diminished secretion by the lacrimal and salivary glands, which results in dry eyes and mouth, and trophic ulceration may be found in the cornea, nose and mouth. The corneal reflex is lost. The distribution of the first division of the fifth nerve is graphically demonstrated in ophthalmic herpes (**1.80**).

If the motor branch is involved, there is weakness and wasting of the muscles of mastication, and if this is unilateral the jaw deviates to the affected side on opening the mouth.

11.15

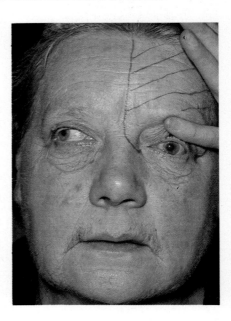

11.15 Trigeminal nerve palsy, affecting the ophthalmic division of the nerve. The distribution of sensory impairment is marked. The palsy results from compression of the fifth nerve by an aneurysm in the cavernous sinus, and it is accompanied by palsy of the third cranial nerve—demonstrated by a failure of adduction of the left eye—and by palsies of the fourth and sixth nerves.

VII Facial nerve

The facial nerve is almost entirely motor in function, supplying all the muscles of the face and scalp except for the levator palpebrae superioris. Paralysis leads to loss of facial expression and movement.

In **supranuclear** paralysis only the lower part of the face is involved because of the bilateral upper motor neuron innervation of the forehead. In **infranuclear** paralysis both the upper and lower parts of the face are involved equally (**11.16, 11.17**).

Bell's palsy is the most common cause of infranuclear paralysis of the facial nerve. The nerve is often involved around the stylomastoid foramen, but symptoms and signs depend on the site of nerve involvement. The onset is usually acute. There is a rapid onset of unilateral paralysis of the muscles of facial expression and occasionally some pain behind the ear. Taste sensation from the ipsilateral anterior two-thirds of the tongue may be lost, and there may be undue sensitivity to sounds (hyperacusis).

On the affected side, there is drooping of the corner of the mouth, with loss of skin creases and folds, particularly the naso-labial fold, and of the furrows on the forehead; the eye will often not close and attempts to close it result in it rolling upwards (Bell's phenomenon). Tears tend to run down the cheek as the lower lid sags and because of paralysis of the lip muscles, saliva dribbles from the corner of the mouth and food collects between the cheeks and gums.

The cause is possibly viral but unknown. Diagnosis is made on clinical grounds, and electromyography may be of some value in detecting interruption in the continuity of nerve fibres.

The disease is usually self-limiting and most patients recover in a few weeks. There is no specific treatment but local measures to prevent exposure keratitis are of value, and local massage and splinting may be of use. Steroids are often prescribed.

Other lesions of the facial nerve may produce similar symptoms and signs, e.g. mononeuritis (7.84), trauma and compression by tumours such as acoustic neuromas.

The **Ramsay Hunt syndrome** (1.82, 11.18) results when herpes zoster affects the geniculate ganglion of the seventh nerve. Patients present with severe pain in the ear and a facial palsy on the same side. There may be a herpes rash in the external auditory meatus and in the pharynx.

11.16

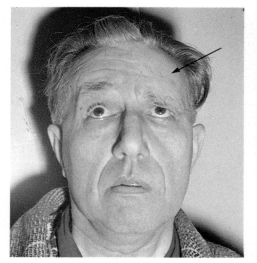

11.17

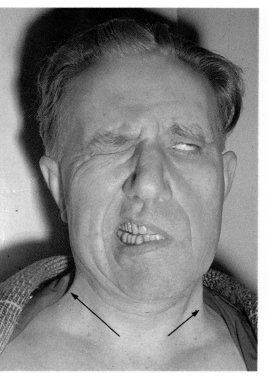

11.18

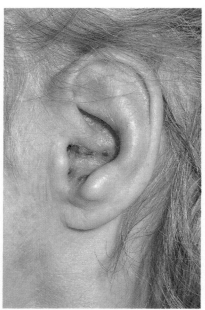

11.18 The Ramsay Hunt syndrome is caused by herpes zoster (shingles) of the geniculate ganglion. The patient had a facial palsy identical to Bell's palsy, and the clinical clue to the diagnosis is the presence of herpetic vesicles in the external auditory meatus (which receives a small sensory branch from the facial nerve).

11.16, 11.17 Lower motor neuron palsy of the facial nerve (Bell's palsy). The face may look almost normal at rest, but the patient is unable to wrinkle his brow on the affected side (**11.16**, arrow). When the patient is asked to close his eyes, show his teeth and contract the platysma muscle (**11.17**, arrows) the difference between the unaffected right side and the affected left side becomes much more obvious. The left-sided facial weakness is severe. In upper motor neuron lesions, the weakness is less evident and the brow muscles function normally.

VIII Vestibulo-cochlear nerve

Two sets of fibres run in this nerve which serves the cochlea (for hearing) and the labyrinth and semicircular canals (for balance). Lesions of the nerve may present with tinnitus, hyperacusis, deafness and dizziness.

Acoustic neurofibromas (neuromas) may develop at the cerebello-pontine angle and present with insidious onset of unilateral deafness, headache, tinnitus, vertigo, ataxia, loss of sensation on the face resulting from trigeminal compression and facial weakness caused by compression of the facial nerve. Signs of a unilateral cerebellar lesion, including nystagmus, soon appear; there may be pressure on the optic nerve with papilloedema. In advanced cases hydrocephalus, long tract signs and coma may develop.

Skull X-ray with special views shows widening of the internal auditory meatus but diagnosis is best made by CT or MRI (**11.19**, **11.48**, **11.114**) which clearly show the site and extent of the lesion.

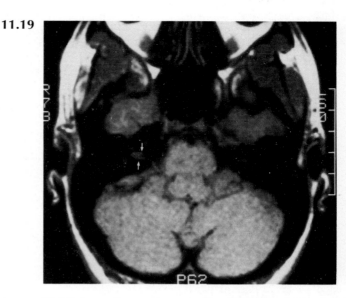

11.19 Acoustic neuroma on the right side (arrowed) demonstrated by axial MRI. The neuroma is intracanalicular.

IX, X and XI Glossopharyngeal, vagus and accessory

These nerves can be considered together. The glossopharyngeal nerve (IX) is predominantly sensory and supplies the posterior third of the tongue, palate, pharynx and fauces. The motor supply to this area is the vagus (X), which also supplies the oesophagus. The accessory nerve (XI) is purely motor, supplying the larynx and pharynx as well as fibres for the sternomastoid and trapezius.

Disorders of these nerves result in paralysis of the soft palate with regurgitation of fluids through the nose, difficulty in swallowing, change in the voice which may become deeper and hoarse, and a diminution of coughing. Palsy of the accessory nerve leads to difficulty in flexion/extension of the neck and in shrugging the shoulders (**11.20**).

The left recurrent laryngeal nerve branch of the vagus is particularly liable to damage as it loops round the aorta and runs a long course back up to supply sensation and motor fibres to the larynx below the level of the vocal cords. Lesions of this branch result in dysphonia (**4.129**) and a 'bovine' cough.

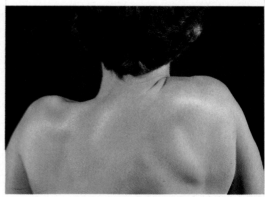

11.20 Accessory nerve palsy. The left trapezius does not contract when the patient shrugs her shoulders, and examination also revealed paralysis of the left sternomastoid muscle. The cause was avulsion of the nerve in a neck injury in a road traffic accident.

XII Hypoglossal

The hypoglossal nerve is wholly motor, supplying the tongue and the depressors of the hyoid bone. Lesions of the nerve result in unilateral paralysis, wasting and fasciculation of the tongue which is pushed over to the paralysed side when put out (**11.21**).

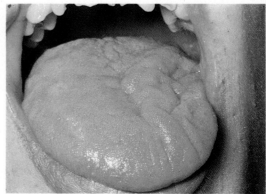

11.21 Hypoglossal nerve palsy. This patient had an isolated left lower motor neuron lesion of obscure cause, with deviation of the tongue to the affected side when it was pushed out, associated with fasciculation and fissuring caused by wasting.

Investigations

As in other systems, investigation of abnormalities in the CNS starts with simple investigations which lead to more specific tests to define the site and nature of the lesion and its consequences. These tests are usually more expensive, more invasive or both, and they must be selected with care.

Haematology

A simple Coulter printout of the profile of absolute values may show evidence of polycythaemia (in a stroke patient), anaemia and macrocytosis (in a patient with subacute combined degeneration), macrocytosis and thrombocytopenia (in alcoholism). A high ESR or plasma viscosity may suggest the possibility of vasculitis, infection or neoplasia.

Biochemistry

Liver function abnormalities may suggest the presence of alcoholism in patients with peripheral neuropathy or coma, or of metastases or liver failure with an associated neurological syndrome. Direct measurement of levels of alcohol or narcotic drugs is of value in patients admitted in coma. Disturbances in serum potassium levels may explain episodes of paralysis; and abnormal thyroid hormone or parathormone/calcium levels are associated with peripheral and central neuron dysfunction. Calcium and glucose levels are of value in patients presenting with epileptic fits. Measurement of levels of creatine kinase (CK) is of value in patients suspected of muscular dystrophy.

The concentration is usually over 100 iu/l, but it must be remembered that mild exertion or an intramuscular injection can raise the level to 300–400 iu/l.

Measurement of myoglobin in the urine gives an indication of muscle necrosis, and high levels may be associated with precipitation in the renal tubules and subsequent renal failure. Under these circumstances exceptionally high levels of CK may be observed.

Optimal control of epilepsy demands monitoring of the serum levels of anticonvulsants to maintain safe and effective therapeutic levels.

Serology

Evidence of infection may be found by the presence of various antibodies, e.g. HIV infection, herpes simplex, neurosyphilis, neuroborreliasis.

Measurement of IgG antibodies to cholinergic receptors in skeletal muscle is of value in confirming the diagnosis of myasthenia gravis.

Biopsies

Biopsy of peripheral nerves may give valuable information which can be both diagnostic and prognostic, and may suggest therapy. The biopsy is best done at the wrist (superficial radial nerve) or at the ankle (distal sural nerve) and should involve partial thickness biopsy to reduce the sensory loss.

Muscle biopsy may be done by needle or open biopsy under local anaesthesia. Enough material should be taken for histology, including electron microscopy, and histochemistry for muscle enzymes. Diagnostic changes are found in muscular dystrophies and inflammatory myopathies. In addition, vessel changes may indicate polyarteritis nodosa.

Brain biopsy is carried out in highly selected patients when there is a possibility that a course of therapy might be indicated, e.g. in suspected brain tumours or in possible herpes simplex encephalitis. It is not justified in dementia as there are currently no therapeutic possibilities, but meningeal biopsy may identify potentially treatable angiitides. If the patient's vision is normal, however, it is likely that the delayed response results from demyelination (11.22).

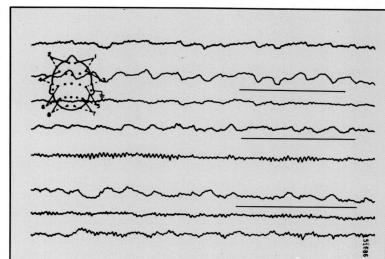

11.22 EEG abnormality caused by a cerebral tumour. This 56-year-old woman presented with late-onset partial seizures and showed a consistent focal abnormality in the left temporal lobe on EEG. Skull X-ray and isotope scan were normal, and the patient was seen before the advent of routine CT or MR scanning, so the EEG was helpful; but it has now been largely replaced by these definitive imaging techniques in the diagnosis of focal lesions.

Nerve conduction studies

Motor and sensory conduction rates can be readily measured in large axons. There are differences in rates of conduction in different nerves and most laboratories apply their own standards. Demyelination greatly reduces conduction, as in the Guillain–Barré syndrome, nerve entrapment or diabetes mellitus; whereas in axonal degeneration, as found in drug-induced neuropathy, conduction velocity is only slightly reduced.

Electromyography

Muscle or nerve action potentials can be recorded with needle or surface electrodes and are used in the differentiation of myopathic or neuropathic processes and in monitoring healing after nerve injury. In myopathies, damage to the motor units produces typical polyphasic responses. The specific cause of a myopathy cannot usually be diagnosed by this technqiue.

Edrophonium (Tensilon) test

This diagnostic test is used in patients with suspected myasthenia gravis (*see* p. 520).

Electroencephalograph (EEG)

The EEG is a record of the spontaneous electrical signals generated within the brain. It is usually recorded from surface electrodes placed on the scalp, but in selected patients additional valuable diagnostic information may be obtained by neurosurgical implantation of sphenoidal, foramen ovale or cortical electrodes. A profile of waves is obtained from the electrodes and these wave patterns reflect the summation of electrical rhythms and are termed alpha, beta, theta and delta. The basic waveforms alter with eye closure, during sleep and with voluntary movements.

The EEG is valuable in detecting general abnormalities in physiological function such as occur in epilepsy, encephalitis or encephalopathies. It can be of value in localising a structural abnormality (**11.22**), but has largely been replaced by CT and MRI. Distinct patterns form the basis of classification of epilepsy. Video-telemetry is sometimes of value in diagnosing patients with 'funny turns' of unknown origin and is particularly important when localising seizure foci before surgery.

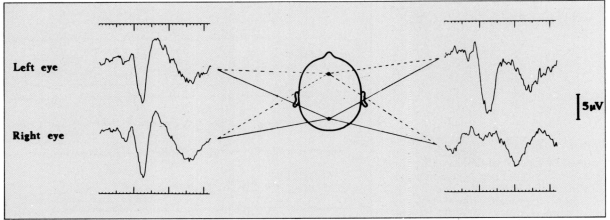

11.23 Visual-evoked response in optic neuritis of the right eye. Visual stimulation with a chequered pattern produces a predictable response on the EEG, and this response is delayed and deformed in this patient (bottom right trace). Optic neuritis is the most common cause of this abnormality and, as damage caused by subclinical or forgotten episodes can be detected, the test is of value; but it is not specific (see text).

Evoked responses

Sensitive scalp electrodes allow the measurement on EEG of cortical responses to controlled stimuli, which may be visual, auditory or somatosensory. Delayed or abnormnal waveforms may provide evidence of physiological dysfunction. Visual-evoked responses are used in the diagnosis of multiple sclerosis, but the test is not specific and abnormalities in any part of the pathway from the eye to the occipital cortex will prolong the response time. If the patient's vision is normal, however, it is likely that the delayed response is caused by demyelination (**11.23**).

Lumbar puncture

Samples of CSF are usually obtained by lumbar puncture at L3–L4 level (**11.24**). The important clinical indications are:

- Probable infections of the central nervous system, including meningitis, encephalitis and neurosyphilis.
- Possible subarachnoid bleeding.
- Possible myelopathies or multiple sclerosis.
- Pressure measurement e.g. in benign intracranial hypertension.

Definite contraindications to lumbar puncture are raised intracranial pressure caused by space-occupying lesions, cord compression, local skin sepsis and any bleeding tendency (including anticoagulant therapy). Access to the subarachnoid space allows the pressure of CSF to be measured—it normally ranges from 80–180 mm of CSF and moves with respiration. Pressure on the jugular vein (Queckenstedt's test) results in a rise of up to 40 mm in CSF pressure. If the pressure does not rise, a block in the spinal canal is possible. This is usually associated with a dense yellow colouration of CSF caused by its protein content (Froin's syndrome).

CSF is collected for cell count, biochemistry and serology. If blood staining is present initially, the CSF should be collected in three tubes to determine if the later tubes clear. Samples should be examined for pus (**1.21**) and blood, and centrifuged to see if the supernatant is xanthochromic (**11.25**). (*See* **Table 11.7** for changes in infection and **Table 11.2** for changes in other conditions.)

Where computed tomography (CT) or magnetic resonance imaging (MRI) is readily available, lumbar puncture is sometimes unnecessary (e.g. subarachnoid haemorrhage can often be diagnosed on CT scan). In all patients with altered consciousness or focal neurological signs CT scanning is advisable before carrying out lumbar puncture.

11.24

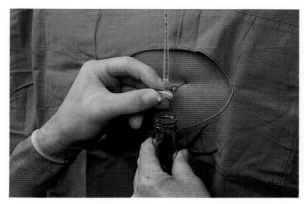

11.24 Lumbar puncture. The patient lies on his side (his head is to the left of the picture). After infiltration with local anaesthetic, the lumbar puncture needle is introduced through the third or fourth lumbar interspace. Its stylet is withdrawn, and a drop of CSF should appear. A manometer and three-way tap allows measurement of the CSF pressure and collection of fluid for examination.

11.25

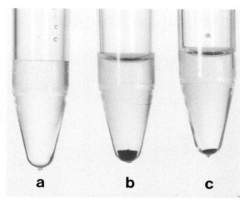

11.25 CSF examination. The fluid has been centrifuged immediately after collection. a) Normal crystal-clear CSF; b) fluid from a 'bloody tap'—there is blood at the bottom of the tube, but the supernatant fluid is clear; c) CSF from a patient with subarachnoid haemorrhage—there is blood at the bottom of the tube and the supernatant is yellow (xanthochromic), as a result of breakdown of blood cells in the CSF before the lumbar puncture.

Table 11.2 Cerebrospinal fluid in disease states.

	Appearance	Pressure (mm CSF)	Cells (per mm³)	Protein (mg/100ml)	Sugar (mmol/l)	Other
Normal	Crystal clear	80–180	0–5 (Lymphocytes)	15–45	3.5–4.5	
Traumatic tap	Bloodstained: clears	Normal	Red cells	Raised	Normal	Supernate clear
Subarachnoid haemorrhage	Bloody	Raised	Red cells	Raised	Normal	Xanthochromia
Multiple sclerosis	Clear	Normal	0–20 (Lymphocytes)	Raised	Normal	Elevated Ig Index
Froin's syndrome	Yellow	Low	Normal	Up to 600 and more	Normal	May clot on standing
Syphilis	Clear	Normal	Up to 50 (Lymphocytes)	Up to 100	Normal	Positive antibody Elevated IgG Index
Viral meningitis	Clear/yellow	Raised	↑ lymphs	Normal	Normal	–
Bacterial meningitis	Clear/yellow	Raised	↑ polys	Raised	Reduced	Bacteria or Gram stain
TB meningitis	Clear/yellow	Raised	↑ lymphs	Raised	Reduced	ZN stain can be negative

Imaging techniques

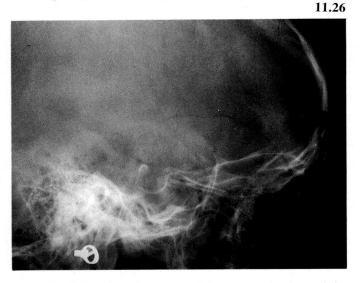

11.26

11.26 Skull fracture shown on plain X-ray. The line of the fracture runs across the middle meningeal artery, so the patient is at high risk of developing an extradural haematoma.

Straight X-rays of the skull are usually of limited value in neurological disease, except where there is a history of direct trauma which may be seen as a fracture (**11.26**) or a foreign body, and in disorders associated with ectopic calcification. Special views of the pituitary fossa, orbit, internal auditory canal, sinuses and spine give valuable additional information.

Computed tomography (CT) is extremely valuable in outlining the anatomy of the brain and skull, especially in defining cerebral haemorrhage, and infarction, space-occupying lesions (**11.27**), subdural haematomas, the presence of hydrocephalus and cerebral atrophy. Structures above the tentorium are better seen than those in the posterior fossa. The spinal canal, disc spaces and cord are also well visualised. Modern techniques allow discrimination down to 5 mm. Intravenous contrast media may be given to enhance imaging.

Magnetic resonance imaging (MRI) is another useful non-invasive technique. Differences between white and grey matter are better demonstrated than with CT and the contents of the posterior fossa and the cranio-cervical region of the spinal canal are well visualised. Brain and spinal cord tumours, vascular abnormalities, anatomical abnormalities (syringomyelia) and demyelinating disorders are particularly well shown (**11.28–11.30**). As with CT, contrast medium injected intravenously may add to the yield of MRI. Dynamic MRI may provide information about blood flow.

11.27

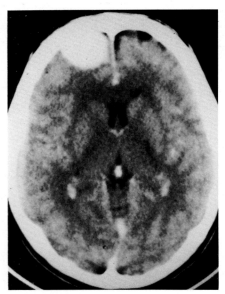

11.27 CT scan showing a right frontal meningioma with a vascular capsule. The contrast-enhancement technique used in this scan demonstrates the classic appearance of a densely enhancing, sharply marginated tumour, tightly against the dura. For MRI views of the same tumour see **11.28** and **11.29**.

11.28

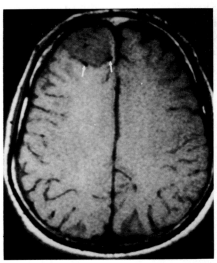

11.28 MRI picture of a right frontal meningioma (same patient as in **11.27**). MRI shows the fissures of the brain more clearly than CT; it shows the tumour well, and parts of its vascular supply appear as hyperdense images (arrows).

11.29

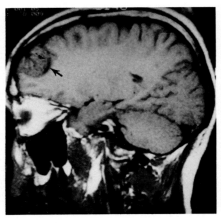

11.29 MRI sagittal view of the patient seen in **11.27** and **11.28**. This view demonstrates the relationship of the meningioma to the dura and skull very clearly, and shows the vascular capsule posteriorly (arrow).

Radionuclide scans have been largely replaced by MRI and CT scans for anatomical localisation, but are still of value in assessing blood flow and in the detection of large ischaemic infarcts, arterio-venous malformations and subdural haematomas. A development of this technique is single photon emission computed tomography (SPECT) scanning. Technetium is given attached to a carrier molecule (hexamethylene propyleneanine oxime, HMPAO) which enters the cerebral cells, and its presence is a reflection of blood flow and cell metabolism. It has a value in the investigation of patients with epilepsy because it may allow localisation of foci. Another radionuclide test involves the use of isotopes of oxygen and glucose which localise in cerebral cells and provide information on local cerebral perfusion and function—positron emission tomography (PET) scans.

Ultrasound and the Doppler flow technique are now widely used to define the waveform, measure blood flow and define anatomical abnormalities in the carotid arteries. The techniques are non-invasive, cheap and readily repeatable and they have transformed the investigation of transient ischaemic attacks and permitted the screening of patients before selection for arteriography.

Cerebral angiography may be carried out by direct injection of contrast into the carotid or vertebral arteries, usually via a catheter inserted into the femoral artery. There is a small morbidity and mortality associated with the procedure. A series of films is taken in two planes to detect arterial and venous obstruction(**11.31**), aneurysms, arterio-venous malformations, tumour circulations and arteritides. An alternative technique is digital subtraction angiography (DSA), in which the injection of contrast may be made intravenously and images of the artery are obtained by computer subtraction of images (**11.32**).

11.30

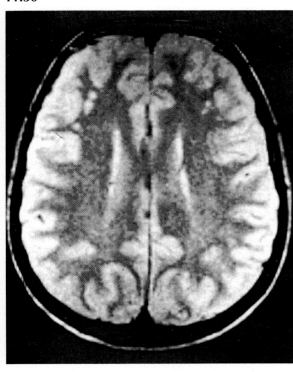

11.30 MRI is useful in many neurological disorders. This patient has systemic lupus erythematosus, and the numerous small white areas represent vasculitic lesions in the brain.

11.31

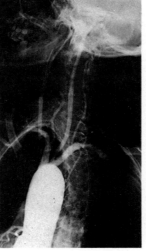

11.31 Aortogram in a patient with unexplained intermittent syncope. The carotid arteries are normal, but on turning her head to the left, the flow of contrast medium through the patient's left vertebral artery is interrupted. This anomaly may also be found in asymptomatic normal individuals.

11.32

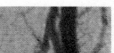
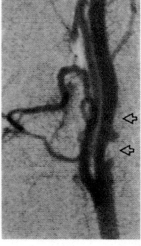

11.32 Digital subtraction angiography of the right carotid arteries. This view shows an extensive atheromatous plaque which has ulcerated in its centre and was the source of emboli in a patient with transient ischaemic attacks (TIAs).

Headache

The most common headaches are tension headaches and migraine. These can usually be distinguished from other causes on the clinical history alone.

Tension headache

This is usually a dull, nagging pain in the frontal, occipital or temporal regions, around the head 'like a band', or pressing on the vertex. There may be tender spots in the scalp and also a throbbing sensation behind the eyes. The headaches may persist for hours, days or weeks, and are often worse at the end of the day. Many, but not all sufferers, recognise a relationship to stress. Tension type headaches are rarely caused by visual refractive errors or hypertension, but these possibilities should be excluded. Tension headaches are benign in nature and respond to reassurance, avoidance of stress and simple analgesics; beta blockers may also help if there is a vascular component and some patients respond to antidepressant therapy.

Migraine

Migraine is an episodic, severe headache which lasts for several hours and presents in association with visual and gastrointestinal symptoms. There may be a prodromal phase in which there are flashing spots (teichopsia) or zig-zag lines (fortification spectra), and vision may be blurred. Additional neurological features may include photophobia, hemianaesthesia, hemiparesis, dysphasia and cranial nerve lesions. There is usually associated nausea and vomiting. Migraine is more common in women than men and is usually familial. There is evidence for vascular mechanisms (altered 5-hydroxytryptamine mechanisms in platelets and blood vessels) and for other abnormal brain mechanisms. Trigger factors often include cheese, shellfish, chocolate, red wine, coffee, smoking, menstruation, menopause, pregnancy, oral contraceptives and minor head trauma. Stress and, paradoxically, relief from stress may also trigger attacks. Some patients describe change in mood, appetite and fluid retention for hours or a day or two before and after the headache. The main classification is:

- **Common migraine.** Usually unilateral but sometimes bilateral throbbing headache, accompanied by nausea, vomiting and photophobia. Sleep may relieve symptoms.

- **Classical migraine.** There is a prodromal visual disturbance such as flashing lights, zig-zag lines, colours, and scotomas. These evolve over 10–30 minutes and are followed by headaches as above. Some variants involve sensory or hemisensory loss, hemiplegia, more complex perceptual changes, or dysphasia. Variants include: **vertebrobasilar system migraine**, associated with brainstem dysfunction and presenting with acute vertigo, diplopia, bilateral weakness, drowsiness or coma; **ophthalmoplegic migraine**, where on ocular palsy persists for hours or days; and **hemiplegic migraine**, which mimicks a stroke, but from which rapid recovery is usual.
- **Complicated migraine.** A very small proportion of migraines are complicated by a true stroke.

The first approach to management is to identify and prevent migraine by eliminating trigger factors. Acute headaches may be treated with bed rest in a darkened room, with ergotamine, aspirin or paracetamol, often with metoclopramide, or with sumatriptan. Prophylactic drugs such as pizotifen, propranolol and amitriptyline may be useful for patients with frequent migraines.

Other forms of headache

Migrainous neuralgia (cluster headache)

Migrainous neuralgia occurs mainly in men as an intense, throbbing, unilateral pain, usually retro-orbital but often spreading to the upper face. It occurs in bouts or 'clusters', with one or more episodes daily, often at regular times including wakening from sleep. Bouts last for days or weeks before clearing for weeks, months or years. There may be associated lacrimation, rhinorrhoea, and a transient Horner's syndrome, but nausea is not a feature. Acute attacks may be prevented with ergotamine; prophylactic treatment with pizotifen, propranolol or lithium carbonate are sometimes successful.

Temporal arteritis

Temporal or cranial arteritis presents in older patients with throbbing or persistent headache and tenderness in the temporal region, or more rarely in the occipital regions or the jaw on chewing. Urgent diagnosis and treatment are essential (*see* p. 150).

Atypical facial pain

The syndrome of 'atypical facial pain' is a nagging, protracted pain in the maxillary region, usually occuring in middle-aged depressed women. The pattern of pain does not usually conform to an anatomical distribution. It may respond to amitriptyline.

Headache of increased intracranial pressure

Increased intracranial pressure (*see* p. 488) is suggested by early morning headache, usually in the occipital region, with exacerbation on coughing or bending. Nausea, vomiting and brief visual disturbance, often on bending, may occur. There are often additional neurological features such as papilloedema, confusion and localising neurological signs. Sixth cranial palsy may occur as a false localising sign.

Meningeal pain

Subarachnoid haemorrhage produces sudden severe headache and neck stiffness, usually with focal signs and/or coma (*see* p. 498). Meningitis also produces headache and neck stiffness together with nausea, vomiting and photophobia (*see* p. 492).

Cervical spondylosis

Cervical spondylosis may cause headaches referred to the occipital region or anteriorly, which are often worse with head movement (*see* p. 511).

Trigeminal neuralgia

Trigeminal neuralgia (tic douloureux) is a disease of unknown origin that presents more commonly in women than in men with excruciating paroxysms of pain over the distribution of the trigeminal nerve. The syndrome may be associated with an aberrant vascular loop and in younger patients may occasionally be an early feature of multiple sclerosis, but usually no cause is found. It is commonest in older patients.

Severe pain occurs in the distribution of the mandibular or maxillary branches of the trigeminal nerve. The brief, agonising bouts are triggered by touch, chewing or cold. Carbamazepine is the drug treatment of choice, but if this fails selective thermocoagulation of trigeminal branches is of value and decompression of the trigeminal nerve may be attempted.

Miscellaneous other headaches

Headaches may occur with cough (cough headache), and in the masticatory syndrome (Costen syndrome), in which there is pain in the maxillary regions and exacerbation with chewing. In patients with severe headache, orbital pain and visual failure, the possibility of acute glaucoma must also be considered.

Dementia

Dementia is a persistent or progressive impairment of intellect, behaviour and personality. The diagnosis requires careful assessment of short- and long-term memory, language, calculation, behaviour, mood, and personality. A relative's history of the patient's decline may be useful in the diagnosis. Dementia differs from acute confusional states that have toxic, metabolic or infective causes.

Alzheimer's disease is the most common cause of slowly progressive dementia over several years. The mental symptoms and signs precede the physical signs by several months to years. Nearly all patients are over 60 years of age, and it is estimated that 5–10% of people over 65 are affected. Pathologically, there are characteristic senile plaques and neurofibrillary tangles.

The most common presentation is with a loss of recent memory, often associated with a personality change, apathy and antisocial behaviour followed by focal signs such as dysphasia, dyslexia, dyspraxia, agnosia and loss of sphincter control. Sleep disturbance is common. Disturbance of gait reduces mobility, but patients are inclined to wander, especially at night, and may injure themselves by falling.

In addition to Alzheimer's disease, a wide range of other conditions may cause dementia (**Table 11.3**). Some are treatable, so investigation is important in younger patients with dementia. Tests should include CT scanning (**11.33–11.35**) or MRI and may also involve full blood count (including serum B_{12} and folate), renal, liver and thyroid function tests, blood sugar, serology for syphilis, chest and skull X-rays, EEG and occasionally CSF examination.

Multi-infarct dementia can be difficult to distinguish clinically from Alzheimer's disease. Sudden deteriorations in neurological status are more in favour of this disorder in which there are multiple small infarcts in the brain, best shown on a CT scan (**11.35**). Clinical examination usually demonstrates physical signs that correspond with the lesions.

Subdural haematoma may produce gradually increasing mental impairment over several weeks or months (*see* p. 499). The initiating head injury may have been slight and unrecognised. It is treated by surgical decompression.

In **normal-pressure hydrocephalus** there is dementia with gait and bladder disorder caused by marked ventricular dilatation. Meningitis, cerebral haemorrhage and trauma are predisposing factors, but it may occur without this history. The surgical creation of a shunt from ventricle to peritoneum may arrest the process.

Alcoholism is a common cause of behavioural change and dementia, and is often complicated by B-group vitamin deficiencies, especially of thiamine (*see* p. 346). Vitamin B_{12} deficiency can produce severe mental impairment; and hypothyroidism can also cause a marked slowing of mental function.

Dementia as a part of **AIDS** is now increasingly common (*see* p. 16); while general paralysis of the insane from **neurosyphilis** (*see* p. 83) is very rare.

In **severe brain damage** from encephalitis, abscess, tumour, cerebral infarction, head injury, severe ischaemia or hypoglycaemia, the cause is usually clear.

Huntington's chorea is a dominantly transmitted condition that is associated with progressive dementia and chorea. The onset of symptoms is usually gradual in the middle years of life. There is usually a family history and, because of knowledge of the outcome, there is a high incidence of depression. The course is progressively downhill over a few years with increasing chorea and dementia. The diagnosis is made on clinical grounds and on the family history. Genetic counselling is mandatory in all adolescents and the availability of a DNA probe aids this process in certain families.

There is no specific treatment for most patients with dementia, but much support for the affected patients and families is required.

11.33

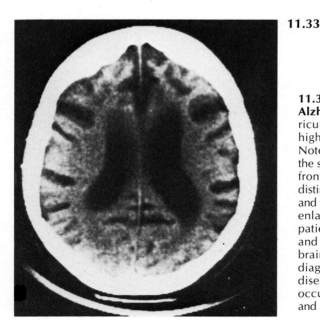

11.34

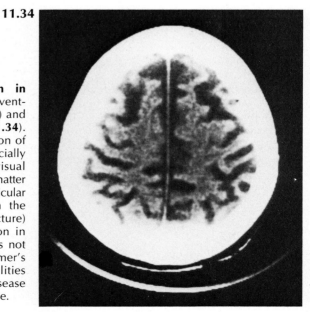

11.33, 11.34 CT scan in Alzheimer's disease at ventricular body level (**11.33**) and high convexity level (**11.34**). Note the marked dilatation of the sulci and fissures, especially frontally, the poor visual distinction between grey matter and white matter, the ventricular enlargement—greater on the patient's left (right of picture) and the general reduction in brain size. The picture is not diagnostic of Alzheimer's disease: similar abnormalities occur in Huntington's disease and Niemann–Pick's disease.

Table 11.3 Causes of dementia.

Unknown	Alzheimer's disease
	Multiple sclerosis
Vascular	Multiple cerebral infarcts
	Diffuse small vessel disease
Metabolic	Uraemia
	Liver failure
	Hypothyroidism
	Vitamin B_{12} deficiency
	Other vitamin B deficiency
	Hypoparathyroidism
	Hypoglycaemia
Physical	Space-occupying lesions (tumour, haematoma)
	Post-head-injury, especially in subdural haematoma
Genetic	Huntington's chorea
Infections	HIV infection
	Tuberculosis
	Toxoplasmosis
	Syphilis
	Creutzfeld–Jakob disease
Toxic	Poisoning with mercury, manganese, carbon monoxide, alcohol, copper

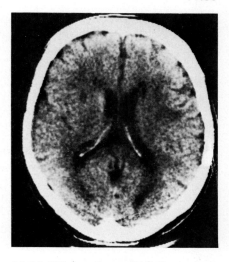

11.35 CT scan in multi-infarct dementia (cut at same level as that seen in **11.33**). The ventricles are normal in size, but there are patchy radiolucencies throughout the white matter. These indicate the presence of demyelinated patches, which result from multiple small infarcts in the brain.

Epilepsy

Epileptic seizures are manifestations of abnormal synchronous activity of populations of neurons in the brain. Even a normal brain can generate such activity given a sufficient stimulus (e.g. electric shock, drug withdrawal). People with epilepsy have a lower 'threshold' for seizure activity, and have epileptic seizures that are unprovoked or reflexly induced (e.g. by flashing lights). Different types of seizures reflect varieties and distributions of synchronous neuronal activity, and are classified according to their clinical and EEG manifestations (**Table 11.4**).

A large number of potential underlying mechanisms contribute to epilepsy, some genetically determined and some acquired. Epileptic syndromes can be broadly divided into those thought to be associated with focal brain pathology, and those associated with a diffuse increase in brain excitability. In many individuals with epilepsy, however, it is likely that there is a combination of underlying mechanisms, explaining, for instance, why one person develops epilepsy after a head injury, while another with an apparently identical injury does not.

A first epileptic seizure can occur at any age. About 1 person in 30 has an epileptic seizure during his/her lifetime, and the prevalence of active epilepsy is 1 in 200. Patients may be seriously injured during attacks (**11.36**), and must be managed carefully during any period of unconciousness or drowsiness that follows them (**11.37**).

An accurate diagnosis of epilepsy is crucial in view of the potential social implications and possible initiation of long-term treatment. Typical attacks are easy to diagnose but the interpretation of odd 'falls and faints' is extremely difficult. The main differential diagnoses are shown in **Table 11.5**. A witnessed account of the attacks is of great importance. It is a common misconception that the EEG (**11.38**, **11.39**) is diagnostic, but it is only rarely so, and the diagnosis is essentially based on an adequate history which may include observed convulsions, unconsciousness, biting the tongue (**11.40**), incontinence and a slow recovery. In adult life, symptomatic partial epilepsy is most common and few clinical signs are found. Investigations usually include CT scanning, which is essential if there are focal signs. It is, however, normal in the majority of patients, and brain tumours are found in fewer than 10% (**11.22**).

A decision to recommend anti-epileptic drug treatment (AEDs) is easy in subjects with recent recurrent seizures, but is controversial in those who have had a single unprovoked seizure or a small number of very infrequent seizures. After a single seizure the risk of a further attack is initially high (about 70%), but it subsequently falls rapidly (about 30% at 2 months). The choice of AED depends on the seizure type(s). Up to 80% will have their seizures controlled, usually by a single AED, once appropriate dose adjustments have been made. Drug-level monitoring is essential with phenytoin, because of saturation kinetics, and can be useful with other drugs to assess compliance and adverse effects.

All anti-epileptic drugs have potential side-effects, and all present risks if taken during pregnancy. A particularly well-recognised side-effect is gingival hyperplasia in patients on phenytoin therapy (**8.20**).

A small proportion of patients with epilepsy uncontrolled by AEDs can be offered neurosurgery (most commonly temporal lobectomy), with a good chance of complete seizure relief.

Discussion of the diagnosis of epilepsy with the patient needs to be clear and detailed. Misconceptions and prejudices remain common (e.g. equating it with mental illness or insanity). The provision of written material is essential, and discussion with other family members is usually important. Areas to be covered include implications for driving, employment, social activities and other interests, what to do when seizures occur, safety precautions, pregnancy, drug interactions and genetic implications.

In many patients who become seizure-free on AED treatment, it is subsequently possible to withdraw their medication. This should be considered after at least 2 years of freedom from seizures, when the statistical risk of further seizures, with or without continued treatment, is approximately one-third.

Table 11.4 A classification of epileptic seizures.

1. **Partial seizures** (arise focally within the brain with variable spread)
   A. *Simple partial seizures* (consciousness not impaired)
      1. With motor signs
      2. With somatosensory or special sensory symptoms
      3. With autonomic symptoms or signs
      4. With psychological symptoms (disturbance of higher cerebral function)
   B. *Complex partial seizures* (with impairment of consciousness)
      1. Simple partial followed by impairment of consciousness
      2. With impairment of consciousness at onset
      Complex partial seizures may be followed by automatism—automatic behaviour of which the patient has no recall.
   C. *Partial seizures evolving to generalized tonic-clonic seizures*

2. **Generalised seizures** (EEG shows widespread bilateral epileptic activity from the onset)
   A 1. Absence seizures (episode in which patient becomes unresponsive for a few seconds, with rapid recovery)
      2. Atypical absence seizures
   B. *Myoclonic seizures* (brief jerks of one or more limbs)
   C. *Clonic seizures* (repetitive jerking of limbs and trunk)
   D. *Tonic seizures* (tonic contraction of muscle causing flexion or hypertension of trunk)
   E. *Tonic clonic seizures* ('grand mal' seizure: tonic followed by clonic phases, which may be associated with salivation, cyanosis, tongue biting and incontinence, and followed by noisy breathing and sleep)
   F. *Atonic seizures* (brief loss of muscle tone)

3. **Unclassified epileptic seizures**

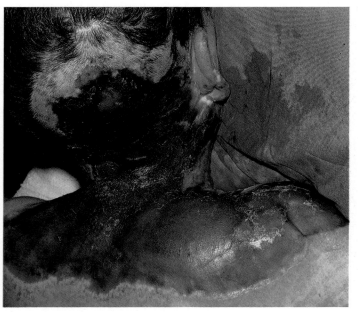

11.36

11.36 Serious injury may occur during generalised seizures in epilepsy. This patient has a large full-thickness burn, sustained when he fell in a fire during a fit.

Table 11.5 Differential diagnoses of epilepsy.

Syncope (including convulsive syncope)
Pseudoseizures
Hypoglycaemia
Parasomnias (sleep walking, sleep talking)
Cataplexy
Transient ischaemic attacks
Migraine

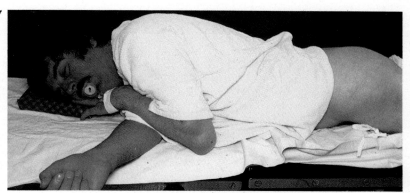

11.37 The correct position for the unconscious patient. Many patients remain unconscious or drowsy for several hours after a generalised seizure. They should be placed in the semi-prone position, and a simple airway should be placed in the mouth. Exactly the same management should be applied to any unconscious patient who does not require cardiac or respiratory support. During epileptic attacks the patient should be protected from harm if possible; but forcible attempts to open the mouth or restrain the patient often do more harm than good.

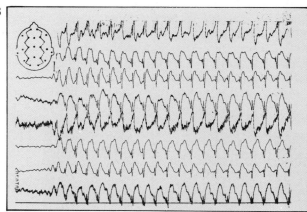

11.38 EEG in a patient with generalised tonic clonic (grand mal) seizures. This shows the typical spike and wave discharge of generalised epilepsy. If the EEG is taken during an attack, this appearance may be diagnostic of epilepsy, but gives no indication of the cause; if spike and wave activity is observed between attacks the appearance does not prove that an episode was epileptic, but the findings support the diagnosis. Ambulatory monitoring of the EEG provides a much more valuable assessment of the relationship of EEG abnormalities to symptoms.

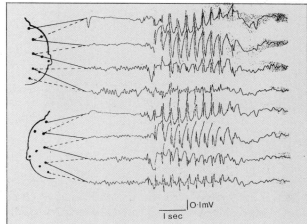

11.39 EEG in a patient with absence (petit mal) seizures. Characteristic 3 Hz spike and wave activity is always present during an attack and is frequently seen in the inter-ictal intervals, so the EEG is a useful tool in the diagnosis of this form of epilepsy.

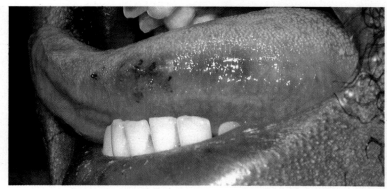

11.40 The bitten tongue as a sign of epilepsy. This patient had nocturnal enuresis and woke up with a sore tongue. This combination of symptoms is strongly suggestive of a nocturnal generalised seizure, and the patient should be further investigated.

Raised intracranial pressure

A rise in the pressure of CSF above 250 mm is usually a reflection of serious neurological disease, caused by a space-occupying lesion, obstruction to the outflow of CSF or obstruction of the venous return.

It is usual to measure CSF pressure by lumbar puncture, but this may not accurately reflect pressure in the brain, e.g. where there is obstruction by spinal tumours or herniation of brain through the foramen magnum. The main causes include tumours, abscesses, hydrocephalus, haematomas and benign intracranial hypertension.

A rise in intracranial pressure is usually associated with headache, especially in the morning, nausea, vomiting and loss of vision and balance. There may be false localising signs, e.g. sixth nerve palsies. The most reliable sign is the appearance of papilloedema (7.7, 11.41), but this is not always seen even when the pressure is high.

Urgent action to reduce pressure is needed in patients with impending herniation of brain through the foramen magnum. This should usually include high doses of dexamethasone and intravenous mannitol. The airway must be maintained and hyperventilation to reduce the $Pa\,CO_2$ may be of transient value. After stabilisation, imaging procedures should be used to establish the underlying diagnosis, which should be treated appropriately.

Benign intracranial hypertension (pseudotumour cerebri) is an unexplained disorder, occuring mainly in pregnant, obese young and middle-aged women, producing headache and papilloedema (11.41); there is increased intracranial pressure as measured on lumbar puncture, without local structural cause. Long-term consequences include blindness from optic nerve atrophy (7.8). Diagnosis is made on lumbar puncture and the CT scan is used to exclude other pathology. Treatment includes weight reduction, diuretics, occasionally a shunt and optic nerve decompression.

11.41

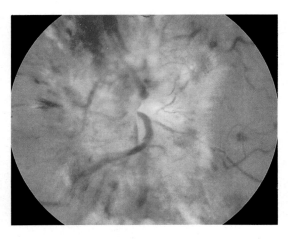

11.41 Chronic papilloedema in the right eye of a middle-aged woman with benign intracranial hypertension. The disc margins are completely blurred, and there are widespread haemorrhages and ischaemic areas in the retina. The appearance of chronic papilloedema should be compared with the less-marked changes seen in early papilloedema (**7.7**).

Hydrocephalus

Hydrocephalus is the enlargement of the cerebral ventricles which is associated with the accumulation of cerebrospinal fluid. This may result from a variety of causes including:

Communicating hydrocephalus
• Excess production of CSF — choroid plexus papilloma.
• Impaired CSF absorption — in meningitis.
• Cerebral dysgenesis or atrophy.

Non-communicating hydrocephalus
• Obstruction to the flow of CSF — intracerebral tumours, aqueduct or foramen stenosis, by blood in subarachnoid haemorrhage.

The clinical features depend on whether the disease process is acute or chronic and whether the process produces complete or partial obstruction. The acute presentation is usually accompanied by severe headache, nausea and vomiting. There are usually no localising symptoms or signs, but there is papilloedema (7.7, 11.41) and there may be a sixth nerve lesion. Neurological signs usually suggest a bilateral upper motor neuron disorder (i.e. bilateral extensor plantar signs and brisk reflexes). There is progressive impairment of higher cerebral functions with loss of memory, impairment of mobility and loss of sphincter control.

CT imaging and MRI show the abnormality of the ventricles (11.42) and may suggest the site of the block (11.116). Lumbar puncture may be of little value as the pressure is often normal.

If the primary lesion is not amenable to treatment, a drainage procedure of the affected ventricles is of value. This involves the surgical creation of a shunt with a valve that allows the one-way drainage of CSF from the ventricles to the peritoneal cavity.

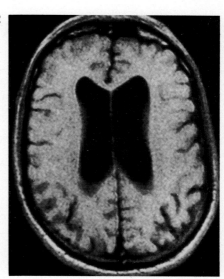

11.42 Hydrocephalus in an active 69-year-old man. This axial MRI at the level of the ventricular bodies shows severe ventricular enlargement, but the sulci of the brain are normal. The patient had communicating (normal pressure) hydrocephalus, associated with minimal memory impairment but no other significant abnormality. Many patients develop the clinical triad of dementia, ataxia and incontinence.

Infantile hydrocephalus

A variety of congenital abnormalities may lead to hydrocephalus which may be present before birth (and hence produce difficulties at birth) or develop during childhood or adult life.

Progressive enlargement of the head is usually obvious, with failure of closure of the fontanelles (**1.178, 11.43**). Milestones of development are delayed and the end result may be mental retardation complicated by epilepsy and motor impairment. CT (**11.44**) or MRI scan may show the abnormality and sometimes the cause, and the early implantation of a shunt may arrest the physical and mental deterioration that would otherwise occur.

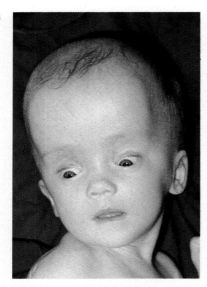

11.43 Infantile hydrocephalus. The head is obviously enlarged and prominent subcutaneous scalp veins are visible. In neglected cases the eyes are displaced downwards (the 'setting sun' sign) so that the upper sclerae are visible. The cranial sutures are widely splayed. This appearance may result from 'internal' (obstructive) or 'external' (communicating) hydrocephalus.

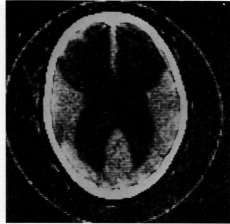

11.44 Severe hydrocephalus. This CT scan shows gross dilatation of the ventricular system and compression of the remaining cortical tissue.

Cerebral tumours

Cerebral tumours represent about 1 in 10 of all tumours. The most common are gliomas, which account for 40–50% of all intracerebral tumours, metastases from tumours of other sites (20–30%) meningiomas (10%), pituitary adenomas (10%) and other tumour types (each about 1–2%).

The usual clinical presentations include:

- Headache, vomiting and papilloedema (7.7, 11.41), i.e. symptoms and signs of raised intracranial pressure.
- Epileptiform seizures.
- Pressure effects on adjacent structures, which produce focal neurological defects.
- Endocrine changes in some pituitary lesions.

These symptoms are also found with other space-occupying lesions, such as intracerebral haematomas, abscesses and subdural haematomas.

Glioma

Gliomas account for 40–50% of all intracerebral tumours and arise from neuroglial cells — usually in the cerebral hemispheres; rarely in the cerebellum. The most common type is the astrocytoma which originates in astrocytes and has a range of degress of malignancy: grade I has a long survival (up to 25 years) and grade IV has a survival of only several months — this rapidly invasive tumour is also known as glioblastoma multiforme. Such tumours rarely metastasise beyond the brain, tending to invade locally in one hemisphere or, less commonly, across the corpus callosum ('butterfly glioma'). In children, the most common sites are the hypothalamus, optic nerve and cerebellum (where they may be cystic and benign). Diagnosis of the space-occupying lesion is by CT scan (11.45) or MRI (11.46), followed by stereotactic biopsy. Solitary low-grade malignant lesions may be amenable to surgery and the more malignant lesions may respond to radiotherapy.

Oligodendrogliomas arise from oligodendroglia and grow extremely slowly. They may sometimes be recognised on a straight skull X-ray by the presence of calcium.

Ependymomas arise from the lining cells of the lateral and fourth ventricles. They tend to occur in the young and are associated with a short survival. They disseminate locally and via the CSF. They may occasionally respond to radiotherapy.

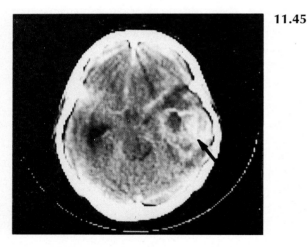

11.45

11.45 Glioma involving most of the left parietal lobe—seen to the right on this axial CT scan (arrow). The appearance is of a cystic tumour, but biopsy and histological confirmation are necessary to be certain of its nature.

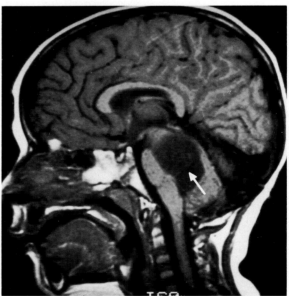

11.46

11.46 Cystic glioblastoma of the brain stem (arrowed), clearly demonstrated by MRI. The sagittal section shows that the tumour involves the posterior part of the brainstem and extends into the cerebellum.

Meningioma

Meningiomas are slowly growing benign tumours that arise from the arachnoid and produce symptoms by compression of adjacent structures. They may arise at any site, even in the spinal canal, but most commonly over the hemispheres. Women over 40 years of age are most commonly affected, and because the tumours are slow growing they may reach a large size before presentation with partial seizures, features of raised intracranial pressure or localised neurological deficits. The tumours have a rich blood supply, may erode bone locally and may calcify. The diagnosis is usually suggested by CT scan (11.27, 11.47) and/or MRI (11.28, 11.29, 11.114) and occasionally localised calcification is seen on the plain X-ray of the skull. Surgery may be curative with early lesions, but local erosion of other structures may make resection extremely difficult, e.g. sphenoidal ridge tumours may envelop the carotid artery and other para-pituitary structures. If incompletely removed, meningiomas tend to regrow. Malignant change is rare. If situated in the spinal canal, they are most likely to occur in the thoracic region where they present with the gradual onset of paraparesis; and surgery carries a good prognosis, because of the earlier presentation.

11.47

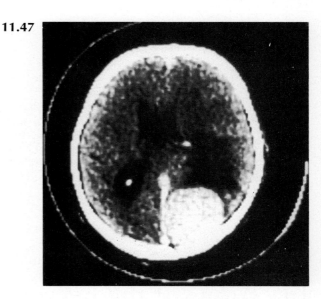

11.47 Meningioma in the occipital lobe, as revealed on contrast-enhanced CT scan. The patient presented with a contralateral homonymous hemianopia.

Pituitary tumours

Pituitary tumours may produce endocrine as well as neurological symptoms (*see also* p. 304). A common presentation is with headache caused by expansion of the tumour, which may erode the clinoid processes and the floor of the pituitary fossa and eventually press on the optic chiasma (7.2–7.5, 7.21). Bitemporal hemianopia results (7.1). Extension laterally into the cavernous sinus affects the oculomotor nerve and the trigeminal nerve. A similar picture may be produced by pressure from aneurysms and meningiomas.

Neuroma

Neuromas are benign tumours that arise from the Schwann cells of the cranial nerves and spinal roots. The most common intracranial site is on the acoustic nerve at the cerebello-pontine angle. The presentation is with progressive deafness and tinnitus, (eighth nerve), loss of sensation on the face (fifth nerve), facial weakness (seventh nerve) and ipsilateral cerebellar signs. Further enlargement produces erosion of the petrous-temporal bone and pressure effects on the brain stem, with long tract symptoms and signs in the arm and leg, followed by hydrocephalus. Diagnosis may be made on a plain X-ray of the skull with tomography, by CT scan (11.48) or by MRI (11.19, 11.114). Partial surgical removal may be all that is possible but early resection may allow conservation of VII/VIII nerve function.

11.48

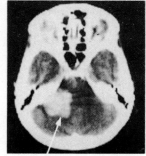

11.48 Acoustic neuroma (arrow), well demonstrated on this enhanced CT scan.

Metastases

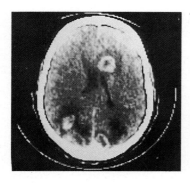

11.49

11.49 Multiple cerebral metastases in a patient with carcinoma of the breast, demonstrated on CT scan. Axial 'cuts' at other levels in the brain demonstrated further lesions.

Metastases account for about a quarter of all cerebral tumours and most frequently arise from lung, breast, kidney, colon, skin and reticulosis. Metastatic lesions may develop in any part of the brain including the cerebellum. Many lesions are found by chance at post-mortem and they tend to be multiple. The diagnosis may be suggested by the development of neurological deficits in patients who have a known malignancy. The clinical course is variable: many patients present with slowly progressive symptoms; while in others an acute presentation may result from haemorrhage within the mass. Diagnosis is most easily made by CT (**4.132, 11.49**) or MRI. Solitary lesions may be amenable to surgical removal with occasional good long-term results. Corticosteroids are of interim value in reducing oedema and temporarily improving clinical status to allow chemotherapy or radiotherapy to be of value.

Infections of the nervous system

Many infections involve the central nervous system. Meningitis, encephalitis and cerebral abscess are considered in this section, and infections considered elsewhere include poliomyelitis (*see* p. 21), herpes zoster (*see* p. 30), rabies (*see* p. 26), neurosyphilis (*see* p. 83) HIV (*see* p. 16) and tetanus (*see* p. 43). The Guillain–Barré syndrome (*see* p. 514) is probably of infective origin, and infection may prove to have a causative role in some patients with dementia and other degenerative diseases of the nervous system.

Meningitis

Meningitis is defined as inflammation of the pia and arachnoid mater and is usually caused by bacteria or viruses; but it may also be caused by fungi, malignant infiltration, blood (subarachnoid haemorrhage) or chemicals (drugs or contrast medium) (**Table 11.6**).

Viruses are the commonest cause of meningitis. They produce a lymphocytic reaction in the CSF, and there may be associated encephalitis. Bacteria are the second most common cause of acute meningitis and they usually provoke a polymorphonuclear leucocytosis in the CSF. A chronic reaction is found in tuberculosis. Fungal infection is uncommon, except in immunocompromised patients, and it may run a chronic or sub-acute course.

The clinical presentation may be with acute or gradual onset of fever, vomiting, headache, lethargy, impaired consciousness (**1.104**) or seizures; signs include a stiff neck, focal signs such as cranial nerve abnormalities (third, fourth, sixth and seventh), hemiparesis, dysphasia, visual field defects and papilloedema. The consequences of infection may also be apparent elsewhere (**1.105, 1.106**). Two important clinical signs of meningitis are dependent on traction of spinal nerves causing pain in the inflamed meninges. These are:

- Kernig's sign — the hip is flexed to 90° with the knee bent; pain is felt on attempting to straighten the patient's leg.
- Brudzinski's sign — flexion of the neck, which causes the legs to be drawn up.

A search must also be made for associated diseases, e.g. mastoiditis, pulmonary tuberculosis or malignancy. Laboratory diagnosis depends on lumbar puncture, which may show a rise in CSF pressure and perhaps a turbid fluid (**1.21**) which should be sent for microbiology, microscopy and biochemistry. These results (**Table 11.7**) will define the infection. If a space-occupying lesion (e.g. abscess) is suspected then CT is essential before undertaking lumbar puncture.

In bacterial meningitis, antibiotic treatment is dictated by the organism found, though treatment will usually be started before culture results are available. Intrathecal antibiotic injection is now rarely used.

Viral meningitis is usually a benign, self-limiting condition.

Table 11.6 Causes of meningitis.

Bacteria	Viruses	Fungi
S. pneumoniae	Echo	Cryptococcus
N. meningitidis	Coxsackie	Histoplasma
H. influenzae	Epstein–Barr	Coccidioides
Streptococci	Polio	Blastomyces
Staphylococci	Mumps	
Listeria monocytogenes	Herpes	
Gram-negative bacilli		
Leptospirosis		
M. tuberculosis		

Table 11.7 Cerebrospinal fluid (CSF) findings in meningitis.

	Cells		Biochemistry		
	Number (per mm)	Type	Protein (mg/100 ml)	Glucose (mmol/l)	Others
Normal	0–5	Lymphocytes	15–45	3.3–4.5	
Viral infection	Up to 2,000	Lymphocytes	Normal range	Normal range	No bacteria on Gram stain
Acute bacterial infection	1,000–50,000	Polymorphs	Elevated	Reduced	Bacteria present on Gram stain or culture
Tuberculosis	Up to 10,000	Lymphocytes	Markedly elevated	Reduced	Fibrin clot forms on standing

Encephalitis

Encephalitis is a generalised non-suppurative inflammation of the brain which is usually caused by infection by a virus but is also found in a variety of bacterial infections. Such infections may also involve the spinal cord, cranial nerves and nerve roots. In the UK encephalitis may follow infection with measles, rubella, chickenpox, influenza virus, herpes simplex and HIV. In the Far East and other parts of the world, epidemic viral encephalitis carries a high morbidity and mortality (*see* p. 23).

The usual clinical features include fever, nausea and vomiting, headache, impairment of the conscious level (**1.57**), the development of focal neurological signs, meningism, and features of raised intracranial pressure. The disease is often followed by complete recovery after a period of weeks.

The EEG may show diffuse or focal abnormalities. CT scan or MRI often show abnormalities (**11.50**). Serology may show a changing level of viral antibody. Lumbar puncture may show a rise in CSF pressure with lymphocytosis, elevated protein content and a normal glucose.

Treatment consists of nursing and supportive care. Acyclovir should be given in all cases of suspected encephalitis because the consequences of untreated herpes simplex encephalopathy in the minority are considerable. In patients who are immunocompromised CMV should also be considered and this responds to gancyclovir.

Acute demyelinating encephalomyelitis presents in a similar manner to encephalitis and is an allergic demyelination disease. It follows some types of vaccination and may follow measles or chickenpox infection after several weeks. A proportion of patients will later develop multiple sclerosis.

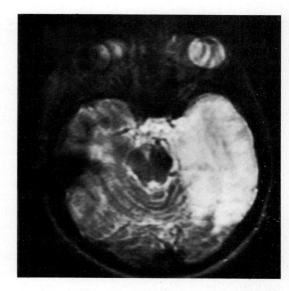

11.50

11.50 Herpes simplex encephalitis. This MRI view shows abnormally increased signal in the left temporal lobe (right of picture). MRI and CT appearances in encephalitis vary; often diffuse or scattered abnormalities are seen.

Brain abscess

Brain abscess is a localised collection of pus in the brain. The infection may be blood borne from a distant site, be introduced by a penetrating head injury or extend from local infections in the head (mastoiditis or sinusitis).

The clinical symptoms are those of infection and of the development of a space-occupying lesion in the brain. There is usually fever, headache, nausea, vomiting, clouding of the conscious level, focal signs and fits. There may be signs of a focus of infection, of an increase in intracranial pressure and of papilloedema. Additional focal signs may occur depending on the anatomical site of the abscess.

The white cell count is elevated and the blood film usually shows a polymorphonuclear leucocytosis. The ESR is elevated. The lesion can be identified on CT scanning (1.33, 11.51, 11.52) as a ring-enhancing lesion, and if there is any doubt about the diagnosis stereotactic biopsy is safer than lumbar puncture.

Treatment is with appropriate antibiotic combinations, corticosteroids to reduce swelling and, in selected patients, neurosurgery. If a predisposing cause has been identified this also requires treatment.

Infections may also localise in the subdural or extradural spaces of both brain and spinal cord. Spinal epidural abscesses present with severe back pain and paraparesis.

11.51
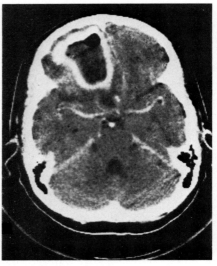

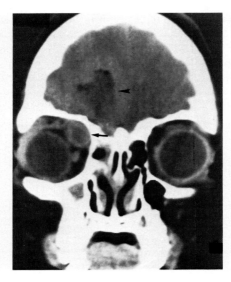
11.52

11.51, 11.52 Cerebral abscess secondary to sinusitis. 11.51 shows an enhanced axial CT scan. A right frontal abscess (left of picture) is seen, and it contains some gas in the anterior region. The coronal CT scan demonstrates the frontal abscess (arrowhead) and also an abscess in the orbit (arrow); both followed infection of the ethmoidal sinuses. Note the soft-tissue density in the ethmoids on this side (below the arrow).

Cerebrovascular disease

Stroke

Completed stroke is defined as a focal loss of neurological function, of presumed vascular origin, which causes death or lasts for over 24 hours. This timescale differentiates it from a transient ischaemic attack (see below). In addition, some clinicians describe a reversible ischaemic neurological deficit (RIND) in which the neurological deficit lasts more than 24 hours and reverses within 3 weeks. Stroke-in-evolution is a condition where the symptoms and signs suggest a focal lesion within the distribution of a major artery and this gradually extends over a period of days or weeks to involve an adjacent motor or sensory site.

Over 90% of strokes result from thrombosis or embolism in a major cerebral artery, and under 10% result from haemorrhage.

The clinical presentations of strokes caused by cerebral thrombosis, embolism and haemorrhage are similar. They involve a combination of features which may include hemiparesis (11.53), hemianaesthesia, loss of speech if the dominant hemisphere is involved and loss of vision. Lesions affecting the non-dominant hemisphere are more likely to be associated with neglect. The clinical onset is often rapid and reaches a maximum within a few hours. The limbs are flaccid and reflexes are initially absent. The patient may have an impaired conscious level because of cerebral oedema, and there may also be papilloedema. Over the next 24-hour period tone increases, some power may return, the tendon reflexes are exaggerated and the plantar response is extensor.

Lacunar infarcts are small lesions around the basal ganglia, thalamus and pons which result in localised motor or sensory deficits. Brainstem infarcts produce complex neurological syndromes, as they involve the long tracts, the cranial nerve nuclei and cerebellar connections.

The signs of acute stroke are usually obvious, but careful examination is necessary to localise the site of damage and the artery involved. CT examination can be used to determine whether the lesion is thrombosis, embolus or haemorrhage (11.54–11.56) and its anatomical site. This is important if any form of anti-thrombotic therapy is contemplated. Haemorrhage is evident immediately on CT examination, whereas infarction may not be evident until 6–8 hours or more after onset.

Immediate examination and investigation should focus on the possibility of a treatable cause of stroke, such as temporal arteritis (*see* p. 150), embolism from the heart (**5.66, 5.74**) or the large arteries (p. 497), or, occasionally, a surgically treatable haemorrhage. No specific treatment is available for most patients with stroke, so their immediate management is supportive. Skilled nursing care prevents the development of pressure sores (**11.57**) and allows adequate nutrition and hydration.

Permanent disability is a common consequence of stroke (**11.58–11.60**). Long-term rehabilitation, with intensive physiotherapy (**11.61**), speech therapy and occupational therapy, should be carefully planned and allows about 25% of stroke patients to return to work or normal retirement. Mortality during the first month is about 40–50% because of extension of the cerebral damage, aspiration pneumonia and deep vein thrombosis with pulmonary embolism.

Secondary prevention by control of cardiovascular risk factors (*see* p. 222) is as important after stroke as in coronary heart disease; and long-term aspirin therapy is usually indicated unless the stroke was haemorrhagic.

11.53

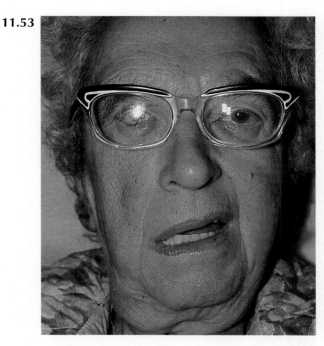

11.53 Right-sided facial palsy resulting from stroke. The patient also had right hemiplegia and complete aphasia. The signs are those of an acute upper motor neuron lesion. The limbs are at first flaccid and areflexic, but after a variable period the reflexes recover and become exaggerated, and an extensor plantar response appears. Weakness in the face and elsewhere may recover gradually over a variable period of time.

11.54

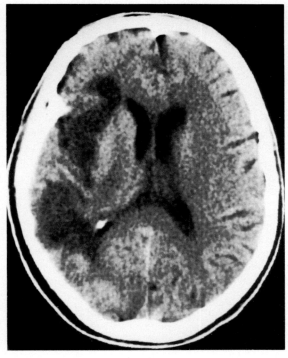

11.55

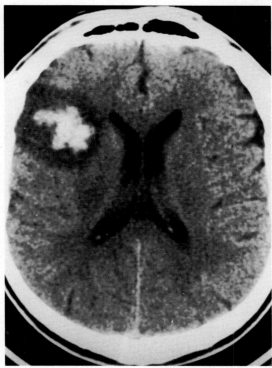

11.54 Extensive right-sided cerebral infarction (left side of picture) demonstrated by unenhanced CT scan, performed 4 days after the onset of stroke. There is no evidence of haemorrhage (cf. **11.55**). High-quality CT scanners allow the diagnosis of cerebral infarction within 6–8 hours of onset.

11.55 Haemorrhagic cerebral infarction demonstrated by unenhanced CT scan one day after the onset of stroke. Note the high-density haemorrhage within the low density of the oedematous, infarcted region in the right hemisphere. Haemorrhage is evident from its onset on CT scanning.

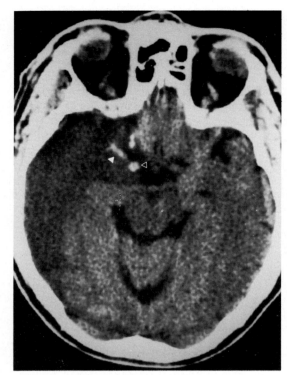

11.56 Cerebral embolism in a patient following cardiac surgery, demonstrated by unenhanced CT scan. The open arrowhead points to a high-density embolus within the distal right internal carotid artery; the filled arrowhead points to a similar embolus in the right middle cerebral artery. There is extensive hypodensity in the right middle cerebral artery distribution, reflecting an extensive area of infarction.

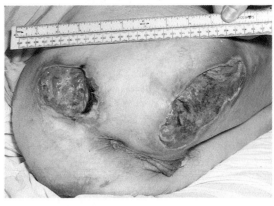

11.57 Severe ischial pressure sores—one of the serious but preventable complications of immobility following stroke.

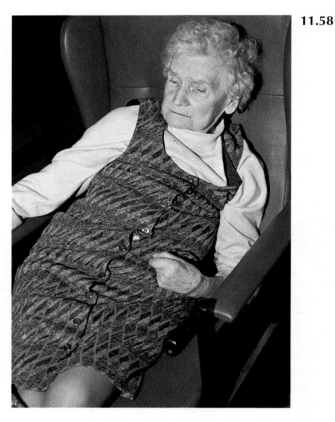

11.58 Loss of postural stability is common following stroke. When the non-dominant hemisphere is involved, walking apraxia and loss of postural control are usually apparent. The patient is unable to sit upright and tends to fall sideways. Appropriate support with pillows or cushions should be provided.

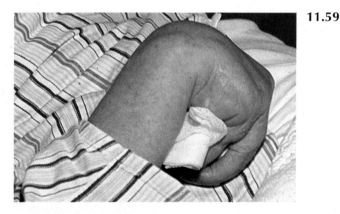

11.59 Permanent flexion contracture of the right hand has occurred in this patient several months after the onset of a dense hemiplegia. This type of disability can be prevented by early and continuing physiotherapy.

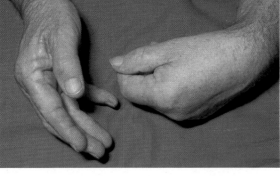

11.60

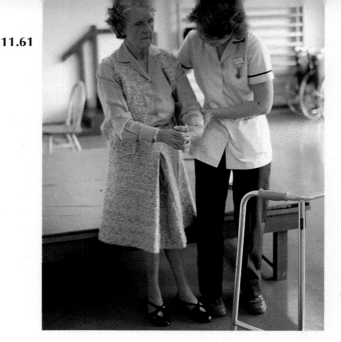

11.61

11.60 Disuse oedema is a common long-term complication of stroke. In this patient, the left hand remains swollen months after the onset of a dense hemiplegia.

11.61 Skilled assistance can greatly aid rehabilitation from stroke. This patient with hemiplegia is being taught to walk without the use of mechanical aids; however, a walking frame (front of picture) can be an important aid in the early stages of rehabilitation.

Transient ischaemic attacks

A transient ischaemic attack (TIA) is defined as sudden focal loss of neurological function, presumed caused by a vascular lesion, which lasts less than 24 hours and leaves no residual signs. Two distinct clinical varieties are described — those where the damage occurs in the territory supplied by the carotid artery and those where the territory of the vertebral arteries is affected. The diagnosis of the attack is made on clinical grounds, but often the actual cause is unknown. Most are assumed to be embolic in origin and the source of these emboli is most commonly a plaque of atheroma, which ulcerates and allows formation of small amounts of platelet-fibrin thrombus that, in turn, break off and produce multiple small emboli. Emboli may be seen in the retina (11.62). Sites of thrombus formation include the internal and common carotid artery, the mitral and aortic valves, the left ventricular wall after acute infarction (*see* p. 227), a dilated fibrillating left atrium, especially when there is mitral stenosis (*see* p. 230), and rarely an atrial myxoma (*see* p. 246). In addition to emboli a search must be made for cardiac arrhythmias, hypertension, bacterial endocarditis, polycythaemia or myeloma — all of which may predispose to TIA.

Carotid territory TIAs (anterior circulation TIAs) present with transient monocular blindness (amaurosis fugax), loss of power or sensation, or loss of speech. Vertebro-basilar TIAs (posterior circulation TIAs) present with loss of balance, staggering, and sensory impairment.

Investigation may include 24-hour monitoring for abnormalities of heart rhythm; echocardiography for thrombus on the left ventricular wall or in the left atrium, mitral valve lesions or vegetations; and routine chest X-ray. A full blood count, ESR, blood sugar and VDRL are also necessary. Ultrasound of the internal carotid artery may show a stenosed origin with altered wave form, and angiography may confirm carotid or vertebral stenosis (11.31, 11.32, 11.63). Treatment is required to reduce the risk of completed stroke which occurs at a rate of 5% per year. Antiplatelet agents such as aspirin and dipyridamole are helpful, as are conventional anticoagulants. Carotid artery surgery may be useful for carotid artery atheroma, but its role is still not fully defined, because results vary greatly between units. Recent multicentre trials suggest that in approximately 70% of highly selected patients surgery may be beneficial.

11.63

11.62

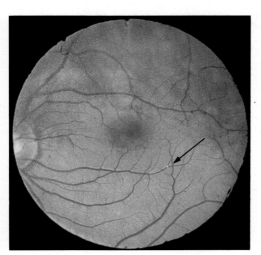

11.62 Retinal embolus in a patient with transient ischaemic attacks. Glistening emboli may sometimes be seen in the retina in patients who have symptoms suggesting TIA. Larger emboli from the carotid territory may even cause transient monocular blindness (amaurosis fugax).

11.63 Carotid angiogram, showing stenosis of the internal carotid artery with thrombosis and ulceration. Carotid or aortic arch angiography can provide accurate information, but is not free of risk. It should be performed only when it will have a clear influence on management.

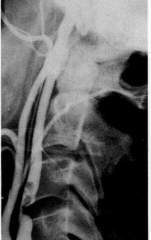

Subarachnoid haemorrhage

Subarachnoid haemorrhage usually results from rupture of an arterial berry aneurysm (70–80%), or leakage from an arteriovenous malformation (5–10%); in 10–20% of cases, no source for the bleeding is found. Berry aneurysms develop at the bifurcations of the intracerebral arteries, probably as a result of an inherited weakness in the vessel wall. They are multiple in about 20% of patients. The common sites are on anterior cerebral artery/anterior communicating artery (30%), the internal carotid and posterior communicating artery (25%), middle cerebral bifurcation (13%), at branches from the internal carotid artery (15%) and on the vertebro-basilar system (5%). Most aneurysms are in the subarachnoid space, so their rupture produces subarachnoid haemorrhage. Aneurysms of the internal carotid artery, when this runs in the cavernous sinus, produce pressure on the adjacent cranial nerves.

The clinical presentation is often dramatic with sudden onset of severe headache, often associated with nausea, vomiting and neck pain. The patient may become unconscious. Focal signs are usually absent. Rarely, an aneurysm may present before rupture, with signs of direct pressure on an adjacent nerve (11.11, 11.12). Examination demonstrates neck stiffness and a positive straight leg raising test. Fundal examination may show papilloedema and occasionally a subhyaloid haemorrhage (11.64).

The investigation of choice is CT scanning, which shows blood in the subarachnoid space (11.65) and CT or MRI may show the aneurysm (11.66). If CT scanning is not available, lumbar puncture can be carried out if there is no evidence of raised intracranial pressure. Within 24 hours of the onset of symptoms there will be uniform blood staining of the CSF; later, xanthochromia develops as a result of haemoglobin degradation (11.25). If the patient is fit, angiography should be carried out to identify the site of the bleeding (11.67) with a view to clipping the aneurysm, ideally within the first 10 days after the incident, because of the highly significant incidence of rebleeding. About 5% of patients rebleed within 24 hours of the initial rupture, and an additional 20% within 2 weeks of the initial event. If untreated, about half the cases will rebleed within 6 months.

The only other treatment of proven value following the diagnosis is use of calcium blockers, which relieve the spasm in adjacent arteries and hence reduce ischaemia in the surrounding brain.

Bleeding from an AV malformation (11.68) tends to be less severe and presents less acutely. There is also a significant incidence of previous epilepsy (see p. 485). Such AV malformations may also be found in the spinal cord and may be difficult to remove safely. Some are amenable to interventional radiology (embolisation procedures) and stereotactic radiotherapy, but both methods may damage the function of adjacent brain.

As this is a disease of young and otherwise fit people and the mortality is so high, consideration should be given to the question of organ donation in those who die.

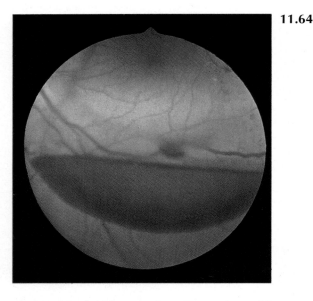

11.64

11.64 Subhyaloid haemorrhage in a patient with subarachnoid haemorrhage. The sudden rise in intracranial pressure may force blood through the retina into the subhyaloid space. The blood collects in large pools, which do not clot; the cells separate from the plasma to produce a 'fluid' level.

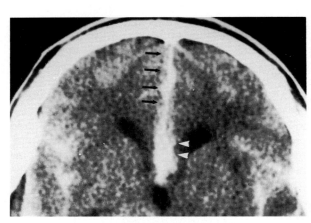

11.65

11.65 Subarachnoid haemorrhage from an anterior communicating artery aneurysm. This uncontrasted CT scan shows areas of increased density representing blood in the interhemispheric fissure (arrows) and the septum pellucidum (arrowheads). A lesser amount of blood is present in the sylvian fissures and the perimesencephalic cistern.

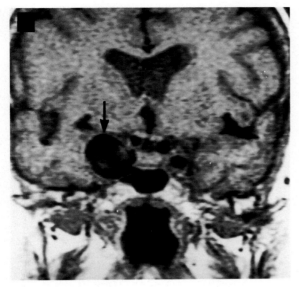

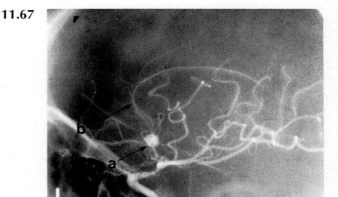

11.67 Berry aneurysm on the anterior communicating artery (a). The angiogram also shows that the anterior cerebral artery (b) is in spasm.

11.66 Right cavernous carotid aneurysm (arrowed), shown on coronal MRI. The signal void at the periphery of the aneurysm represents flowing blood, while the intensity in the central portion may represent either a clot or slowly flowing blood. MRI may demonstrate aneurysms clearly, but is much less successful than CT at demonstrating the presence or absence of blood in the subarachnoid space.

11.68

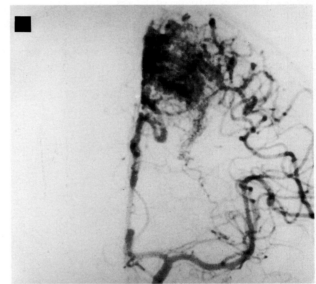

11.68 Left parietal arteriovenous malformation, shown in an anteroposterior view of an internal carotid angiogram. Bleeding from AV malformations is usually less severe than that from aneurysms, but their size may lead to other symptoms including epilepsy.

Subdural and extradural haematomas

Subdural haematoma is the accumulation of blood in the potential subdural space (i.e. the dura-arachnoid interspace). It often results from a deceleration head injury, as in a fall (**11.69**) or a road traffic accident, but may also occur spontaneously, especially in the elderly. About 40% of patients also have a skull fracture. The diagnosis is often missed because of the slow development of symptoms. These include headache, intermittent fluctuation of conscious level, confusion and coma. There are often no immediate focal signs, but pupillary size may be asymmetrical. CT (**11.70**) or MRI (**11.71**) confirm the diagnosis. Later in the course, hemiparesis and hemisensory loss may occur.

A **chronic subdural haematoma** is one that has been present for over 3 weeks. These occur particularly in the aged, often after a trivial injury, so insignificant that it is not remembered. About 20% are bilateral. In only a few cases (about 5%) is there X-ray evidence of a fractured skull. In the long term, if untreated, these chronic subdural haematomas may calcify (**11.72**). CT and MRI appearances reflect the location, extent and age of the haemorrhage.

Extradural haematoma is often caused by rupture of the middle meningeal artery, associated with skull fracture resulting from direct injury. A haematoma forms and expands between the dura mater and the calvarium. The patient may have a 'lucid interval' after awakening from the unconscious state following trauma. The rapidly accumulating haematoma compresses the hemisphere and produces coma and death. An abnormal pupillary response may be the only focal sign early in the disease. The diagnosis is confirmed by CT scan (**11.73**) and the haematoma is removed surgically.

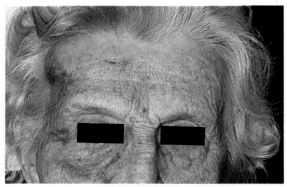

11.69 Subdural haematoma often follows a fall in an elderly patient, as in this woman who developed suggestive symptoms within a few days of a fall, despite the absence of skull fracture. The diagnosis is often missed because of the slow development of symptoms.

11.70 Large acute subdural haemorrhage (arrows) revealed by CT scan at the level of the lateral ventricles. The haemorrhage has resulted in midline shift, with marked compression and displacement of the right lateral ventricle (arrowheads). Because of the brain distortion and obstruction of CSF outflow, the left lateral ventricle is dilated (wavy arrows).

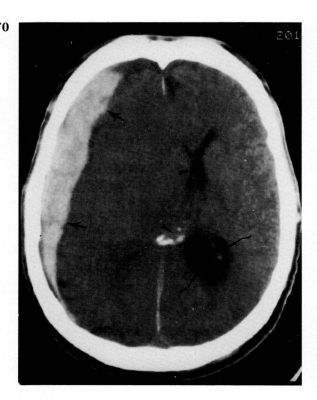

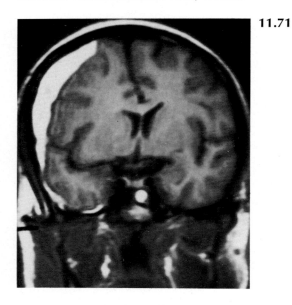

11.71 Right subdural haemorrhage revealed by MRI. The high intensity (white) haemorrhage has dissected under the temporal lobe, and the midline has been displaced to the left. Note the skull fracture overlying the haematoma.

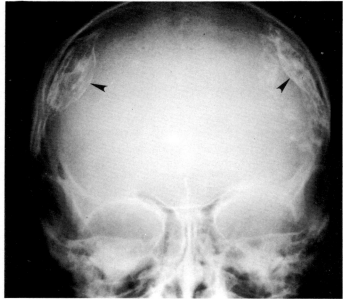

11.72 Chronic bilateral subdural haematoma. This skull X-ray shows areas of calcification adjacent to the inner table of both parietal bones (arrows). The diagnosis was confirmed by CT.

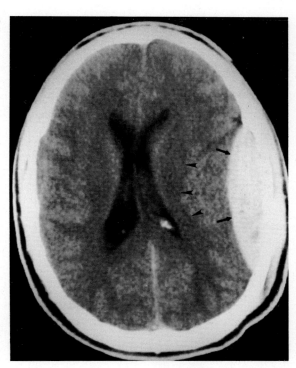

11.73 Extradural haematoma. A well-defined biconvex collection of blood (arrows) compresses the left cerebral hemisphere. There is inward displacement of the grey-white junction (arrowheads) and slight rightward displacement of the left lateral ventricle.

Cerebral venous sinus thrombosis

Thrombosis in the large dural venous sinuses is almost always associated with spread of infection from an adjacent focus, with obstruction caused by focal malignancy or with a thrombotic tendency. The lateral sinus, cavernous sinus and superior sagittal sinus may be involved. The common sites of initial infection are the middle ear, the maxillary sinus, the nose and the periorbital region. Infection of the sagittal venous sinus may result from extension of thrombophlebitis from other dural veins or venous sinuses.

The presenting features are often acute, with abrupt onset of fever, rigors, headache, coma or paresis. Cavernous sinus thrombosis may cause severe eye manifestations (11.74) and there may be papilloedema with visual loss. Occasionally the adjacent cranial nerves may be involved (fifth, sixth).

The diagnosis may be made by a digital subtraction angiogram which defines the thrombus, or by MR (11.75) or CT imaging.

Treatment is with antibiotics. Most physicians are reluctant to anticoagulate the patient because of fear of bleeding into the brain, but such therapy may be used if there is an evolving neurological deficit.

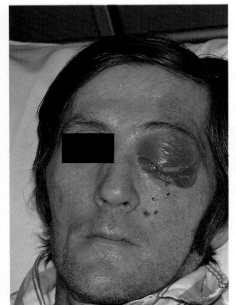

11.74

11.75

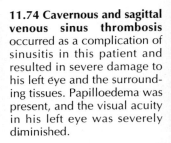

11.74 Cavernous and sagittal venous sinus thrombosis occurred as a complication of sinusitis in this patient and resulted in severe damage to his left eye and the surrounding tissues. Papilloedema was present, and the visual acuity in his left eye was severely diminished.

11.75 Acute right sigmoid sinus thrombosis (arrows) demonstrated by MRI.

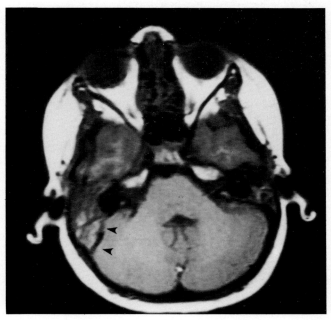

Cerebral palsy

Cerebral palsy is the end result of brain damage caused by a range of disorders which may have been present in the growing fetus, at birth or in early infancy. The most common factors are hypoxia, intracerebral bleeding, trauma, kernicterus, hypoglycaemia and cerebral infection.

The result is a degree of mental retardation, motor and sensory impairment and epileptic fits, all of which produce social and behavioural problems as the child grows. The most common defects are motor: spastic hemiplegias and paraplegia are often compounded by choreo-athetosis and dystonia (11.76, 11.77). There is a wide range of other neurological defects. Such children need careful assessment so that they may be given the opportunity to develop their residual mental and physical skills. Special schooling is often required. These children are now encouraged to lead independent and productive lives, and control of fits and surgical correction of muscle and joint abnormalities are important.

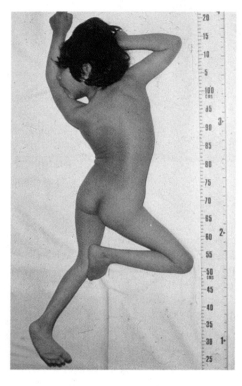

11.76

11.76 Spastic quadriplegia in cerebral palsy. Note the asymmetrical spasticity, with flexion of all limbs, the trunk and the neck. Flexion contractures commonly develop. In this severely affected child, the spasticity was complicated by uncontrollable choreo-athetoid movements.

11.77

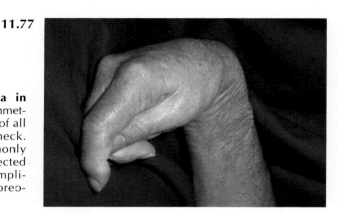

11.77 The spastic hand in cerebral palsy. This common deformity includes pronation of the forearm, flexion of the wrist, the 'thumb in palm' position and flexion of the metacarpophalangeal joints.

Extrapyramidal disorders

Parkinson's disease

Parkinson's disease is a progressive degenerative disease of the extrapyramidal system which results from loss of the functional dopaminergic neurons that radiate from the substantia nigra to the caudate nucleus and putamen. This loss results in bradykinesia, a resting tremor, restricted mobility resulting from muscular rigidity (cogwheel rigidity) and postural instability. Symptoms usually first appear over the age of 50. A slow (3–4 Hz) tremor of the hands, often unilateral, is the most common initial sign (11.78). This is typically 'pill-rolling' in form and it diminishes on voluntary movement. It is usually bilateral, and may involve the upper and lower limbs and the jaw. Slowness of movements is often noticed first by the family rather than the patient. Rigidity compounds this slowness and leads to abnormalities in posture, which is typically stooped (11.1, 11.2, 11.79) and to gait abnormalities (a 'shuffling' or 'festinant' gait—11.3, 11.79). The patient often has a mask-like face (11.80), dribbles saliva because of difficulty in swallowing, and has monotonous speech, caused by dysarthria and dysphonia; writing is also impaired, often with micrographia. Parkinson's disease is a major cause of disability and increased mortality results from aspiration pneumonia, bed sores and urinary tract infections.

Diagnosis is made on the clinical picture, which is usually characteristic but a careful history and examination are required to exclude identifiable causes of parkinsonism (*see* **Table 11.8**).

The mainstay of treatment is levodopa, which dramatically improves the symptoms of Parkinson's disease, especially akinesia, but not survival. Small doses are now used to minimise side effects, often with concomitant therapy with a decarboxylase inhibitor or with an anticholinergic agent for tremor. After treatment for some years a number of disabling problems may develop. Levodopa effects may become shorter-lasting with deterioration at the end of each dose period.

Increasing periods of rapid dyskinetic movements or longer-maintained dystonias may occur with a variable relationship to the doses of levodopa. Periods of unpredictable immobility, the 'on-off' phenomenon, may occur many times a day. These complications are best treated with small, frequent levodopa doses, dopamine receptor agonists (bromocriptine, lysuride) and, occasionally, selegeline.

11.78

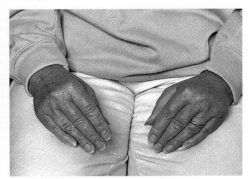

11.78 Tremor in Parkinson's disease is usually worst at rest, and can be observed while talking to the patient with her hands in her lap. The tremor usually lessens or disappears with the arms outstretched, and it is absent when the patient touches her nose. It is usually bilateral.

11.79

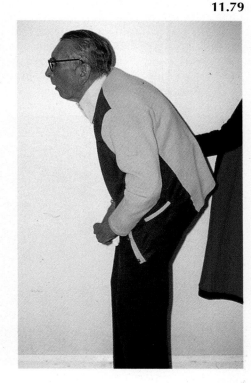

11.79 Parkinson's disease—typical posture and gait (*see also* **11.1–11.3**).

Table 11.8 Identified causes of parkinsonism.

Secondary causes:
- Drugs: phenothiazines, reserpine, methyldopa
- Infections: post-encephalitic
- Toxins: carbon monoxide, manganese and MPTP (1-methyl-4- phenyl-1-2-3-6-tetrahydropyridine) —a synthetic opiate by-product
- Hypoparathyroidism:
- Vascular: cerebrovascular disease
- Trauma: eg in boxers

Parkinsonism in combination with:
- Progressive supranuclear palsy (Steele–Richardson) (MSA)
- Alzheimer's disease
- Shy–Drager syndrome (primary autonomic failure) (MSA)
- Normal pressure hydrocephalus
- Huntington's chorea
- Hepato-lenticular degeneration
- Athetoid cerebral palsy

11.80

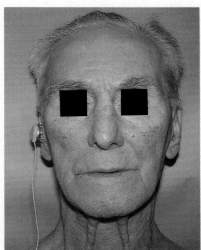

11.80 Parkinson's disease is characteristically associated with a mask-like face, devoid of emotion despite changes in circumstance. The patient often dribbles saliva, and commonly has monotonous speech.

Involuntary disorders of movement

A number of involuntary disorders of movement may occur.

Physiological tremor at about 10 Hz is normal, but increases to a noticeable level in anxiety and thyrotoxicosis.

Postural tremor, usually at about 6–7 Hz, may occur spontaneously as an essential tremor or in families as a familial tremor. This is seen in the outstretched hands and during movement. Stress increases it and alcohol inhibits it. Beta blockade with propranolol is the treatment of choice.

Chorea is a rapid, semipurposeful movement seen in levodopa toxicity (dyskinesia), and also in Huntington's disease (*see* p. 484), and other disorders such as Sydenham's chorea (*see* p. 230), pregnancy chorea, systemic lupus erythematosus and drug-induced chorea (**11.81**).

Hemiballismus is a unilateral disorder with dramatic, wild flailing of the limbs. It is attributed to a lesion, usually vascular, in the subthalamic nucleus.

Dystonias are a group of disorders in which spasm may be restricted to one area, e.g. in the neck (spasmodic torticollis, **11.82**), in the facial muscles around the eyes (blepharospasm) or in the hand (writer's cramp). Dystonias may rarely be widespread as a grossly disabling disorder which includes the trunk (torsion dystonia, **11.83**).

Tardive dyskinesias are involuntary movements of the face and tongue (oro-facial dyskinesias), and of the limbs, caused by treatment with phenothiazines and butyrophenones. They are common in treated patients with chronic schizophrenia.

11.81 **11.82**

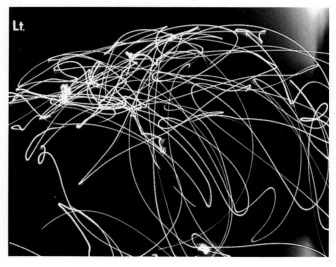

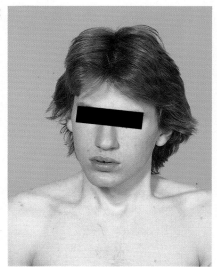

11.81 Chorea. A light tracing, obtained by following movements of lights held in both extended hands in a dark room for 30 seconds. Note the great extent of purposeless movement in this condition.

11.82 Spasmodic torticollis. In this condition, the head turns spasmodically as a result of asymmetrical contraction of the neck muscles. The condition is not usually associated with any other pathology.

11.83

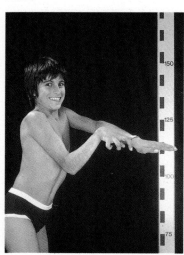

11.83 Torsion dystonia. This congenital condition is associated with severe fixed posturing of the hands, arms, neck and trunk. It is difficult or impossible to treat.

Multiple sclerosis

Multiple sclerosis is the most common disorder of myelin affecting the central nervous system, but there are many other acquired and inherited leucodystrophies (Table 11.9).

It is a disease of unknown cause in which there is patchy demyelination in brain and spinal cord. The acute lesions are infiltrated by lymphocyte and plasma cells and may have an immunological basis. The end result of recurrent acute lesions is a chronic disease with relapses and remissions, but with the development of progressive neurological deficit. The disease has a definite geographical predilection, being rare in equatorial countries and increasing in incidence further away from the equator. In the UK, there is a higher incidence in the Northern Isles of Orkney and Shetland compared to the south of England. It affects mainly young adults and is the commonest neurological disorder of early adult life. The clinical features take many forms (Table 11.10).

Optic neuritis (11.84) is one of the most common early presentations of multiple sclerosis, but is not always followed by further features of progressive disease. It is usually unilateral, and is associated with loss of visual acuity, loss of colour vision and, sometimes, with pain in the eye. These symptoms may come on suddenly and progress rapidly to a central scotoma (11.7). Examination shows the extent of visual loss and the presence and size of a scotoma. There is a defective pupillary response (afferent pupillary defect). The retina may show papilloedema (or papillitis) in the early stages. Most patients show rapid resolution of the acute symptoms but residual signs often remain, such as visual impairment or even optic atrophy (7.8).

Sensory impairment is also common at onset with numbness and paraesthesiae. Involvement of the pyramidal tracts usually occurs later. It is usually bilateral, and the patient

Table 11.9 Some disorders of myelin in the CNS.

Multiple sclerosis	Acute or chronic perivenular demyelination; multiple sites
Schilder's diease	Massive monophasic demyelination
Acute disseminated demyelination	Acute post-viral or post-vaccinal encephalomyelitis
Binswanger's disease	Demyelination associated with ischaemia, especially hypertension
Progressive multifocal leucoencephalopathy	Associated with immune depression; papovaviruses in oligodendroglia
Subacute sclerosing panencephalitis	Follows measles (see p. 24); slowly progressive
AIDS leucoencephalopathy	AIDS-linked progressive disorder (see p. 19)
Central pontine malnutrition, myelinolysis	Associated with alcoholism, severe hyponatraemia

Table 11.10 Clinical features of multiple sclerosis.

Site	Features
Optic neuritis (retrobulbar neuritis)	Pain on ocular movement, loss of central vision, sometimes papillitis
Brainstem lesions, III, IV, VI nerves	Diplopia
Cerebellum and its brainstem connections	Ataxia, dysarthria, oscillopsia
Subcortex, brainstem, spinal cord	Paraesthesiae, numbness, impaired position sense, trigeminal or other acute pain syndromes
Pyramidal tract	Limb or bulbar weakness, spasticity, clonus, brisk tendon reflexes, extensor plantar responses, urgency, frequency, or urinary retention
Subcortical demyelination	Dementia, euphoria, depression

presents with motor, sensory, and bladder function abnormalities. Brisk reflexes are usual with an extensor plantar response.

Brainstem involvement may present as sixth nerve palsy (11.14), as internuclear ophthalmoplegia (11.85, 11.86) or with nystagmus. Involvement of the cerebellum results in ataxia and dysarthria. Subcortical involvement results in dementia and euphoria. Depression is also a common feature at all stages of the disorder.

There is no definitive diagnostic test, and sometimes the diagnosis only becomes clear clinically over the course of years, because of the relapsing nature of the neurological findings. Evoked responses — visual (11.23), auditory or somatosensory — may be of value; they depend on the demonstration of delayed nerve conduction. Lumbar puncture shows a raised CSF total protein, with a selective rise in IgG and oligoclonal bands on electrophoresis. The most sensitive methods of demonstrating the areas of demyelination are CT (11.87) and MRI (11.88).

There is no specific treatment but high dose intravenous steroids have a place in the acute episode. Dietary manipulation and hyperbaric oxygen have been used, but there is little evidence of their efficacy. Physiotherapy, psychotherapy and family counselling and support are mandatory. Depression should be actively treated and spasticity may respond to baclofen. Pain and troublesome paraesthesiae may respond to carbamazepine. Urinary retention and incontinence are treated symptomatically; and care must be taken to avoid pressure sores (11.57) as the patient becomes immobile.

11.84

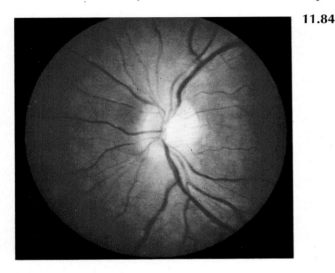

11.85

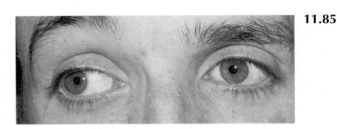

11.86

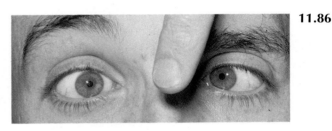

11.84 Retrobulbar neuritis is a common initial presentation of multiple sclerosis. In the early stages the disc appears normal. Later, it may become pale, with a clearly defined margin—as in the right half of this disc. Subsequently, the patient may develop the complete pallor of optic atrophy; or the disc may return to a normal appearance.

11.85, 11.86 Internuclear ophthalmoplegia may be a presenting feature of brain stem involvement in multiple sclerosis. On lateral gaze to the right, adduction of the left eye is incomplete (11.85). On convergence, eye movement is normal (11.86). The third nerve and the medial rectus muscle must be intact. so the lesion must lie in the left medial longitudinal bundle—between the nucleus in the pons and the third nerve nucleus on the opposite side.

11.87

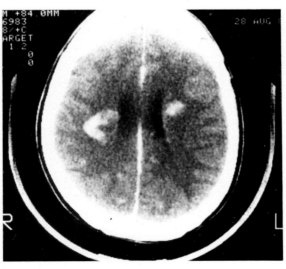

11.87 Multiple sclerosis. This contrast-enhanced CT scan shows multiple areas of abnormal enhancement, each of which represents an area of demyelination.

11.88 Multiple sclerosis. This MRI picture shows multiple 'high signal' lesions in the white matter of both hemispheres. Again, these represent multiple areas of demyelination.

11.88

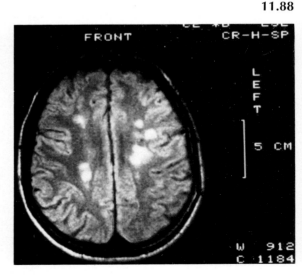

Motor neuron disease

Motor neuron disease is a rare, progressive degenerative disease of the upper and lower motor neurons which mainly affects the elderly. There is no impairment of intellect, sensation, sexual/bowel/bladder function or balance. Frontal lobe dementia may occur. No cause has been found, although there is, on occasion, a family history. Clinical presentation may be in one of three patterns:

- **Progressive muscular atrophy (PMA)** presents as wasting of the small muscles in one hand (**11.89**), rapidly followed by wasting in the other and proximal spread to involve the arms. The feet may be similarly involved. Symptoms usually include weakness, easy fatigability, muscle cramps and lack of muscle strength. The main signs are muscle wasting with loss of power and fasciculation. Tendon reflexes may be absent.
- **Amyotrophic lateral sclerosis (ALS)** presents with features of degeneration of the upper motor neuron and the lateral corticospinal tracts. There is usually an associated progressive muscular atrophy, so that the clinical picture is of combined upper and lower motor neuron degeneration.
- **Progressive bulbar palsy** mainly affects women; patients have involvement of the cranial nerves with upper and lower motor neuron lesions. The dominant and distressing features are dysarthria and dysphonia, difficulties in chewing and swallowing, and regurgitation of food and fluids via the nose because of palatal palsy. The tongue may be wasted (**11.90**) and fasciculation is obvious. Paralysis of the respiratory muscles is also apparent. Aspiration pneumonia is a common complication and, with hypoventilation, causes death.

The diagnosis may be made on clinical grounds alone but EMG may provide evidence of denervation. The CSF is normal. Cervical and lumbar spondylosis and motor neuropathies must be excluded, as they also cause amyotrophy (**7.85**). There is no specific treatment and most patients are dead in 3 years.

11.89

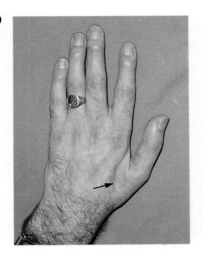

11.89 Motor neuron disease. This patient has progressive muscular atrophy, which presented with fasciculation and wasting of the muscles between the thumb and the index finger on the dorsal (arrow) and palmar surfaces. Wasting in the left hand was followed by the development of similar wasting in the right hand, and subsequently by progressive wasting and fasciculation elsewhere.

11.90

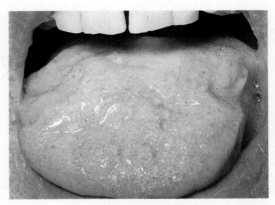

11.90 Motor neuron disease. This patient had progressive bulbar palsy. An early feature was fasciculation of the tongue, followed by progressive wasting, with furrowing of the surface. Progressive difficulties in chewing, swallowing and respiration accompanied this sign.

Disorders of the spinal cord

Syringomyelia

Syringomyelia results from the formation of a 'syrinx' in the spinal cord. This is a cavity filled with CSF that probably arises during development, when it may be associated with an Arnold–Chiari malformation. Less commonly it occurs after trauma. The syrinx may extend all the way down the central canal of the cord, but is usually most prominent in the upper cervical cord and in the brainstem (syringobulbia). As the cavity enlarges there is progressive neurological impairment, starting with the decussating fibres of the spino-thalamic tract, which carry pain and temperature, and resulting in disassociation sensory impairment of the trunk and upper limbs. This impairment results in the development of painless ulcers of the hands from unrecognised trauma and burns (**11.91**) and later to Charcot's joints in the upper limb (**11.92**). Later, the anterior horn cells are affected, leading to wasting of the small muscles of the hand (**11.91**) and arms with absent reflexes. Extension to the corticospinal tracts produces a spastic paraplegia. A syrinx in the brainstem (syringobulbia) results in loss of cranial nerve motor function with dysphagia and dysarthria, impairment of hearing and loss of fifth nerve sensation or a Horner's syndrome (**11.10**).

The diagnosis is made by showing the presence of a cervical expansion of the cord on myelography; or — most commonly now — by demonstrating the presence of the cavity on CT scanning or MRI (**11.93**).

Treatment is surgical by posterior decompression of the foramen magnum.

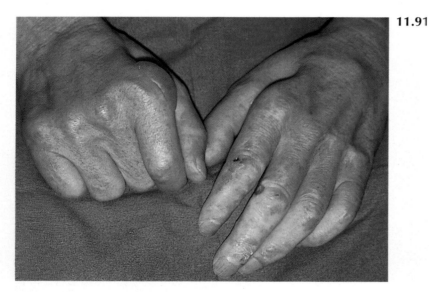

11.91

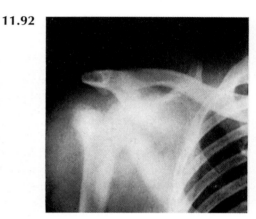

11.92

11.92 Charcot's joint in syringomyelia. The shoulder joint has been destroyed, and the radiological appearance is confused by new bone formation. This painless joint destruction is the result of sensory loss. In syringomyelia it is usually confined to the upper limbs, but similar changes may occur in the upper or lower limbs in diabetes, leprosy and tertiary syphilis (*see* **1.236, 1.237**).

11.91 Syringomyelia. The patient has severe wasting of the small muscles of both hands. He has also sustained a painless burn at the base of the right index finger—a result of the sensory loss associated with the condition.

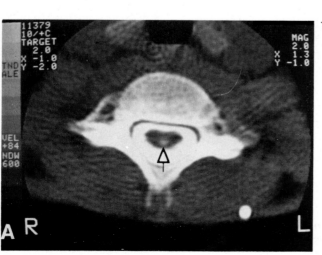

11.93

11.93 Syringomyelia. This picture, obtained by a combination of CT and myelography, demonstrates a flattened cord, and shows the presence of contrast in its enlarged central canal (arrow).

Friedreich's ataxia

Friedreich's ataxia is an autosomally transmitted (both dominant and recessive) form of spino-cerebellar degeneration. The disease usually presents between the ages of 5 and 10 years, with clumsiness in walking. This progresses inexorably and is associated with loss of proprioception and vibration sense, which produces lower limb atrophy and loss of tone. Tendon reflexes are lost and the plantar responses are extensor. The degenerative process moves upwards with time to affect speech and eye movements.

In addition to the neurological defect, there are skeletal abnormalities, notably pes cavus (**11.94**), scoliosis, and a high-arched palate. There may also be conduction defects in the heart, cardiomegaly and heart failure.

Rare associated nerve defects include retinal degeneration, deafness, mental retardation and lower motor neuron degeneration.

Diagnosis is made on clinical finding and family history. Genetic counselling is important.

Treatment is purely supportive.

11.94

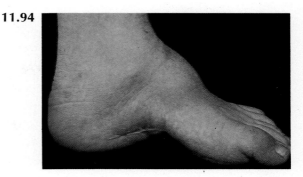

11.94 Pes cavus is a characteristic finding in Friedreich's ataxia. Both feet are usually more or less symmetrically high-arched and stubby.

Spina bifida

Spina bifida results from defective fusion of the vertebral arches. The most common site is in the lumbar region. Spina bifida occulta may be found in asymptomatic people who are X-rayed for some other reason (**11.95**). In some patients, there may be an associated tuft of hair over the lower back (**11.96**) or tethering of the cord with a 'dimple' in the skin. Spina bifida occulta is a benign complaint which usually requires no treatment.

In the severe form of spina bifida, the meninges may protrude through the bony defect (meningocele) and may include neural elements (meningomyelocele). These abnormalities are often associated with hydrocephalus (**11.97**) and usually there is impairment of leg and bladder function. Surgery is required to cover the defect and shunting is necessary for hydrocephalus.

11.95

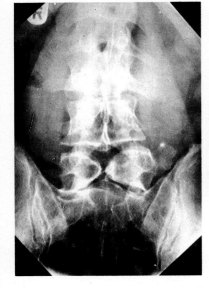

11.95 Occult spina bifida, discovered by chance on X-ray. The fifth lumbar and first sacral vertebrae have failed to fuse posteriorly in the midline, but the patient had no symptoms.

11.96

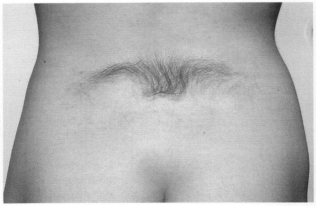

11.96 Occult spina bifida may be suggested by the presence of a tuft of hair over the base of the spine. This is usually a harmless anomaly.

11.97

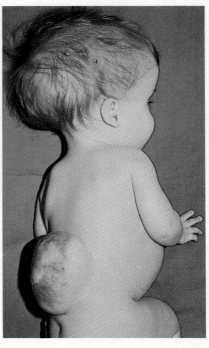

11.97 Meningomyelocele and hydrocephalus in a neonate. This combination is likely to result in severe neurological disability despite any possible surgical treatment.

Paraplegia

Paraplegia is paralysis of both lower limbs and may be acute or chronic. The limbs are flaccid in the acute phase and become spastic later. There is loss of bladder control. A large number of diseases may produce similar clinical features (**Table 11.11**).

Investigations should include a full blood count, sedimentation rate, plain X-rays, myelography and CT or MRI scan. A neurosurgical or orthopaedic opinion is urgently required in paraplegia of acute onset.

Table 11.11 Causes of paraplegia.

Skeletal diseases	Disc prolapse
	Spondylosis
	Metastatic carcinoma
	Paget's disease
	Rheumatoid arthritis
Spinal tumours	Neurofibromas
	Meningiomas
	Secondary carcinoma/lymphoma
	Ependymoma
Infections	Abscess (pyogenic)
	Tuberculosis (Pott's spine)
	Myelitis
	HIV
	Syphilis
Demyelination	Multiple sclerosis
Blood disorders	Bleeding disorders
(spinal haematoma)	Anticoagulants
Vascular occlusion	Emboli
	Thrombosis
Trauma	Falls, road traffic accidents
Metabolic	Vitamin B_{12} deficiency

Neoplasms of the spinal cord

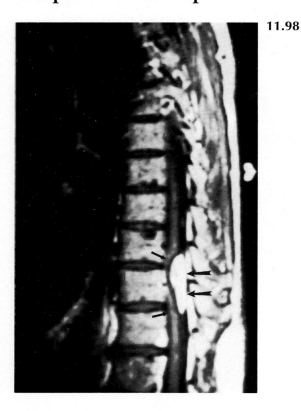

11.98

11.98 Subdural lipoma demonstrated by MRI in sagittal section. The lipoma (large arrows) is severely compressing the spinal cord (small arrows).

Primary neoplasia causing nerve root or cord compression may arise from any of the tissues in the area, and metastases from distant organs may also involve the spinal cord, nerve plexi or surrounding structures. The lesions may therefore be paravertebral, extradural, or intradural or intramedullary. Symptoms may be produced by direct invasion, by compression or, more rarely, by ischaemia resulting from invasion of the nutrient arteries. The process is usually insidious, with local pain that may radiate along a dermatome and may produce motor signs such as muscle wasting (**4.127**), sensory signs and occasionally autonomic changes (anhidrosis, hyperhidrosis or Horner's syndrome, **4.128**, **11.10**). Cord compression may result in lower motor neuron features at the level of the lesion, coupled with sensory loss and progressive features of upper motor signs below. Pain may be local or referred. Dysfunction of the bowel and bladder may be prominent early features. Occasionally, patients may present acutely with paraplegia.

Myelography will demonstrate most tumours and CSF examination usually reveals xanthochromia, a yellow cerebrospinal fluid rich in protein. Queckenstedt's test may be positive and malignant cells may rarely be found. The diagnosis may also be made on straight X-ray or by CT or MRI (**11.98**).

Treatment is dependent on the diagnosis. If the patient has suffered from previous malignancy, especially of lung or breast or a lymphoma, treatment may be possible with radiotherapy and /or appropriate chemotherapy. Biopsy may be necessary to establish a diagnosis and surgical resection to relieve cord or nerve root compression.

Spondylosis

Spondylosis is the term applied to chronic degenerative changes that occur with ageing in the intervertebral discs and the associated changes in the adjacent ligaments and vertebral bodies, including the outgrowth of osteophytes. In most instances changes are found incidentally on a routine examination and do not produce symptoms. However, in the cervical and lumbar spine there may be sufficient new growth to cause pressure on nerves or on the cord itself. Symptoms and signs are usually slowly progressive in contradistinction to those of a disc protrusion which are acute. Radicular compression produces pain, which may be referred, and there may be associated muscle spasm. Lower motor neuron weakness and wasting may also occur in the same distribution. Spinal movement may be reduced, and movement may exacerbate pain. The patient may be aware of 'creaking' or 'clicking' on movement. If the cord is involved, there may be myelopathy with progressive upper motor neuron weakness of the upper and lower limbs, with sensory signs, including loss of vibration sense and proprioception, and with sphincter disturbance.

Osteophytic outgrowth may also involve the vertebral canal, so that movements of the neck constrict the vertebral arteries and produce cerebellar ischaemia. These patients present with dizziness or drop attacks ('vertebro-basilar syndrome').

Straight X-ray of the cervical spine shows the typical degenerative changes with osteophyte formation (11.99, 11.100). Of more importance is an assessment of the diameter of the spinal canal in cases where myelopathy is present. This is best done by myelography or CT scan (11.101). In the cervical canal, a reduction to 10 mm is diagnostic of cord compression caused by spondylosis — a diameter greater than 15 mm suggests that spondylosis is not the cause of the myelopathic symptoms.

Spontaneous resolution of symptoms of radiculopathy and myelopathy occurs frequently in cervical spondylosis and treatment with a collar and analgesia is often helpful. Some patients benefit from bed rest with neck traction. Progression of the symptoms and signs of myelopathy requires urgent surgery for decompression.

11.99

11.100

11.101

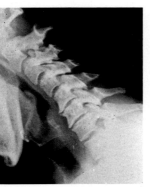 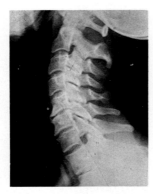

11.99, 11.100 Cervical spondylosis at the most common level (C5/6) demonstrated by X-rays taken in full flexion and extension. Note the narrowing of the intervertebral spaces and the prominent osteophyte formation, which leads to obvious abnormalities in the shape of the vertebral bodies. This appearance is very common in patients over the age of 50, and it is often asymptomatic.

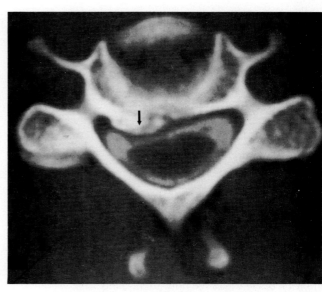

11.101 Cervical spondylosis. A CT scan demonstrates that spur formation (arrow) is distorting the thecal sac; but although the spinal cord is slightly displaced, it is not compressed.

Herniated intervertebral discs

Herniation of an intervertebral disc is one of the most common neurological lesions and low back pain attributed to 'slipped disc' is the single commonest cause of time lost from work. Accurate diagnosis and treatment therefore has financial and social, as well as medical, implications.

The material from the central portion of the disc (nucleus pulposus) may herniate through the annulus in two directions: lateral to the posterior longitudinal ligament, to compress the spinal roots; or posteriorly, to compress the cord or the cauda equina. The acute protrusion may follow trauma, abnormal movement or weight-bearing, but other factors such as degeneration of the disc, spondylosis or congenital abnormalities of the vertebrae may also be relevant. The common sites affected are the cervical and lumbar spine and the signs and symptoms depend on the site(s) and extent of the disc protrusion. If the protrusion is large, several adjacent nerve roots may be affected.

In the cervical spine, the most common sites are between C5/C6 and C6/C7. In the lumbar spine, the common sites are L4/L5 and L5/S1. Thoracic disc herniations are not common.

Local pain is common and may be exacerbated by movement, coughing or sneezing. There is usually associated local muscle spasm and the patient resists all movements. Compression of the associated nerve results in pain referred along its distribution. Stretching of the nerve root exacerbates the pain and this forms the basis of the straight leg raising test (11.102). Local pain may also be induced by pressing over the back. Sensory and motor symptoms and signs may identify the root involved. Herniation of the disc into the cord may produce remarkably few local signs, and the patient may present with symptoms and signs of cord compression — muscle weakness, sensory loss and upper motor neuron signs.

Diagnosis is usually made on clinical examination and straight X-ray of the spine. CT and MRI may help to identify more accurately the size and site of the herniation (11.103) and these have replaced myelography as the investigations of choice.

Most physicians agree that bed rest on a firm mattress, and adequate analgesia are the most important form of treatment. Local injection of steroids, manipulation and traction may all have a place. Surgery is indicated for intractable pain, or when the cord is involved, and consists of removal of the central portion of the disc. An alternative to surgery is the injection of proteolytic enzymes into the disc space.

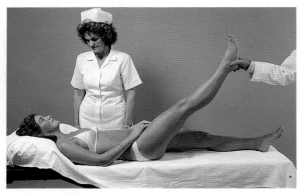

11.102

11.102 Straight leg raising is a test that stretches the sciatic nerve roots. The patient is asked to relax, and the heel is lifted by the examiner with the knee kept straight until pain is felt. If pain is felt in the back or buttock, a central disc prolapse may be the cause. If pain is felt at the back of the thigh, the only abnormality may be tight hamstrings. If pain is felt below the knee, its location may correspond to the lumbo-sacral dermatomes and forms an important localising sign. If pain is felt in the opposite leg as well, this may be an indication of abnormalities within the spinal canal. In the absence of spinal or hip abnormality, straight leg raising may usually be carried to the vertical position without pain.

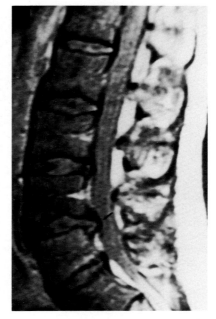

11.103

11.103 Central L4–5 disc herniation, demonstrated by sagittal MRI. The herniated disc is compressing the cord and causing symptoms.

Disorders of peripheral nerves (neuropathies)

Many disease processes produce peripheral neuropathy (**Table 11.12**). Most present with features of lower motor neuron involvement and sensory changes, but sometimes also or predominantly with motor changes. The cranial nerves may be affected by the same processes (*see* p. 471). The condition may be symmetrical or localised to one side. There are great variations in the degree of defects and their distribution. Motor involvement is associated with wasting and loss of power (**7.91, 11.104, 11.105**). Sensory features include numbness, paraesthesiae or hyperaesthesiae, pain and impaired temperature sensation. There may be associated skin ulceration and loss of skin hair. The tendon reflexes are absent.

Autonomic neuropathy typically presents with orthostatism and may have associated dysphagia, gastric atony with vomiting, diarrhoea and gustatory sweating (**7.92**). There is usually retention of urine with overflow incontinence and failure of erection. Hypotension may occur on standing (postural hypotension).

11.104

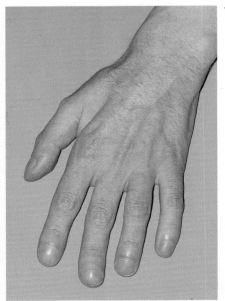

11.105

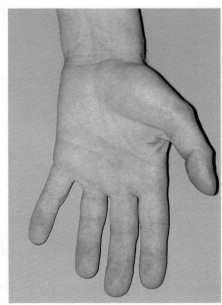

11.104, 11.105 Wasting of the hand as a consequence of ulnar neuropathy. Note the marked wasting of the interosseous muscles, especially the first dorsal interosseous. This patient also had early finger clubbing, and he proved to have a bronchial carcinoma.

Table 11.12 Causes of peripheral polyneuropathies.

Metabolic	Endocrine—diabetes (*see also* p. 333), thyroïd, acromegaly Renal failure Chronic liver failure Vitamin deficiency—B_1, B_6, nicotinic acid, B_{12}, vitamin E Amyloid Acute intermittent porphyria
Infections	Diphtheria exotoxin Leprosy Herpes zoster HIV
Toxic	*Alcohol* *Drugs,* e.g. lithium, isoniazid, gold, phenytoin, vincristine, chlorambucil, cisplatin *Heavy metals*—lead, arsenic, thallium *Organic solvents*—trichlorethylene, ethylene oxide, organophosphates, n-Hexane, tri-orthocresyl phosphate
Autoimmune disorders	Systemic lupus erythematosus
Neoplasia	A variety of cancers especially carcinoma of lung and myeloma
Hereditary disorders	Fabry's disease, Refsum's disease Charcot–Marie–Tooth disease
Idiopathic	Guillain–Barré syndrome

Immune polyneuropathy

Guillian–Barré syndrome (acute infectious polyneuropathy, AIP) is thought to be an immune polyneuropathy as it appears 2–3 weeks after a virus infection of the upper respiratory or gastrointestinal tract. It may affect all ages, but is most commonly found in the middle years of life. There may be a range of prodromal symptoms, including pyrexia, headache, nausea and vomiting; these are followed by back and limb pain, with a gradual onset of ascending motor neuropathy starting in the limbs, then involving the truncal muscles, cranial nerves and muscles of respiration. Sensory changes may be present early in the disease and dysaesthesia may be severe. Autonomic involvement may also be present and associated with postural hypotension and arrhythmias. Death may occur from respiratory impairment or from arrhythmias.

The diagnosis is made on the clinical picture, and it may be substantiated by finding a normal cell count in the CSF, with normal pressure but a high protein level which may give a deep yellow colour to the CSF. There may be evidence of delayed nerve conduction velocities.

The natural history of the disease is of a progressive neuropathy over several days, a period of stable neuropathy and then gradual recovery of normal function in the majority of cases. Intensive respiratory support may be required at any stage if the respiratory muscles are involved. In the early stages of the disease, plasmapheresis has been used with benefit. Steroids may be of value in chronic inflammatory demyelinating polyneuropathy.

Direct injury and compression neuropathy

Acute

Acute damage to peripheral nerves can result from direct penetrating or non-penetrating trauma, and may involve any nerve or plexus. The result is loss of motor and sensory function, and atrophy of muscle and skin in the areas supplied. The most common types of injury include acute stretching resulting from road traffic accidents (**11.106**); and compression, from coma resulting from alcohol, drugs, during general anaesthesia or simply from lying or sitting in a cramped position for a prolonged period. Penetrating injuries include bullet or knife wounds and ill-placed intramuscular injections. The most common such lesion is that involving the radial nerve which is usually injured as it winds round the back of the humerus (Saturday night palsy—as a result of alcoholic coma—**11.107**). Other examples are the peroneal nerve which may be compressed as it passes over the head of the fibula (**11.108**) and the ulnar nerve at the elbow (producing signs similar to those in **7.91**).

11.106

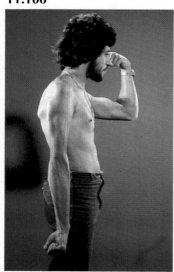

11.106 Right upper brachial plexus palsy (C5/6) following a motor cycle accident. The patient has been asked to make the same movement with his right arm and hand as with his left, but is unable to do so. He has paralysis of shoulder abduction, and external rotation of elbow flexion and of forearm supination. He also has sensory loss over the shoulder. This palsy is commonly known as Erb's palsy, or the porter's tip position.

11.107

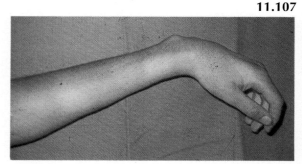

11.107 Radial nerve palsy. The patient is unable to extend the wrist and the metacarpophalangeal joints of the fingers or thumb—he has 'wrist drop'. Compression is a common cause of this injury; laceration of the nerve is another possible cause.

11.108

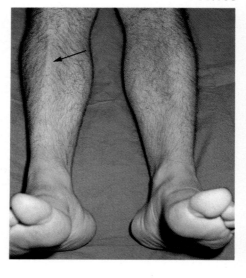

11.108 Peroneal nerve palsy. The common peroneal nerve has been compressed as it winds around the head of the fibula. Wasting of the anterior tibial muscles has occurred, revealing the ridge at the anterior border of the tibia (arrow). The condition is provoked by working in a squatting position or sitting for long periods with crossed legs.

Chronic

Carpal tunnel syndrome is commonest in middle-aged women, and results from compression of the median nerve as it passes through the carpal tunnel deep to the flexor retinaculum. The cause is often unclear, but sometimes a predisposing disorder is present (**Table 11.13**). The main complaints are of pain, numbness and paraesthesiae in the fingers supplied by the median nerve. The symptoms are often worse on awakening. Pain may radiate up the arm to the elbow, and it may be relieved by elevation of the hand or by gentle shaking of the hand in the air (Flick test). Use of the hand leads to loss of the symptoms. Examination shows sensory loss over the distribution of the median nerve—usually the thumb, index and middle fingers and half the ring finger (**11.109, 11.110**). There may be power loss in the thumb, both in abduction and adduction (i.e. abductor pollicis brevis, flexor pollicis brevis and opponens) and there may be wasting of the thenar eminence (**11.111**).

Additional tests include:

- Tinel's sign which is elicited by tapping with a finger over the carpal tunnel—this produces paraesthesiae in the hand and travelling up the arm.
- Phalen's test is similar to the above, but the stimulus is flexion of the wrist for 60 seconds. A positive test is the production of paraesthesiae.
- Tourniquet test is the testing of sensation deficit resulting from application of an upper arm tourniquet.

Nerve conduction studies are also of value in early diagnosis.

Management depends on the cause. If this is temporary (e.g. pregnancy), then simple measures such as splints or diuretics may buy enough time for spontaneous resolution to occur after delivery Steroid injection into the carpal tunnel gives symptomatic relief and is sometimes curative. Otherwise surgical decompression is required; this leads to return of motor function and usually to some sensory recovery.

In the **thoracic outlet syndrome** there is compression of the lower trunks of the brachial plexus as they pass over an abnormal cervical rib (**5.147**) or fibrous band, or over the normal first rib and muscle. Damage is usually confined to the C8, T1 fibres. Patients present with paraesthesiae, weakness, numbness of the ulnar fingers and wasting of the small muscles of the hand, especially the thenar muscles. There may be coincidental obstruction of the arterial supply of the limb (*see* p. 260). Symptoms are usually more apparent when the arm is abducted. Treatment is by removal of the fibrous band or rib.

Ulnar nerve damage (entrapment) is usually caused by recurrent trauma to the nerve in its shallow groove at the back of the medial condyle of the humerus. It can also occur following fracture of the condyle and subsequent healing. There is usually weakness and atrophy of the interossei with clawing of the fingers and difficulty with fine movements. Sensory loss may be detected in the small finger and the adjacent half of the ring finger and it may be possible to elicit sensory complaints by compressing the nerve at the elbow.

Compression of the lateral cutaneous nerve of the thigh may occur as it passes under the inguinal ligament, especially in grossly obese individuals wearing a tight belt or corset. Paraesthesiae occur in the nerve distribution, i.e. the lateral surface of the thigh as far down as the knee. Symptoms may be brought on by change in posture, especially by sitting. Resolution of symptoms can be produced by advice about clothing and by weight control and some patients require surgical decompression.

11.109　**11.110**

11.109, 11.110 Carpal tunnel syndrome. The common areas of sensory impairment are marked in this patient. Note that they usually extend round the fingertips on to the nail area in the affected fingers and even further over the extensor surface on the thumb.

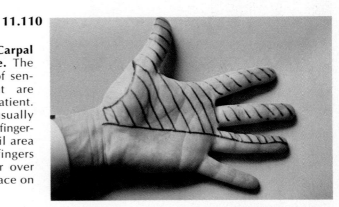

Table 11.13 Causes of the carpal tunnel syndrome.

Idiopathic
Pregnancy
Hypothyroidism
Diabetes mellitus
Acromegaly
Rheumatoid arthritis
Trauma to wrist

11.111

11.111 Carpal tunnel syndrome in the right wrist, with wasting of the thenar eminence, demonstrated by opposing the thumb. The abductor pollicis brevis muscle is weak and wasted. Compare the appearance with the normal left hand. The patient has already undergone surgical decompression on the right.

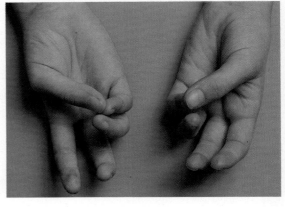

Neurocutaneous syndromes

Sturge–Weber syndrome

This congenital condition, with a diffuse capillary haemangioma of the face, forehead and anterior crown, in the distribution of the ophthalmic division of the trigeminal nerve (**11.112**), is associated with similar ipsilateral angiomas of the pia mater and underlying cortex, typically in the parieto-occipital region. This combination is associated with the development of epilepsy—usually generalised seizures—with associated mental retardation and/or hemiparesis. Straight X-ray of the skull or CT scan (**11.113**) show calcification in the deep layers of the cortex.

Treatment is by drug control of epilepsy and cosmetic covering of the facial lesions.

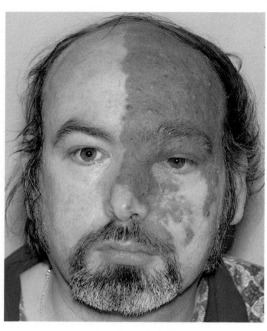

11.112

11.112 Sturge–Weber syndrome. This patient has a classic diffuse capillary haemangioma in the distribution of the ophthalmic and nasociliary branches of the trigeminal nerve. The lesion extends backwards over the anterior two-thirds of the crown of the head. The patient has had mental retardation, epilepsy and a right spastic hemiparesis with hypoplasia since infancy.

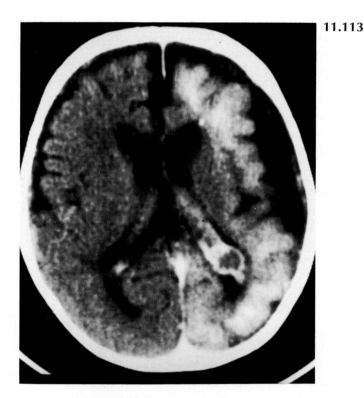

11.113

11.113 Sturge–Weber syndrome. This enhanced CT scan shows increased density throughout the atrophic left cerebral hemisphere, probably representing a combination of calcification and enhancement of the pial angiomas. There is enhancement of an enlarged left ventricular choroid plexus, which is again angiomatous. The right frontal lobe also shows some atrophy, and this patient may have bilateral involvement.

Neurofibromatosis (von Recklinghausen's disease)

This is a rare disease with an autosomal dominant transmission, in which multiple neurofibromas develop in peripheral and cranial nerves, and in which central nervous system tumours also appear (gliomas and meningiomas). There is also a rare association with the development of phaeochromocytomas (*see* p. 315). Two distinct types are now recognised:

- **Type I** (abnormality on chromosome 17) is generally associated with peripheral lesions—papillomas of skin, multiple cutaneous neurofibromas (**2.72**), café-au-lait spots, pigmented hamartomas of iris (Lisch nodules), axillary freckling, spinal and autonomic neurofibromas, phaeochromocytomas and optic gliomas.
- **Type II** (abnormality on chromosome 22) is generally associated with central lesions—bilateral acoustic neurofibromas, multiple intracranial meningiomas (**11.114**), schwannomas of cranial nerves and a few cutaneous lesions.

Diagnosis is readily confirmed by biopsy. Excision of peripheral lesions that rapidly change in size is important, because sarcomatous change may occur. Gene markers are of value in antenatal diagnosis and subsequent counselling is required.

11.114

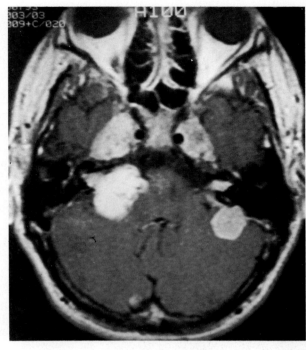

11.114 Neurofibromatosis (Type II). This patient has multiple cerebral tumours, as demonstrated by gadolinium-enhanced MRI. This scan shows bilateral eighth nerve tumours, a meningioma along the left petrous bone and bilateral parasellar meningiomas.

Tuberous sclerosis (epiloia)

11.115

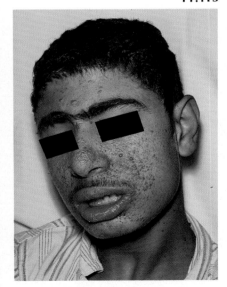

11.115 Adenoma sebaceum of the face—a marker of tuberous sclerosis (epiloia). The lesions are angiofibromas and in tuberous sclerosis they are associated with mental retardation, epilepsy and sometimes with other skin changes.

This is inherited as an autosomal dominant trait and presents in childhood with mental retardation, epilepsy and typical facial lesions (adenoma sebaceum, **11.115**). These lesions are angiofibromas. The diagnosis is usually clinically obvious. There may also be nodules in the retina (phakomas). Skin changes in addition to those on the face include white oval patches on the thorax (ash leaf patches), fibromas under the nails and naevi at the base of the spine (shagreen patches). There is a rare association with intracranial gliomas and hamartomas of the kidney. X-ray of the skull or CT scan may show calcification in the walls of the lateral ventricles (**11.116**).

Treatment involves control of epilepsy. Genetic counselling is important.

11.116

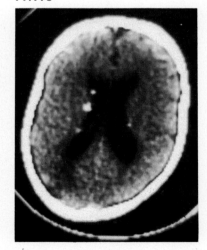

11.116 Tuberous sclerosis. This CT scan shows calcified periventricular lesions. These are hamartomatous tubers, containing both neurons and astrocytes. The patient also shows bilateral ventricular enlargement (hydrocephalus) which probably results from the presence of tubers near the foramen of Munro, causing CSF obstruction.

Disorders of muscle

Muscular dystrophies

Muscular dystrophies are a large group of poorly understood genetic disorders in which there is progressive degeneration of selected muscle groups. They usually present with progressive muscle weakness in the early years of life.

One of the most common is **Duchenne dystrophy**, which is transmitted as an X-linked recessive disorder and affects males. The syndrome is caused by deletion of the dystrophin gene on the X chromosome. Symptoms and signs become obvious at the age of about 2 years, with weakness of the pelvic and shoulder girdle muscles, and the first signs are commonly difficulty in walking, abnormal gait, frequent falling and difficulty in climbing steps and in getting off the floor (11.117, 11.118). Some muscle groups—especially in the calf—become hypertrophied. The course is inexorably downhill and by adolescence the boy is often deformed and invariably in a wheelchair (11.119, 11.120). The commonest cause of death is hypostatic pneumonia associated with failure of the muscles of respiration.

The diagnosis is usually obvious clinically and from the family history. There is usually massive elevation of the serum creatine kinase.

11.117

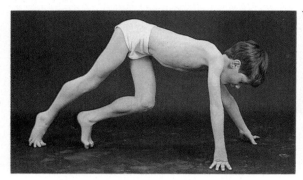

11.118

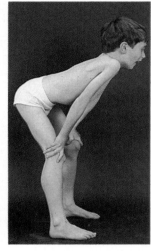

11.117, 11.118 Duchenne muscular dystrophy leads to great difficulty in getting up from a prone position. To reach the stage shown in **11.117**, this boy rolled over and 'walked' his hands and feet towards each other. He then walked his hands to his feet and up the front of his legs to reach the position shown in **11.118**. From here, he reaches an upright position by releasing his grip on his knees and swinging his arms and trunk sideways and upwards. This manoeuvre is known as Gowers' sign. Note the prominence of the calf muscles, especially in **11.117**. This boy was 10 years old, but many patients have lost the ability to get up from the floor by this age.

11.119

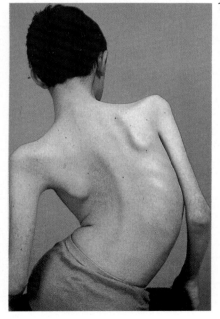

11.120

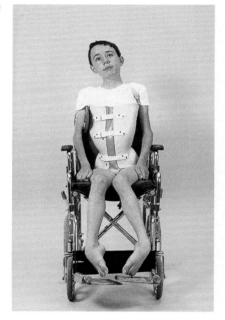

11.119, 11.120 Duchenne muscular dystrophy. This 15-year-old boy has severe scoliosis and an equinovarus deformity of the feet. A fair degree of improvement in the scoliosis, which was still relatively mobile, was achieved with a spiral brace. By this stage in the disease, patients are invariably confined to a wheelchair.

No treatment will alter the course of the disease. Genetic counselling for the family and psychosocial support are important.

A number of less common dystrophies include:

- **Becker muscular dystrophy,** a milder X-linked disease than Duchenne dystrophy, in which the patients live well into adult life.
- **Limb-girdle dystrophy** is an autosomal recessive disorder that affects the pelvic and shoulder girdle of boys and girls and is progressive in symptomatology (**11.121**).
- **Facio-scapulo-humeral dystrophy** is an autosomal dominant disease that affects the muscles of the face, neck and shoulders; these atrophy to give characteristic winging of the scapulae and atrophy of the deltoids and pectoralis major (**11.122**). Scoliosis occurs because of loss of support from weak truncal muscles. The pelvic girdle muscles may be similarly affected. The history is of progressive muscle weakness and atrophy.

11.121

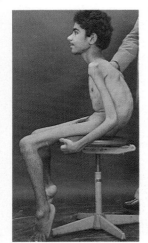

11.122

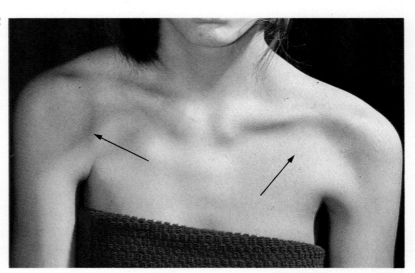

11.121 Limb-girdle dystrophy. This 18-year-old boy showed severe signs, with extreme proximal muscle wasting and weakness, and a prominent kyphosis.

11.122 Facio-scapulo-humeral dystrophy in a 13-year-old girl. This view shows wasting of the deltoids and pectoral muscles (arrows), and she also had facial weakness, winging of the scapulae and kyphoscoliosis.

Myotonic dystrophy

Myotonia is increased spasm of muscle fibres which results from abnormalities of the muscle membrane producing a delay in relaxation. The most common myotonic disorder is **myotonic dystrophy** (dystrophia myotonica), which is transmitted as an autosomal dominant disorder and presents in the age range 20–30 years with weakness of the limb muscles associated with myotonia. This becomes apparent as failure to relax a grip. There is also cranial muscle involvement, often with ptosis, difficulty in whistling and dysarthria. There is associated wasting of the temporalis, masseter and sternomastoid muscles. A variety of other signs may occur, including the development of cataracts, frontal baldness (in men) and testicular or ovarian atrophy. The facies is very typical (**11.123**). There may be associated cardiomyopathy with arrhythmias; and there may occasionally be mental retardation.

The diagnosis is made on clinical grounds. Treatment is generally unsatisfactory and is directed at the myotonia (e.g. procainamide). Genetic counselling is important. **Myotonia congenita (Thomsen's disease)** is a rare myotonic disorder, which may be dominant or recessive and is characterised by muscle hypertrophy and a milder degree of myotonia which is provoked by cold weather and improves with exercise.

11.123

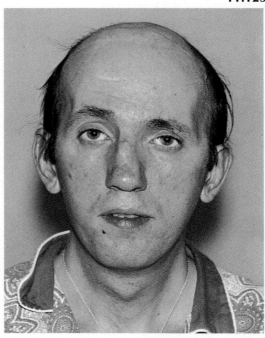

11.123 Myotonic dystrophy in a 35-year-old man. The characteristic facies includes bilateral ptosis, facial weakness, atrophy of the sternomastoids and frontal baldness, which produces a 'monk-like' appearance.

Myopathies

Myopathy occurs in a number of systemic disorders, including dermatomyositis, polymyalgia rheumatica and a number of endocrine disorders including Cushing's syndrome, Addison's disease, thyrotoxicosis and hypothyroidism; and it may occur as a remote effect of malignant tumours. A number of other rare forms of myopathy also occur.

Periodic paralysis

Disorders in this group are often familial, being transmitted as an autosomal dominant trait. Repeated attacks of generalised muscle weakness are associated with either a high or low serum potassium. The symptomatology usually starts in adolescence and is often provoked by hard physical exercise. The limb muscles are usually affected and weakness may last for many hours before spontaneously improving. In the hypokalaemic variant, attacks may also be precipitated by a carbohydrate meal. Examination of the patient often shows very little except in the acute phase where there may be myotonia and a positive Chvostek's sign.

The diagnosis may be confirmed by finding a low potassium (2.5–3.5 mEq/l) or a high potassium (6–7 mEq/l). It is important to exclude thyrotoxicosis and diuretic therapy as causes. Occasionally, the potassium levels are normal.

Remission of the condition may occur spontaneously after the age of 30 years. In the acute hypokalaemic attack, an infusion of potassium chloride will terminate the symptoms, and in the hyperkalaemic variant, intravenous calcium gluconate is effective.

Myasthenia gravis

Myasthenia gravis is a disease in which a reduction in the available functional nicotinic receptors at the neuromuscular junction is associated with increased fatiguability and weakness of striated muscles. It may appear at any time of life and affects women more commonly than men.

The cause is not known, but it is an autoimmune condition with evidence of IgG antibodies to acetylcholine receptor protein in 90% of patients. There is an increased incidence of other autoimmune disorders, such as rheumatoid arthritis, pernicious anaemia and systemic lupus erythematosus in patients with myasthenia gravis. Some patients have a thymoma.

The common presentation is with muscle weakness and fatiguability. This commonly involves the ocular muscles but any group may be affected. Ptosis and diplopia are common manifestations and get worse during the course of the day. Similarly affected are the muscles of mastication, swallowing and speech. Muscle bulk is usually maintained until late in the disease.

The diagnostic test is the Tensilon (edrophonium) test (11.124, 11.125). Electromyography shows a declining response to repeated stimuli. The presence of circulating antibodies to acetylcholine receptors is diagnostic but antibody-negative forms are recognised. A search for a thymoma should be made by X-ray (11.126) or thoracic CT scanning.

Drug treatment is with a long-acting anti-cholinesterase which is usually symptomatically effective. Thymectomy may also result in long-term improvement and immunosuppression with prednisolone and azathioprine may be beneficial, as is plasma exchange in severe cases.

The course of the disease is variable but progressive, and death may result from aspiration pneumonia.

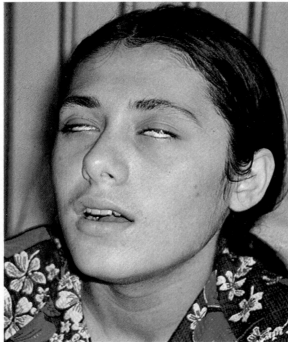

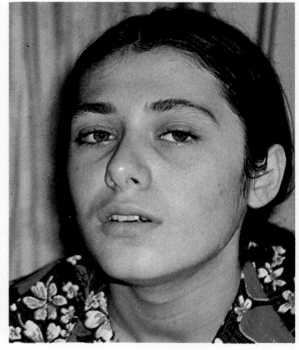

11.124, 11.125 Myasthenia gravis. The edrophonium (Tensilon) test can be used to confirm the diagnosis. Facial weakness is provoked by repeated facial movements (**11.124**). Edrophonium chloride, a short-acting anticholinesterase, is then injected intravenously—initially, 2 mg as a test dose, followed after one minute by a further 8 mg if there are no adverse effects. In myasthenia gravis the facial weakness is rapidly relieved by this test (**11.125**). Objective testing of muscular power elsewhere in the body will reveal similar responses.

11.126

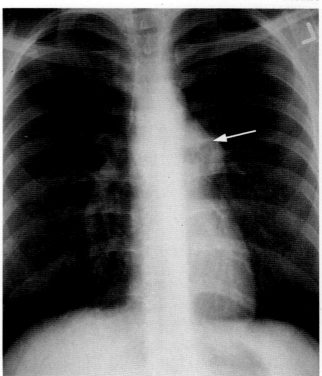

11.126 Thymoma (arrow) in a patient with myasthenia gravis. A lateral film confirmed that this mass was in the anterior mediastinum. The differential diagnosis of this appearance includes lymphadenopathy, retrosternal thyroid tissue or a dermoid tumour; but in the presence of myasthenia gravis, thymoma is the most likely diagnosis. Thymectomy may result in cure or great improvement in the myasthenia.

INDEX

Numbers in normal type are page numbers; numbers in **bold** are caption numbers.